Pulmonary Disease Diagnosis and Therapy

A Practical Approach

Pulmonary Disease Diagnosis and Therapy

A Practical Approach

M. Gabriel Khan, MD,
FRCP(London), FRCP(C), FACC, FACP
Associate Professor of Medicine
University of Ottawa
Ottawa, Canada

Joseph P. Lynch III, MD
Professor of Internal Medicine
Division of Pulmonary and Critical Care Medicine
University of Michigan
Ann Arbor, Michigan

Editors

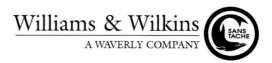

Williams & Wilkins
A WAVERLY COMPANY

BALTIMORE • PHILADELPHIA • LONDON • PARIS • BANGKOK
BUENOS AIRES • HONG KONG • MUNICH • SYDNEY • TOKYO • WROCLAW

Editor: Jonathan W. Pine, Jr.
Managing Editor: Molly L. Mullen
Marketing Manager: Daniell T. Griffin
Production Coordinator: Carol Eckhart
Copy Editor: Karen M. Ruppert
Illustration Planner: Wayne Hubbel
Cover Designer: Julie Burrie
Typesetter: Maryland Composition Co., Inc.
Printer and Binder: RR Donnelley & Sons Company

351 West Camden Street
Baltimore, Maryland 21201-2436 USA

Rose Tree Corporate Center
1400 North Providence Road
Building II, Suite 5025
Media, Pennsylvania 19063-2043 USA

Accurate indications, adverse reactions and dosage schedules for drugs are provided in this book, but it is possible that they may change. The reader is urged to review the package information data of the manufacturers of the medications mentioned.

Printed in the United States of America

Library of Congress Cataloging-in-Publication Data

Pulmonary disease diagnosis and therapy : a practical approach / M.
Gabriel Khan, Joseph P. Lynch III., editors.
    p.   cm.
    Includes index.
    ISBN 0-683-04613-6
    1. Respiratory organs—Diseases. I. Khan, M. I. Gabriel.
II. Lynch, Joseph P.
    [DNLM: 1. Lung Diseases—diagnosis. 2. Lung Diseases—therapy.
WF 600 P98342 1997]
RC731.P835 1997
616.2′4—dc20
DNLM/DLC
for Library of Congress   96-43620
                                           CIP

The publishers have made every effort to trace the copyright holders for borrowed material. If they have inadvertently overlooked any, they will be pleased to make the necessary arrangements at the first opportunity.

To purchase additional copies of this book, call our customer service department at **(800) 638-0672** or fax orders to **(800) 447-8438**. For other book services, including chapter reprints and large quantity sales, ask for the Special Sales department.

Canadian customers should call **(800) 665-1148**, or fax **(800) 665-0103**. For all other calls originating outside of the United States, please call **(410) 528-4223** or fax us at **(410) 528-8550.**

Visit Williams & Wilkins on the Internet: **http://www.wwilkins.com** or contact our customer service department at **custserv@wwilkins.com.** Williams & Wilkins customer service representatives are available from 8:30 am to 6:00 pm, EST, Monday through Friday, for telephone access.

98 99 00 01
2 3 4 5 6 7 8 9 10

Preface

Two excellent textbooks on pulmonary disease are currently available in the marketplace. These are large texts, however—each over 2,000 pages—and are suitable only for pulmonologists and as reference textbooks. Of the two medium-sized textbooks available, one is directed mainly at pulmonologists who care for patients in intensive care units.

Thus we offer here a medium-sized pulmonary disease textbook that emphasizes diagnosis and therapy. This book is written for internists; family physicians; residents in internal medicine, pulmonology, and family medicine; senior medical students; and critical care nurses.

The chest radiograph is the single most important diagnostic tool used by pulmonologists and physicians caring for patients with a pulmonary illness. The pulmonology books currently available for internists and trainees do not appear to cover the topics of interpretation of the chest radiograph, and formal training sessions in the appropriate interpretation of the chest radiograph are not included in the curriculum of teaching hospitals. Consequently, trainees often appear puzzled when asked to interpret an abnormal chest radiograph.

Because we believe that practicing physicians and medical residents do not require the repetition of topics covered in preclinical years, we have omitted discussion of the anatomy and physiology of the lungs and the mechanics of respiration. Omission of these topics, then, allowed us to expand the discussion of areas such as pulmonary function testing, the diagnosis and therapy of pleural diseases, acute respiratory distress syndrome, acid base disturbance, asthma, and restrictive lung disease.

The chapter on interpreting the chest radiograph is extensive and includes 120 radiographs that cover a range of pulmonary disease. The chapters on bacterial pneumonia and on fungal, mycobacterial, and viral pulmonary infection are highly detailed. True to its title, the text throughout concentrates on relevant pathophysiology, diagnosis, and therapy and covers the core knowledge in these three areas for board examinations in internal medicine and pulmonology.

We are pleased that Williams & Wilkins has provided us with an interior book design that allows ready access to the wealth of clinical information contained within and that highlights our emphasis on diagnosis and therapy. It is appropriate, therefore, to extend our appreciation to the excellent production team at Williams & Wilkins: Jonathan W. Pine Jr, Senior Executive Editor; Molly L. Mullen, Senior Managing Editor; Carol Eckhart, Production Coordinator; and Karen M. Ruppert, Book Project Editor. With the invaluable assistance of our contributors, our book should be like a tree of wisdom that seeks to reach beyond the horizon to all those who care for those who ail—"a tree that looks at God all day and lifts its leafy arms to pray."

M. Gabriel Khan
Joseph P. Lynch III

Contributors

Sidney S. Braman, MD
Professor of Medicine
Department of Medicine
Brown University School of Medicine
Director
Division of Pulmonary, Sleep, and
  Critical Care Medicine
Rhode Island Hospital
Providence, Rhode Island

Bartolome R. Celli, MD
Professor of Medicine
Tufts University
Chief, Pulmonary and Critical Care
St. Elizabeth's Medical Center
Boston, Massachusetts

**Conway Don, MB, BS, FRCP, FRCPC,
  DMRD, FRCR**
Professor of Radiology
University of Ottawa
Radiologist
Ottawa General Hospital
Ottawa, Ontario, Canada

Mari M. Goldner, MD
Research Fellow
Department of Pulmonary and Critical
  Care Medicine
University of Minnesota
St. Paul, Minnesota

D. Ian Hammond, MD, FRCP
Professor and Chairman
Department of Radiology
University of Ottawa
Ottawa, Ontario, Canada

**M. Gabriel Khan, MD, MB BCh,
  FRCP(Lond), FRCP(C), FACP**
Associate Professor of Medicine
University of Ottawa
Ottawa General Hospital
Ottawa, Canada

Richard W. Light, MD
Professor of Medicine
University of California, Irvine
Veterans Administration Medical Center
Long Beach, California

Joseph P. Lynch III, MD
Professor of Internal Medicine
Division of Pulmonary and Critical Care
  Medicine
University of Michigan
Ann Arbor, Michigan

John J. Marini, MD
Director
Pulmonary and Critical Care Medicine
St. Paul Ramsey Medical Center
St. Paul, Minnesota

Paul L. Marino, MD, PhD, FCCM
Clinical Associate Professor of Medicine
University of Pennsylvania
Director
Critical Care Academic Program
Department of Surgery
The University of Pennsylvania Health
  System
Philadelphia, Pennsylvania

Fernando J. Martinez, MD
Associate Professor
Department of Internal Medicine
University of Michigan
Ann Arbor, Michigan

Borna Mehrad, MD
Fellow in Pulmonary and Critical Care
    Medicine
Division of Pulmonary and Critical Care
    Medicine
Department of Internal Medicine
University of Michigan Medical Center
Ann Arbor, Michigan

David R. Moller, MD
Assistant Professor of Medicine
Division of Pulmonary and Critical Care
    Medicine
Director
Sarcoidosis Clinic
The Johns Hopkins University School of
    Medicine
Baltimore, Maryland

David M. Nierman, MD, FCCP
Assistant Professor of Medicine and
    Surgery
Director
The Gaisman Medical Intensive Care
    Unit
Department of Medicine
Mt. Sinai Medical Center
New York, New York

Lucy B. Palmer, MD
Assistant Professor
Pulmonary and Critical Care
SUNY at Stony Brook New York
Stony Brook, New York

Thomas W. Shields, MD, DSc (Hon)
Professor Emeritus of Surgery
Department of Surgery
Northwestern University Medical School
Chicago, Illinois

Galen B. Toews, MD
Professor of Internal Medicine
Chief
Division of Pulmonary and Critical Care
    Medicine
University of Michigan Medical Center
Ann Arbor, Michigan

John G. Weg, MD
Professor of Internal Medicine
Pulmonary and Critical Care Medicine
    Division
Department of Internal Medicine
University of Michigan Medical Center
Ann Arbor, Michigan

Contents

1 Interpretation of the Chest Radiograph

D. Ian Hammond, Conway Don,
M. Gabriel Khan

THE NORMAL POSTEROANTERIOR (PA) CHEST RADIOGRAPH

The PA chest radiograph (Figs. 1.1–1.3) is taken at full inspiration with a 6-foot distance between the x-ray tube and the film to minimize magnification and increase sharpness of detail, with the front of the patient's chest pressed against the film cassette.

It is important to analyze the chest film systematically, despite the temptation to focus on an obvious lesion.

The routine used to ensure systematic examination varies with the individual, but analysis of the film in the following order is suggested:

- Check for patient rotation, as this causes asymmetry of the soft tissue shadows that may produce apparent increased density in one lung (Fig. 1.4) and may also simulate or disguise mediastinal shift;
- Soft tissues and bones;
- Lung fields;
- Hila;
- Tracheobronchial tree;
- Cardiac shadow;
- Vascular pedicle;
- Thoracic aorta;
- Diaphragm and costophrenic angles.

NORMAL LATERAL CHEST RADIOGRAPH

The lateral chest radiograph (Figs. 1.5–1.6) is also taken at a 6-foot distance, in full inspiration. A left lateral position (i.e., with the left side nearer to the film) is preferred, as in this situation the right hilum is projected in front of the left, allowing differentiation of the hila. In the right lateral position, the hila are superimposed.

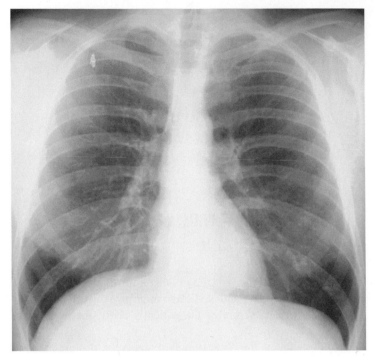

Figure 1.1. Normal PA radiograph of the chest.

It is important that the lateral radiograph is also analyzed systematically, and this applies particularly to the divisions of the mediastinum because certain lesions have preferential locations in the various divisions.

There is a variety of classifications of the mediastinum; the simplest and most effective is the long-established anatomic classification (Fig. 1.7).

A suggested routine for systematic evaluation is as follows:

- Soft tissues and bones, particularly the thoracic spine;
- Anterior mediastinum;
- Middle mediastinum;
- Posterior mediastinum;
- Diaphragm and posterior costophrenic angles;
- Superior mediastinum.

ABNORMAL SIGNS ON THE PA CHEST RADIOGRAPH

1. Soft Tissues and Bones

The soft tissues and bony structures of the thorax should be examined before analyzing the lungs to detect lesions of the chest wall, such as rib metastases (Fig. 1.8).

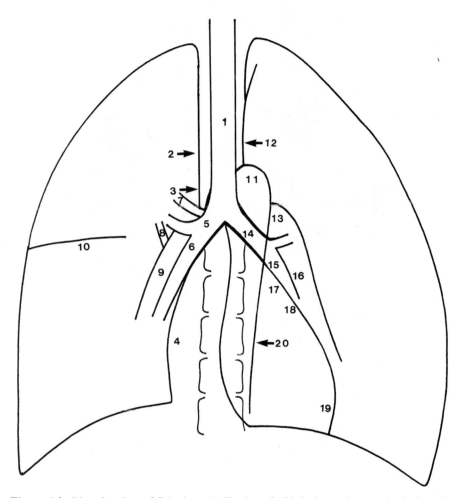

Figure 1.2. Line drawing of PA chest. 1, Trachea. 2, Right innominate vein. 3, Superior vena cava (SVC). 4, Right atrium. 5, Right main bronchus. 6, Intermediate bronchus. 7, Right upper lobe artery. 8, Right upper lobe vein. 9, Descending branch of right pulmonary artery. 10, Lesser fissure. Usually lies between the anterior ends of the third and fourth ribs. Horizontal disposition, commonly smoothly convex superiorly. 11, Aortic knuckle. 12, Left subclavian artery. 13, Left pulmonary artery. 14, Left main bronchus. 15, Left lower lobe bronchus. 16, Left lower lobe artery. 17, Main pulmonary artery. 18, Left auricular appendage (not seen as a separate bulge in normal hearts). 19, Apex of left ventricle. 20, Descending aorta.

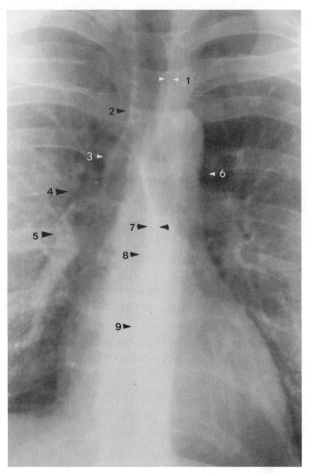

Figure 1.3. Mediastinal detail. 1, Posterior junction line, formed by the two lungs coming in contact behind the trachea. Terminated inferiorly by the aortic arch, which separates the two lungs. 2, The right paratracheal stripe. It should not exceed 4 mm in diameter. 3, Azygos vein. It should not exceed 6 mm in diameter. 4, Upper converging point. 5, Lower converging point. 6, Aortopulmonary window. Usually concave; may be straight. Convexity implies a ductus adenopathy. 7, Anterior junction line, formed by the two lungs meeting in the anterior mediastinum; has to start below the level of the clavicles and usually runs downward and to the left. 8, Upper portion of the azygo-esophageal recess; should be smoothly concave to the right. 9, Lower half of the azygo-esophageal recess; should be smoothly convex to the right.

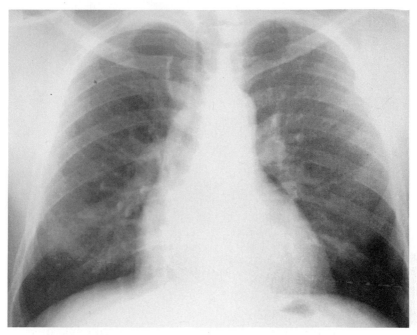

Figure 1.4. Rotated PA chest. Notice from the position of the clavicles and the trachea in relation to the thoracic spine that the patient is rotated to the right. This has displaced the heart to the right and has caused asymmetric density of the lung fields, the left lung field appearing denser than the right.

Chest wall lesions as well as normal variants may give the false impression of pulmonary disease. Abnormalities of the chest wall may alter the density of a hemithorax (see "Unilateral Hyperlucency of the Lung"). A mastectomy, the commonest of such causes, produces ipsilateral hyperlucency. Conversely, a chest wall mass may increase the density of the ipsilateral hemithorax.

Normal Variants on the Chest Wall That May Be Confused with a Pulmonary Nodule

- Sclerotic or hypertrophic anterior costal cartilages, especially in the first rib;
- Sclerotic foci (bone islands) in the ribs;
- Nipple shadow (Fig. 1.9).

2. Lung Fields

Because of the multiplicity of abnormal signs in the lung fields, they are discussed individually later in this chapter (see "Lung Parenchyma").

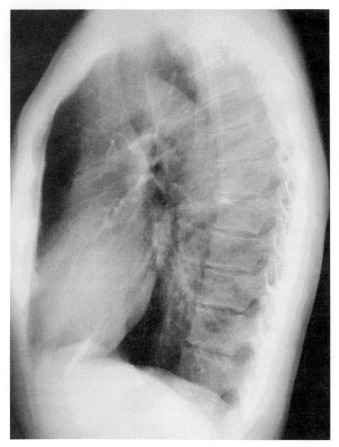

Figure 1.5. Normal lateral chest radiograph.

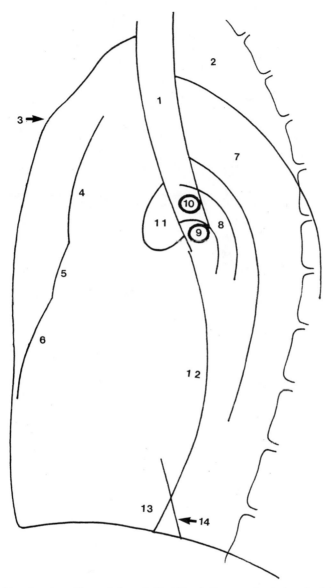

Figure 1.6. Line drawing of lateral chest. 1, Trachea. 2, Retrotracheal triangle. 3, Manubriosternal junction (Angle of Louis). 4, Ascending aorta. 5, Main pulmonary artery. 6, Right ventricle. 7, Posterior aspect of arch of aorta. 8, Left pulmonary artery. 9, Origin of left upper lobe bronchus. 10, Origin of right upper lobe bronchus. 11, Right hilum. 12, Left atrium. 13, Left ventricle. 14, Inferior vena cava.

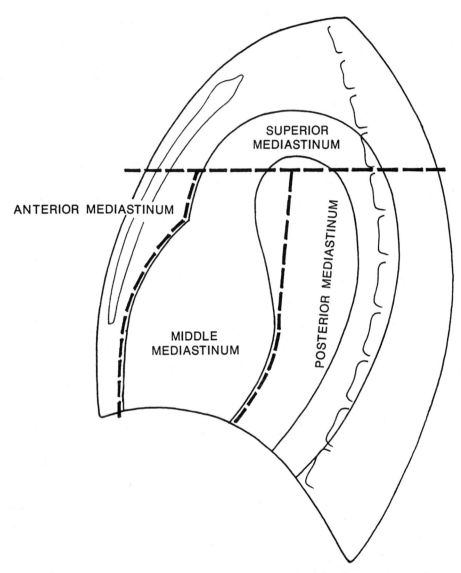

Figure 1.7. Divisions of the mediastinum. This is the long-established anatomic classification used in this text.

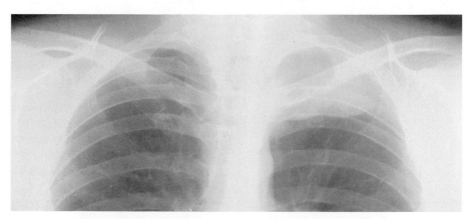

Figure 1.8. Rib metastases from renal adenocarcinoma causing a soft tissue mass at the left apex with destruction of the left third rib posteriorly.

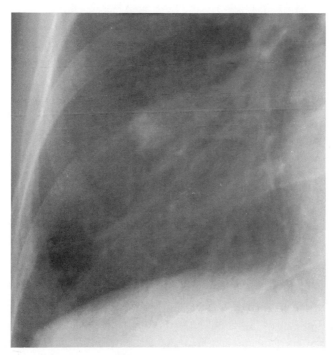

Figure 1.9. This nipple is well-defined on its lateral aspect but its medial border fades imperceptibly. When present, this sign distinguishes the nipple from a pulmonary nodule, which is well-defined in its complete circumference.

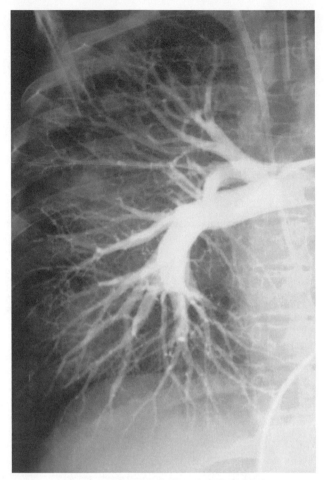

Figure 1.10. Right selective pulmonary arteriogram, demonstrating how the right pulmonary artery divides inside the mediastinum into the right upper lobe artery (truncus anterior) and the descending pulmonary artery, producing two converging points.

3. The Hila

The radiographic hila are composed primarily of vascular shadows, predominately the pulmonary arteries.

- The right pulmonary artery (Fig. 1.10) divides inside the mediastinum, into the upper lobe artery (truncus anterior) and the descending pulmonary artery. This produces two components or converging points at the right hilum.
- The lower converging point, corresponding to what is normally described as the right hilum, is composed of the descending branch of the right pulmonary artery

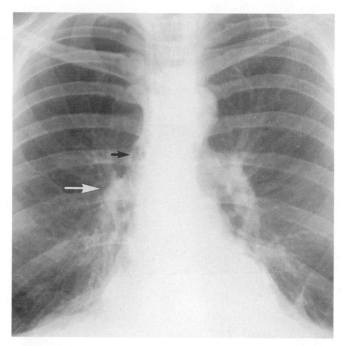

Figure 1.11. Single right converging point (*white arrow*) as a result of long-standing complete collapse of the right upper lobe. The upper converging point is not present, and the remains of the collapsed right upper lobe can just be seen as the bronchiectatic ring shadows superimposed on the lower end of the right paratracheal stripe (*black arrow*). This patient suffered from ciliary dyskinesia syndrome. The blurring of the right heart border is the result of bronchiectasis in the middle lobe, and the blurring of the left heart border is the result of bronchiectasis in the inferior segment of the lingula.

applied to the lateral aspect of the intermediate and lower lobe bronchi, and supplemented by the branches of the middle lobe artery and the artery to the superior segment to the lower lobe.
- A contributory shadow is that of the superior pulmonary vein, which crosses the descending pulmonary artery at this level.
- The upper converging point produced by the right upper lobe artery is much less conspicuous (Fig. 1.3), but it is visible in 95% of normal chest radiographs.
- Absence of one of the two converging points on the right is a significant finding and implies either resection or collapse of one of the two major lobes of the right lung (Fig. 1.11).
- The left pulmonary artery enters the lung as a single vessel (Fig. 1.12) and divides inside the lung. Thus there is only one converging point on the left (Fig. 1.3).
- The lower converging point of the right hilum lies below the level of the single left converging point in 97% of patients and never lies above it. The upper converg-

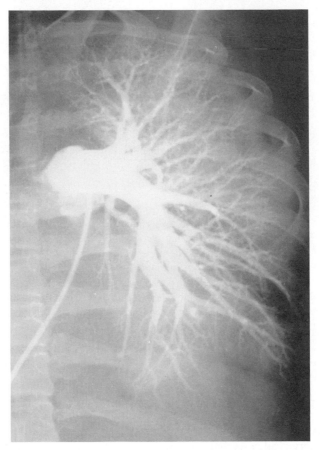

Figure 1.12. Left selective pulmonary arteriogram, showing the left pulmonary artery passing over the left main bronchus and entering the lung undivided. This produces only a single converging point on the left.

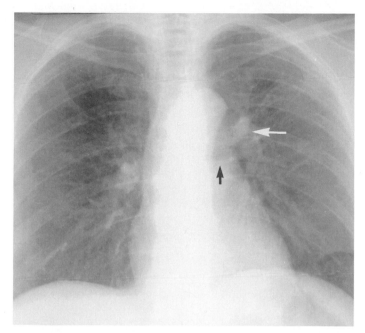

Figure 1.13. Marked elevation of the left hilum (*white arrow*) from radiation fibrosis in the left upper lobe. Note also that the left main bronchus is not straight but terminates in an upward curve (*black arrow*) from this elevation of the left hilum.

ing point lies above that of the left in 87% of patients and only occasionally lies below it.
- Displacement of the hila is common in collapse, fibrosis, or resection of the lung and is estimated from the disturbance of this normal relationship (Fig. 1.13).

Enlarged Hila

- Enlarged but otherwise normal hila occur with dilatation of the pulmonary arteries. Dilatation is an index of increased pulmonary artery pressure or of increased pulmonary artery flow, and the commonest causes are congenital heart disease with left to right shunt (Fig. 1.14), cor pulmonale (Fig. 1.18, *A–B*), and severe pulmonary hypertension.
- Increased caliber of the pulmonary arteries is most easily estimated from the descending branch of the right pulmonary artery, which has a constant position lateral to the intermediate bronchus (Fig. 1.3), and it should not exceed 16 mm in diameter.
- The caliber of the left pulmonary artery is not so easily estimated, as it runs partly lateral and partly posterior to the left lower lobe bronchus.
- Unilateral enlargement of a pulmonary artery may occur in massive embolization, in which the artery becomes distended by thrombus (Fig. 1.15).

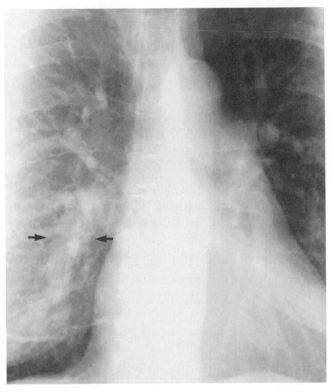

Figure 1.14. Enlarged hila from increased pulmonary arterial flow in an atrial septal defect. Note the mild prominence of the main pulmonary artery. The width of the right descending pulmonary artery (*arrows*) is 20 mm (normal maximum is 16 mm).

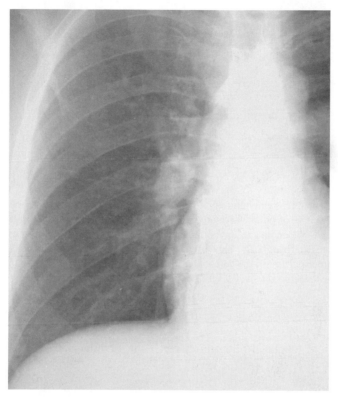

Figure 1.15. Enlargement of the right hilum from distension of the descending right pulmonary artery from a massive pulmonary embolus. The transverse diameter of the pulmonary artery is 22 mm. The distension is not the result of raised pulmonary artery pressure proximal to the clot but of distension by thrombus. Note the abrupt change of caliber in the descending pulmonary artery, which is accompanied by diminished vascularity in the lower lobe.

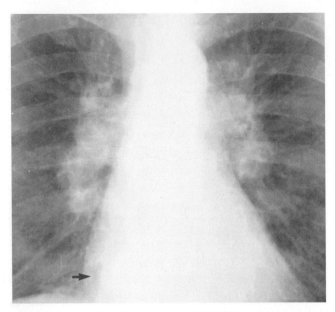

Figure 1.16. Bilateral symmetric enlargement and lobulation of the hila from adenopathy. Although suggestive of pulmonary sarcoidosis, this enlargement was the result of metastasis from melanoma. Melanoma and hypernephroma are particularly likely to produce this type of hilar metastasis. There is also subcarinal adenopathy causing increased density and deviation of the upper portion of azygo-esophageal recess. Note also the 2.5-cm intrapulmonary metastatic mass behind the lower right heart border (*arrow*).

- Enlarged and lobulated hila are characteristic of hilar adenopathy (Figs. 1.16, 1.24A).

Diminished Hila

- Just as the hilar arteries increase in size with increased pulmonary arterial pressure or flow, they decrease in size with reduced arterial pressure or flow.
- Common causes are congenital heart disease with pulmonary stenosis (Fig. 1.17) and Swyer-James syndrome.

Blurred Hila

- Perihilar haze is an early occurrence in interstitial pulmonary edema; estimation of this is likely subjective.
- A valuable early and reliable objective sign is blurring of the normally sharp lateral border of the descending pulmonary artery (Fig. 1.18, *A–B*).

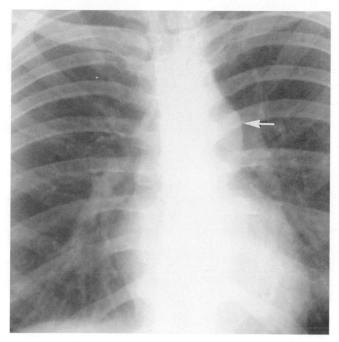

Figure 1.17. Small hila from diminished pulmonary artery pressure and flow in congenital pulmonary valve stenosis. Note also the poststenotic dilatation of the left pulmonary artery (*arrow*).

The Dense Hilum

The density of the hilar shadows on the two sides is symmetric, and a valuable sign is the presence of increased density of one hilum (Fig. 1.19). If a hilum is not enlarged and does not show calcification, intrinsically it cannot be denser than normal; there must therefore be an intrapulmonary density superimposed on it. This is a not infrequent sign in carcinoma of the bronchus.

4. The Tracheobronchial Tree

A. Trachea

- The trachea is normally straight and lies in the midline of the chest as judged by its relationship to the upper thoracic spinous processes and to the medial ends of the clavicles.
- In the root of the neck, the trachea may be bowed, commonly by thyroid enlargement (Fig. 1.20), but sometimes by enlarged cervical nodes (Fig. 1.26).
- Between the sternal notch and the aortic arch, tracheal bowing is common, the

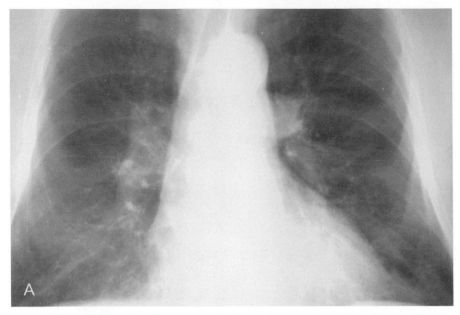

Figure 1.18A. Patient with COPD and marked cor pulmonale, as evidenced by the dilatation of the hilar arteries.

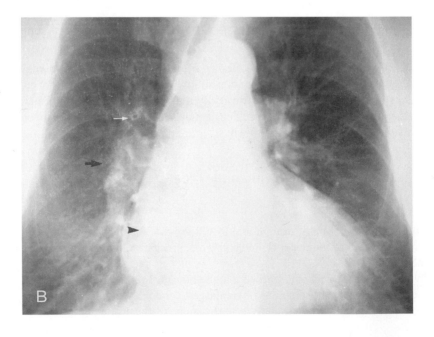

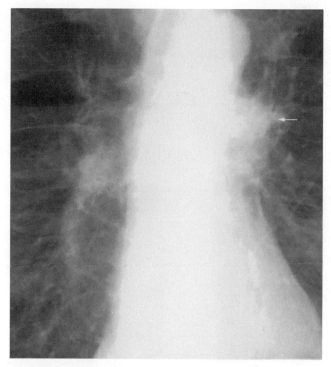

Figure 1.19. Comparison with the right hilum shows a distinct increased density of the left hilum (*arrow*). This indicates a density superimposed on the hilum and is not an infrequent sign in the small peripheral bronchial carcinoma. In this case, the carcinoma was a peripheral lesion in the superior segment of the left lower lobe.

Figure 1.18B. The patient in Figure 1.18*A* has developed heart failure, a common and not infrequently clinically unrecognized occurrence in COPD. The upper lobe veins are somewhat more prominent, but a striking feature of interstitial pulmonary edema is the blurring of the lateral border of the descending right pulmonary artery (*black arrow*). Note the thickened and ill-defined bronchial wall superimposed on the right upper hilum, that of the anterior segmental bronchus of the upper lobe (*white arrow*). This thickening is not the result of peribronchial edema, as commonly stated, but of edema of the entire bronchial wall. The heart has increased in size with left ventricular dilatation. The double density behind the right side of the heart (*arrowhead*) is the result of confluence of the right pulmonary veins.

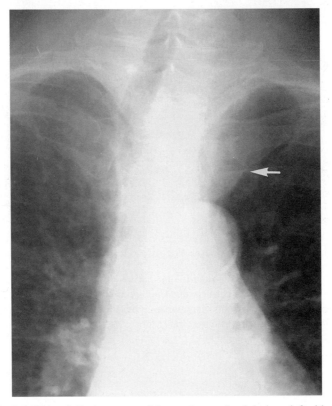

Figure 1.20. Bowing and displacement of the trachea to the right by a left-sided goiter. The soft tissue mass of the goiter can just be distinguished extending down to just above the aortic knuckle (*arrow*).

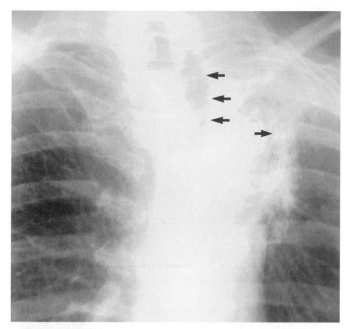

Figure 1.21. Gross contracture of the left upper lobe following radiotherapy for carcinoma of the bronchus. The loss of volume has caused considerable bowing of the trachea to the left (*three arrows*). Note also the gross elevation of the left hilum (*single arrow*).

trachea being either pushed by a mass or pulled by loss of volume in the adjacent lung (fibrosis, atelectasis, or resection) (Fig. 1.21).

- At the level of the aortic arch, tracheal displacement to the right is almost invariable in older patients because of unfolding of the aorta.
- Bowing to the left at this level is invariably abnormal. In the absence of any lung disease, suspect a right-sided aortic arch (Fig. 1.22).
- Uniform displacement of the trachea, as opposed to localized bowing, occurs with mediastinal shift when there is any major change of lung volume, particularly following collapse or resection of the lung.
- In patients with severe chronic obstructive pulmonary disease (COPD), a smoothly tapered symmetric narrowing of the intrathoracic portion of the trachea may occur (Fig. 1.23). Termed the "sabre sheath trachea," it has no clinical significance other than indicating COPD, but it is important to recognize to avoid consideration of bilateral extrinsic compression of the trachea from a mediastinal lesion.

B. Right Paratracheal Stripe

- The right paratracheal stripe is produced by contact of the lung with the right lateral border of the trachea.
- It is a well-defined thin line, which should not exceed 4 mm in width, and is commonly seen ending at the azygos vein (Figs. 1.3, 1.24*B*).

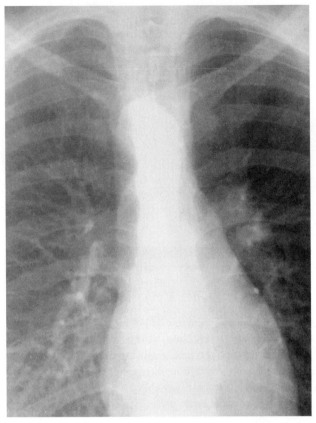

Figure 1.22. Displacement and slight bowing of the trachea to the left by a right-sided aortic arch. The aortic knuckle can be clearly seen lying to the right of the trachea. An additional sign of right aortic arch is the absence of sufficient space to the left of the trachea to accommodate the normal left arch.

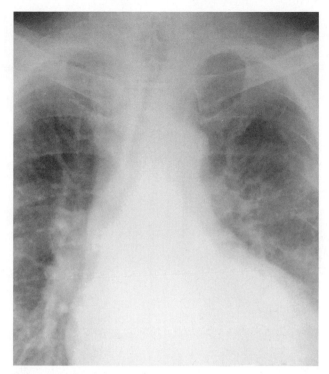

Figure 1.23. A "sabre sheath trachea." Note the considerable diffuse symmetric narrowing of the trachea extending from the thoracic inlet to the aortic arch. This a sign of severe COPD and is accompanied by increased sagittal diameter of trachea on the lateral view. It is important not to confuse this with tracheal compression from a mediastinal lesion.

- In the absence of disease in the adjacent lung or pleura, blurring of this stripe, particularly when accompanied by increased density or a convex bulge, is a significant sign (Figs. 1.24A, 1.34).
- Causes of blurring of the paratracheal stripe are detailed in Table 1.1.

C. Tracheal Bifurcation Angle

- The left main bronchus is longer than the right and usually has an angle of around 45° from the vertical. The right main bronchus is shorter and more vertical than the left and is usually oriented around 30° from the vertical.
- The tracheal bifurcation angle is variable but in 95% of normal patients falls between 45° and 80°.
- An angle of 90° or greater is abnormal and requires investigation (Fig. 1.25).
- Causes of increased tracheal bifurcation angle are listed in Table 1.2.

D. Azygo-esophageal Recess

- Subcarinal masses will produce another sign on the PA chest film: deviation of the azygo-esophageal recess.

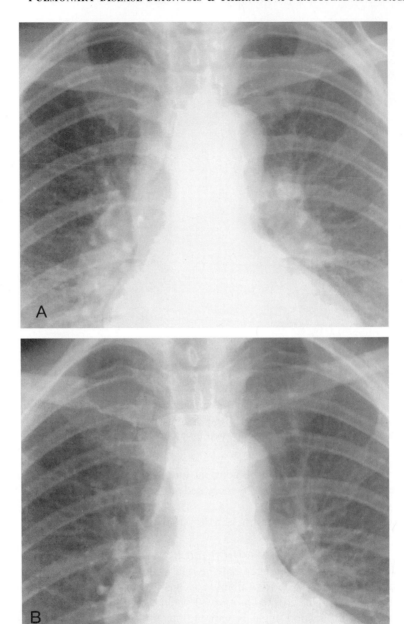

Figure 1.24. A, A patient with bilateral symmetric hilar adenopathy of sarcoid. Note that the right paratracheal stripe is blurred, and there is a subtle increased density in the azygos area. These latter findings are the result of enlargement of the azygos node. **B,** Normal radiograph of the same patient as in Figure 1.24A before the development of the right paratracheal and hilar adenopathy. Note the clarity of the thin right paratracheal stripe, ending in the azygos vein.

Table 1.1. Causes of Blurring of the Right Paratracheal Stripe

Hemorrhage	Iatrogenic	Catheter insertion
		Postmediastinoscopy
	Traumatic	Particularly rupture of aorta
Adenopathy		
Adjacent lung consolidation or pleural effusion		

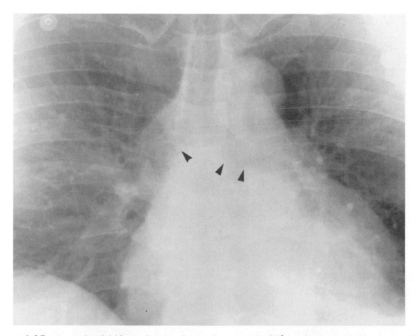

Figure 1.25. A tracheal bifurcation angle rarely exceeds 80° in the normal; an angle of 90° or greater requires explanation. In this case the angle of a little over 90° was the result of pericardial effusion (two *arrowheads* on inferior margin of left main bronchus, single *arrowhead* on inferior margin of right main bronchus).

Table 1.2. Causes of Increased Tracheal Bifurcation Angle

Left auricular enlargement particularly as a result of mitral valve disease
Subcarinal adenopathy
Pericardial effusion (pericardial fluid does not collect posteriorly, but pushes the left auricle
    posteriorly into the tracheal bifurcation)
Bronchogenic cyst
Carcinoma of the esophagus

- The normal azygo-esophageal recess is the impression of the medial border of the right lung on the mediastinum, below the level of the azygos vein. It is normally mildly concave to the right in the upper half and mildly convex to the right in the lower half (Fig. 1.3).
- Subcarinal masses will reverse this subcarinal concavity, producing a convex bulge, and often will produce a recognizable increased density (Figs. 1.16, 1.26).
- Retrocardiac masses arising in the posterior mediastinum behind the heart will cause marked convex bulging to the right of the lower aspect of the recess (Fig. 1.27).

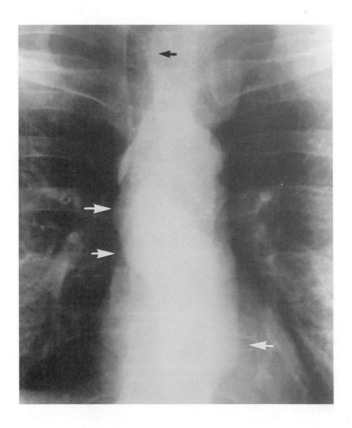

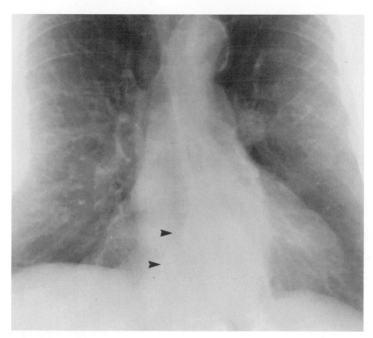

Figure 1.27. Marked convex bulging of the lower margin of the azygo-esophageal recess (*arrowheads*) from hiatus hernia.

- The most common cause of a retrocardiac mass is an esophageal lesion, particularly a hiatus hernia, and much less frequently a benign or malignant tumor of the esophagus.

5. Cardiac Shadow

The anatomic composition of the heart borders is illustrated in Figure 1.2. Generalized enlargement of the heart and specific chamber enlargement are not discussed in this section.

The narrow transverse diameter of the heart that occurs in COPD and the prominence of the main pulmonary artery that occurs in primary or secondary pulmonary hypertension may be important considerations in patients who have pulmonary symptoms.

◀————————————————————————————————

Figure 1.26. Marked convexity to the right of the upper azygo-esophageal recess, which should be concave, together with increased subcarinal density from subcarinal adenopathy (*two white arrows*). This was metastatic disease from a hypernephroma. There is also lobulation of the lateral margin of the lower descending thoracic aorta from para-aortic adenopathy (*single white arrow*) and marked displacement of the trachea to the right by a mass of left cervical nodes (*black arrow*).

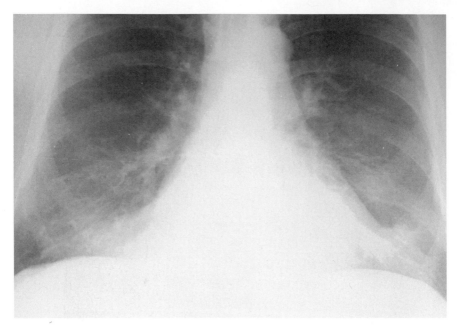

Figure 1.28. Blurring of the lower aspect of both cardiac borders by pericardial fat.

- The clarity of the heart borders is an important consideration in localizing pulmonary disease, arising from the significance of the "silhouette sign."
- This sign stems from the fact that any intrathoracic opacity that obliterates the normally sharp border of the heart, aorta, or diaphragm must lie in contact with the tangential plane of that structure. Correspondingly, structures in front of or behind the tangential plane will not obliterate the margin.
- The heart borders are uniformly sharp except that the lower aspects of the heart borders in the cardiophrenic angles may be blurred by pericardial fat. A left pericardial fat pad blurring the border is common; bilateral fat pads are less common (Fig. 1.28), and an isolated right pericardial fat pad is rarest.
- Blurring of the left heart border is characteristic of lingular disease (Fig. 1.29).
- Middle lobe disease will blur the right heart border (Fig. 1.30).
- Blurring of the right heart border, however, is a common finding in depressed sternum (Fig. 1.31). A clue to this on the PA view is that the posterior ribs are more horizontal than normal and the anterior ribs are more vertical.

6. Vascular Pedicle

- The heart may be thought of as suspended in the mediastinum by the great systemic vessels, and these vessels have been termed the vascular pedicle.
- It is best measured radiologically from the lateral border of the innominate vein or superior vena cava (SVC) on the right to the origin of the subclavian artery on

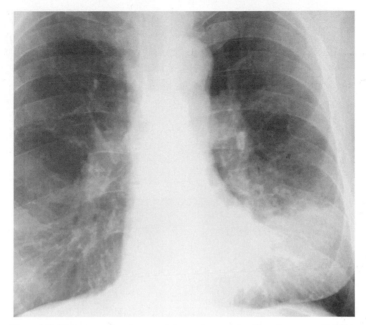

Figure 1.29. Blurring of the left heart border by lingular consolidation.

the left (Fig. 1.32A) and normally does not exceed 5.4 cm in diameter on a 6-foot upright PA radiograph.

- The right border, being venous, distends with increased blood volume. The left border, being arterial, does not.
- Increase of the width of the vascular pedicle is thus a good index of fluid retention in renal dialysis (Fig. 1.32, A–B), although increased transverse diameter of the heart shows an even better correlation with increased blood volume. Surprisingly, there is a poor correlation with increased right atrial pressure.
- Increased width will also occur in heart failure, but it is an inconstant sign.

7. Thoracic Aorta

- The right upper border of the mediastinum above the right atrium is a straight edge formed by the SVC, but an unfolded ascending aorta from atherosclerosis may project beyond the SVC, producing a convex bulge.
- The lateral border of the ascending aorta should not project beyond a vertical line tangential to the right atrium, and if it does so, this should raise consideration of poststenotic dilatation in aortic stenosis or of aortic aneurysm.
- Intimal calcification of the aorta is common in older people (Fig. 1.27). Calcification in the aortic knuckle allows the thickness of the aortic wall to be determined and it should not be more than 6 mm. Figure 1.33 shows an obvious aneurysm of the aortic arch, and the intimal calcification shows that the thickness of the aortic wall is 16 mm. This indicates a dissecting aneurysm of the aorta.

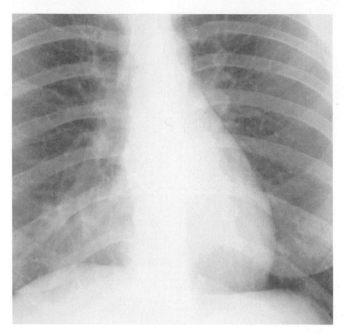

Figure 1.30. Blurring of the right heart border by consolidation in the medial segment of the middle lobe. On the original film, the lesser fissure was in normal position (between the anterior ends of the third and fourth ribs) and was completely sharp, indicating the lateral segment was not involved.

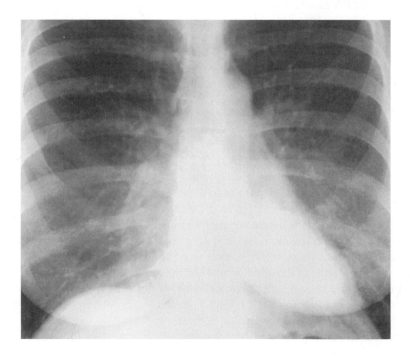

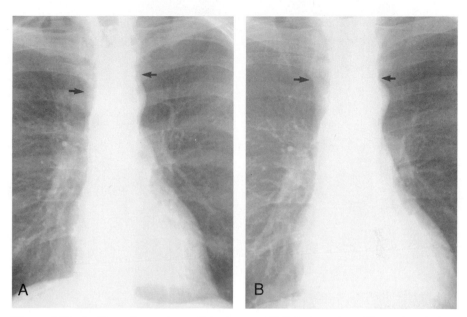

Figure 1.32. A, Normal vascular pedicle in a renal dialysis patient. The patient is in a satisfactory volemic state following dialysis, and the vascular pedicle (*arrows*) measures 5.2 cm. The transverse diameter of the heart is 13 cm. **B,** The same patient as in Figure 1.32*A,* predialysis. The vascular pedicle (*arrows*) has increased to 6.0 cm, which exceeds the normal limit of 5.3 cm, and there had been a distinct increase in the transverse diameter of the heart to 15 cm. Both are signs of fluid retention.

Figure 1.31. Blurring of the right heart border from depressed sternum. Note the characteristic configuration of the ribs that commonly occurs in depressed sternum. The posterior aspects of the ribs are more horizontal than normal and the anterior aspects more sharply declining.

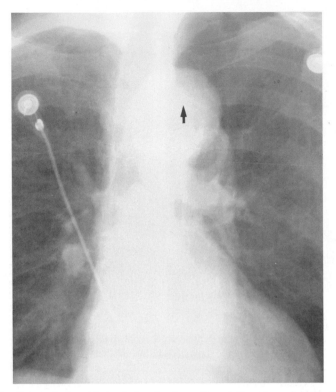

Figure 1.33. The aortic knuckle is obviously circumferentially enlarged, indicating an aneurysm of the aortic arch. In addition, intimal calcification can be seen (*arrow*), and this allows the thickness of the aortic wall to be measured. The aortic wall is markedly thickened (1.6 cm), indicating a dissecting aneurysm.

- In children and younger adults, the descending aorta lies predominately in front of the vertebral column. As the patient ages, the aorta becomes tortuous and comes to lie increasingly to the left of the vertebral column, producing a double density behind the heart. This can be confusing if the continuity of the shadow with the upper descending aorta is not appreciated (Fig. 1.34).
- The lateral margin of the descending aorta is smooth and uniformly sharp. Blurring of the margin (Fig. 1.35) is an example of the silhouette sign, and, other than from obvious pleural effusion, usually indicates consolidation in the adjacent left lower lobe.
- Lobulation of the lateral margin (Fig. 1.26) is evidence of enlargement of the para-aortic lymph nodes.
- The aortopulmonary window, the space between the aortic knuckle and the left pulmonary artery, is normally concave (Fig. 1.3), although it occasionally may be straight. Convexity is a good indication of enlargement of the ductus node (Fig. 1.36).

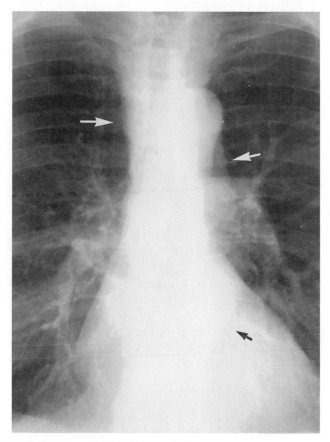

Figure 1.34. The left paravertebral soft tissue shadow behind the left side of the heart (*black arrow*) could be mistaken for a paravertebral soft tissue swelling if the continuity of the margin with the upper descending aorta (*white arrow*) is not recognized. Note also the right paratracheal bulge and loss of the paratracheal stripe from enlarged nodes (*white arrow*).

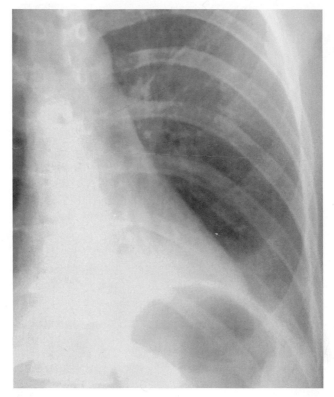

Figure 1.35. The lateral margin of the descending aorta can be identified down to the level of the lower margin of the left main bronchus and is then obliterated, from atelectasis in the left lower lobe. This is a common finding, particularly in the ICU and in the postoperative patient.

8. The Diaphragm and Costophrenic Angles

The radiologic custom is to refer to the right and left hemidiaphragms as the right and left diaphragms.

- Both diaphragms, the costophrenic angles and the cardiophrenic angles, are normally well-defined except that pericardial fat may blur the cardiophrenic angles. Blurring of the diaphragm implies either pleural fluid or disease in the adjacent lung field.
- The dome of the right diaphragm is normally up to 1 cm higher than the left, although the right and left cardiophrenic angles are usually at about the same level.
- The outline of the right diaphragm is lost as it reaches the right heart border.
- The left diaphragm is visible medially as far as the vertebral column.
- A weakened and elevated anteromedial flange of the diaphragm is common, particularly on the right.

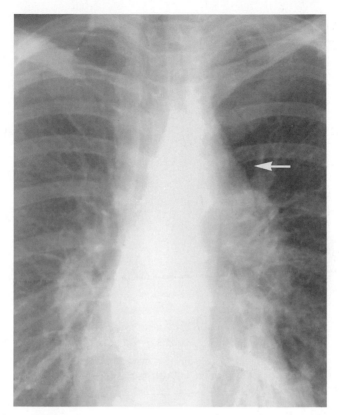

Figure 1.36. Convexity of the aortopulmonary window (*arrow*) indicating ductus node enlargement in a patient with lymphoma. Note also bilateral hilar adenopathy (more marked on the left), displacement of the trachea to the right by massive left cervical node enlargement, and increased tracheal bifurcation angle (90°) and subcarinal density from subcarinal adenopathy.

- When weakening is extensive and involves most of the diaphragm, it is termed eventration of the diaphragm. Eventration is distinguishable from a paralyzed diaphragm by a costophrenic angle that remains at the normal level in eventration (Fig. 1.37).

Pleural Effusion

- A trace of fluid in the costophrenic angle will merely blunt the angle.
- A minimal pleural effusion will obliterate the angle, but the margins will be ill-defined (Fig. 1.38).
- A larger effusion will cause an obvious homogeneous density with an ill-defined margin extending upward and inward from the costophrenic angle, and extending along the axillary border of the lung (Fig. 1.38).

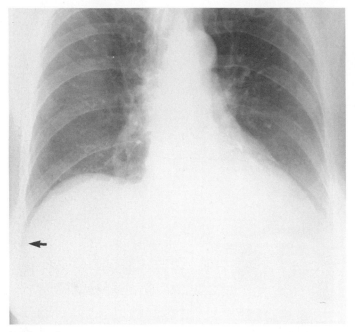

Figure 1.37. Eventration of the right diaphragm. This is distinguished from an elevated diaphragm, whether from phrenic paresis or other cause, in that the costophrenic angle is not elevated but lies at the same level as the left (*arrow*).

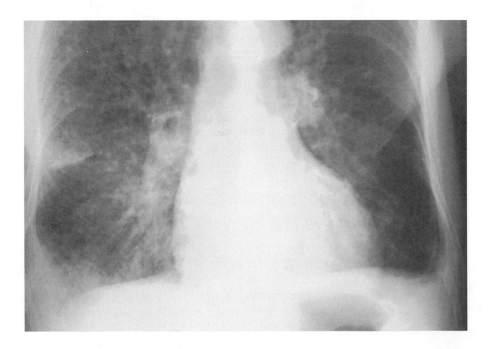

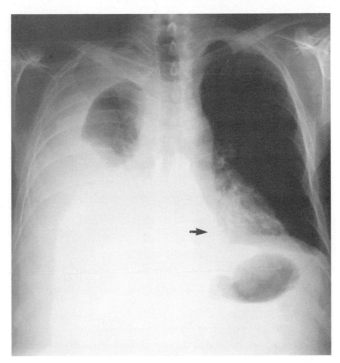

Figure 1.39. Massive right pleural effusion, extending over the apex of the lung onto the mediastinal aspect of the upper lobe. There is no mediastinal shift because of the complete collapse of the middle and lower lobes. The left paravertebral opacity (*arrow*) is the result of right pleural effusion bulging the azygo-esophageal recess to the left of the midline.

• Massive effusions extend over the apex of the lung onto the mediastinal aspect of the apex (Fig. 1.39) and will usually cause mediastinal shift to the opposite side. Large effusions commonly cause compression atelectasis of the underlying lung (particularly of the basal segments), however, and if the atelectasis is sufficient, no mediastinal shift will be produced.

• Particularly large effusions may cause depression of the diaphragm, and on the right will commonly displace the azygo-esophageal recess to the left of the midline (Fig. 1.39).

• A lateral decubitus film is of value in confirming that the obliteration is the result

Figure 1.38. Bilateral pleural effusions in a patient with metastatic nodules scattered throughout both lungs, primary unknown. There is a small left pleural effusion obliterating the left costophrenic angle, with an ill-defined margin. There is a larger right pleural effusion, also with an ill-defined margin, extending along the axillary margin of the lung. There is a little atelectasis in the anterior segment of the right upper lobe, abutting on the outer aspect of the lesser fissure.

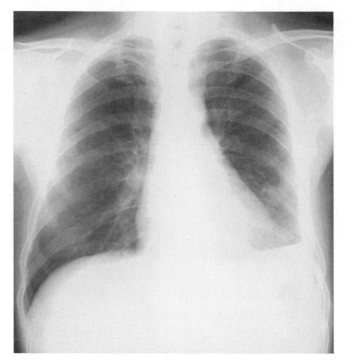

Figure 1.40. Old pleural thickening obliterating the left costophrenic angle. Note the considerable lateral elevation and straightening of the left diaphragm, and the sharpness of the costophrenic angle, indicating an old pleural reaction with adhesions from fibrosis.

of fluid and not pleural adhesions and in giving an index of the volume of the effusion.

- Costophrenic angle blunting or obliteration may be produced by flattening of the diaphragm in COPD or by fibrous adhesions from previous effusion; these can usually be distinguished from fluid in that the costophrenic angle is sharp and well-defined in these two circumstances.
- An additional sign of old pleural adhesions rather than recent effusion is straightening of the diaphragm with elevation of the lateral aspect (Fig. 1.40). Because of the fibrous adhesions, the lateral aspect does not descend with the rest of the diaphragm on inspiration, impairing the normal "piston action" of the diaphragm.
- Occasionally pleural fluid collects under the lung, the subpulmonary or infrapulmonary effusion. It has a characteristic appearance on both PA (Fig. 1.41) and lateral views (Fig. 1.55). In the normal PA view, the dome of the diaphragm lies in the medial third, whereas in infrapulmonary effusion it is displaced to the lateral third and there is usually a minimal effusion in the costophrenic angle.
- A further sign is that the normal vascular pattern is not seen behind the dome of the diaphragm, a result of the usually associated posterior costophrenic effusion.
- On the left side, infrapulmonary effusion is easier to diagnose because of the

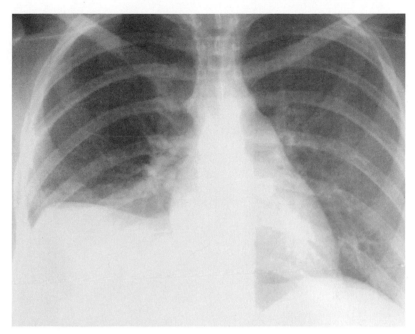

Figure 1.41. Right intrapulmonary effusion. The dome of the apparently elevated right diaphragm, actually the infrapulmonary fluid, is markedly displaced laterally, and there is slight blurring of the costophrenic angle indicating a trace of fluid. This configuration is characteristic of infrapulmonary fluid on the PA view.

increased space between the gastric air bubble and the apparent dome of the diaphragm.

- Infrapulmonary effusion is easily confirmed with a lateral decubitus view (Fig. 1.42).
- Calcification of the diaphragmatic pleura is a frequent finding in asbestosis and is usually accompanied by pleural thickening and possibly calcification in the midaxillary regions. Diaphragmatic pleural calcification can also follow empyema, tuberculous pleurisy, and hemothorax. Occasionally an asymptomatic idiopathic diaphragmatic calcification is seen.

ABNORMAL SIGNS ON THE LATERAL CHEST RADIOGRAPH

Anterior Mediastinum

- This space lies between the sternum anteriorly and the heart and aorta posteriorly, and extends from the level of the manubriosternal junction above to the diaphragm below (Fig. 1.7).

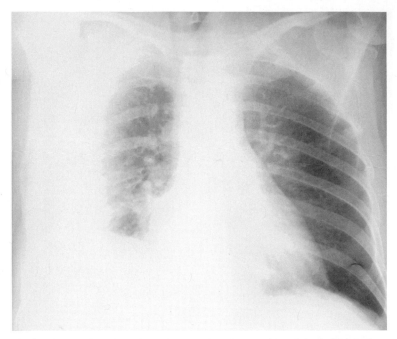

Figure 1.42. Right lateral decubitus film showing the layering of the infrapulmonary fluid, which moves freely out of its infrapulmonary position to extend along the axillary border of the lung to the apex. In the erect position, the fluid returns to the infrapulmonary site.

- The retrosternal space is usually of the same translucency as the retrocardiac space, but undue amounts of anterior mediastinal fat will make the retrosternal space more opaque.
- Normally the right ventricle is in contact with the lowest third of the anterior chest wall, measured from the manubriosternal junction to the diaphragm. This contact is decreased in emphysema (Fig. 1.43) and is increased in right ventricular hypertrophy (Fig. 1.44).
- Enlargement of the prevascular lymph glands in the anterior mediastinum occurs particularly in lymphoma. The anterior mediastinal mass merges with the aortic and cardiac shadows (Fig. 1.45).
- Internal mammary adenopathy occurs, particularly in carcinoma of the breast. The nodal mass merges anteriorly with the sternum, but it stays separate from the vascular shadows (Fig. 1.46).
- The most common primary anterior mediastinal tumors are thymomas (Fig. 1.47) and germ cell neoplasms, particularly teratomas. These tumors usually do not merge with the sternum, but the malignant varieties commonly merge with the heart and aortic shadows.

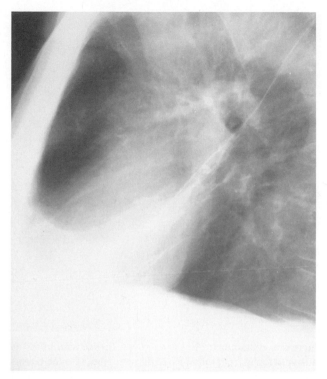

Figure 1.43. Diminished contact between the heart and the sternum in a patient with severe COPD. Note the flattening of the diaphragm from the COPD.

Middle Mediastinum

- The middle mediastinum extends posteriorly from the anterior mediastinum to the vertical extent of the posterior limit of the pericardium (Fig. 1.7). It thus includes the distal trachea and the hila, as well as the heart.
- The most common abnormality other than cardiac seen in the middle mediastinum is hilar adenopathy. Figure 1.48 shows the characteristic lobulated enlargement of both right and left hilar nodes.

Posterior Mediastinum

- Although, according to the strict definition, the posterior mediastinum ends prevertebrally, in clinical practice there is a general consensus that it extends paravertebrally to the level of the ribs.
- Normally there is an even gradation of density in the thoracic spine that gradually decreases in whiteness as one descends inferiorly. Reversal of this gradation indicates an overlying density, and the commonest pulmonary cause is collapse or consolidation in one of the lower lobes (Fig. 1.49).

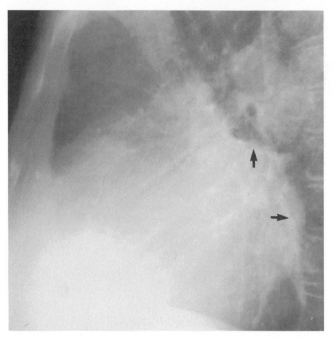

Figure 1.44. Increased contact between the heart and the sternum in a patient with severe right ventricular hypertrophy from mitral valve disease. Note also the considerable posterior bulging of the heart border (*arrow*) and the posterior and upward displacement of the left lower lobe bronchus (*arrow*) from the considerable left atrial enlargement.

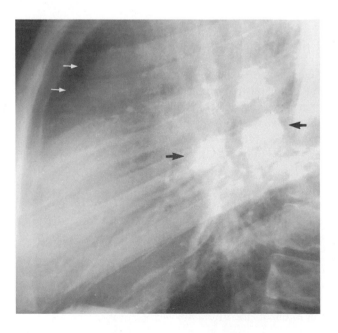

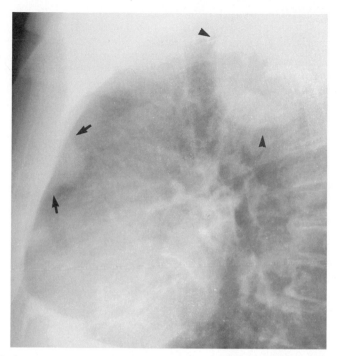

Figure 1.46. An enlarged internal mammary node in a patient with metastatic hypernephroma. The mass merges with the sternum anteriorly and has a well-defined posterior margin distinct from the vascular shadows. The angles of the contact with the sternum (*arrows*) are convex, indicating that the mass is extrapulmonary in origin. Note the 6.5-cm pulmonary metastasis lying behind the trachea (*arrowheads*).

Figure 1.45. A mass of anterior mediastinal prevascular enlarged lymph nodes (*white arrows*) in lymphoma encroaching on the upper anterior mediastinal space, separate from the sternum but merging posteriorly with the vascular shadows. This patient with lymphoma also has markedly enlarged left hilar and right hilar (*black arrows*) adenopathy.

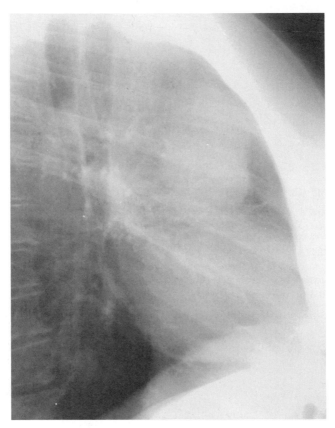

Figure 1.47. One of the two most common anterior mediastinal primary tumors, a thymoma. It is distinct from the sternum anteriorly and merges with the vascular shadow posteriorly.

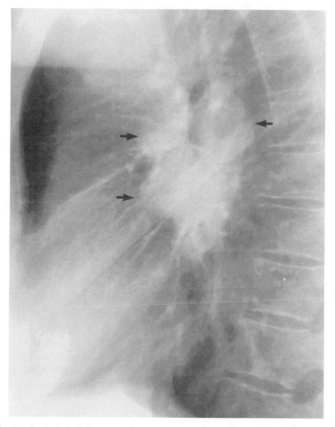

Figure 1.48. Marked right hilar and left hilar (*arrows*) node enlargement in a patient with non-Hodgkin's lymphoma.

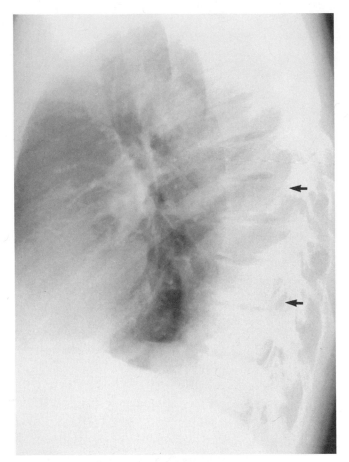

Figure 1.49. Reversal of the normal in density gradient of the thoracic spine (*arrows*) in partial collapse of the left lower lobe. Note the obliteration of the outline of the posterior aspect of the left diaphragm from contact with the collapsed lobe. Note also that in this left lateral film, the posterior aspect of the right ribs, which lie further from the film, are larger and less well-defined than the left. The diaphragm reaching the right posterior costophrenic sulcus is obviously the right diaphragm. The collapse must therefore be of the left lower lobe.

- The intervertebral foramina show a similar gradation of density, and reversal also indicates an overlying opacity (Fig. 1.50).
- Aneurysms of the descending aorta usually can be clearly seen in the posterior mediastinum on the lateral view (Fig. 1.51).
- The most common primary tumor in the posterior mediastinum is a neurogenous tumor, but the most common opacity seen in clinical practice is a hiatus hernia. If the characteristic air bubble of the hernia is missing (Fig. 1.52), the appearance may be confusing.

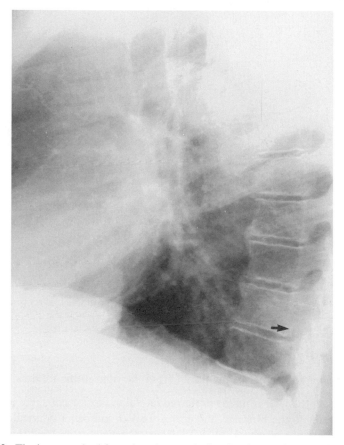

Figure 1.50. The intervertebral foramina show a similar density gradient, as do the vertebral bodies, and there is reversal of this density gradient at one of the lower foramina (*arrow*). In addition to this lesion, there is considerable overlying pleural thickening. This is a case of round atelectasis.

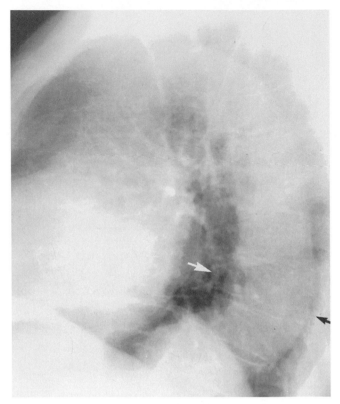

Figure 1.51. Mild aneurysmal dilatation of the lower thoracic aorta (*arrows*).

The Diaphragm

The left diaphragm can be distinguished from the right in the following ways:

- Assuming a left lateral film, the preferred lateral in most centers, the left posterior ribs are nearer to the film and, therefore, smaller and better defined than are the right. The left ribs also tend to lie in front of the right ribs, and the diaphragm terminated at the left ribs is obviously the left diaphragm, and vice versa (Fig. 1.49).
- The left diaphragm tends to end at the posterior cardiac border, whereas the right diaphragm usually extends through the heart shadow toward the anterior chest wall (Fig. 1.49).
- If the gastric air bubble can be clearly identified as being applied to one diaphragm, this identifies it as the left diaphragm.
- The posterior costophrenic angles are normally sharp. They become obliterated or blurred in pleural effusions (Fig. 1.53).
- The posterior costophrenic angles can also be obliterated by either pleural adhesions (Fig. 1.54) or diaphragmatic flattening in COPD.

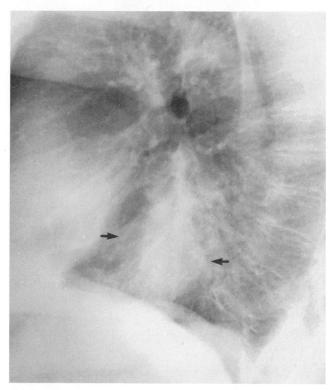

Figure 1.52. A fixed hiatus hernia (*arrows*) visible behind the heart. With the lack of the characteristic air bubble, this could be confused with a solid space-occupying lesion (such as a large esophageal tumor) or, in a patient following splenectomy for blood dyscrasia, with extramedullary hematopoiesis.

- Infrapulmonary effusion has a characteristic appearance on the lateral view as well as on the PA view. This fluid resembles an elevated diaphragm but with a sharply declining straight anterior border continuous with the major fissure (Fig. 1.55). There is usually blurring of the posterior costophrenic sulcus from the small effusion, which usually occurs in association with the infrapulmonary fluid.

Superior Mediastinum

- The superior mediastinum extends from the thoracic inlet above to a line drawn between the lower border of the fourth thoracic vertebra posteriorly and the manubriosternal junction anteriorly (Fig. 1.7).
- In the anterior aspect of the superior mediastinum, in front of the trachea, the most common abnormality is an intrathoracic goiter, which if large enough will cause an anterotracheal density and posterior displacement of the trachea (Fig. 1.56).

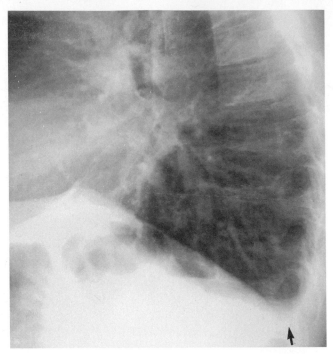

Figure 1.53. Obliteration and blurring of both posterior costophrenic angles (*arrow*) in small bilateral pleural effusions.

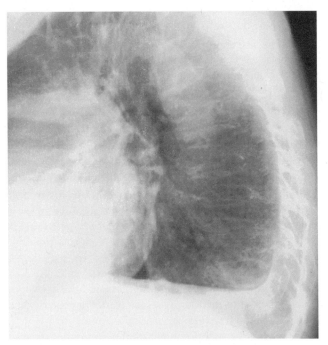

Figure 1.54. Obliteration of the left costophrenic angle by adhesions. The sharp interface would suggest that this is not the result of recent effusion.

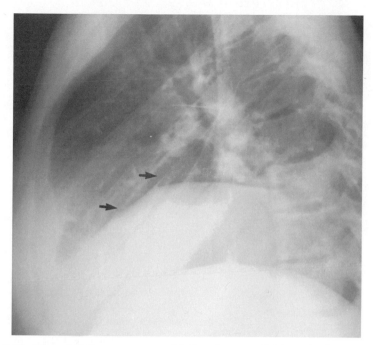

Figure 1.55. Characteristic appearance of infrapulmonary fluid on the lateral view. The shadow of the apparently elevated diaphragm is the result of infrapulmonary fluid. The anterior margin of the diaphragm declines sharply in a linear fashion and is continuous superiorly with the major fissure (*arrows*). Note also the obliteration and lack of definition of the posterior costophrenic sulcus by a small costophrenic effusion, which usually accompanies infrapulmonary fluid. Note also the minor fluid in both major fissures and in the lesser fissure.

- The space behind the trachea is termed the retrotracheal triangle. Its boundaries are the posterior wall of the trachea anteriorly, the superior wall of the aorta inferiorly, the upper four thoracic vertebrae posteriorly, and the thoracic inlet superiorly (Figs. 1.5–1.6). It is a unique triangle in that it is defined as having four sides! A carcinoma of the esophagus may produce a visible mass in the triangle (Fig. 1.57).
- The most common abnormal structure in the retrotracheal triangle is an intrathoracic goiter, of which approximately 25% are retrotracheal. It will produce a mass abutting on the posterior wall of the trachea (Fig. 1.58). Another clinically rare abnormality in this triangle is a right-sided aorta.
- The inferior portion of the superior mediastinum is occupied by the horizontal portion of the aortic arch. The anterior aspect of the superior aortic margin is not well-defined (Fig. 1.5) because the great vessels prevent the left lung from providing a sharp interface with the aorta. The posterior aspect, however, is often clearly visible, particularly in older people. An aneurysm of the aorta, with or without calcification, may give a characteristic appearance (Fig. 1.59).

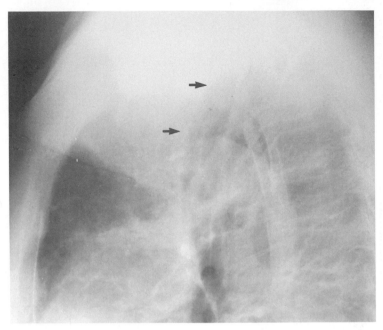

Figure 1.56. Posterior bowing and displacement of the trachea in the superior mediastinum (*arrows*) by an intrathoracic goiter lying in front of the trachea.

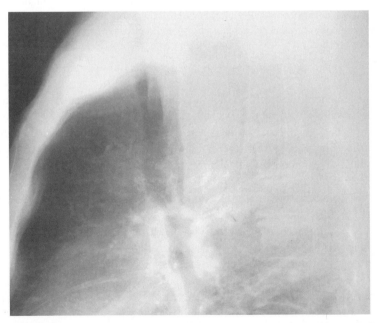

Figure 1.57. Obliteration of the retrotracheal triangle by a mass formed by a carcinoma of the esophagus with a tracheo-esophageal fistula.

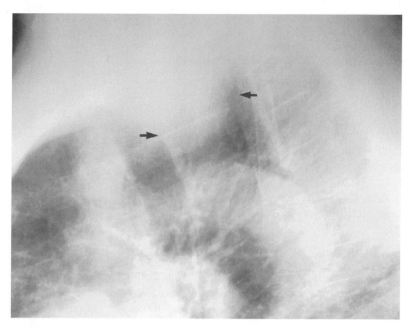

Figure 1.58. A 4-cm mass in the anterior aspect of the retrotracheal triangle (*arrows*) from a large retrotracheal intrathoracic goiter.

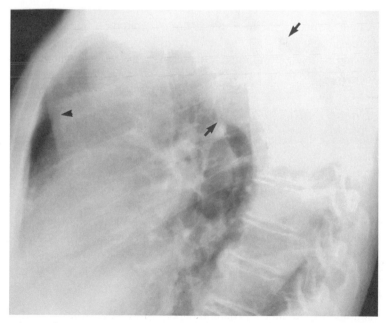

Figure 1.59. Moderate fusiform aneurysmal dilatation of the posterior aspect of the aortic arch and upper descending aorta (*arrows*). Note also the encroachment on the superior aspect of the anterior mediastinum from involvement of the anterior arch (*arrowhead*).

LUNG PARENCHYMA

This section discusses diseases of the lung parenchyma:

• Unilateral hyperlucency of the lung;
• Airspace disease;
• Atelectasis;
• Pulmonary edema;
• Emphysema;
• Bronchiectasis;
• Pulmonary masses;
• Cavitation;
• Diffuse interstitial lung disease.

Unilateral Hyperlucency of the Lung

Normally each hemithorax attenuates the radiographic beam to roughly the same degree, and the two lungs appear of equal density. Many conditions may render one hemithorax more translucent (or, conversely, more opaque) than the other, leading to the appearance of unilateral hyperlucency.

Radiographic Technique

• If the patient is rotated, the lung that is farther from the film may appear darker or more translucent (Fig. 1.4).
• On a bedside radiograph, improper alignment of the radiographic grid may lead to unequal exposure of the two hemithoraces.

Chest Wall Abnormalities

• Any reduction in the thickness of the chest wall on one side can produce ipsilateral hyperlucency.
• Mastectomy, the clue to which is the absence of the normal curve of the inferior aspect of the breast, is a common cause.
• Congenital deficiency of the pectoral muscles (Poland's syndrome) is a rare cause of ipsilateral hyperlucency.
• A large unilateral chest wall mass increases the density of the ipsilateral hemithorax such that the normal side may appear falsely hyperlucent.

Pleural Abnormalities

• Pneumothorax may produce ipsilateral hyperlucency (Fig. 1.60). Identification of the visceral pleural line is required for the absolute diagnosis of a pneumothorax.
• In the supine patient, a pleural effusion layers posteriorly, increasing the density of the ipsilateral hemithorax so that the contralateral lung may appear hyperlucent.

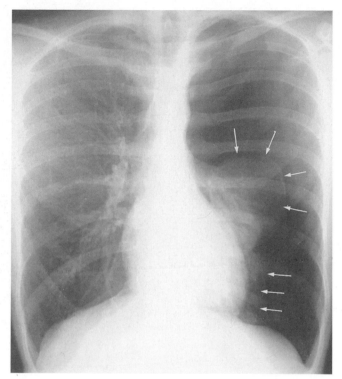

Figure 1.60. Large left pneumothorax causing an increase in the lucency of the left hemithorax. Note the visceral pleural margin of the collapsed lung (*arrows*).

Lung Abnormalities

- An increase in the translucency of one lung can result from a decrease in its blood flow, a decrease in its interstitial tissue, an increase in its aeration, or a combination of these factors. True hyperlucency of both lungs can occur for identical reasons, but its recognition is difficult. Because of the identical density of the two lungs, there is no "control" side with which to compare. More commonly, a technical aberration leading to an increase in the overall blackening of the film gives the spurious appearance of bilateral hyperlucency.
- Unilateral hyperlucency from aspiration of a foreign body into a main bronchus is more common in children than in adults—atelectasis usually occurs in adults.
- Asymmetric pulmonary emphysema in adults may lead to relative hyperlucency of the more severely affected lung.
- Lobar resection results in compensatory overinflation of the remaining lung, which may appear hyperlucent.
- In Swyer-James (MacLeod's) syndrome, the hyperlucent lung has a small hilum

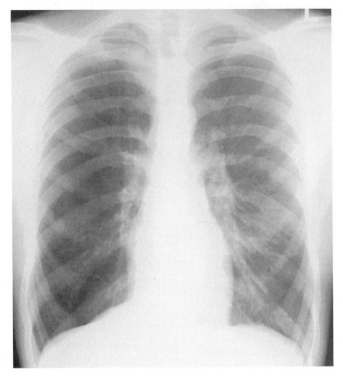

Figure 1.61. Hyperlucent right lung with diminished vascularity in Swyer-James (Mac-Leod's) syndrome.

and traps air in expiration (Fig. 1.61); an identical appearance can occasionally result from a partially occluding neoplasm in a main bronchus.
- Obstruction of a main pulmonary artery by an embolus or a neoplasm may render the ipsilateral lung hyperlucent.

Airspace Disease (Alveolar Disease, Parenchymal Consolidation)

Consolidation refers to replacement of the air in the pulmonary acini by fluid, cells, or both. Because fluid and cells attenuate an x-ray beam to the same degree, a similar appearance may result regardless of the material that fills the acini—edema fluid, inflammatory exudate, blood, or neoplastic cells. Because consolidation affects primarily the airspaces of the lung, rather than the pulmonary interstitium, the radiographic appearance of consolidation is known commonly as the airspace or alveolar pattern.

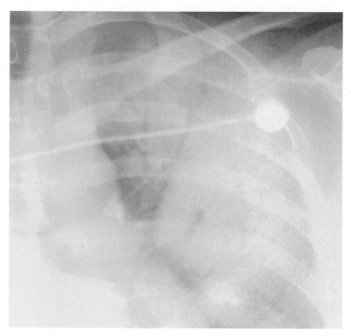

Figure 1.62. Pulmonary hemorrhage in Goodpasture's syndrome, showing air bronchograms in the left upper lobe.

Signs of Parenchymal Consolidation

- Air bronchogram. Because the bronchial tree is not occluded in consolidation, the larger conducting airways will be visible as dark, tubular, branching structures within the opaque areas of consolidation (Fig. 1.62).
- Acinar shadows. Poorly marginated nodular opacities 4–10 mm in diameter representing consolidated acini, if seen, denote filling of the peripheral airspaces (Fig. 1.63).
- Coalescence. As the consolidation spreads, groups of involved acini merge, forming coalescent or confluent areas of opacification (Figs. 1.64–1.65).
- Poor margination. Unlike a mass that typically has discrete margins, an area of consolidation is usually poorly marginated, except where it abuts a fissure, because of the random superimposition of consolidated and normal groups of acini (Figs. 1.66–1.67). Rarely, pneumonia will result in a spherical, well-defined opacity resembling a mass (Fig. 1.68).
- Butterfly pattern of distribution. This bilateral perihilar pattern, also known as the bat wing pattern, is indicative of consolidation, usually resulting from pulmonary edema or pulmonary hemorrhage (see ''Pulmonary Edema'').
- Normal lung volume. Because the acinar air is replaced by fluid or tissue, marked

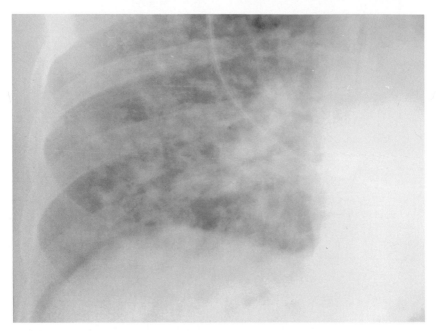

Figure 1.63. Acinar shadows in *Pneumocystis carinii* pneumonia. Detailed view of the right lower lung zone showing ill-defined nodular shadows with diameters in the 10-mm range.

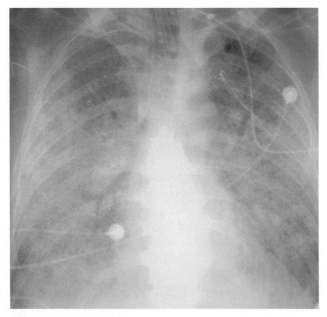

Figure 1.64. Diffuse bilateral consolidation from combined *Pneumocystis carinii* and cytomegalovirus infection in an AIDS patient.

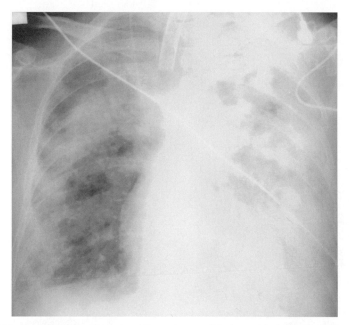

Figure 1.65. *Legionella* pneumonia. Bilateral consolidation with marked confluence in the left lung.

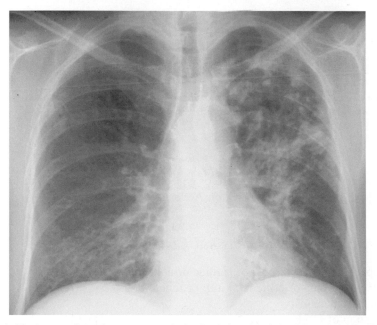

Figure 1.66. Acute tuberculous pneumonia in the left upper lobe. Note that the disease is poorly marginated and fades imperceptibly into the normal lung.

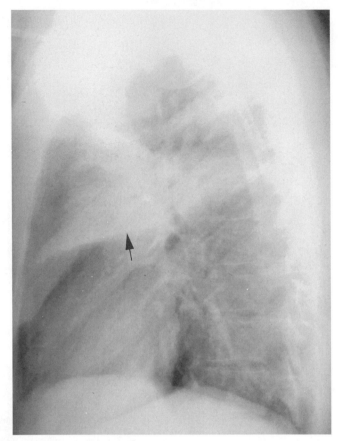

Figure 1.67. Acute right upper lobe pneumonia demonstrating the sharp inferior margination of the consolidation by the minor fissure (*arrow*).

volume loss is not a usual feature of consolidation unless there is obstruction of a major bronchus (see "Resorption Atelectasis").

Causes of Parenchymal Consolidation

• Alveolar pulmonary edema of cardiac or noncardiac origin;
• Acute pneumonia of bacterial, viral, or fungal origin;
• Pulmonary hemorrhage;
• Aspiration of fluid;
• Bronchoalveolar carcinoma or lymphoma;
• Alveolar proteinosis.

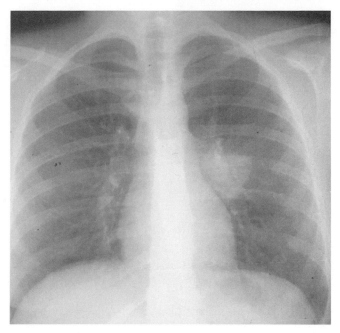

Figure 1.68. Round pneumonia pattern. Acute pneumonia in a 17-year-old woman producing a well-defined spherical opacity in the superior segment of the left lower lobe.

Atelectasis (Collapse, Loss of Volume)

Some forms of atelectasis increase the radiographic density of the affected lung tissue, but this is not essential to the diagnosis (e.g., in the presence of a pneumothorax, the atelectatic lung is usually of normal density).

Types of Atelectasis

- **Resorption** atelectasis caused by bronchial obstruction is the most common form. An air bronchogram is not present in resorption atelectasis because of the bronchial occlusion. Obstructive pneumonitis or drowned lung refers to the consolidation that develops in a lobe following the occlusion of its lobar bronchus by an endobronchial neoplasm. There is usually no infection, the lung being filled with retained bronchial secretions.
- **Passive** (relaxation) atelectasis occurs in the presence of a space-occupying process, such as a pneumothorax, a pleural effusion, or a large mass.
- **Cicatrization** atelectasis results from pulmonary fibrosis (e.g., old granulomatous infection, radiation fibrosis).
- **Adhesive** atelectasis denotes alveolar collapse with patent airways and appears to

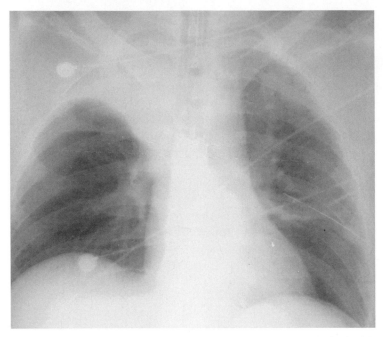

Figure 1.69. Right upper lobe collapse from mucous plugging. The smooth curvilinear inferior margin of the opaque lung represents the minor fissure. Absence of air bronchograms indicates occlusion of the lobar bronchus.

result from a deficiency of surfactant. Air bronchograms can be seen in passive, cicatrization, and adhesive atelectasis because of airway patency in these processes.
- **Discoid** (plate) atelectasis, generally seen at the lung bases, is thought to result from hypoventilation.
- **Round** atelectasis is an unusual type of atelectasis that is associated with pleural fibrosis and that leads to a masslike lesion (Fig. 1.50).

Radiographic Signs of Atelectasis

- Displacement of lobar fissures, the most reliable sign (Fig. 1.69);
- Displacement of the pulmonary hila (refer to ''The Hila'');
- Shift of the mediastinum;
- Elevation of the hemidiaphragm;
- Compensatory overinflation of nonatelectatic lung;
- Narrowing of the rib interspaces, the least reliable sign.

Atelectasis of the various lobes of the lung, alone or in combination, produces distinct patterns (Figs. 1.30, 1.70–1.72), the recognition of which can be a guide to appropriate therapy.

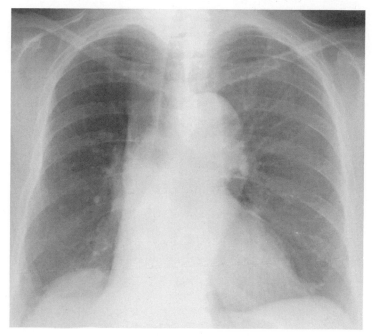

Figure 1.70. Right lower lobe collapse resulting from bronchogenic carcinoma. The collapsed lobe forms a wedge-shaped opacity inferomedially, increasing the density of the right paraspinal region. Note also the displacement of the upper mediastinum to the right and the small right hilum, which are additional signs of lower lobe collapse.

Pulmonary Edema

In general, pulmonary edema may result from elevated pressure in the pulmonary microvasculature (hydrostatic or cardiogenic pulmonary edema), from increased permeability of the alveolar-capillary membrane (noncardiogenic or increased permeability pulmonary edema), or from a combination of both. The ability to distinguish cardiogenic from noncardiogenic edema based on the appearance of the chest radiograph is a subject of disagreement. The radiologic signs of cardiogenic pulmonary edema are:

Vascular Redistribution (Pulmonary Venous Hypertension)

As the pressure rises in the pulmonary venous system, redistribution of blood flow to upper zonal vessels occurs, leading to vascular enlargement in the upper lobes. The sign is most reliable when serial radiographs demonstrate the development of vascular redistribution. This sign is not valid in two situations:

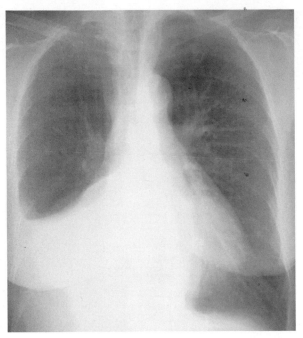

Figure 1.71. Combined collapse of the right middle and lower lobes from a carcinoma arising in the intermediate bronchus. The combined collapse of these two lobes can be mistaken for a right pleural effusion if the hilar anatomy is not analyzed carefully (see also Figure 1.11).

- In the normal patient examined in the supine position;
- In the presence of any disease that alters vascular compliance so as to increase the perfusion of the upper lobes (e.g., basal emphysema, mitral stenosis).

Interstitial Edema

Transudation of fluid initially occurs into the interstitial spaces of the lung, producing the following signs:

- Loss of the sharp definition of the pulmonary vessels;
- Thickening of the interlobular septa (A and B lines of Kerley, Fig. 1.73);
- Bronchial wall thickening;
- Thickening of the interlobar fissures;
- Haziness of the pulmonary hila.

Airspace (Alveolar) Edema

Continued transudation of fluid results in filling of the pulmonary airspaces, producing some of the signs associated with parenchymal consolidation (Fig. 1.74):

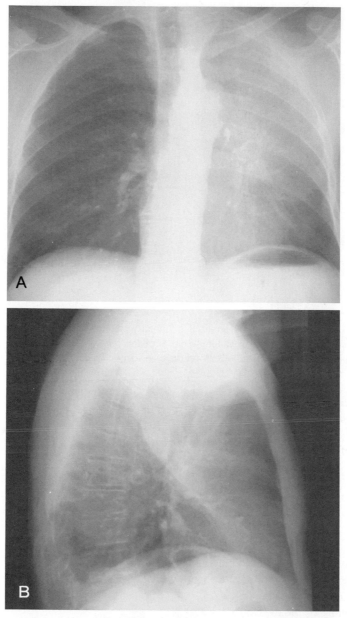

Figure 1.72. A, Atelectasis of the left upper lobe from bronchogenic carcinoma. The obstructed lobe forms a diffuse opacity that fades inferiorly and that obliterates the left cardiac border. **B,** Lateral view of same patient showing posterior bowing of the superior part of the left major fissure from the obstructing carcinoma. Obstructive pneumonitis prevents complete collapse of the lobe.

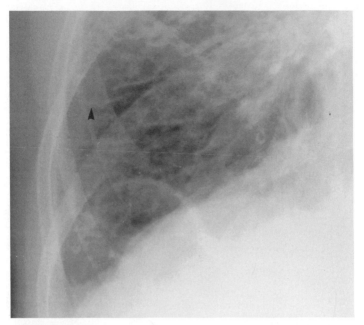

Figure 1.73. Kerley B lines in interstitial pulmonary edema. These are short opaque lines (*arrowhead*) seen best along the lateral aspects of the lungs. Thickened interlobular septa from lymphangitic spread of tumor can produce an identical appearance.

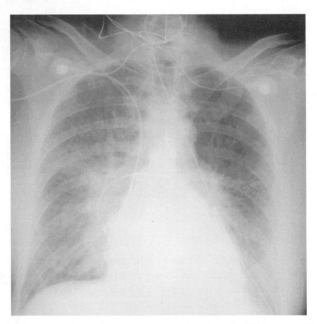

Figure 1.74. Diffuse alveolar pulmonary edema showing ill-defined opacification in both lungs that is most prominent in the perihilar regions.

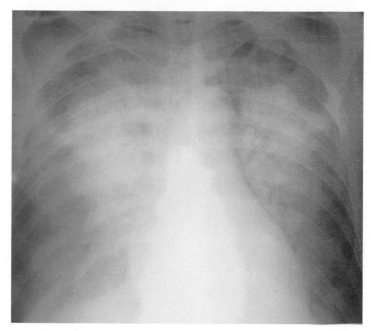

Figure 1.75. Classical butterfly (bat wing) pattern of pulmonary edema in a uremic patient.

- Diffuse, bilateral, poorly marginated opacities;
- Acinar shadows;
- Butterfly pattern of distribution (Fig. 1.75).

Cardiac enlargement, widening of the vascular pedicle, and pleural effusions are commonly but not always present in cardiogenic pulmonary edema. Signs that have been suggested to favor the diagnosis of increased-permeability pulmonary edema are normal heart size, normal vascular pedicle, absence of Kerley A or B lines, absence of pleural effusions, peripheral distribution of the edema, and the presence of air bronchograms.

Pulmonary Emphysema

The plain radiographic signs of pulmonary emphysema include the following:

Overinflation of the Lungs (Fig. 1.76)

- Flattening of the diaphragm;
- Increased size of the retrosternal airspace;
- Anteriorly bowed sternum with increased thoracic kyphosis;
- Infracardiac translucency.

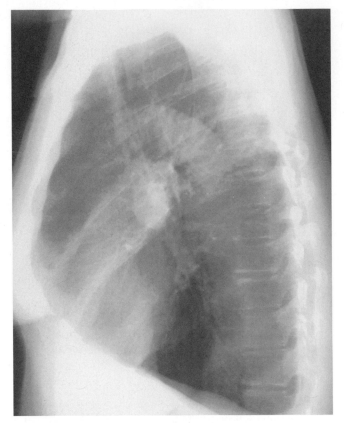

Figure 1.76. Emphysema. Lateral radiograph in severe emphysema showing a flattened diaphragm and an enlarged retrosternal airspace, with loss of contact between the heart and the sternum.

Altered Pulmonary Vascularity (Fig. 1.77)

- Focal or generalized areas of reduced vascularity (oligemia);
- Vascular shunting to less severely affected areas.

Bullae (Fig. 1.78)

- Thin-walled air-filled spaces;
- Multiple or single;
- Varying size from 1 cm in diameter to replacement of an entire lung;
- May acquire an air-fluid level if they become infected.

The combination of these features tends to give the distinctive appearance of the overinflated chest with exceptionally clear lungs and a long, narrow heart. Computed

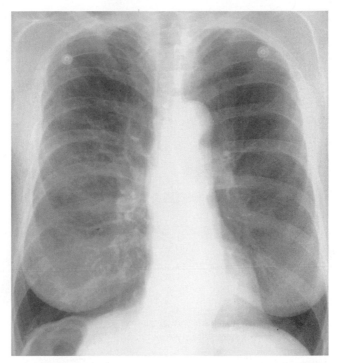

Figure 1.77. Emphysema. PA view of the same patient as in Figure 1.76; note the relatively oligemic left lung with vascular shunting to the more compliant right lung.

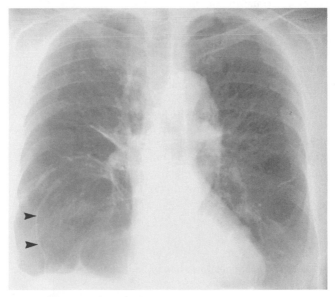

Figure 1.78. Large emphysematous bullae (*arrowheads* on lateral margin) at the right base in a patient with α_1-antitrypsin deficiency.

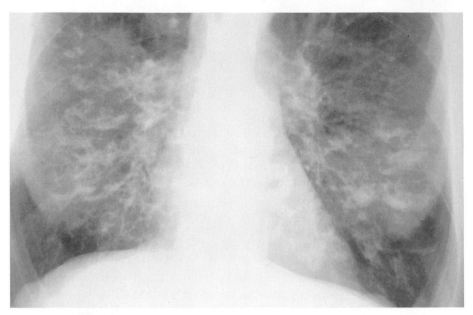

Figure 1.79. Bronchiectasis. Note the saccular spaces in the lower lobes, many of which contain air-fluid levels. This patient with dyskinetic cilia does not have dextrocardia.

tomography (CT) can be useful in clarifying the presence of emphysema and is more sensitive than the plain radiograph in this regard.

Bronchiectasis

Although bronchiectasis is variable in location, the basal segments of the lower lobes are affected most commonly. Bronchography or CT (see "Computed Tomography of the Chest with Radiographic Correlation") is confirmatory but the following signs on the plain film are suggestive of bronchiectasis:

• Dilated, thick-walled segmental bronchi (tram lines);
• Crowded lung markings and displaced hila resulting from atelectasis;
• Mucous-filled bronchi forming tubular fingerlike opacities;
• Saccular air-filled spaces containing air-fluid levels if there are retained secretions (Fig. 1.79).

Cystic Fibrosis

This common cause of bronchiectasis has typical radiographic manifestations (Fig. 1.80).

• Generalized overinflation of the lungs;
• Diffuse bronchial wall thickening;

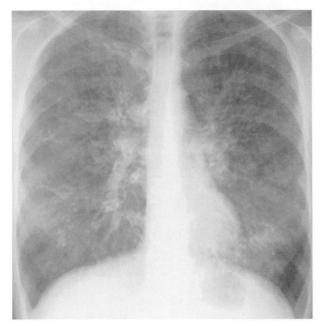

Figure 1.80. Cystic fibrosis showing large lung volumes, patchy bilateral parenchymal opacities, and bronchial wall thickening. Bilateral hilar enlargement is suspected.

- Diffuse bilateral, ill-defined, patchy opacities;
- Hilar and mediastinal lymphadenopathy in more severe cases.

Pulmonary Masses

The Fleischner Society distinguishes between a nodule (diameter < 3 cm) and a mass (diameter > 3 cm), whereas others use the words interchangeably. In general, solitary lesions larger than 3 cm in diameter are likely malignant (Fig. 1.81). A peripheral bronchogenic carcinoma cannot usually be detected on a chest radiograph until it has achieved a diameter of at least 9 mm. In the evaluation of a solitary pulmonary nodule, certain observations present strong evidence that the lesion is benign (see Chapter 15).

Signs of a Benign Solitary Pulmonary Nodule

CALCIFICATION

- Central, uniform, and concentric calcification is characteristic of infectious granulomas (Fig. 1.82);
- "Popcorn" calcifications are typical of hamartomas;
- Eccentric calcification does not rule out the possibility of a bronchogenic carcinoma but makes it extremely unlikely.

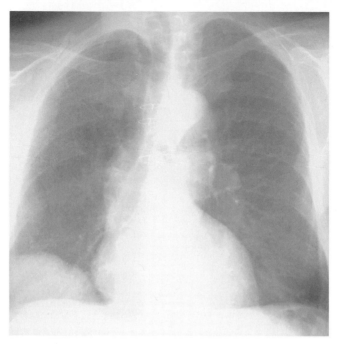

Figure 1.81. Large cell bronchogenic carcinoma. Right lower lobe mass is 9 cm in diameter. The diagnosis was established by fine needle aspiration biopsy.

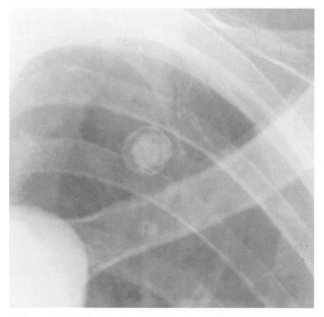

Figure 1.82. Presumed histoplasmoma. Left apical nodule with laminated calcification (dot and ring calcification) characteristic of an infectious granuloma.

GROWTH RATE

- A documented lack of growth of a solitary pulmonary nodule over a 2-year period is a generally accepted sign that the lesion is benign;
- This points out the importance of obtaining previous radiographs for comparison.

There are no other criteria that distinguish reliably a benign from a malignant solitary pulmonary nodule except for the unequivocal demonstration of a feeding artery and draining vein in the case of an arterio-venous malformation, which is a rare cause of a solitary nodule (see "Computed Tomography of the Chest with Radiographic Correlation"). Although the goal of cancer detection is to identify primary carcinoma of the lung at the stage of the small solitary nodule, this disease can on occasion be multifocal (particularly the bronchoalveolar type), and the presence of more than one lesion does not exclude the diagnosis of primary lung cancer.

Multiple Masses or Nodules

Although the differential diagnosis of multiple pulmonary nodules is long, the majority are caused by metastases and infectious granulomas.

- Metastases are commonly variable in size and have smooth borders.
- Multiple calcified nodules indicate a benign etiology, with the exception of metastases from osteosarcoma or chondrosarcoma, which may be calcified.

Cavitation

A cavity can be defined as a gas-filled space within a zone of consolidation or within a mass or a nodule. Cavitation in a lesion is usually the result of tissue necrosis with expulsion of the necrotic material into a bronchus. Although both benign and malignant lesions may undergo cavitation, the presence of cavitation in a solitary well-defined mass is suggestive of malignancy.

- Most cavities in which the thickest part of the wall is 4 mm or less are benign.
- Most cavities in which the thickest part of the wall is 15 mm or greater are malignant.
- A nodular inner cavity wall suggests primary lung cancer (Fig. 1.83).
- Occasionally, squamous cell carcinoma, primary or secondary, can result in thin-walled cavities.

Diffuse Interstitial Lung Disease

In diffuse, bilateral pulmonary disease there may be radiographic clues as to the predominate location of the abnormality—the pulmonary airspaces (see "Airspace Disease") or the pulmonary interstitium. Analysis of these clues is known as pattern recognition, an approach of considerable merit, but one that is sometimes difficult and not without its limitations. For example, airspace disease can hide underlying interstitial disease, mixed patterns are common, and the radiographic patterns do

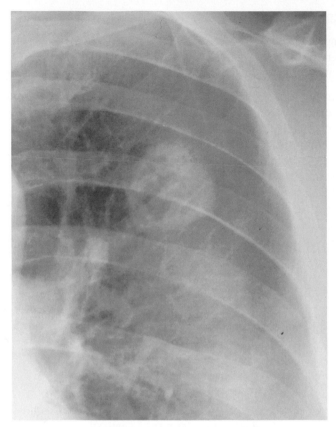

Figure 1.83. Bronchogenic carcinoma. Solitary thick-walled left upper lobe cavity with inner nodularity characteristic of bronchogenic carcinoma.

not always correlate with the histologic findings. With the relatively recent advent of high-resolution CT scanning of the lung, new insights have been gained into diffuse infiltrative pulmonary disease. This technique is more sensitive than the conventional chest radiograph in detecting diffuse disease and can guide the clinician to the site and type of biopsy (transbronchial versus open) that is more likely to yield the diagnosis (see Chapter 6).

Several patterns have been described for diffuse interstitial lung disease:

Reticular or Linear Pattern

- Resembles a net, with thin linear shadows surrounding air-containing spaces;
- As with a screen or a sieve, the net may be fine, medium, or coarse;
- The honeycomb pattern is a specific type of coarse reticular pattern;
- Septal lines (Kerley A or B lines) are an example of linear shadowing (Fig. 1.73);

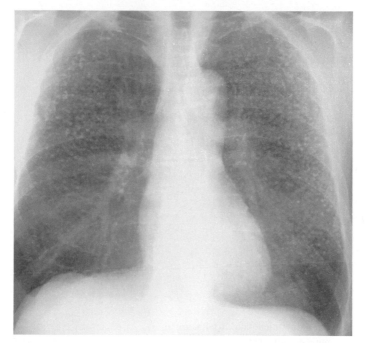

Figure 1.84. Nodular pattern. Diffuse small-to-medium nodularity resulting from silicosis in a gold miner.

- If chronic, common causes include interstitial pulmonary fibrosis and lymphangitic carcinomatosis.

Nodular Pattern

- Interstitial nodules are usually clearly defined (Fig. 1.84);
- They can be classified according to size as micronodular (diameter < 1 mm), small (1–3 mm), medium (3–5 mm), or large (greater than 5 mm);
- Common causes are granulomatous disease and diffuse metastases.

Reticulonodular Pattern

- This denotes an admixture of the reticular pattern and the nodular pattern (Fig. 1.85);
- Common causes are sarcoidosis, lymphangitic carcinomatosis, and some varieties of pneumoconiosis.

CHEST RADIOLOGY IN THE CRITICAL CARE SETTING

This section will concentrate on those principles of interpretation that are relatively unique to the critically ill patient.

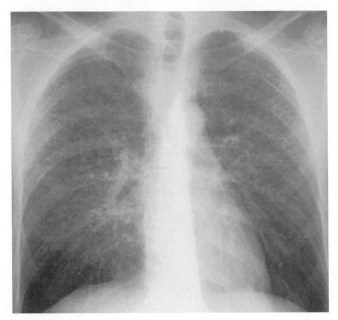

Figure 1.85. Reticulonodular pattern with upper zone predominance in sarcoidosis. Compared with the purely nodular pattern in Figure 1.84, nodules and a netlike appearance are both present.

General Principles

Radiography is usually performed at the bedside in the anteroposterior (AP) projection with a portable x-ray unit. The patient is often supine and breathing with low lung volumes. This can create problems in interpretation, particularly with regard to congestive heart failure (CHF), in which the traditional radiologic signs may not be helpful or may be difficult to detect.

Limitations of Bedside Radiography

- There is magnification of the cardiac shadow because of the shortened distance between the x-ray tube and the film and because of the AP projection; on an AP film, a cardiothoracic ratio of 0.56 corresponds to a normal ratio of less than 0.5 on a conventional PA radiograph.
- In the supine position, there is a physiologic redistribution of blood flow to the upper lobe pulmonary vessels and therefore assessment of vascular redistribution is not possible.
- In the supine position, there may be an increase in the width of the upper mediastinum by 10–40% compared with the upright position, which can, for example, lead to difficulty in the assessment of the patient in whom there is concern of mediastinal hemorrhage.

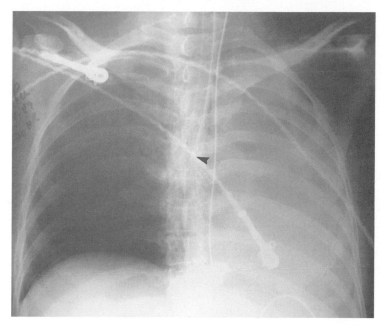

Figure 1.86. Collapse of the left lung following placement of the endotracheal tube in the right main bronchus (*arrowhead* at tip of tube). Ipsilateral mediastinal shift distinguishes this from a large left pleural effusion.

• These physiologic changes are accentuated by the low lung volumes at which the chest radiograph is often obtained in the critically ill patient; on an expiratory film in a normal subject, the pulmonary vessels are closer together, the lungs more opaque, and the heart and upper mediastinum wider than on an inspiratory film obtained at the same time.

• Pneumothoraces and pleural effusions are more difficult to detect in the supine patient.

Tubes and Monitoring Devices

Film interpretation should begin with an evaluation of the position of tubes and intravascular lines. It is wise to obtain a chest radiograph after the insertion of a new tube or catheter to ensure its proper placement and to exclude a complication of its insertion.

ENDOTRACHEAL TUBE

The tip of the tube should be above the carina; with the patient's head in neutral position, the tip should be in the midtrachea, approximately 5–7 cm from the carina.

• Flexion of the head causes the tube to descend by up to 2 cm, extension of the head causes it to ascend by up to 2 cm;

• Intubation of a main bronchus will lead to collapse of the contralateral lung (Fig. 1.86).

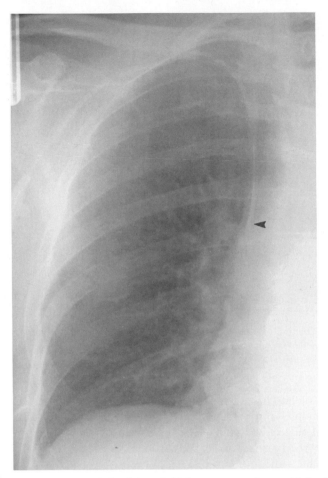

Figure 1.87. Correct placement of a right subclavian venous catheter with its tip in the mid-SVC (*arrowhead* at tip of catheter).

CENTRAL VENOUS CATHETER

As a rule of thumb, the subclavian and internal jugular veins meet to form the brachiocephalic veins at the level of the sternoclavicular joints; the two brachiocephalic veins unite to form the SVC at the level of the first right intercostal space, which is roughly the same level as the inferior aspect of the aortic knob; the SVC enters the right atrium at the upper margin of the right heart border.

- The tip of the subclavian catheter, internal jugular catheter, or peripherally placed central venous pressure catheter should lie beyond the most central venous valves, which are located in the subclavian and internal jugular veins approximately 2 cm from the origins of the brachiocephalic veins (Fig. 1.87).

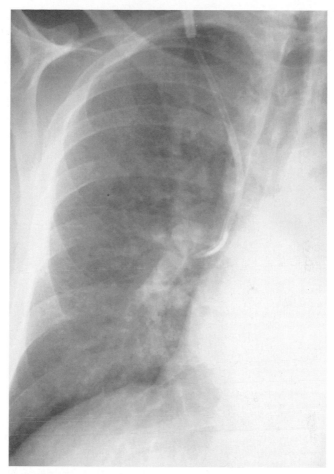

Figure 1.88. Inadvertent placement of an internal jugular venous catheter into the right pleural space. Note that the course of the catheter does not conform to expected venous anatomy and that its tip angles abruptly laterally.

- Long-term venous access catheters are optimally placed in the distal SVC to dilute the infused substances; because the SVC normally has a smooth vertical course, any abrupt deviation of the catheter is suggestive of malplacement (Fig. 1.88).
- A left-sided SVC is seen in 0.3% of the normal population and is usually accompanied by a right-sided SVC; the left SVC drains into the right atrium via the coronary sinus (Fig. 1.89).

SWAN-GANZ CATHETER

Ideal placement with the balloon deflated is in the right or left pulmonary artery (Fig. 1.90).

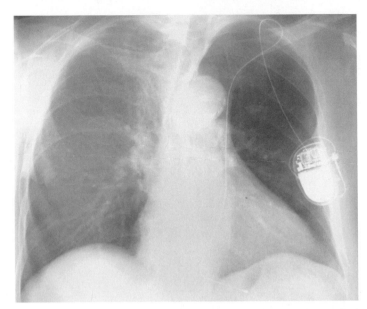

Figure 1.89. A cardiac pacemaker wire in a left-sided SVC entering the heart via the coronary sinus.

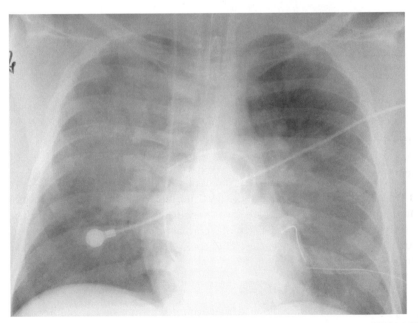

Figure 1.90. Swan-Ganz catheter in the right interlobar pulmonary artery. Positioning distal to this point increases the likelihood of pulmonary infarction or vessel rupture.

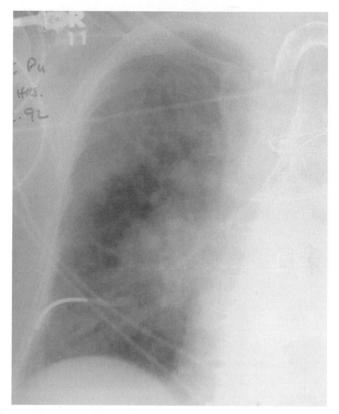

Figure 1.91. Inadvertent placement of a nasogastric feeding tube in the bronchial tree. Note the opaque tip of the tube in the periphery of the right lung.

NASOGASTRIC TUBE

The degree of radiopacity of various nasogastric tubes differs, and visualization is sometimes difficult. The tip of the tube should be in the stomach or proximal duodenum. Inadvertent insertion into the tracheobronchial tree is not uncommon in sick patients whose gag reflexes are depressed (Fig. 1.91).

- In the appropriate clinical setting, deviation of the nasogastric tube to the right may indicate mediastinal hemorrhage resulting from traumatic aortic laceration.
- In a patient who has sustained thoraco-abdominal trauma, visualization of the stomach (as outlined by the nasogastric tube) in the thorax indicates rupture of the left hemidiaphragm.

Atelectasis

Retained secretions in the critically ill are probably the commonest cause of pulmonary opacities. These secretions may form focal evanescent areas of increased density

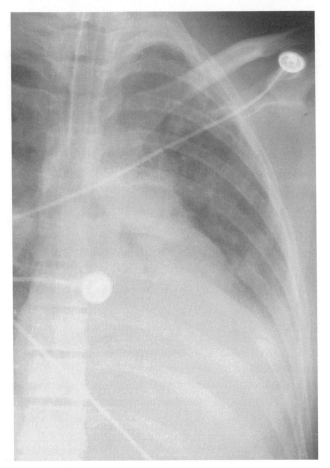

Figure 1.92. Collapse of the basal segments of the left lower lobe leading to opacification of the lung behind the heart and loss of the border of the descending aorta and the left hemidiaphragm (silhouette sign).

representing small zones of atelectasis or may lead to lobar collapse requiring therapeutic bronchoscopy.

- Collapse of the basal segments of the left lower lobe is common in patients in the intensive care unit (Fig. 1.92).
- Absence of air bronchograms in the area of collapse suggests that the lobar bronchus is occluded and that the patient will benefit from bronchoscopy to clear the obstruction (Fig. 1.69).
- Conversely, the presence of air bronchograms indicates that the atelectasis is not the result of central bronchial obstruction and is unlikely to respond to bronchoscopy.

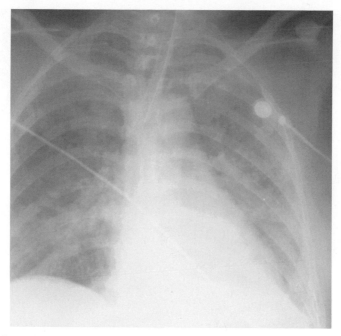

Figure 1.93. Diffuse opacification of the lungs in a patient who was observed to aspirate gastric fluid prior to intubation (Mendelson's syndrome).

Pulmonary Edema

As mentioned, the traditional signs of CHF may be difficult to detect on a bedside radiograph. Although the ability of the portable chest radiograph to distinguish cardiac from noncardiac pulmonary edema remains a subject of debate, cardiomegaly, Kerley lines, and pleural effusions usually indicate edema of cardiac origin. In patients with pulmonary edema who are receiving assisted ventilation, continuous positive airway pressure (CPAP) and positive end-expiratory pressure (PEEP) can by themselves lead to increased lung volumes and clearing of areas of lung opacification.

- Other conditions in the critically ill patient may result in a radiographic appearance resembling cardiogenic pulmonary edema. These include:
    Fat embolism;
    Pulmonary hemorrhage;
    Massive aspiration of gastric contents of low pH, Mendelson's syndrome (Fig. 1.93);
    Severe bacterial or viral pneumonia;
    Adult respiratory distress syndrome (ARDS).
- In ARDS, the chest radiograph is usually normal for the first 12 hours after the onset of clinical symptoms; from 12–24 hours, patchy areas of opacification de-

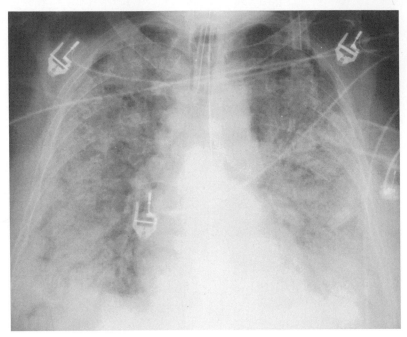

Figure 1.94. ARDS. Note the widespread generalized opacification in both lungs, extending from the chest wall to the mediastinum.

velop that may be indistinguishable from pulmonary edema of cardiac origin or from diffuse pneumonia; after 24 hours, there is severe diffuse airspace consolidation, which typically shows no change for several days (Fig. 1.94).

Atypical Patterns of Pulmonary Edema

Although pulmonary edema is usually a diffuse bilateral process, atypical patterns of distribution, including unilateral pulmonary edema, are not uncommon. Some causes of unilateral pulmonary edema are:

- Rapid expansion of the lung following treatment of a large pneumothorax or hydrothorax;
- Prolonged lateral decubitus position;
- Preferential perfusion of one lung as a result of contralateral pulmonary emphysema or pulmonary embolism;
- Recent pneumonectomy or lobectomy (Fig. 1.95).

Extravascular Fluid

- Pleural fluid in the supine patient gravitates posteriorly and leads to an overall increase in lung density without a corresponding loss of visualization of the pulmo-

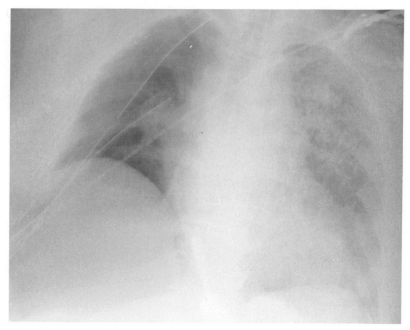

Figure 1.95. Unilateral pulmonary edema of the left lung following right upper lobectomy for lung cancer.

nary vessels; a lateral decubitus film or an erect film will show the fluid more clearly, but ultrasound may also be useful to confirm the presence of pleural fluid and to assist with thoracentesis (Fig. 1.96).

• On occasion, patients with clinical evidence of fluid overload will show clear lungs; examination of the soft tissues of the chest wall may demonstrate subcutaneous edema, indicating that the excess fluid has accumulated in the "third space" (Fig. 1.97, *A–B*).

Pneumonia

Although the chest radiograph plays an essential diagnostic role in the diagnosis of community-acquired pneumonia, the portable radiograph in the critical care setting is not accurate in predicting nosocomial bacterial pneumonia, particularly in patients on mechanical ventilation. This is largely because of the similar radiographic appearances of focal opacities that may result from retained secretions, bland aspiration, atypical cardiogenic pulmonary edema, pulmonary hemorrhage, pulmonary embolism, asymmetric ARDS, and pneumonia.

Abnormal Air Collections

Subcutaneous emphysema is often the initial manifestation of barotrauma in patients on mechanical ventilation and, if extensive, may obscure a concomitant pneumothorax or pneumomediastinum.

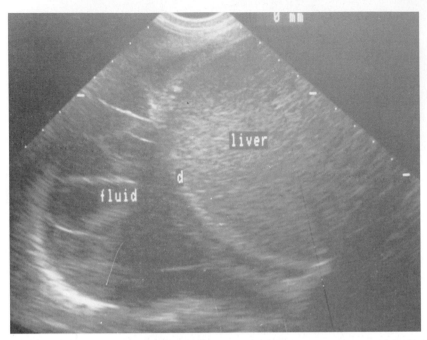

Figure 1.96. Bedside ultrasound scan of the right lower chest showing a pleural effusion with internal septations, proven to be an empyema (*d*, diaphragm).

- In the supine patient, a small pneumothorax may be difficult to detect and is commonly overlooked; in this situation, air in the pleural space rises to the anterior and inferior aspect of the thorax (Fig. 1.98) rather than to the lung apex as in the upright subject.
- Among the clues to the presence of a pneumothorax in the supine patient are a deep lateral costophrenic sulcus, visualization of the normally invisible anterior costophrenic sulcus (Fig. 1.99), and the clear visualization of a pericardial fat pad (Fig. 1.100).
- A skin fold may be mistaken for the visceral pleural line of a pneumothorax; it may be necessary to repeat the radiograph or to obtain a lateral decubitus film to make the correct diagnosis (Fig. 1.101).
- In pneumomediastinum, the air can collect in many sites but is often seen best along the left heart border and around the aortic knob (Fig. 1.102).

Pulmonary Embolism (PE)

The large multicenter PIOPED study demonstrated that the chest radiographic findings are poor predictors of pulmonary embolism. The chest radiograph remains essential, however, in the investigation of suspected PE for two reasons:

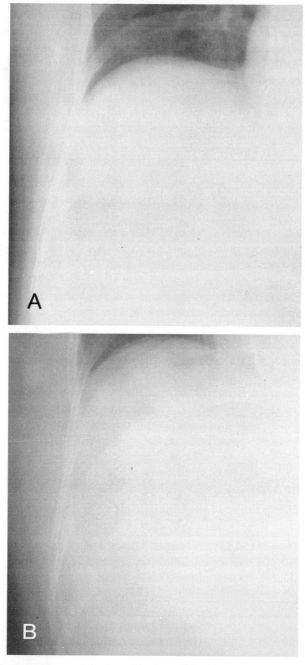

Figure 1.97. **A,** Soft tissues of the lateral body wall in a burn patient. **B,** Three days later, there has been a marked increase in the thickness of the soft tissues from the accumulation of fluid in the third space.

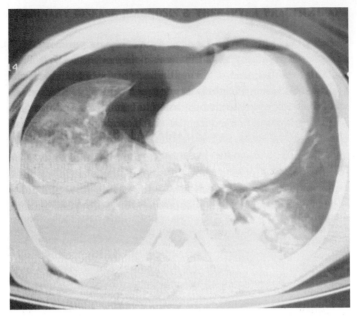

Figure 1.98. CT scan in a supine patient with a right pneumothorax. Note that the air lies in the anterior aspect of the pleural cavity near the lung base.

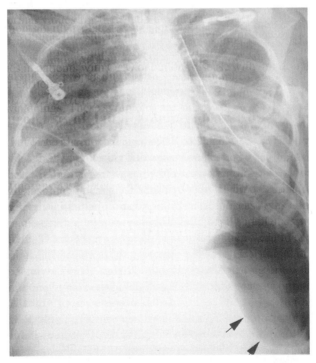

Figure 1.99. Left pneumothorax in a supine patient producing a deep radiolucent anterior costophrenic sulcus (*arrows*).

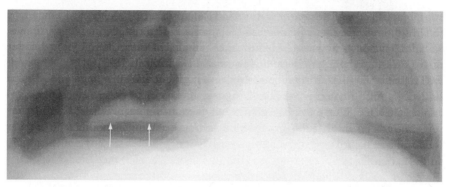

Figure 1.100. Visualization of a pericardial fat pad (*arrows*) at the right base from a small pneumothorax.

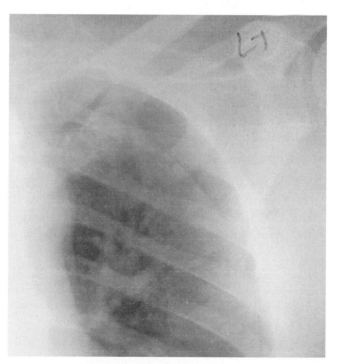

Figure 1.101. Skin fold on the upper left chest wall mimicking the visceral pleural line of a pneumothorax; repeat radiograph was normal.

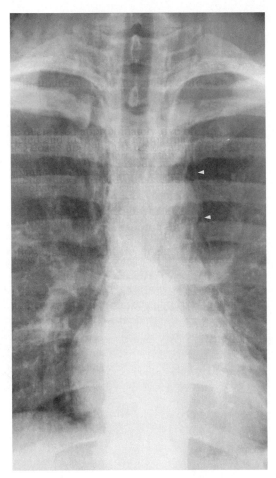

Figure 1.102. Pneumomediastinum secondary to penetrating pharyngeal trauma, with air adjacent to the left cardiac border and aortic knob. The thin opaque line (*arrowheads*) represents the pleura of the left lung, which has been lifted away from the mediastinum. Note the subcutaneous emphysema in the neck.

- To permit interpretation of the ventilation-perfusion lung scan;
- To exclude other diseases, such as pulmonary edema, pneumonia, or pneumothorax, that may mimic the clinical features of PE.

Radiographic Findings in PE Without Infarction

- Normal chest radiograph (12% of proven cases in the PIOPED study);
- Prominent central pulmonary artery (Fleischner sign) (Fig. 1.15);
- Oligemia distal to a large vessel occluded by a PE (Westermark's sign);
- Elevated diaphragm.

Radiographic Findings in PE With Infarction (Fig. 1.103)

- Increased size and abrupt tapering of the feeding artery;
- Parenchymal opacification;
- Pleural-based opacity (Hampton's hump);
- Pleural effusion;
- Elevated diaphragm.

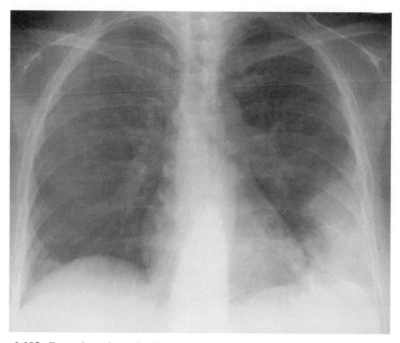

Figure 1.103. Parenchymal opacity in the left lower lung zone and prominent left pulmonary artery in a patient with left-sided chest pain, hypoxia, and lower limb deep vein thrombosis. The ventilation-perfusion lung scan showed high probability for PE.

COMPUTED TOMOGRAPHY (CT) OF THE CHEST WITH RADIOGRAPHIC CORRELATION

CT has become the most useful imaging technique in the evaluation of chest disease after the plain chest radiograph. CT produces thin cross-sectional images of the thorax, 1–10 mm in thickness, whose contrast range can be manipulated by the operator to enhance the visualization of normal structures and lesions. The contrast resolution (the ability to distinguish differences in brightness or density) of CT exceeds that of the chest radiograph and this feature, coupled with its tomographic capability, enables it to distinguish lesions that cannot be identified on the routine chest film. Atelectatic lung, for example, can be distinguished clearly from pleural fluid, a distinction that may be impossible on a conventional radiograph. The extent to which tissues attenuate the x-rays used to create the CT images can be measured and expressed in units (commonly called Hounsfield units, in recognition of the scientist who invented CT).

High-resolution CT (HRCT) is a technique that optimizes spatial resolution by use of very thin sections (1–2 mm) and a high-spatial frequency reconstruction algorithm. HRCT improves the visualization of diffuse lung parenchymal disease and bronchial abnormalities. It has replaced bronchoscopy in the assessment of bronchiectasis.

Indications for Chest CT

Mediastinum and Hila

- Confirmation and evaluation of mediastinal and hilar masses suspected on the chest x-ray, including aneurysms and vascular anomalies;
- Staging of lung cancer;
- Search for occult thymic lesions (myasthenia gravis);
- Assistance in percutaneous biopsy;
- Evaluation of suspected traumatic aortic laceration (still controversial).

Lungs and Airways

- Search for pulmonary neoplasms (primary or secondary);
- Determination of calcification in a pulmonary lesion;
- Confirmation and assessment of chronic restrictive lung disease (HRCT);
- Assessment for lung biopsy (percutaneous or transbronchial);
- Evaluation of hemoptysis;
- Evaluation of bronchiectasis (HRCT);
- Evaluation of pulmonary emphysema.

Pleura and Chest Wall

- Evaluation of complex pleural effusions;
- Differentiation between lung abscess and empyema;
- Assessment of asbestos-related pleural disease;
- Evaluation of pleural neoplasms;
- Assessment of chest wall invasion by neoplasm or infection (MRI is superior).

It is customary to use a standard CT protocol that provides information about the lungs, mediastinum, hila, pleura, and chest wall. Patients are usually scanned in a supine position during suspended respiration at full lung volume. Depending on the indication for the examination, the patient may receive intravenous contrast media to opacify the heart, the systemic thoracic vessels, and the pulmonary vessels. Images are routinely reconstructed and filmed at two different ''window'' settings, known as mediastinal windows and lung windows. If the patient does not expand the lungs to the same degree for each tomographic section, the misregistration of sequential images can result, which may lead to small lesions being missed. Volumetric scanning (also known as spiral or helical scanning) is a relatively new technical advancement that enables the scanner to examine the entire thorax during a single breath hold, thereby eliminating this problem. Volumetric scanning has been shown to improve the detection of nodules, the assessment of the airways, and the visualization of the intrathoracic vessels. It is beyond the scope of this chapter to provide a comprehensive overview of CT of the thorax; some representative cases are shown together with some correlative chest radiographs (see Figs. 1.104–1.116).

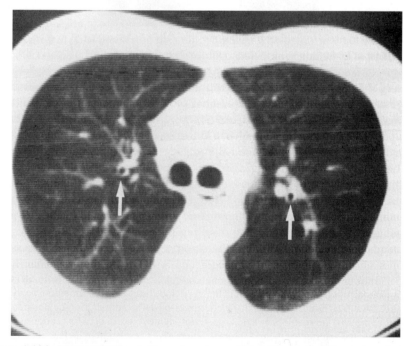

Figure 1.104. Upper hilar level. Normal anatomy. CT at the level of the carina shows the apical segmental bronchus (*arrow*) of the right upper lobe in cross-section, with several adjacent vessels of similar size. On the left, the apical posterior segmental bronchus (*arrow*) of the left upper lobe and associated arteries and veins have a similar appearance. (From Webb WR, Brant WE, Helms CA. Fundamentals of body CT. Philadelphia: WB Saunders, 1994:64. Reprinted with permission.)

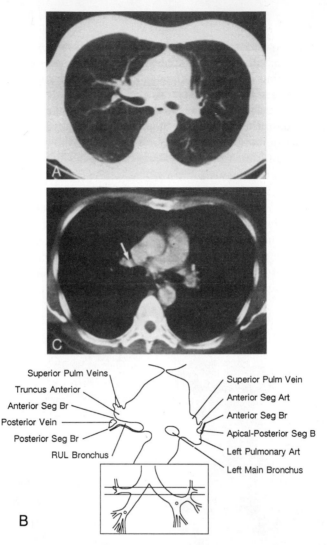

Superior Pulm Veins
Truncus Anterior
Anterior Seg Br
Posterior Vein
Posterior Seg Br
RUL Bronchus

Superior Pulm Vein
Anterior Seg Art
Anterior Seg Br
Apical-Posterior Seg B
Left Pulmonary Art
Left Main Bronchus

B

Figure 1.105. A-C. Right upper lobe bronchus and left upper lobe segments level. Normal anatomy. Right hilum: The right upper lobe bronchus is visible along its length, along with its anterior and posterior segmental branches. The truncus anterior (*arrow*, **C**) is anterior to the right upper lobe bronchus. An upper lobe vein branch (posterior vein) lies in the angle between anterior and posterior segmental branches; the superior pulmonary veins result in some lobulation anterior to the truncus anterior. The posterior wall of the upper lobe bronchus appears smooth and is 2–3 mm in thickness. Left hilum: On the left side, the apical-posterior and anterior segmental bronchi of the left upper lobe are visible. The apical-posterior segment is seen in cross-section as a round lucency, while the anterior segment is directed anteriorly. These bronchi lie lateral to the main branch of the left pulmonary artery, which produces a large convexity in the posterior hilum, and lateral to the superior pulmonary vein, which results in an anterior convexity. The artery supplying the anterior segment of the left upper lobe is seen medial to the anterior segmental bronchus. (From Webb WR, Brant WE, Helms CA. Fundamentals of body CT. Philadelphia: WB Saunders, 1994:66. Reprinted with permission.)

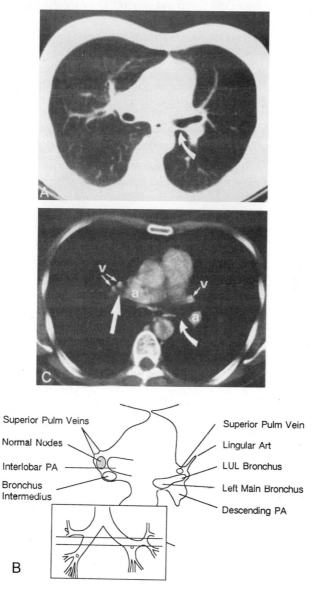

Figure 1.106. A–C. Normal bronchus intermedius and left upper lobe bronchus level. The bronchus intermedius is visible as an oval lucency, with its posterior wall sharply outlined by lung. Anterior and lateral to the bronchus, the hilum is made up of the interlobar pulmonary artery and superior pulmonary veins. Normal lymph nodes and fat (*straight arrow*) are visible in the anterolateral hilum, between the opacified pulmonary artery (*a*) and veins (*v*). On the left, the upper lobe bronchus is usually seen along its axis, extending anteriorly and laterally from its origin. The left superior pulmonary vein (*v*) is anterior and medial to the bronchus, and the descending branch of the left pulmonary artery (*a*) forms an oval soft tissue density posterior and lateral to it. The left posterior bronchial wall (*curved arrows*) is outlined by lung at this level. (From Webb WR, Brant WE, Helms CA. Fundamentals of body CT. Philadelphia: WB Saunders, 1994:68. Reprinted with permission.)

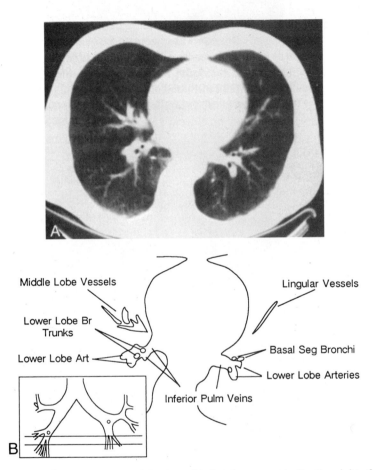

Figure 1.107. A-B. Normal lower lobe bronchi (basal segments). On the right, the right lower lobe bronchus has bifurcated. On the left, three branches are seen. The inferior pulmonary veins are posterior and medial, and pulmonary artery branches accompany the bronchi. (From Webb WR, Brant WE, Helms CA. Fundamentals of body CT. Philadelphia: WB Saunders, 1994:75. Reprinted with permission.)

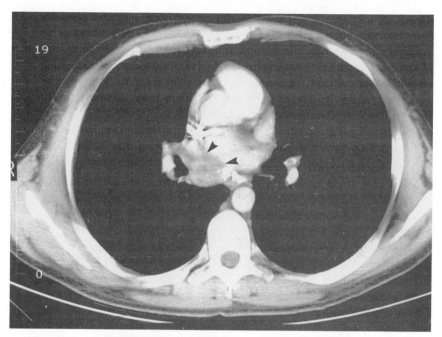

Figure 1.108. Right subcarinal lymphadenopathy (*arrowheads*) in Castleman's disease (giant lymph node hyperplasia). Note that the use of intravenous contrast medium helps to distinguish the lymphadenopathy from the adjacent cardiac chambers.

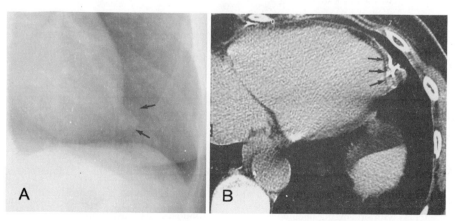

Figure 1.109. Nodule adjacent to left cardiac border (**A**, *arrows*). Based on the plain radiograph, malignancy could not be excluded, but the CT scan shows thick, irregular calcification (**B**, *arrows*) suggestive of a benign lesion. Surgical excision was therefore deferred.

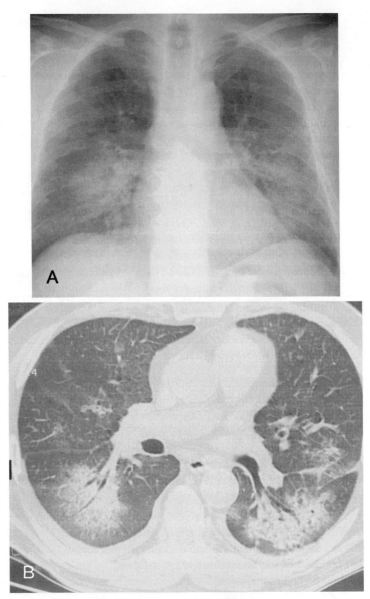

Figure 1.110. Plain radiograph (**A**) and HRCT (**B**) showing airspace consolidation (note air bronchograms) in both lower lobes of a patient on chemotherapy. Transbronchial biopsy was performed, guided by the location of the disease on the CT scan, and revealed bronchiolitis obliterans with organizing pneumonia (BOOP) attributed to carmustine toxicity.

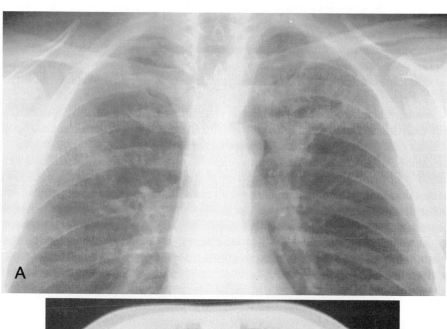

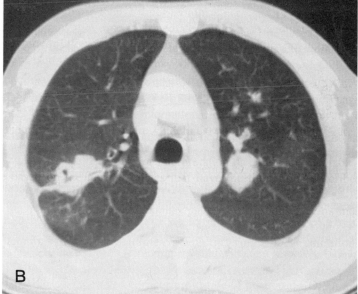

Figure 1.111. Plain radiograph (**A**) and CT scan (**B**) showing bilateral upper lobe pulmonary masses in a heavy cigarette smoker. Fine needle aspiration biopsies, guided by the CT scan, revealed bilateral synchronous bronchogenic carcinomas.

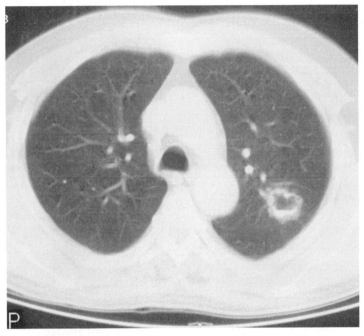

Figure 1.112. Left upper lobe cavity with thick nodular wall (same patient as in Figure 1.83) in primary squamous cell carcinoma. The CT scan was done principally to evaluate the mediastinum, not the obvious pulmonary lesion.

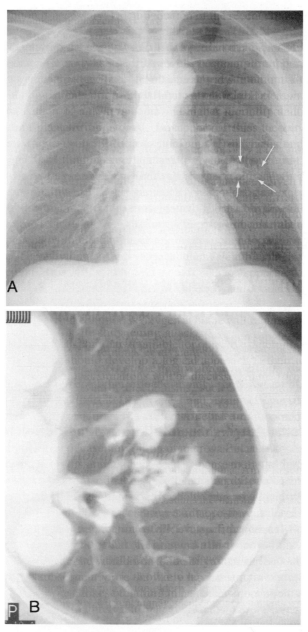

Figure 1.113. Plain radiograph (**A**, *arrows*) and CT (**B**) showing tortuous tubular opacities characteristic of pulmonary arterio-venous fistulae in a patient who presented with septic cerebral emboli following dental surgery. CT confirms the diagnosis in this case.

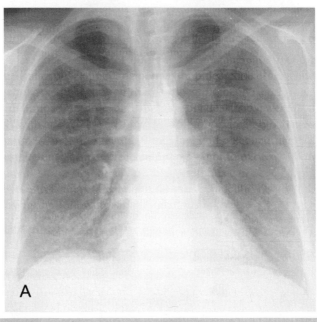

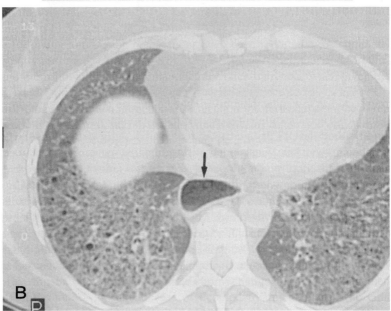

Figure 1.114. A, Plain radiograph of a patient with CREST syndrome showing bibasilar reticulonodular disease. **B**, HRCT shows that the pattern is actually one of small cysts or honeycombing. Note the dilated air-filled esophagus (*arrow*).

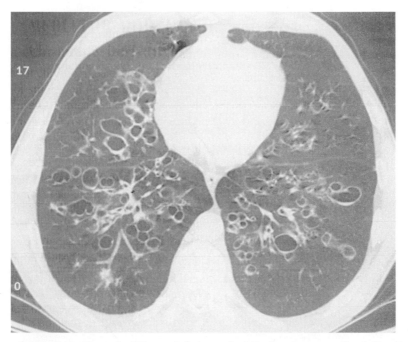

Figure 1.115. Bronchiectasis. CT scan inferior to the hila showing generalized dilatation of the segmental and subsegmental bronchi in a patient with bronchiectasis resulting from dyskinetic cilia syndrome.

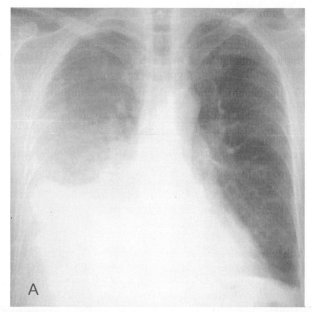

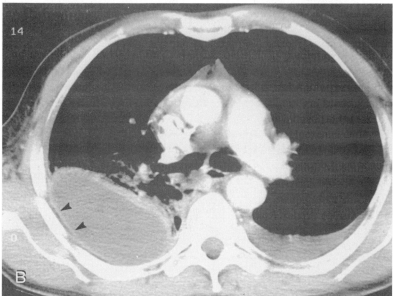

Figure 1.116. Plain radiograph (**A**) and CT scan (**B**) in a man with right-sided streptococcal pneumonia and empyema. Note the lentiform shape of the pleural fluid collection and the thin enhancing pleural wall (*arrowheads*) on the CT scan, which are characteristic of empyema.

BIBLIOGRAPHY

Aberle DR, Wiener-Kronish JP, Webb WR, Matthay MA. Hydrostatic versus increased permeability pulmonary edema: diagnosis based on radiographic criteria in critically ill patients. Radiology 1988;168:73–79.

Armstrong P, Wilson AG, Dee P. Imaging of diseases of the chest. St. Louis: Mosby Year Book, 1990.

Burke M, Fraser RS. Obstructive pneumonitis: a pathologic and pathogenetic reappraisal. Radiology 1988;166:699–704.

Calenoff L, Kruglik CD, Woodruff A. Unilateral pulmonary edema. Radiology 1978;126:19.

Don C, Burns K, Levine D. Body fluid volume status in hemodialysis patients: the value of the chest radiograph. JCAR 1990;41:123–126.

Don C, Hammond DI. The vascular converging points of the right pulmonary hilus and their diagnostic significance. Radiology 1985;155:295–298.

Don C, Johnson R. The nature and significance of peribronchial cuffing in pulmonary edema. Radiology 1977;125:577–582.

Don C, Kalapos P. Post-mediastinoscopy chest film changes. JCAR 1988;39:270–272.

Fleischner Society: Glossary of terms for thoracic radiology. Recommendations of the nomenclature committee of the Fleischner Society. AJR 1984;143:509–517.

Fraser RS, Pare JAP, Fraser RG, Pare PD. Synopsis of diseases of the chest. 2nd ed. Philadelphia: WB Saunders Co, 1994.

Goodman LR, Putman CE, ed. Critical care imaging. 3rd ed. Philadelphia: WB Saunders Co, 1992.

Groskin SA. Heitzman's the lung. 3rd ed. St. Louis: Mosby Year Book, 1993.

Keats TE. Atlas of normal roentgen variants that may simulate disease. 4th ed. Chicago: Year Book Medical Publishers, 1988.

Lefcoe MS, Fox GA, Leasa DJ, et al. Accuracy of portable chest radiography in the critical care setting. Chest 1994;105:885.

Milne ENC. A physiological approach to reading critical care unit films. J Thorac Imaging 1986;1:60–90.

Slinger P. Perioperative fluid management for thoracic surgery: the puzzle of postpneumonectomy pulmonary edema. J Cardiothorac Vasc Anesth 1995;9:442–451.

Winer-Muram HT, Rubin SA, Ellis JV, et al. Pneumonia and ARDS in patients receiving mechanical ventilation: diagnostic accuracy of chest radiography. Radiology 1993;188:479.

Worsley DF, Alavi A, Aronchick JM, et al. Chest radiographic findings in patients with acute pulmonary embolism: observations from the PIOPED study. Radiology 1993;189:133–136.

2 Pulmonary Function Testing

Fernando J. Martinez

Pulmonary function testing (PFT) is useful in the diagnosis and management of respiratory disease because it allows both objective monitoring of the respiratory system and the identification of abnormalities in lung function that may otherwise be overlooked. Varying combination of tests describe the function of the airways, pulmonary parenchyma, pulmonary vasculature, and respiratory muscles. In this regard, PFT is clinically valuable in a range of situations, many of which are enumerated in Table 2.1.

As with any diagnostic studies, the user must be aware of the testing limitations prior to interpretation and clinical use. These caveats apply to PFT whether one is using simple spirometry or more complicated cardiopulmonary exercise testing. Factors that must be assessed include the adequacy of patient effort, the level of training and skill of the technician performing the study, the type of equipment used, and appropriate calibration and quality control.

SPIROMETRY

Measurements

Spirometry is the simplest and most widely used pulmonary function study.

- For this test, the subject inhales maximally to total lung capacity (TLC) and then exhales fully;
- Expired volume or flow is measured;
- The test slowly yields a measure of the vital capacity (VC) (Fig. 2.1).

Although reproducible and relatively sensitive, the VC is nonspecific because decreases can be seen with restrictive lung disease (decreased TLC, as described subsequently) or with obstructive diseases.

If the spirometric maneuver is performed forcefully and maximally, a typical tracing of volume versus time is generated, as illustrated in Figure 2.2. The forced vital capacity (FVC) represents the total volume exhaled during the maneuver.

- Timed components measured include the FEV_1, which represents the volume expired during the first second of the maneuver.
- This dynamic volume is the measurement most commonly used in conjunction with the FVC. The average forced expiratory flow, which is meant to reflect the most effort-independent portion of the curve, is represented by the forced expired flow between 25% and 75% of the VC (FEF_{25-75}).

107

Table 2.1. Indications for Pulmonary Function Testing

Diagnostic	*Monitoring disease activity*
Symptoms	Effectiveness of bronchodilator
dyspnea	medications
cough	Effectiveness of therapeutic
wheezing	intervention in interstitial lung
orthopnea	disease
chest pain	Document natural course of disease
Signs	Assess effect of occupational
hyperinflation	exposure
thoracic deformity	Assess possible toxicity of
decreased breath sounds	medications
wheezing	*Disability evaluation*
rales/crackles/crepitations	
expiratory slowing	
cyanosis	
Abnormal laboratory tests	
polycythemia	
hypercarbia	
hypoxemia	
abnormal chest radiograph	
Preoperative assessment	
Assess prognosis	
Screen individuals at risk for pulmonary disease	

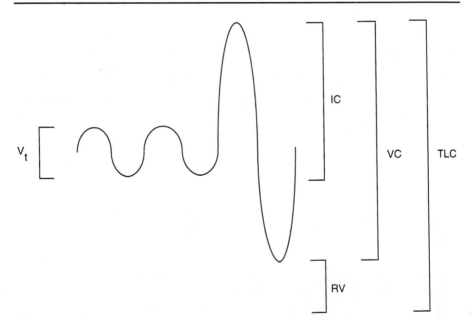

Figure 2.1. Expired volumes during a voluntary spirometric maneuver are illustrated. In this fashion tidal volume (V_T) and inspiratory capacity (IC) can be measured. During a maximal exhalation, vital capacity (VC) is measured. Residual volume (RV) and total lung capacity (TLC) cannot be measured in this fashion.

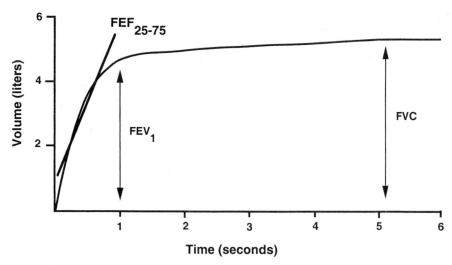

Figure 2.2. A forceful spirometric maneuver yields a typical plot of volume versus time. This allows measurement of forced vital capacity (*FVC*), forced expired volume in one second (*FEV$_1$*), and the forced expired flow between 25 and 75% of the vital capacity (FEF$_{25-75}$).

Techniques

Since the late 1970s the major source of variability in spirometric results has changed from the instrumentation to the improper performance of the tests. The American Thoracic Society (ATS) has recently revised the recommended minimum standards for spirometers. Individuals wishing to acquire equipment to perform spirometric studies should ensure that the instruments meet or exceed these ATS guidelines, which establish specific criteria for instruments meant predominantly for diagnostic studies compared with those meant simply to be used for monitoring. A 1990 evaluation of spirometers demonstrated that only 57% of spirometers tested met the ATS guidelines for accuracy.

Given the importance of patient effort and cooperation in achieving reproducible and valid results, strict recommendations have been made regarding the performance and reporting of spirometric results. These recommendations include adequate training for personnel to include at least 6 months of supervised training prior to conducting spirometry and 1 year of supervised training if troubleshooting is to be part of the technician's responsibilities. The subject must be tested using a standard posture (sitting or standing if possible) and instructed to inhale fully and then exhale fully and forcefully with little delay. Spirometric maneuvers should be repeated until at least three acceptable forced expiratory curves are recorded. Criteria used to determine acceptable curves are enumerated in Table 2.2. Once these goals are achieved, the largest FVC should be reported from the acceptable curves. Similarly, the largest FEV$_1$ should be recorded (not necessarily from the same curve). FEF$_{25-75}$ should be reported from the single curve, which meets acceptability criteria and gives the largest sum of FVC and FEV$_1$.

Table 2.2. Criteria for Acceptability and Reproducibility of Spirometric Maneuvers

---

Acceptability criteria
Curve is free from artifacts
Maneuver demonstrates a "good start"
Maneuver demonstrates a satisfactory exhalation (at least 6 seconds and/or plateau in volume-
   time curve)
Reproducibility criteria
After three acceptable maneuvers are recorded
   Two largest FVC are within 0.2 L of each other
   Two largest FEV_1 are within 0.2 L of each other
Or
   A total of eight tests have been performed
Or
   The patient/subject cannot continue with testing

Reference Values

Interpretation of spirometric results is largely based on establishing a variation from normal, expected values for a specific individual. The ATS recently reviewed the source of biologic variation in spirometric indices in an effort to standardize interpretative strategies. This report describes intraindividual variation that includes diurnal and seasonal factors, which are small. More important are interindividual differences. In this regard, sex, age, height, ethnic differences, and weight account for up to 70% of variation in FEV_1 or FVC among adults. In general, normal values are based on regression equations that take these factors into account. None of the currently available equations represent adequate numbers of subjects in all the groups determining interindividual biologic variability. Each laboratory must understand the limitations of these regression equations and use those that most resemble the patients being tested.

   Once an appropriate reference equation has been chosen, limits of the "normal range" must be established. Ideally, values below the fifth percentile are considered to be below the expected range while those above the fifth percentile are within the normal range. More commonly, values of FEV_1 and FVC below 80% of predicted are considered to be below the normal range. This has clinical limitations, with shorter, older subjects more likely to be classified as "abnormal" and taller, younger subjects more likely to be classified as "normal." These limitations must be remembered when applying interpretative strategies in individuals with "borderline" spirometric indices. When analyzing flow rates, such as the FEF_{25-75}, it is important to understand the much greater biologic variability in this value. The lower limits of normal for these values are closer to 50% of predicted. Defining an absolute $FEV_1/$FVC ratio as a lower limit of normal is now considered incorrect given the biologic variability in this parameter, particularly with age. The use of regression equations is advised when interpreting this parameter.

Interpretative Strategies

Spirometry is most useful in defining an obstructive ventilatory defect. A disproportionate decrease in FEV_1 compared with FVC (decrease in the FEV_1/FVC ratio) is used to define airflow obstruction. In some younger, fit individuals the values of FVC may be relatively larger than those for FEV_1, resulting in a lower FEV_1/FVC ratio than predicted. Defining airflow obstruction in this setting (usually in the setting of normal absolute levels of FEV_1 and FVC) must be made with caution. Isolated decreases in FEF_{25-75} were once considered early predictors of airflow obstruction. More recent recommendations caution against this practice, given the poor specificity and broad variability of this parameter.

• A restrictive defect is inferred when FVC is decreased but FEV_1/FVC is normal or increased. Restriction is defined by a decrease in measured TLC. Definitive characterization of a restrictive ventilatory defect requires measurement of lung volumes (see below).

Response to bronchodilators in the pulmonary function laboratory is usually assessed by the change in spirometric parameters after the administration of a short-acting bronchodilator (such as a beta$_2$-agonist). To accurately define "bronchodilation" one must be aware of the within-individual variability in response to different bronchodilators and the "normal" range of response to bronchodilators in large population studies. The most recent ATS recommendations consider bronchodilation to have occurred when the FVC and/or FEV_1 rise by at least 12% and when the absolute volume also rises by more than 200 mL. The clinical importance of bronchodilation in the pulmonary function laboratory can be questioned because there are clear benefits to bronchodilator medications that may be independent of acute changes noted in the laboratory. Similar considerations exist when interpreting changes in spirometry over time. The ATS has clarified these changes in the recommendations as enumerated in Table 2.3.

Table 2.3. Change in Spirometric Indices over Time

	Percent Change Required To Be Significant		
	FVC	FEV_1	FEF_{25-75}
Within a day			
Normal subject	≥ 5	≥ 5	≥ 13
Patient with CAO	≥ 11	≥ 13	≥ 23
Week to week			
Normal subject	≥ 11	≥ 12	≥ 21
Patient with CAO	≥ 20	≥ 20	≥ 30
Year to year	≥ 15	≥ 15	

Determination of disease severity is in many respects arbitrary. General guidelines have been published that include determination of severity in obstructive lung disease based predominantly on the FEV_1 as a percent of predicted and not on the FEV_1/FVC ratio.

The FEV_1 appears to be the most useful test in determining mortality in obstructive disorders, and a commonly used system defines airflow obstruction as follows:

• Mild obstruction as an FEV_1 between 70 and 80% predicted;
• Moderate obstruction as an FEV_1 between 50 and 70% predicted;
• Severe airflow obstruction as an FEV_1 less than 50% predicted.

In such a fashion, the ATS has recently recommended staging chronic obstructive pulmonary disease (COPD) in three stages based on FEV_1:

• Stage I, FEV_1 more than 50% predicted with little impact on health-related quality of life;
• Stage II, FEV_1 between 35 and 49% predicted in which the impact on quality of life and health care expenditures are higher;
• Stage III, with FEV_1 less than 35% predicted in which mortality is highest and health care expenditure is significantly increased.

Clinical Use

• Because of its simplicity, reproducibility, and widespread availability, spirometry is the most widely used of pulmonary function tests. It has a clear role in defining airflow obstruction.

Badgett et al. defined the sensitivity of physical examination and history in identifying chronic airflow obstruction (CAO). The authors identified a history of 70 or more pack/years of cigarette smoking and a decrease in breath sounds as the most useful variables. These variables yielded a sensitivity of 67% but a specificity of 98%. Spirometry was used as the "gold standard" to define the presence of CAO.

• FEV_1 remains the most accurate physiologic variable to define the severity of airflow obstruction.

The routine use of spirometry in these patients at each visit remains controversial. Owen and colleagues examined the role of routine spirometry in 150 consecutive patients (75 with obstructive disease and 26 with mixed restriction/obstruction). A clinical management plan was formulated based on initial history and physical examination. The addition of spirometric results altered plans in only 5% of patients. Those with severe (FEV_1, FVC, or FEV_1/FVC ≤ 40% predicted values) disease and/or a deterioration in clinical status were the most likely to benefit from routine spirometry.

Spirometry is central to the management of patients with restrictive disorders (see below and also Chapter 6). In sarcoidosis, the FVC has been recommended as an optimal method of providing follow-up data, with a 10% change generally considered significant. Certainly this datum must be used in conjunction with clinical and radio-

graphic parameters for optimal clinical management. In idiopathic pulmonary fibrosis (IPF), the literature is less certain, with most authors advocating the use of
multiple pulmonary function and clinical and radiographic parameters.

• The VC has served as a standard test to monitor function in patients with neuromuscular disease. A decreasing VC, particularly if it drops below 10–15 mL/kg or
three times the tidal volume, may identify progressive respiratory failure. Early
institution of mechanical ventilation in this setting has been shown to decrease
morbidity and mortality. Finally, spirometry is central to the evaluation of operative
risk and in the determination of impairment and disability, discussed subsequently.

FLOW-VOLUME STUDIES

With improved electronic pulmonary function equipment, it has become common
to record expired and inspired flows during a spirometric maneuver. During this
study the patient is asked to exhale fully and maximally from TLC to residual volume
(RV) followed by a rapid, maximal inhalation. The data are usually represented as
in Figure 2.3. Maximal expiratory flow is achieved during the first 25% of the VC;
this peak expiratory flow rate (PEFR) depends mainly on the effort of the subject
and the resistance in the upper airway. Additional parameters include the forced
expired flow at 50% of the VC (FEF_{50}) and forced inspired flow at 50% of the VC
(FIF_{50}). Diffuse airway obstruction, such as seen with emphysema, produces a typical

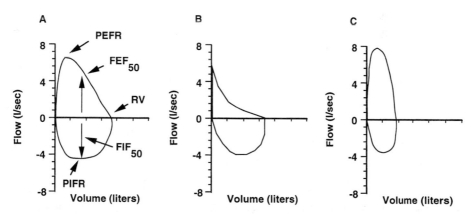

Figure 2.3. Maximal spirometric maneuver with data expressed as flow (*y* axis) versus lung
volume (*x* axis), a flow-volume loop. **A,** Normal subject. Parameters measured include: peak
expiratory flow rate (*PEFR*), peak inspiratory flow rate (*PIFR*), forced expired flow at 50%
of vital capacity (*FEF_{50}*), and forced inspired flow at 50% of vital capacity (*FIF_{50}*). Residual
volume (*RV*) is shown for reference. **B,** Flow-volume loop in an individual with airflow
obstruction, such as emphysema. Note concavity in expiratory flows. **C,** Flow-volume loop
in an individual with restrictive lung disease, such as interstitial pulmonary fibrosis. Peak
flows are preserved but loop is "narrowed" because lung volume is decreased.

abnormality in the flow-volume loop as shown in Figure 2.3*B*. Restrictive lung diseases (such as pulmonary fibrosis) are associated with ''narrowed'' loops as shown in Figure 2.3*C*.

Flow-volume loops are invaluable in detecting upper airway obstructions (UAO). Understanding the determinants of airflow allows us to apply the flow-volume loop to the diagnosis of UAO. The elasticity of the upper airway significantly influences airflow during respiration (Fig. 2.4). The airway outside the thorax (extrathoracic airway) is surrounded by pressures close to atmospheric. During inspiration, negative intratracheal pressures cause the airway to collapse. During expiration, the opposite occurs in the extrathoracic portion of the airway. The airway within the thorax (intrathoracic airway) is surrounded by pleural pressures and responds differently. During forced expiration, the transmural pressure tends to collapse this intrathoracic portion of the trachea. The location of an abnormality along the length of the upper airway will exert varying effects on airflow.

The nature of the lesion in the upper airway will also affect the airflow resulting from respiratory maneuvers. ''Variable obstructions'' are those in which airway geometry varies with transmural pressure. Examples include vocal cord paralysis in the extrathoracic airway and tracheomalacia in the intrathoracic airway. The aperture of such variable lesions depends on their location in the airway as a result of the different transmural pressures (Fig. 2.4). A variable intrathoracic lesion affects flow predominantly during expiration, while a similar lesion in the extrathoracic airway affects flow predominantly during inspiration. A lesion whose geometry is little

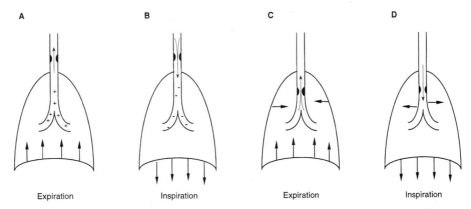

Figure 2.4. Elasticity of the upper airway is illustrated. The effect of a variable extrathoracic obstruction (**A-B**) and intrathoracic obstruction (**C-D**) are shown. The effect on flow-volume loops is illustrated in Figure 2.5. **A,** Effect of forceful expiration in a patient with a variable extrathoracic obstruction. Preservation of expiratory flow is illustrated. **B,** Effect of forceful inspiration in a patient with a variable extrathoracic obstruction. Impairment of inspiratory flow is illustrated. **C,** Effect of a forceful expiration in a patient with a variable intrathoracic obstruction. Impairment of expiratory flow is illustrated. **D,** Effect of a forceful inspiration in a patient with a variable intrathoracic obstruction. Preservation of inspiratory flow is illustrated.

affected by transmural pressure changes (a "fixed" lesion, such as a fibrotic or malignant tracheal stricture) will affect both inspiratory and expiratory flow regardless of its location in the airway. Greater degree of obstruction should result in progressive abnormalities of inspiratory flow, expiratory flow, or both. The location of a variable obstruction would give rise to specific abnormalities of inspiratory or expiratory flow. This was proven in the classic work of Miller and Hyatt and is illustrated in Figure 2.5, which demonstrates the features of a variable extrathoracic (Fig. 2.5A), intrathoracic (Fig. 2.5B), and fixed obstruction (Fig. 2.5C). Additional spirometric parameters that should raise suspicion of a UAO include $FIF_{50} \leq 100$ L/min, $FEF_{50}/FIF_{50} \geq 1$, $FEV_1/PEFR \geq 1.5$, $FEV_1/FEV_{0.5} > 1.5$, and $MVV/FEV_1 < 25$.

There are limitations to the use of flow-volume loops. In patients with severe CAO, the flow-volume loop shows significant alteration as a result of the peripheral airflow obstructions, and superimposed upper airway lesions may be difficult to detect. Spirometric criteria as enumerated in the previous paragraph may be useful. Garcia-Pachon et al. studied 137 patients of whom 23 had a UAO and CAO; 54, only UAO; 60, only CAO. The presence of three or more spirometric abnormalities or an FEF_{50}/FIF_{50} more than 1 or MVV/FEV_1 less than 25 suggested the presence of additional UAO. Additional studies may be needed in difficult situations. Changes in flows while the patient breathes a low density gas (such as Helium, which decreases airway resistance because of the lower gas density) may be useful in diagnosing UAO in patients with underlying CAO. Unfortunately, the marked within-subject variability during these studies limits their widespread applicability.

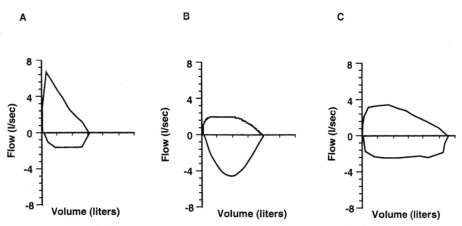

Figure 2.5. Flow-volume loops in disorders with varying upper airway obstruction. **A,** Impaired inspiratory flow in a patient with a variable extrathoracic obstruction (corresponding to Figure 2.4, **A-B**). **B,** Impaired expiratory flow in a patient with a variable intrathoracic obstruction (corresponding to Figure 2.4, **C-D**). **C,** Impaired inspiratory and expiratory flow in a patient with a fixed obstruction or with simultaneous variable extrathoracic and intrathoracic obstructions.

PEAK EXPIRATORY FLOW RATE (PEFR)

The measurement of PEFR has been extensively used in managing patients with asthma. The availability of inexpensive and portable devices has markedly increased the use of this study. PEFR (see Fig. 2.3) is highly dependent on effort and is associated with greater variability. Its major role is as a monitoring tool. Appropriate teaching and assurance of an accurate device are crucial. Some widely used peak flow meters lose accuracy with repeated use. This will have clear implications on clinical decision-making, and intermittent spirometry must be performed to confirm the extent of airflow obstruction.

BRONCHOPROVOCATION TESTING

Spirometry can also be used during bronchoprovocation studies, in which multiple spirometric maneuvers are performed before and after exposure to varying stimuli. Stimuli that may elicit bronchospasm in susceptible patients may be nonspecific (e.g., methacholine, histamine, cold air) or specific (e.g., aspirin, antigen, or bisulfate). Decrements in pulmonary function after exposure that resolve after an inhaled bronchodilator suggest bronchial hyperreactivity. Guidelines for testing have been established. To ensure safety and validity of measurement, relative contraindications to testing have been published (Table 2.4).

Table 2.4. Relative Contraindication to Bronchoprovocation Testing

Ventilatory impairment at time of study
  $FEV_1 < 80\%$ of previous best values
  $FEV_1/FVC < 70\%$
  $SG_{AW} < 0.09s^{-1}$ cm H_2O^{-1}
  $FEV_1 < 1.0$ L in adults
Significant response to the diluent ($> 10\%$ fall in FEV_1 from baseline)
Inability to perform acceptable (reproducible) spirometry
Upper or lower respiratory infection within prior 6 weeks
Specific antigen exposure within previous week
Exposure to high atmospheric pollution within previous week
Pregnancy
Failure to withhold medications that may affect reactivity and including:
  Beta$_2$-adrenergic agonists within 12 hours
  Anticholinergic aerosols within 12 hours
  Disodium cromoglycate within 8 hours
  Oral beta$_2$-agonists within 12 hours
  Theophylline within 48 hours
  H^1-receptor antagonists within 72–96 hours
  Beta blockers (may increase response)
Ingestion of caffeine or theobromine-containing substance (colas, coffee, etc.)

Methodology for Bronchial Provocation Testing

A baseline FEV_1 is obtained and the patient breathes diluent. The subsequent FEV_1 serves as the control. The agent to be inhaled is delivered by a Wright nebulizer or by a dosimeter designed to deliver a constant amount of solution from a DeVilbiss nebulizer. Both of these methods appear to yield comparable results. A widely used abbreviated study has been proposed. Two concentrations of methacholine are used, 5 mg/mL and 25 mg/mL. After the saline diluent, FEV_1 is established and the subject inhales one breath of 5 mg/mL. A repeat spirometry is obtained. If no significant change has occurred, four breaths of 5 mg/mL are then inhaled. If no change occurs in spirometry, the subject inhales one breath of 25 mg/mL and finally four breaths of 25 mg/mL, with monitoring of FEV_1. The histamine challenge is performed in a similar manner. Cold air hyperventilation is safe, specific for asthma, and easy to perform but requires expensive and more sophisticated equipment, which is not readily available.

The pulmonary function parameter to be used in defining bronchial reactivity is controversial. The indices usually measured include the FEV_1 and the specific airway conductance (SG_{AW}). The SG_{AW} is more sensitive, but has a greater variability and lower specificity and is more difficult to measure. The FEV_1 is less sensitive but more reproducible. The optimal method of measurement depends on the clinical scenario. In many laboratories, both the FEV_1 (20% drop) and SG_{AW} (40% drop) are measured.

Clinical Use

Bronchoprovocation testing is a useful clinical study that is underused. The study is most often used to establish the diagnosis of asthma. In this context, bronchial hyperreactivity is sensitive but not specific because several other conditions may be associated with hyperreactivity (Table 2.5). A recent study assessed methacholine challenge in 51 patients with suspected asthma. The physician's clinical diagnosis of asthma was compared with objective measurement of methacholine responsiveness. Disagreement occurred in 20 patients (39%). Bronchoprovocation was normal in 13 patients with suspected asthma (on clinical grounds); 7 had abnormal hyperresponsiveness despite negative clinical diagnosis. Published data have correlated the response to bronchoprovocation testing with the clinical severity of asthma.

Table 2.5. Disorders Associated with Bronchial Hyperactivity

Asthma	Congestive heart failure
Chronic obstructive pulmonary disease	Near drowning
Cystic fibrosis	Sarcoidosis
Bronchiolitis	Chemical irritant exposure
Upper respiratory infections	Foreign body aspiration
Hay fever	Postadult respiratory distress syndrome
Smoke inhalation	

Bronchoprovocation is an excellent diagnostic study to evaluate chronic cough and unexplained dyspnea. Irwin et al. confirmed the value of methacholine challenge testing in patients who coughed for more than 3 weeks. These authors reported a sensitivity of 100% for hyperactive airways disease but a specificity of only 67%. Pratter et al. prospectively performed methacholine challenge on 85 patients presenting with dyspnea in whom findings and history were nonspecific. Bronchoprovocation had a 95% positive predictive value and a 100% negative predictive value for asthma, the most common diagnosis encountered in their series. DePaso et al. noted a similar utility in the evaluation of 72 patients with unexplained dyspnea. Bronchoprovocation testing was particularly useful in patients younger than age 40, with intermittent dyspnea and normal resting arterial oxygenation. Bronchoprovocation testing clearly has great value as a diagnostic study in patients with respiratory symptoms.

MAXIMUM VOLUNTARY VENTILATION (MVV)

Maximum voluntary ventilation represents the maximal volume of air a subject can breathe rapidly and deeply within 12–15 seconds. This test depends on adequate respiratory muscle function and endurance, as well as on airway resistance. The MVV is a sensitive but nonspecific indicator of respiratory muscle dysfunction and increased airway resistance. In addition, MVV/FEV_1 ratio less than 25 may suggest UAO even in the presence of both CAO and UAO. MVV may be estimated by multiplying FEV_1 by 40. Unfortunately, the MVV is extremely effort-dependent and its clinical utility is limited.

LUNG VOLUME MEASUREMENT

Spirometry measures FVC (Fig. 2.1) but provides no information on the volume of air remaining in the lungs after a maximal forced expiration (RV or TLC). RV and TLC measurement requires additional techniques. Direct measurement of TLC is important because a decrement in TLC is the definition of restrictive disease, while a decrement in VC can be caused by elevation of RV or a decrement in TLC.

Three methods have been used to measure lung volumes: chest radiography (which will not be discussed further), gas dilution, and body plethysmography. Dilutional methods use a physiologically inert gas that is poorly soluble in alveolar blood and tissue. Dilutional techniques include open circuit (nitrogen (N_2) washout) and closed circuit (Helium (He) dilution).

Dilutional Lung Volume Measurement
Open Circuit (N_2 Washout)

In this technique, the subject inhales 100% O_2, and all exhaled gas is collected. The test is usually started from the end-tidal position, thus measuring functional residual capacity (FRC). This method assumes the initial N_2 concentration in the lungs is 0.81, and the rate of N_2 elimination from blood and tissue is approximately 30 mL/min; the volume of N_2 in the subject's lung is equal to the volume in the collection system at the end of the test.

The nitrogen washout method is simple and permits assessment of the uniformity of ventilation by analyzing the slope of the change in N_2 concentration over consecutive exhalations. Unfortunately, this method is sensitive to leaks in the system and measures only the volume of air communicating freely with the airways.

Closed Circuit (He Dilution)

The closed circuit method is based on a similar concept. The patient rebreathes from a spirometer with a known volume of inert gas (He). The CO_2 generated is recovered and oxygen replenished with 100% O_2 to maintain constant volume. After equilibration, the concentration of He is decreased in direct proportion to the volume added to the system by the patient's lung volume. The lung volume measured in this fashion depends on the point at which the patient is connected to the spirometer, usually the end-expiratory position, FRC.

The closed circuit method is also sensitive to leaks in the system and measures only the communicating lung volume. The lung volume in patients with severe maldistribution, such as severe obstruction or bullous disease, is underestimated. Burns and Scheinhorn measured TLC by He dilution and radiographic techniques in 79 patients with varying degrees of airflow obstruction. They confirmed that He dilution progressively underestimated TLC with increasing airflow obstruction. The role of dilutional lung volume measurement to determine coexisting restriction in patients with CAO is clearly limited.

Body Plethysmography

Despite its greater complexity, body plethysmography is the most accurate method for measuring absolute lung volumes. The technique is based on Boyle's law, which holds that the product of pressure and volume is constant if the temperature is unchanged. The subject sits in a large, air-tight chamber with a pneumotachograph to measure flow at the mouth, a pressure transducer to measure mouth pressure and box pressure, and a shutter to close the mouthpiece. While the subject sits in the box breathing through the mouthpiece, the door is closed and the temperature is allowed to equilibrate. Panting is performed lightly against the closed shutter, thereby compressing and decompressing the thorax. Change in the lung volume can be calculated because the change in thoracic volume is reflected in the change in box pressure and thoracic pressure (reflected by mouth pressure). As this usually is performed at the end of expiration, the thoracic gas volume measured is FRC.

The major limitations of body plethysmography are its complexity and the expense of the equipment. Recent studies suggest that body plethysmography may overestimate lung volumes in subjects with CAO, largely as a result of the compliance of the upper airway and high airway resistance. Shore and colleagues studied three normal subjects and 10 patients with severe CAO in a body plethysmograph. The frequency of panting was varied. Frequencies greater than 1 Hz resulted in artifactual increases in TLC. The authors also showed that supporting the cheeks during lung volume measurement decreased the artifactual overestimation of TLC. Strict attention to the technique of plethysmography is vital to obtain accurate data in patients with airflow obstruction.

Normal Values

Measurement of lung volumes is usually employed to achieve the following:

- A low VC or to establish a baseline;
- Quantify the level of impairment;
- Follow a patient serially or establish response to therapy;
- Screen for early disease, which may yield specific patterns of abnormality.

The variability of lung volume measurement must be kept in mind while one considers normalcy. Normal predictive values for lung volumes differ considerably. In addition, the upper and lower limits of normal vary with the study. Crapo et al. defined normal as values within a single 95% confidence interval. Viljanen et al. established 95% confidence ranges for TLC (80–125% of predicted) and RV (60–160% of predicted for men and 65–155% of predicted for women). Each laboratory must use those values most representative of their patient population and confirm appropriate normal values for their laboratory. Data establishing the degree of variability in lung volume measurement are more limited. In general, variability with plethysmography and He dilution have ranged from 4 to 7%. The underestimation of lung volumes in patients with CAO or bullous disease with dilutional measurement was described earlier.

Clinical Use of Lung Volume Measurement

Measurement of TLC is accepted as the "gold standard" in defining a restrictive ventilatory defect. Data supporting TLC measurement as a support to VC measurement are remarkably limited, however. In fact, studies of biopsy-proven interstitial lung disease suggest that TLC is less sensitive than VC in detecting restriction. The sensitivity and specificity of spirometry in restrictive disease was addressed by Gilbert and Auchincloss, who defined restriction on clinical and plethysmographic criteria in 211 patients. Definition of restriction by spirometry criteria included a low FVC with normal FEV_1/FVC. Using a lower limit for FEV_1/FVC of 70%, the spirogram was 93% sensitive but only 82% specific for detecting or excluding a restrictive defect. Combining spirometry, TLC, and clinical features is optimal in detecting restrictive diseases.

The value of TLC measurement in detecting restriction superimposed on CAO is controversial. The opposite effects of restriction and obstruction on TLC have formed the basis for this consideration. Lanier and Olsen examined spirometry and Helium dilution lung volumes in 58 patients with CAO, 18 of whom had undergone various forms of pulmonary resection (superimposed restriction). Using 80% of predicted as the lower limit of normal, 61% of patients with mixed obstruction/restriction would have been missed. The absolute TLC was lower in patients who had undergone pulmonary resection. Barnhart et al. studied 41 patients with asbestosis by history and chest radiograph, 17 of whom had concomitant airflow obstruction (decreased FEV_1/FVC). The TLC in those with "mixed" disease was higher (104% of predicted) compared with uncomplicated asbestosis (TLC 87% of predicted). There was significant overlap between both groups, however. Sole use of PFT to diagnose a mixture of restrictive and obstructive lung disease is unwise. A final decision must be based on additional clinical and radiographic data. Given their limitations in CAO, dilutional lung volumes should not be used in defining restriction superimposed on CAO.

With the known variability in lung volume measurement, it is difficult to assign a specific assessment of severity based solely on pulmonary function data. A typical arbitrary assessment is illustrated in Table 2.6. In IPF, TLC values correlate poorly with pathologic indices of disease severity. Conversely, in two recent studies a lower TLC on presentation was associated with increased mortality from IPF. A single measure of lung volume cannot be used to assess clinical severity in IPF but does provide useful prognostic information. Results are similar in sarcoidosis, in which no single lung volume measurement can accurately predict histologic severity. Disease severity in CAO is best judged by the level of FEV_1 as a percent of predicted values. Measures of RV or TLC add little in this respect.

Given the variability in measurement and the limited ability to predict histologic severity, the role of serial lung volume measurement in the follow-up of patients with restrictive lung disease of parenchymal origin (IPF and sarcoidosis) is controversial. In IPF no single parameter is ideal. Raghu et al. noted significant discordance between changes in FVC, TLC, and DL_{CO} during a clinical trial of immunosuppressive therapy in IPF. Conversely, Schwartz et al. noted an independent contribution to changes in TLC during therapy of IPF as clinical response to therapy. It is unlikely that sole monitoring of one individual lung volume will be optimal in the follow-up of patients with IPF. The approach of Watters et al. offers a good compromise. In this fashion, multiple clinical (dyspnea), radiographic, and pulmonary function parameters (including lung volume) are used serially to monitor response to therapy in IPF. In sarcoidosis a similar conclusion can be reached, as no single parameter can serve to determine clinical response to therapy.

Understanding the determinants of each of the absolute lung volumes allows one to use lung volume measurement to identify patterns of abnormality. Such an approach is illustrated in Table 2.7. For example, a decrease in TLC with an increase

Table 2.6. Arbitrary Assessment of Severity Based on Lung Volume Measurement

Lung Volume	Mild Defect	Moderate Defect	Severe Defect
TLC	70–80%	60–70%	< 60%
	120–130%	130–150%	> 150%
RV	55–65%	45–55%	< 45%
	135–150%	150–250%	> 250%

Table 2.7. Pattern of Lung Volume Abnormality in Restrictive Lung Disease

Disease	FVC	TLC	FRC	RV
Alveolar filling/loss	⇓	⇓	⇓	⇓
Interstitial	⇓	⇓	↓	N/↓
Neuromuscular				
Inspiratory	⇓	⇓	N	N
Expiratory	⇓	N	N	⇑
Both	⇓	⇓	N	⇑
Thoracic cage				
Kyphoscoliosis	⇓	⇓	⇓	↓
Ankylosing spondylitis	⇓	⇓	⇑	⇑
Pleural disease	N/⇓	N/⇓	N/⇓	N/⇓

N, normal; ⇓, decreased; ↓, mildly decreased; ⇑, increased.

in RV may suggest respiratory muscle weakness. Owens et al. recently identified the value of isolated decrements in RV (less than 65% of predicted). Sixty-three of sixty-nine patients had clinical conditions that could account for the lung volume abnormality. These included both parenchymal abnormalities and chest wall abnormalities. Furthermore, change in RV coincided with changes in clinical condition. As such, measurement of lung volumes in patients with restrictive disease can serve a diagnostic purpose.

In patients with CAO, the value of lung volume measurement is limited. The pattern of lung volume measurement may be useful in identifying asthma, chronic bronchitis, and emphysema. This, however, is likely of little clinical value. The finding of an isolated RV elevation has been addressed by Vulterini et al. In 14 subjects with isolated RV elevation but no airflow obstruction by spirometry, a reduction in elastic recoil suggesting occult emphysema was identified. Measuring noncommunicating lung volume (''trapped gas'') or the difference between plethysmographic and dilutional lung volumes may have value when considering surgical management for emphysema. The physiologic contribution of a large bulla may be inferred prior to bullectomy. Similar data has been employed in evaluating patients for volume reduction surgery (pneumectomy). Although some have advocated lung volume measurement (usually RV) in detecting patients with CAO at particularly high risk for thoracic resection, recent data have confirmed that lung volume measurement has little role in preoperative evaluation. Spirometry, DL_{CO}, and exercise testing (see below) have become more widely accepted in this clinical setting.

DIFFUSING CAPACITY FOR CARBON MONOXIDE (DL_{CO})

Measurement of the DL_{CO} dates to 1914 when Marie Krogh first performed the measurement to dispute the theory that oxygen was secreted actively in the lung. Since that time the DL_{CO} has become an invaluable, widely used pulmonary function test.

Methodology

The DL_{CO} is a measure of the ability of gases to diffuse from the alveoli to the pulmonary capillary blood. Carbon monoxide is used because of its high solubility in blood compared with lung tissues and because of its great affinity for hemoglobin (210 times greater than oxygen). Determination of DL_{CO} requires measuring the amount of CO that is transferred from the alveolar gas to blood per minute, the alveolar CO pressure, and the mean pulmonary capillary CO pressure. Five methods can measure DL_{CO}, but the single breath is most widely used and will be the only technique discussed in this chapter.

During the test the subject exhales to RV and inhales quickly to TLC a mixture of 21% O_2, 10% He, 0.3% CO, and the balance N_2. The breath is held for 10 seconds during which time CO diffuses into the capillary blood. Subsequently enough gas is exhaled to wash out mechanical and anatomic dead space. DL_{CO} is then calculated from the total alveolar volume (V_A), breath hold time, and the initial and final concentration of CO. The advantages of this method include wide availability, simplicity, and relative insensitivity to back pressure of CO in capillary blood.

Careful attention to technique is crucial, as an interlaboratory coefficient of variation of 12.7% has been reported. Recent comparison of DL_{CO} measurements on five individuals at 13 laboratories revealed individual values ranging from 20.6 to 54.2. The source of this great variability includes errors in gas concentration measurement, breath hold time, inspired volume, and the computation algorithms chosen. Measurement of DL_{CO} should abide by recently published guidelines.

Normalcy

Multiple other factors can affect the DL_{CO}. The coefficient of variability in normal subjects ranges from 5 to 9% but may be higher in patients with CAO. The accepted variability is ± 10% or 3 mL CO (STPD)/min/mm Hg. DL_{CO} can change with hemoglobin concentration; polycythemia will increase DL_{CO} and anemia will decrease it. The DL_{CO} should be corrected for hemoglobin using the following equations:

Hemoglobin adjusted DL_{CO} = observed DL_{CO} (10.22 + Hgb)/1.7 Hgb

(for adolescents and adult males adjusted to Hgb 14.6 gm/dL)

Hemoglobin adjusted DL_{CO} = observed DL_{CO} (9.38 + Hgb)/1.7 Hgb

(for children under the age of 15 years and women adjusted to Hgb 13.4 gm/dL)

Carboxyhemoglobin (HbCO) will decrease DL_{CO} by approximately 1% for each 1% increased in HbCO. A recommended equation for this correction is:

HbCO adjusted DL_{CO} = measured DL_{CO} (1 + [%HbCO/100])

Additional factors that can affect DL_{CO} include cigarette smoking, which can decrease DL_{CO} independent of HbCO, body position (supine > sitting > standing), diurnal variation, and pregnancy. Although these are minor factors, the interpreting physician must keep them in mind as serial comparisons of DL_{CO} are made in a given individual.

Because the total capillary membrane surface is dependent on the patient's lung volume, this parameter has been noted to be a large source of variability in DL_{CO} measurement. Thus the DL_{CO} is often corrected for the V_A, the DL_{CO}/V_A. This parameter may be more useful than the DL_{CO} alone. As discussed subsequently, DL_{CO} is a useful screening test; DL_{CO}/V_A adds complementary information.

Reference equations for DL_{CO} vary widely and may be confining. Most reference equations use height, sex, and age to predict DL_{CO}. Additional equations are available that predict DL_{CO}/V_A. Most studies are based on Caucasians, with little data available in other ethnic groups. One abstract suggested African-Americans had lower DL_{CO} compared with Caucasians, but DL_{CO}/V_A were similar. Each laboratory should select 15–20 normal subjects and examine reference equations for that which produces the sum of residuals closest to zero. This variability must also be kept in mind when comparing values of DL_{CO} among different laboratories. Normal values are best defined by 95% confidence intervals and not as $\pm$ 20% of predicted. These normal values have been published for several reference equations. Similarly, assessment of disease severity by DL_{CO} is arbitrary, and no generally accepted guidelines exist.

Clinical Use

Despite obvious limitations, DL_{CO} is an extremely valuable clinical tool that is most often used in the evaluation of patients with respiratory symptoms, CAO, interstitial lung disease, in determination of disease severity, and in serial evaluation during therapy. DL_{CO} is highly sensitive but has less specificity. In patients with unexplained dyspnea, DL_{CO} may direct the subsequent evaluation. Table 2.8 illustrates typical diagnostic considerations for abnormal values of DL_{CO}.

The major considerations for decreases in DL_{CO} include:

• Interstitial lung diseases;
• Emphysema;
• Pulmonary vascular diseases.

The DL_{CO} is particularly useful in evaluating restrictive lung diseases. DL_{CO} may be useful in patients with normal chest radiographs and high resolution computed tomography of the chest or normal biopsy-proven interstitial lung disease. DL_{CO} may be normal, however, in over 25% of patients with diverse various interstitial lung disorders. This can be seen, but is less common, in patients with IPF. Serial measurements of DL_{CO} have been used by many investigators to follow patients with IPF during treatment. Clearly, DL_{CO} can provide prognostic information in these individuals. Correlations between histologic severity and DL_{CO} are poor, however, and use of DL_{CO} as a sole indicator of clinical course is problematic. A better approach is to include DL_{CO} in a battery of physiologic, clinical, and radiographic parameters in determining response to therapy or the natural history of IPF.

In patients with scleroderma, DL_{CO} may identify patients at higher risk for pulmo-

Table 2.8. Diagnostic Possibilities in Patients with Abnormal DL_{CO}

Abnormality in DL_{CO}	Diagnostic Possibilities
⇑ DL_{CO}	Left to right shunt
	Exercise
	Altitude
	Supine position
	Polycythemia
	Alveolar hemorrhage
	Asthma
⇓ DL_{CO}	
with normal or ⇓ V_A (low DL/V_A)	Anemia
	Emphysema
	Pulmonary vascular diseases
with low V_A (low, normal, or high DL/V_A)	Lung resection
	Pulmonary alveolar proteinosis
	Interstitial lung diseases
	Neuromuscular disease
	Thoracic cage disorders

⇑, increase; ⇓, decrease.

nary mortality and morbidity. Peters-Golden noted an increase in mortality with DL_{CO} below 40% of predicted. Steen et al. noted a high frequency of isolated DL_{CO} reduction (19% of patients) in systemic sclerosis with a subgroup demonstrating pulmonary hypertension and severely reduced survival. The latter was more likely if the DL_{CO} was less than 55% of predicted and the ratio of FVC (percent predicted)/ DL_{CO} (percent predicted) was more than 1.4. Significant variability exists, however. In the setting of systemic sclerosis, measurement of DL_{CO} appears to have prognostic value and can identify scleroderma patients deserving aggressive therapy and close follow-up.

DL_{CO} measurement in sarcoidosis is useful but with limitations. Correlations between DL_{CO} and histologic severity have been, in general, poor, although a lower DL_{CO} is usually associated with greater histologic abnormality. The DL_{CO} appears to be less sensitive to change with therapy than the VC. We recommend obtaining a baseline measurement of DL_{CO} and repeating measurements during follow-up when the clinical course is not adequately reflected by chest radiography.

In CAO, a decrement in DL_{CO} is frequently used to separate emphysema from chronic bronchitis and asthma. Reductions in DL_{CO} have been shown in asymptomatic individuals who are noted to have emphysema in lung biopsies taken for other purposes. Decreases in DL_{CO} are more sensitive for emphysema than is examination of lung compliance. These data are of little practical value, as treatment for the various obstructive diseases is similar and disease severity is best determined by spirometric changes. DL_{CO} may identify individuals at high risk for postoperative complications or limited ventilatory reserve after bullectomy or thoracic resection. Predicted postoperative DL_{CO} is the strongest predictor of risk of complications and mortality after lung resection and should be routinely measured prior to thoracic resection. A DL_{CO} below 50% of predicted may identify individuals at high risk for exercise-induced desaturation.

Patients with chronic thromboembolic disease usually demonstrate a decrease in DL_{CO}. A decrease in DL_{CO} was noted in 5 of 6 patients with chronic thromboembolic pulmonary hypertension (CTPH) and in 9 of 15 patients with primary pulmonary hypertension (PPH). The reduction in DL_{CO} was the sole pulmonary function abnormality in four patients with PPH and in two patients with CTPH. Burgess noted frequent abnormalities in DL_{CO} in patients with "pure inflow obstruction," such as PPH and CTPH, compared with individuals with pulmonary hypertension associated with valvular heart disease. The specificity of a decrease in DL_{CO} is low, while the sensitivity in pulmonary hypertension remains undefined. A normal DL_{CO} is seen with relative frequency in both CTPH and PPH. Data in acute pulmonary embolism are limited. Wimalaratna and colleagues measured the DL_{CO} within 72 hours of admission in 20 consecutive patients with pulmonary embolism diagnosed by ventilation-perfusion lung scan ($\dot{V}/\dot{Q}$ scan). DL_{CO} was decreased in all subjects (less than 75% predicted) and persisted for up to 3 years despite resolution of perfusion abnormalities on $\dot{V}/\dot{Q}$ scan. Wimalaratna et al. suggested that a normal DL_{CO} excludes significant pulmonary embolism. Given the small number of patients in the study, this conclusion must be accepted with caution.

The change in DL_{CO} with left ventricular dysfunction is controversial. Naum et al. reported pulmonary function data, including DL_{CO}, in patients with chronic, severe cardiomyopathy prior to heart transplantation. Most patients had abnormal pulmonary function, with low DL_{CO} being common. Pulmonary capillary wedge pressure correlated *positively* with DL_{CO}. Siegel et al. noted a correlation between DL_{CO} and left ventricular ejection fraction only in those patients with rales on physical examination. Changes in DL_{CO} are common in left ventricular dysfunction but depend on the chronicity and stability of the clinical condition.

RESPIRATORY MUSCLE TESTING

Pulmonary function observations that may be observed with respiratory muscle weakness include:

- A decrement in FVC (which is nonspecific);
- An increased RV/TLC ratio with a decreased TLC (of unknown specificity);
- A decrease in MVV out of proportion to FEV_1.

Methods of Assessing Respiratory Muscle Function

Black and Hyatt described a method to measure inspiratory (PI_{max}) and expiratory (PE_{max}) pressures, among a group of 120 normal subjects. Decreasing pressures were noted in those subjects over 55 years of age.

To measure PE_{max}, the patient inspires forcefully against an occluded airway and maintains the pressure for 1–2 seconds. Multiple factors, in addition to loss of muscular capacity, can affect these measurements. These measures are voluntary efforts, and patient cooperation is crucial for valid and reproducible results. Technical factors include the mouthpiece used for the measurements. In young subjects who are highly motivated, a simple tube mouthpiece provides the highest values. The more popular flanged mouthpiece gives consistently lower values, particularly in PE_{max}. Recruitment of facial muscles can lead to inappropriately elevated mouth pressures. For this reason, a 1–2-mm leak should be maintained in the system.

An additional, major factor is the lung volume at which the measurement is made. Inspiratory pressure depends on lung volume because the function of the diaphragm is highly dependent on thoracic volume and diaphragm length. Most data for PI_{max} have been recorded from RV to maximize diaphragm length and pressure generation. To minimize the effect of respiratory system recoil and to simplify the maneuver, some authorities argue measurement from FRC. Measurement of PE_{max} is generally performed from TLC.

Mouth pressures provide a view of global respiratory muscle function that may be difficult to reproduce. A low PI_{max} suggests that inspiratory muscle function is depressed. In this setting, measurement of esophageal pressure as an estimate of pleural pressure (Ppl) may be useful. Similarly, measurement of transdiaphragmatic pressure (Pdi), the difference between Ppl and gastric pressure, can provide further information. Maximal diaphragm function can be measured during a Müller maneuver (Pdi_{max}) or during a sharp sniff maneuver (Pdi_{sniff}). The Müller movement is more difficult and variable.

Normal Values for Respiratory Muscle Function

Data on normal values for respiratory pressures are more limited. The different techniques used and patient populations studied have resulted in various regression equations for PI_{max} and PE_{max}, with wide normal ranges. Until recently this was particularly problematic in elderly patients. Enright and colleagues examined PI_{max} and PE_{max} in a large cohort of elderly subjects (65 years of age or older) studied as part of the Cardiovascular Health Study. These authors reported mean values of 57/116 for PI_{max}/PE_{max} for women and 83/174 for men. Lower limits of normal were 45 to 60% of mean predicted values. Regression equations were provided. Race was not a significant factor after sex, age, and weight were taken into account. Normal ranges for Pdi are lacking, as published data are limited. Most laboratories establish normal ranges for the populations most likely to be encountered. Recent work has confirmed decreases in Pdi with aging.

Clinical Use

Respiratory muscle testing is indicated in patients with unexplained dyspnea, particularly when associated with lung volume restriction or decrements in MVV (out of proportion to FEV_1). Measurement of PI_{max} and PE_{max} is simple, inexpensive, and feasible. Pi_{max} and PE_{max} may be useful in patients with CAO and dyspnea out of proportion to spirometry. In this setting, hyperinflation influences PI_{max} but not PE_{max}. As such, PE_{max} remains invaluable.

More commonly, PI_{max} and PE_{max} are used in the initial evaluation and follow-up of patients with neuromuscular disease. Black and Hyatt first described the greater sensitivity in measurement of maximal static respiratory pressures compared with spirometry in 15 patients with neuromuscular disease alone and in 5 with additional cardiopulmonary disease. Griggs et al. confirmed this and suggested that PE_{max}, with its greater range, may be the most sensitive marker in patients with neuromuscular disease. Even in mild to moderate neuromuscular disease, decrements in respiratory pressures are the earliest and most pronounced abnormality.

PE_{max} and PI_{max} are especially valuable in individuals with labile neuromuscular conditions, such as polymyositis, Guillain-Barré syndrome, and myasthenia gravis. In these illnesses, FVC and respiratory muscle pressure measurement are monitored frequently, particularly during the early acute illness. Respiratory failure generally occurs when PI_{max} drops below one-third of predicted values. It is standard practice to monitor FVC and PI_{max} frequently during the acute illness. Initiation of mechanical ventilation must be considered when the FVC drops below 10–15 mL/kg or PI_{max} drops below 20–25 cm H_2O. A PE_{max} below 40 cm H_2O predicts a poor cough and increased respiratory complications.

EXERCISE TESTING

Significant limitations of exercise testing include the nonuniformity of established normal ranges for exercise parameters and interpretation algorithms. Cardiopulmonary exercise testing (CPET) is distinct from "cardiac stress testing" in that emphasis is placed not only on parameters of cardiac function but also on the interaction of cardiac and pulmonary function during exercise. Pulmonary exercise testing can be thought of as proceeding from the simplest to the most complex and invasive testing:

- Exercise oximetry;
- Noninvasive CPET;
- Invasive CPET;
- CPET with pulmonary arterial catheter (will not be discussed further).

Exercise Oximetry

Methodology

Pulse oximetry has largely replaced nonpulse oximetry. These oximeters are more portable and have simplified exercise testing. They exhibit similar accuracy (95% confidence interval of 3–5%) at saturation above 70% while at rest. HbCO can lead to spurious results because pulse oximeters tend to read approximately the sum of HbO_2 + HbCO. This is problematic with HbCO levels greater than 4–4.9%. Methemoglobinemia leads to underestimation of O_2 saturation. Anemia is associated with greater error as hypoxemia increases. Skin pigmentation influences saturation readings. Nail polish, particularly blue polish, may affect accuracy of readings and should be removed. Similarly, bright ambient light can provide spurious results. Motion artifact is evident with some of the commercially available pulse oximeters. A poor pulse correlation between the pulse oximeter and ECG recordings may help identify signals producing spurious saturation readings. Finally, and of the most concern, Hansen and Casaburi studied 14 patients with an ear oximeter during exercise. Readings were falsely low in the five patients, with cardiovascular limitation and saturation overestimated in two patients with interstitial lung disease. Pulse oximeters correlate with trends in oxygen saturation, but their ability to predict the PaO_2 or O_2 saturation during exercise is limited, particularly with increasing hypoxemia.

Clinical Use

Exercise oximetry has a role in detecting desaturation during ambulation in patients with pulmonary disease. The long-term value of O_2 administration during exercise in patients who desaturate during exercise but have adequate saturation at rest has not been proven. Because right ventricular dysfunction occurs with nocturnal desaturation in patients with sleep disorders, it seems logical that exercise-induced desaturation could result in a similar phenomenon. The limitation of pulse oximetry in this regard was highlighted by Carlin and colleagues. These investigators noted that oxygen saturation could not determine the need for O_2 supplementation in a large group of patients with cardiopulmonary disease. This may have been related in part to the format of exercise testing used by these investigators. As long as one remembers the limitations of pulse oximetry during exercise, the level of accuracy is likely acceptable during a test simulating the patient's usual activity level.

The value of oximetry in patients with respiratory symptoms is more limited. Artifactual changes may be of greater clinical significance at higher work loads, thereby decreasing specificity of pulse oximetry during exercise. Sensitivity is also limited by the measurement of oxygen saturation and not PaO_2. Given the hemoglobin-O_2 dissociation curve, a major drop in PaO_2 (from 100 to 70, for example) can occur with only minor changes in oxygen saturation as measured by oximetry. A drop of more than 4% or a saturation of 88% are considered to be clinically significant with pulse oximetry during exercise.

Noninvasive CPET
Methodology

Continued improvements in sensor technology and computer software have markedly enhanced the ability to measure expired gases for airflow and volume, O_2 concentration, and CO_2 concentration. This allows measurement of minute ventilation ($\dot{V}_E$), O_2 consumption ($\dot{V}O_2$) and CO_2 production ($\dot{V}CO_2$). During CPET, work load can be increased on a treadmill, bicycle ergometer, or arm ergometer. A work protocol can be used that will result in a symptom-limited, maximal exercise study in 10–15 minutes. Blood pressure and ECG are monitored in addition to expired gases. Oximetry is recorded as described above.

From these data we can determine aerobic capacity or maximal achieved $\dot{V}O_2$. This forms the basis for most interpretation algorithms for CPET. The cardiac response can be defined by several major $\dot{V}O_2$ relationships, including $\dot{V}O_2$ versus power, O_2 pulse ($\dot{V}O_2$/heart rate), and heart rate (HR) versus $\dot{V}O_2$. The $\dot{V}O_2$ at which anaerobic metabolism supplements aerobic metabolism is defined as the anaerobic threshold (AT). This may be detected noninvasively by examining the $\dot{V}O_2/\dot{V}_E$ relationship (the breakpoint of $\dot{V}_E/\dot{V}O_2$) or the slope of the $\dot{V}O_2$ and $\dot{V}CO_2$ relationship (V-slope method).

Ventilatory response is defined mechanically by the maximal $\dot{V}_E$ ($\dot{V}_{Emax}$) as a percentage of maximal ventilation, usually estimated by the MVV. The breathing reserve (BR) is defined as $1-\dot{V}_{Emax}$/MVV. The pattern of breathing (tidal volume, V_T, and respiratory rate, f_b) are often used to define abnormal patterns of ventilation during exercise. Oxygenation is monitored using oximetry.

Normal Values

Before considering interpretation algorithms we must consider the range of normal values for the most commonly used parameters measured during a noninvasive CPET. The normal range for $\dot{V}O_2$max is wide because many factors affect the aerobic response to exercise. These factors include age (decreases with increasing age), sex (greater in males than in females), body size (increases with increased weight), and the exercise format (treadmill > bicycle ergometer > arm ergometer). Any regression equation used must represent the patient population being studied and the type of exercise being performed. A value of 84% predicted $\dot{V}O_2$max is often used as the lower limit of normal.

Peak HR declines with age. Well-validated formulas exist to predict this, including:

$$\text{Peak HR} = 220 - \text{age (years)} \quad \text{or peak HR} = 210 - 0.65 \text{(age)}$$

The O_2 pulse predicted can be calculated from the predicted values for $\dot{V}O_2$ and HR. Normal values for AT are more loosely established, varying with age and type of exercise. The values for AT range from 41 to 54% of predicted maximal $\dot{V}O_2$ in adults. The lowest values were found in sedentary, middle-aged men at 40% of peak $\dot{V}O_2$. This level is used by many as the lower limit of normal. The variability and limited data supporting these predicted ranges must be remembered as we proceed with interpretation.

Ventilatory response is initially described as a function of MVV. The latter, however, is not representative of the pattern of respiratory muscle recruitment during exercise, which limits the applicability of this determination. In normal subjects the $\dot{V}_{Emax}$/MVV has a wide range but usually does not exceed 70–75%. This value has been used by many as the normal threshold. Similar difficulties are encountered when defining normal values for V_T and f_b during exercise. It is more valuable to examine ventilation as a pattern of response than to rely heavily on arbitrary normal ranges.

The efficiency of ventilation is in part related to the degree of dead space ventilation. This can be estimated, noninvasively, by examining the ventilatory equivalents for $\dot{V}CO_2$ ($\dot{V}_E/\dot{V}CO_2$). For practical purposes, the nadir of this value occurs at the AT, with normal values reported by Hansen et al. Elevated values of $\dot{V}_E/\dot{V}CO_2$ can be caused by alveolar hyperventilation or an increase in dead space. When examined in the context of end-tidal CO_2 (PETCO$_2$), one can better surmise the reason for the increase in $\dot{V}_E/\dot{V}CO_2$.

Invasive CPET

Methodology and Normal Ranges

An invasive CPET includes sampling of arterial or venous blood for arterial blood gas analysis and/or lactate measurement. The former allows a more accurate assessment of oxygenation. These samples are optimally obtained through the use of an indwelling arterial catheter. A resting arterial blood gas and one obtained within 20 seconds of terminating exercise, however, may suffice. The P(A-a)O$_2$ can be accurately calculated as the R quotient ($\dot{V}CO_2/\dot{V}O_2$) is measured. The P(A-a)O$_2$ usually increases with exercise in relation to the work load but rarely rises above 35. The measured PaCO$_2$ can be used to measure physiologic dead space, V_D/V_T. Lactate measurement allows a more accurate measurement of the lactate threshold. The clinical value of these invasive parameters remains unsettled. Resnikoff et al. suggested that invasive measurements may alter the interpretation of CPET in 23.6% of patients undergoing CPET for the evaluation of dyspnea. In diagnostic CPET we recommend the routine measurement of arterial blood gases.

Interpretation Strategies

Multiple widely used algorithms for interpretation of CPET are available. Most of these are based on the normal ranges that have the limitations described earlier. They are useful for interpretation of CPET as illustrated in Figure 2.6. An approach that uses such an algorithm but examines patterns of response seems most useful. Such an approach has been described by Weisman and Zeballos. Table 2.9 describes typical alterations in exercise parameters with differing clinical conditions.

Clinical Use

Despite the limitations of CPET, the information obtained is valuable. This is particularly true when used in conjunction with clinical information. In evaluating unexplained dyspnea, CPET can frequently prove diagnostic. DePaso et al. and Pratter et al. have documented a limited role of CPET in chronic dyspnea, particularly if resulting from a psychogenic cause. Martinez et al. confirmed the ability of CPET to detect pulmonary and cardiac disease in patients with unexplained dyspnea. The

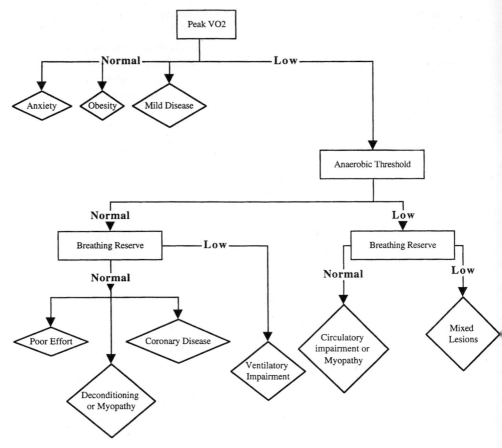

Figure 2.6. Typical algorithm used in the interpretation of cardiopulmonary exercise tests at our institution. The text provides further detail.

Table 2.9. Patterns of Exercise Response by Disease Category

Variable	Respiratory Disease	Cardiac Disease	Poor Conditioning
$\dot{V}O_{2max}$	$\Downarrow$	$\Downarrow$	$\Downarrow$
Anaerobic threshold	N (if present)	$\Downarrow$	N or $\Downarrow$
O_2 pulse	N	$\Downarrow$	N
HR reserve (1-peak HR)	$\Uparrow$	N	N
$\dot{V}O_2$/work rate slope	N	$\Downarrow$	N
Breathing reserve	$\Downarrow$	N	N
Saturation	May $\Downarrow$	N	N

$\Uparrow$, increase; $\Downarrow$, decrease.

limitation of CPET in differentiating between cardiac disease and poor conditioning was also evident.

CPET has been used widely in patients with left ventricular dysfunction. The data are limited in supporting the ability of CPET to predict the extent of left ventricular dysfunction or diagnose early disease. There has been ample support of measuring maximal $\dot{V}O_2$ to predict prognosis in left ventricular dysfunction. This has become routine in evaluating patients prior to heart transplantation. Patients with a maximal achieved $\dot{V}O_2$ less than 14 mL/kg/min have a higher mortality and are candidates for immediate transplant listing.

Over the past 15 years the value of CPET in the diagnosis and follow-up of patients with interstitial lung disease has been proven. Although not as valuable in sarcoidosis, measures of gas exchange ($P(A-a)O_2$ in particular) are the best predictors of histologic abnormality in IPF. Sequential evaluation of gas exchange has been valuable during the treatment of patients with IPF. In addition, CPET data have become widely used in the determination of impairment and in the preoperative evaluation of patients with cardiopulmonary disease prior to pulmonary resection.

APPLICATION OF PULMONARY FUNCTION TESTING IN CLINICAL PRACTICE

With understanding of the techniques available for objective determination of pulmonary function, the reader should develop a logical approach to their use in common clinical settings. These clinical situations will be discussed in the form of commonly asked clinical questions.

What Is the Source of Pulmonary Symptoms?
Chronic Exertional Dyspnea

Multiple studies have confirmed that chronic exertional dyspnea is most commonly caused by pulmonary or cardiac disease. PFT should play a central role in the evaluation of this complaint, in addition to selective cardiac testing. A diagnostic algorithm demonstrating the possible application of PFT in such patients is shown in Figure 2.7. The routine measurement of lung volumes as illustrated in this figure remains controversial. If excluded, one would fail to identify those individuals with isolated RV decrement who subsequently are shown to have restrictive lung disease.

Chronic Cough

Several authors have defined a logical, diagnostic algorithm to evaluate patients with chronic cough. As occult asthma is frequently seen in this setting, PFT is used by all clinicians in the early phase of the evaluation of chronic cough. Bronchoprovocation is cost-effective as an early diagnostic study if spirometry is normal and if postnasal drainage is excluded or treated without relief of cough.

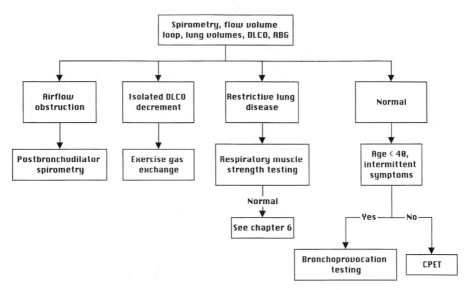

Figure 2.7. Diagnostic algorithm applicable to the evaluation of a patient presenting with chronic dyspnea. The text provides further detail. (*ABG,* arterial blood gas.)

What Is the Role of PFT in Asthma Evaluation and Follow-up?

The management of asthma is discussed at greater length in Chapter 4. The role of PFT has assumed a much greater role as a result of the summary recommendations of several expert panels. These authors have based these recommendations largely on the inherent difficulties encountered in the initial diagnosis of asthma. Spirometry (before and after bronchodilator administration) is recommended in the initial evaluation of patients with a clinical suspicion of asthma. PEFR can be used but is not ideal because it has greater variability, effort dependency, and tends to underestimate FEV_1. Bronchoprovocation testing may be necessary in more difficult diagnostic settings.

Evaluation of disease severity is difficult for patients and even more so for physicians. PFT (spirometry or PEFR) is able to objectively demonstrate the severity of airflow obstruction and the response to therapy. This form of monitoring is effective in managing acutely ill individuals. As the emphasis on patient self-management of asthma has increased, so has reliance on home monitoring with spirometry or PEFR. Some investigators have shown dramatic improvements in asthma management with home PEFR monitoring and the use of detailed treatment plans. The Grampian Asthma Study of Integrated Care (GRASSIC) prospectively studied 569 patients randomized to self-monitoring with PEFR measurement or conventional management. Both groups were carefully instructed in optimal asthma management; no significant differences in outcome between the groups were noted. The authors concluded that routine PEFR was unnecessary. Close attention to education was optimal and PEFR monitoring was helpful in the most severe asthmatics.

Is the Patient Physically Impaired from Lung Disease?

Disability is defined as ''an alteration of an individual's capacity to meet personal, social, or occupational demands or statutory or regulatory requirement because of an impairment. Disability refers to an activity or task the individual cannot accomplish.'' Disability is determined by administrative bodies partly on the basis of a physician's determination of physical impairment. Several national and international agencies have recommended 12 different systems to grade impairment from respiratory disease, as summarized by Smith. The ATS has published a widely used system that is illustrated in Figure 2.8.

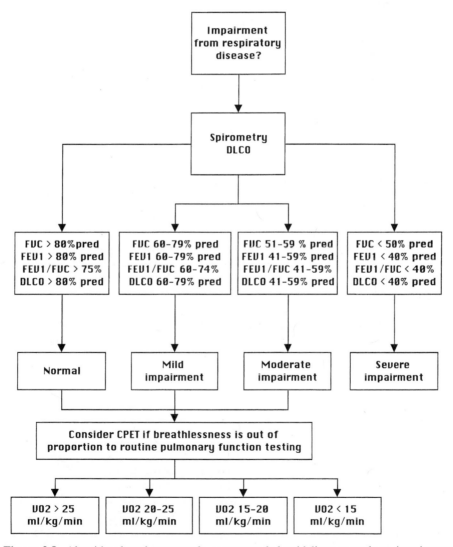

Figure 2.8. Algorithm based on recently recommended guidelines to evaluate impairment in an individual with pulmonary disease.

These systems use arbitrary ranges for normal that may not be applicable to all. Cotes and colleagues performed maximal CPET on 157 patients who met criteria for respiratory impairment by ATS criteria. Using measured $\dot{V}O_2$max, 44 of these patients had no disability and 31 had only a slight disability. Several groups of investigators have confirmed the value of CPET in detecting frequent, unexpected cardiac limitation in patients evaluated for impairment from lung disease. As a result, we recommend that routine PFT be the first line of investigation in determining pulmonary impairment. CPET should be more widely used if breathlessness seems out of proportion to initial testing.

The ATS has published specific recommendations for evaluating impairment in patients with asthma. These guidelines rely heavily on confirmation of disease severity using spirometry before and after the administration of a bronchodilator. If the findings are inconclusive, bronchoprovocation testing is recommended. Optimal treatment is delivered before a final determination is made to ensure as much reversal as possible with aggressive medical therapy. To determine an impairment score, the postbronchodilator FEV_1, percent reversibility after a bronchodilator, degree of bronchial hyperresponsiveness, and minimum medication needed are tabulated. This total score is used to grade the level of impairment.

Is the Patient at Higher Risk of Perioperative Pulmonary Complications?

Pulmonary complications are frequent following major surgery, particularly in thoracic and upper abdominal surgery. The use of PFT in predicting which patients will be at higher risk of pulmonary complications has been recently reviewed, but the data are contradictory. Current recommendations are for limited testing in higher risk groups as enumerated in Table 2.10. Spirometry and arterial blood gas analysis are the minimal studies indicated in patients undergoing head and neck surgery, coronary artery bypass grafting, or upper abdominal procedures.

The data supporting preoperative PFT are solid for patients undergoing thoracic resections. Marshall and Olsen have reviewed these data in detail. Most investigators now recommend preoperative spirometry, DL_{CO}, and arterial blood gases as the minimal diagnostic testing. Exercise testing may add independent information in selected cases. From these data an algorithm as illustrated in Figure 2.9 can be followed.

Table 2.10. High Risk Groups for Postoperative Pulmonary Complications

Patients undergoing	Patients with
thoracic resections[a]	history of cigarette smoking
coronary artery bypass grafting[b]	history of lung disease
upper abdominal surgery[b]	planned operative procedure requiring prolonged
head and neck surgery[b]	anesthesia

[a] Pulmonary function testing indicated in all routinely.

[b] Pulmonary function testing indicated at least in high risk by initial history/physical.

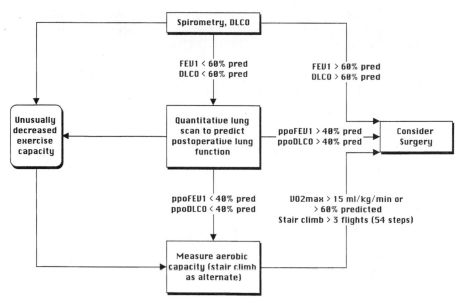

Figure 2.9. Algorithm based on recently published data to establish candidacy for thoracic resection in an individual with pulmonary disease.

BIBLIOGRAPHY

Spirometry

American Thoracic Society. Lung function testing: selection of reference values and interpretative strategies. Am Rev Respir Dis 1991;144:1202–1218.

American Thoracic Society. Standardization of spirometry. 1994 Update. Am J Respir Crit Care Med 1995;152:1107–1136.

American Thoracic Society. Standards for the diagnosis and care of patients with chronic obstructive pulmonary disease. Am J Respir Crit Care Med 1995;152(supp 5):S77–S120.

Badgett R, Tanaka D, Hunt D, Jelley L, Feinberg L, Steiner J, Petty T. Can moderate chronic obstructive pulmonary disease be diagnosed by historical and physical findings alone? Am J Med 1993;94:188–196.

D'Angelo E, Prandi E, Marazzini L, Milic-Emili J. Dependence of maximal flow-volume curves on time course of preceding inspiration in patients with chronic obstruction pulmonary disease. Am J Respir Crit Care Med 1994;150:1581–1586.

Garcia-Pachon E, Casan P, Sanchis J. Indices of upper airway obstruction in patients with simultaneous chronic airflow obstruction. Respiration 1994;61:121–125.

Knudson R, Lebowitz M, Holberg C, Burrows B. Changes in the normal maximal expiratory flow-volume curve with growth and aging. Am Rev Respir Dis 1983;127:725–734.

Owen M, Anderson W, George R. Indications for spirometry in outpatients with respiratory disease. Chest 1991;99:730–734.

Pickering R, Martinez F. PFT Corner "41: Helium flow-volume loop in an asthmatic patient. Respir Care 1991;36:1157–1159.

Watters L, King T, Schwarz M, Waldron J, Stanford R, Cherniack R. A clinical, radiographic, and physiologic scoring system for the longitudinal assessment of patients with idiopathic pulmonary fibrosis. Am Rev Respir Dis 1986;133:97–103.

Peak Expiratory Flow Rate (PEFR)

Cross D, Nelson H. The role of the peak flow meter in the diagnosis and management of asthma. J Allerg Clin Immunol 1991;87:120–128.
Shapiro S, Hendler J, Ogirala R, Aldrich T, Shapiro M. An evaluation of the accuracy of Assess and miniWright peak flow meters. Chest 1992;99:358–362.
Sheffer A. Guidelines for the diagnosis and management of asthma. J Allerg Clin Immunol 1991;88:425–534.

Bronchoprovocation Testing

DePaso W, Winterbauer R, Lusk J, Dreis D, Springmeyer S. Chronic dyspnea unexplained by history, physical examination, chest roentgenogram, and spirometry. Analysis of a seven-year experience. Chest 1991;100:1293–1299.
Irwin R, Curley F, French C. Chronic cough. The spectrum and frequency of causes, key components of the diagnostic evaluation, and outcome of specific therapy. Am Rev Respir Dis 1990;141:640–647.
Pratter M, Curley F, Dubois J, Irwin R. Cause and evaluation of chronic dyspnea in a pulmonary disease clinic. Arch Intern Med 1989;149:2277–2282.
Shrake K, Blonshine S, Brown R, Ruppel G, Wanger J, Kochansky M. American Association for Respiratory Care. Clinical practice guideline. Bronchial provocation. Respir Care 1992; 37:902–906.

Lung Volumes

American Association for Respiratory Care. AARC Clinical Practice Guideline. Static lung volumes. Respir Care 1994;39:830–835.
Barnhart S, Hudson L, Mason S, Pierson D, Rosenstock L. Total lung capacity. An insensitive measure of impairment in patients with asbestosis and chronic obstructive pulmonary disease. Chest 1988;93:299–302.
Burns C, Scheinhorn D. Evaluation of single-breath helium dilution total lung capacity in obstructive lung disease. Am Rev Respir Dis 1984;130:580–583.
Cherniack R, Colby T, Flint A, Thurlbeck W, Waldron J Jr, Ackerson L, Schwarz M, King T. Correlation of structure and function in idiopathic pulmonary fibrosis. Am J Respir Crit Care Med 1995;151:1180–1188.
Gilbert R, Auchincloss J. What is a "restrictive" defect? Arch Intern Med 1986;146: 1779–1781.
Lanier R, Olsen G. Can concomitant restriction be detected in adult men with airflow obstruction? Chest 1991;99:826 830.
Martinez F, Paine R III. Medical evaluation and management of the lung cancer patient prior to surgery, radiation, or chemotherapy. In: Pass H, Mitchell J, Johnson D, Turrisi A, eds. Lung cancer: principles and practice. Philadelphia, PA: Lippincott-Raven Publishers, 1995: 511–534.

Owens M, Kinasewitz G, Anderson W. Clinical significance of an isolated reduction in residual volume. Am Rev Respir Dis 1987;136:1377–1380.

Raghu G, DePaso W, Cain K, Hammar S, Wetzel C, Dreis D, Hutchinson J, Pardee N, Winterbauer R. Azathioprine combined with prednisone in the treatment of idiopathic pulmonary fibrosis: a prospective double-blind, randomized, placebo-controlled clinical trial. Am Rev Respir Dis 1991;144:291–296.

Ries A. Measurement of lung volumes. Clin Chest Med 1989;10:177–186.

Schwartz D, Helmers R, Galvin J, vanFossen D, Frees K, Dayton C, Burmeister L, Hunninghake G. Determinants of survival in idiopathic pulmonary fibrosis. Am J Respir Crit Care Med 1994;149:450–454.

Shore S, Huk O, Mannix S, Martin J. Effect of panting frequency on the plethysmographic determination of thoracic gas volume in chronic obstructive pulmonary disease. Am Rev Respir Dis 1983;128:54–59.

Viljanen A, Viljanen B, Halttunen P, Kreus K. Body plethysmographic studies in nonsmoking healthy adults. Scand J Clin Lab Invest 1981;41(suppl 159):35–50.

Vulterini S, Bianco M, Pellicciotti L, Sidoti A. Lung mechanics in subjects showing increased residual volume without bronchial obstruction. Thorax 1980;35:461–466.

Diffusing Capacity (DL$_{CO}$)

Burgess J. Pulmonary diffusing capacity in disorders of the pulmonary circulation. Circulation 1974;49:541–550.

Crapo R, Forster R II. Carbon monoxide diffusing capacity. Clin Chest Med 1989;10:187–198.

Ferguson M, Reeder L, Mick R. Optimizing selection of patients for major lung resection. J Thorac Cardiovasc Surg 1995;109:275–281.

Mohsenifar Z, Collier J, Belman M, Koerner S. Isolated reduction in single-breath diffusing capacity in the evaluation of exertional dyspnea. Chest 1992;101:965–969.

Morrison N, Abboud R, Ramadan F, Miller R, Gibson N, Evans K, Nelems B, Muller N. Comparison of single breath carbon monoxide diffusing capacity and pressure-volume curves in detecting emphysema. Am Rev Respir Dis 1989;139:1179–1187.

Moser K, Auger W, Fedullo P, Jamieson S. Chronic thromboembolic pulmonary hypertension: clinical picture and surgical management. Eur Respir J 1992;5:334–342.

Naum C, Sciurba F, Rogers R. Pulmonary function abnormalities in chronic severe cardiomyopathy preceding cardiac transplantation. Am Rev Respir Dis 1992;145:1334–1338.

Peters-Golden M, Wise RA, Hochberg MC, Stevens MB, Wigley FM. Carbon monoxide diffusing capacity as predictor of outcome in systemic sclerosis. Am J Med 1984;77:1027–1034.

Rubin L. Primary pulmonary hypertension. Chest 1993;104:236–250.

Siegel J, Miller A, Brown L, DeLuca A, Teirstein A. Pulmonary diffusing capacity in left ventricular dysfunction. Chest 1990;98:550–553.

Society AT. Single-breath carbon monoxide diffusing capacity (Transfer factor). Recommendations for a standard technique—1995 update. Am J Respir Crit Care Med 1995;152:2185–2198.

Steen V, Graham G, Conte C, Owens G, Medsger TJ. Isolated diffusing capacity reduction in systemic sclerosis. Arthritis Rheum 1992;35:765–770.

Wanger J, Irvin C. Comparability of pulmonary function results from 13 laboratories in a metropolitan area. Respir Care 1991;36:1375–1382.

Wimalaratna H, Farrell J, Lee H. Measurement of diffusing capacity in pulmonary embolism. Respir Med 1989;83:481–485.

Respiratory Muscle Testing

Black L, Hyatt R. Maximal static respiratory pressures in generalized neuromuscular disease. Am Rev Respir Dis 1971;103:641–650.

Black L, Hyatt R. Maximal respiratory pressures: normal values and relationship to age and sex. Am Rev Respir Dis 1969;99:696–702.

Enright P, Kronmal R, Manolio T, Schenker M, Hyatt R, C.H.S. Group. Respiratory muscle strength in the elderly. Correlates and reference values. Am J Respir Crit Care Med 1994; 149:430–438.

Gibson G. Diaphragmatic paresis: pathophysiology, clinical features, and investigation. Thorax 1989;44:960–970.

Gibson G. Measurement of respiratory muscle strength. Respir Med 1995;89:529–535.

Griggs R, Donohue K, Utell M, Goldblatt D, Moxley R. Evaluation of pulmonary function in neuromuscular disease. Arch Neurol 1981;38:9–12.

Kelly B, Luce J. The diagnosis and management of neuromuscular diseases causing respiratory failure. Chest 1991;99:1485–1494.

Mier-Jedrzejowics A, Brophy C, Moxham J, Green M. Assessment of diaphragm weakness. Am Rev Respir Dis 1988;137:877–883.

Exercise Testing–Oximetry

Escourrou P, Delaperche M, Visseaux A. Reliability of pulse oximetry during exercise in pulmonary patients. Chest 1990;97:635–638.

Hansen J, Casaburi R. Validity of ear oximetry in clinical exercise testing. Chest 1987;91: 333–337.

Mengelkoch L, Martin D, Lawler J. A review of the principles of pulse oximetry and accuracy of pulse oximeter estimates during exercise. Phys Ther 1994;74:40–49.

Servinghaus J, Koh S. Effect of anemia on pulse oximeter accuracy at low saturation. J Clin Monitor 1990;6:85–88.

Shrake K, Blonshine S, Brown R, Ruppel G, Wanger J, Korchansky M. American Association for Respiratory Care. Clinical practice guideline. Exercise testing for evaluation of hypoxemia and/or desaturation. Respir Care 1992;37:907–912.

Noninvasive Cardiopulmonary Exercise Testing (CPET)

Weisman I, Zeballos R. An integrated approach to the interpretation of cardiopulmonary exercise testing. Clin Chest Med 1994;15:421–445.

Invasive Cardiopulmonary Exercise Testing

DePaso W, Winterbauer R, Lusk J, Dreis D, Springmeyer S. Chronic dyspnea unexplained by history, physical examination, chest roentgenogram, and spirometry. Analysis of seven-year experience. Chest 1991;100:1293–1299.

Eschenbacher W, Mannina A. An algorithm for the interpretation of cardiopulmonary exercise tests. Chest 1990;97:263–267.

Mahler D, Horowitz M. Clinical evaluation of exertional dyspnea. Clin Chest Med 1994;15: 259–269.

Martinez F, Stanopoulos I, Acero R, Becker F, Pickering R, Beamis J. Graded, comprehensive, cardiopulmonary exercise testing in the evaluation of dyspnea unexplained by routine evaluation. Chest 1994;105:168–174.

Resnikoff J, Covin R, Harper P, Martinez F. Cardiopulmonary exercise testing (CPET) in the evaluation of dyspnea: the need for routine invasive testing. Am J Respir Crit Care Med 1994;151(suppl 4):A548.

Applications of Pulmonary Function Testing in Clinical Practice

American Thoracic Society. Evaluation of impairment/disability secondary to respiratory disorders. Am Rev Respir Dis 1986;133:1205–1209.

American Thoracic Society. Guidelines for the evaluation of impairment/disability in patients with asthma. Am Rev Respir Dis 1993;147:1056–1061.

Bolliger C, Jordan P, Soler M, Stulz P, Gradel E, Skarvan K, Elsasser S, Gonon M, Wyser C, Tamm M, Perruchoud A. Exercise capacity as a predictor of postoperative complications in lung resection candidates. Am J Respir Crit Care Med 1995;151:1472–1480.

Cotes J, Zejda J, King B. Lung function impairment as a guide to exercise limitation in work-related lung disorders. Am Rev Respir Dis 1988;137:1089–1093.

Grampian Asthma Study of Integrated Care (GRASSIC). Effectiveness of routine self monitoring of peak flow in patients with asthma. BMJ 1994;308:564–567.

Kamp D. Physiologic evaluation of asthma. Chest 1992;101(suppl 6):396S–400S.

Pratter M, Bartter T, Akers S, DuBois J. An algorithmic approach to chronic cough. Ann Intern Med 1993;119:977–983.

Smith D. Pulmonary impairment/disability evaluation: controversies and criticisms. Clin Pulmonary Med 1995;2:334–343.

Zibrak J, O'Donnell C. Indications for preoperative pulmonary function testing. Clin Chest Med 1993;14:227–236.

3 Bronchodilators in Lung Disease

John G. Weg

Bronchodilators address the problem of airflow obstruction caused by:

- Increased airways smooth muscle tone—"bronchospasm";
- Increased mucosal edema, congestion, and mucus secretion;
- Airways inflammation.

The clinical settings encompass a broad spectrum of diseases, such as asthma, asthmatic bronchitis, chronic bronchitis, bronchiectasis, cystic fibrosis, and the response to inhaled irritants (including inhaled aerosols, such as distilled water, hypertonic solutions, and even normal saline).

Bronchodilators are classified by their basic mechanism of action:

- Beta adrenergic agents (particularly beta$_2$ agents);
- Anticholinergic (antimuscarinic) agents;
- Theophylline;
- Agents that modify mediator release;
- Antiinflammatory agents.

In claims of one drug over another, especially if they are from the same class, it is important to carefully evaluate the validity of each claim and its supporting data. The following criteria should be met:

- In vitro finding appropriately supports in vivo conclusion;
- Animal study has valid human application;
- Efficacy comparisons account for routes of administration—aerosol, oral, subcutaneous, intramuscular, or intravenous;
- Equipotent doses are compared (not by weight);
- Side effects are compared at equipotent doses;
- Comparisons start with similar baseline data, especially with crossover studies;
- Improvement from baseline is likely (e.g., forced vital capacity in one second (FEV_1) that is $\leq 70\%$ of predicted);
- Percent improvement is clinically important (e.g., an improvement in FEV_1 from 300 mL to 360 mL is a 20% improvement that may not be important);
- The most appropriate test should be used (e.g., FEV_1 may not change but 6-minute walk distance increases);
- The cost to the patient at actual doses used should be similar;
- If the cost of a drug is much greater, the benefits should be worth the difference.

In evaluating an individual patient's response to bronchodilators, there are three indicators (in descending order of utility):

143

- Clinical response—the history;
- A 6-minute walking distance;
- Spirometric response.

The clinical response is usually the most reliable. Questions concerning dyspnea with specific activities, e.g., dressing, distance walked on level ground at the pace of peers or slowly, climbing a flight(s) of stairs, are necessary. Obtain information concerning the frequency, time, and circumstances of dyspnea, wheezing, and/or coughing. The 6-minute walk will provide objective evidence of low level exercise capability. The patient can be asked to rate his or her dyspnea on a Borg Scale (a 10-cm line with no markings other than "no breathlessness" at the left end and "greatest breathlessness" at the right end) before and after the walk. An increase in forced vital capacity (FVC) and/or forced expired volume at one second (FEV_1) of 15% or greater also indicates effective bronchodilation. Patients may experience important clinical improvement or an increased 6-minute walking distance without spirometric improvement, however, which is common with chronic obstructive pulmonary disease (COPD).

ROUTE OF DELIVERY

The currently used bronchodilators can be delivered most effectively to the respiratory tree by inhalation, except for theophylline and oral or IV corticosteroids.

Aerosols are suspensions of liquid droplets or particles in air. Particles from current aerosol generators are of varying size, heterodispersed. Respirable particles have an aerodynamic diameter of $\leq 5\ \mu$. They are deposited primarily by sedimentation or diffusion; a modest number of submicron particles ($< 0.5\ \mu$) can be deposited by diffusion. A particle impacts when its inertia does not allow it to continue in the airstream or when the airstream changes direction, such as at airway bifurcations. Impaction is greater the larger the particle and the greater the air velocity. Sedimentation occurs when particles $< 5\ \mu$ settle onto the airway surface by the force of gravity as airflow slows, and particularly with breath holding. When aerosols are water-soluble they absorb moisture and increase in size (hydroscopic growth).

Means of Delivery
Metered Dose Inhalers

Metered dose inhalers (MDIs) are currently available in many models. They may be activated by finger compression of a valve or be breath actuated during inspiration. Breath-actuated devices may be multidose or single dose using capsules. The drugs they contain may be suspended or dissolved in a liquid propellant. While chlorofluorocarbons (CFCs) are the most common vehicle currently used, vehicles without CFCs are under development. The drug may also be in a dry powder form.

Each of these devices delivers a specified dose per actuation (puff). Although the dose delivered at the mouthpiece is usually only slightly less than the dose released from the canister or capsule, the difference is substantial for some products. The convention in the United States is to report the dose delivered at the mouthpiece; in Europe and in some other countries, it is the dose released from the canister. Deposition in the lungs ranges between 10 and 25% of the drug released at the mouthpiece. This compares favorably with small volume nebulizers (SVNs), in which the dose deposited ranges from 1% or less to perhaps 10%.

Available data indicate that deposition is *enhanced* by:

- *Synchronized inspiration with MDI actuation;*
- *A slow inspiratory flow rate;*
- *Breath holding at end inspiration;*
- *Initiating inspiration from end-expiratory tidal volume;*
- *Holding the MDI approximately 4 cm (2.5 inches) from the open mouth* and aiming it directly at the pharynx (not at the teeth, tongue, or roof of the mouth); some clinicians recommend holding it at or by the lips;
- Perhaps allowing a couple of minutes between puffs.

Achievement of these recommendations requires the patient to practice under the careful tutelage of a trained care provider who is patient, clearly designated to perform this duty, and has adequate time to coach until the patient "gets it right." Such training often requires repeated sessions. It is also prudent to check patient competence at routine intervals (e.g., 3 or 6 months). Ideally, this responsibility should be assigned to a respiratory therapist or nurse. Have the patient practice in front of a mirror; technique is often better maintained and improved when the MDI is used while observing in the mirror (e.g., morning and evenings).

The generally recommended flow rate is approximately 0.5 L/second. When an individual begins inspiration at end-expiratory tidal volume, the inhalation includes the tidal volume and the inspiratory reserve volume—the inspiratory capacity. The sitting inspiratory capacity in the average man is approximately 2,700 mL and in the average woman approximately 2,100 mL. Therefore, the recommended *time* of inspiration is approximately 3–5 seconds. Using the *time of inspiration* rather than a flow rate in L/sec (or the more obtuse L/min) allows the trainer and the patient to seek a recognizable and measurable goal. A breath-holding time of 5–10 seconds is most effective and generally achievable. A delay between puffs theoretically allows the bronchodilation from the prior puff to enhance subsequent deposition. It carries the disadvantage of prolonging medication administration, which may negatively affect patient compliance.

A spacer is more effective in patients who are unable to synchronize finger activation with the initiation of inspiration despite repeated practice efforts; a breath-activated device is an alternative. Spacers range from a simple tube with a volume of approximately 100 mL (e.g., a pulmonary function mouthpiece) to chambers with volumes up to 1.5 liters, some with valves controlling inspiration and expiration. They may increase deposition in the lung by 10 to 15% and reduce deposition in the oropharynx by approximately 50%. A series of single puff into the spacer followed by a breath is more effective than multiple puffs followed by a single breath. Spacers reduce oral candidiasis with inhaled steroids. Likely candidates for such devices are patients with physical disabilities affecting the hands (such as arthritis) or those with neurologic disorders. Young children or elderly patients who cannot successfully coordinate inspiration and actuation are also likely to benefit.

MECHANICAL VENTILATION

Delivery of bronchodilators during mechanical ventilation by SVNs is inefficient—only 1–3% of the drug is delivered beyond the endotracheal tube. In contrast, delivery of drug from an MDI through a chamber adapter in the inspiratory limb just prior to the Y connector increases delivery to approximately 30%. In-line and elbow adapters are less effective.

Small Volume Nebulizers

SVNs are based on the Bernoulli principle. Compressed air or oxygen flows through a narrow tube at high velocity, creating a decreased pressure at the tube opening that causes the liquid in the nebulizer reservoir to rise to the tube opening, where airflow over baffles turns the liquid into droplets that are then inhaled. These devices are inefficient; lung deposition ranges from less than 1% to 10%. Thus, less than 0.2 mg of a 2.5-mg dose of albuterol is delivered as the respirable mass—the amount of the aerosol available to the patient. This approximates the 0.180 mg delivered by two puffs of an MDI. The respirable mass does not address the most important issue: the actual amount and site of deposition of the drug in the airways. In a bench evaluation of albuterol delivered by various brands of nebulizers, there was a threefold difference in the respirable mass. Whether this translates into the effectiveness of bronchodilator delivery awaits clinical study. A majority of the medication impacts on the nebulizer's inner surfaces and is never delivered. This dead volume can be ameliorated by increasing the volume of diluent to 5 mL while increasing the flow rate to 10 L/min. With continuous-flow SVNs, the medication delivered during exhalation and pauses between inspirations is wasted in the atmosphere; this can be minimized by using a finger-controlled device that limits nebulization to the time of inspiration.

Other Inhaled Delivery Modes

Ultrasonic nebulizers (USNs) had been used frequently in the past to deliver increased fluid (so-called bland aerosols) to the lungs in hopes of liquefying secretions. Efficacy of such efforts has not been documented. A USN offers no advantage in delivering bronchodilators. Large volume nebulizers or adapted SVNs are used to deliver bronchodilators by continuous nebulization. To our knowledge, there are no prospective randomized trials documenting any advantage other than one study in 17 pediatric patients. These patients, however, were not well matched at baseline (FIO_2 continuous .5 versus intermittent .93 ($p < 0.001$)), and the intermittent group probably had more bronchodilator left in the nebulizer dead space. Bronchodilators have also been given via an intermittent positive-pressure breathing (IPPB) machine, although no advantage has ever been documented. IPPB may be of value in highly selected patients who have an inadequate inspiratory capacity.

Selection of Means of Inhaled Delivery

There are many prospective randomized controlled trials documenting that MDIs with or without a spacer are at least equivalent to delivery by SVNs. These studies have been performed on patients with acute exacerbations of asthma and COPD, as well as in the chronic maintenance of patients with asthma and COPD. Because supervised delivery of a treatment by SVN takes 15–20 minutes for respiratory care or other personnel, dramatic reductions in hospital costs occur with the use of MDIs because treatment is delivered in a few minutes. Reports have estimated reduction in costs in the range of $253,000 or in charges of 75 to 80%. MDIs also reduce the time required to give bronchodilators to patients requiring mechanical ventilation. In addition, use of MDIs provides an extended opportunity for patient training by respiratory care personnel (RCP).

We developed clear-cut indications for bronchodilator therapy along with a change to MDIs in our hospital more than five years ago. Written protocols were developed empowering RCPs to select the means of bronchodilator delivery. Indications for bronchodilator therapy were defined as wheezing, measured decreased airflow, known COPD, or asthma. MDIs were designated as the standard delivery mode for bronchodilators. Able patients who received detailed instruction in MDI use were put into a self-administered program without difficulty; the patient and RCP shared documentation responsibilities. The use of SVNs was limited to patients who were:

- Not alert;
- Uncooperative;
- In severe respiratory distress (e.g., respiratory rate > 30/min);
- Unwilling to try MDI therapy;
- Not responding appropriately to MDI with a spacer.

Attending physicians could override the protocol after consultation with a respiratory care supervisor or the Medical Director of Respiratory Care Services (very rarely required). The utilization of strict criteria resulted in a reduction in bronchodilator treatments from a high of 118,000 per year to 78,000 per year despite an increased number of admissions, increased patient days, and unchanging severity of illness. Compliance with indications increased from 55–60% to 98–100%. Cost savings over the six-year period of 1989–1990 to 1994–1995 have amounted to approximately $400,000, allowing a reduction in 8.7 FTE RCPs. Currently 80% of the 78,000 bronchodilator treatments are given by MDIs; 20% of these are self-administered.

Oral or Systemic Delivery

Many beta agonists are available in oral form, and some are available for subcutaneous injection. There is a marked increase in side effects by either route in equipotent doses. Often a patient can only tolerate a dose that has a potency of approximately

50% of an inhaled dose. Therefore, they are generally not recommended. A possible exception is in the treatment of very young children who are unable to learn how to take the drug by inhalation. In such children, oral or systemic beta agonists are used by some physicians even though side effects are greater. Subcutaneous epinephrine, which has both alpha and beta activity, may also be of value in acute exacerbations in these youngsters.

BETA ADRENERGIC AGONISTS
Types and Actions

Beta agonists are subtyped as $beta_1$ and $beta_2$. $Beta_1$ agonists increase the force of myocardial contraction, cardiac rate, and A-V node conduction velocity. $Beta_2$ agonists produce bronchial smooth muscle relaxation; they also produce vascular, gastrointestinal, and genitourinary muscle relaxation. The effects of adrenergic agonists are determined by the type and number of receptors in various organs. Although $beta_2$ agonists primarily affect bronchial smooth muscle with its large numbers of $beta_2$ receptors, $beta_2$ receptors are also present in the myocardium and striated muscle.

Mechanism of Action

Adrenergic agonists produce their effects by binding with receptors and protein recognition sites in the cell membrane. These complexes activate G proteins, leading to an increase in adenyl cyclase. This results in an increase in intracellular adenosine $3',5'$-cyclic monophosphate (cAMP). This, in turn, causes bronchial wall smooth muscle relaxation. Alpha receptors and G_q cause vascular smooth muscle contraction by activation of various Ca^{2+} sensitive protein kinases, which increase intracellular Ca^{2+} (Fig. 3.1).

In addition to relaxation of smooth muscle, beta agonists have been shown to increase mucociliary transport, mucus secretion from submucosal glands, ion and water transport, and NO_2 (endothelium-derived relaxing factor), inhibit bronchial wall edema and cholinergic neurotransmission, decrease airway hyperresponsiveness, and prevent mediator release from mast cells, macrophages, and eosinophils.

Unwanted effects of beta agonists include tachycardia and palpitations. These effects, however, occur infrequently with currently used inhaled $beta_2$ selective agonists. Muscle tremors caused by activation of $beta_2$ receptors in striated muscle are usually associated with oral or systemic administration. They are rarely associated with inhaled $beta_2$ agonists in the usual doses.

Beta agonists also have metabolic effects. They may cause a very modest and generally unimportant decrease in serum potassium. They may effect increases in serum insulin, glucose, glycerol, lactate, pyruvate, nonesterified fatty acids, and high-density lipoprotein cholesterol.

Beta agonists can cause a transient modest decrease in arterial oxygen tension (i.e., 5–6 torr) before bronchodilation is achieved. They block the local alveolar

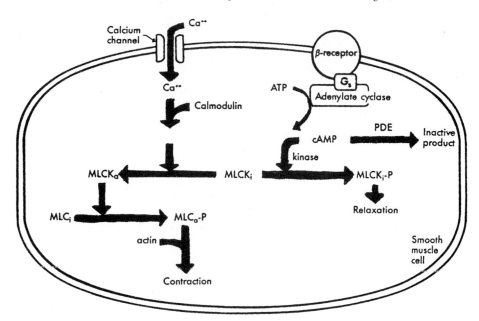

Figure 3.1. Possible mechanisms of contraction and relaxation in vascular smooth muscle. Contraction is initiated by the Ca^{++}-calmodulin complex, which activates myosin light-chain kinase (MLCK). The latter phosphorylates myosin light chain (MLC), leading to contraction. Relaxation by β-adrenergic agonists that increase cAMP and cAMP kinase activity results in phosphorylation of MLCK to give an inactive phosphorylated form. Subscripts: a, active; I, inactive; MLC_i, inactive myosin light chain; $MLCK_a$, active myosin light-chain kinase; PDE, phosphodiesterase; MLC_a-P, active phosphorylated myosin light chain. (From Wingard LB Jr, et al. Human pharmacology: molecular to clinical. St. Louis: Mosby Year Book, 1991: 226. Reprinted with permission.)

hypoxic reflex, allowing an increase in blood flow to poorly ventilated or unventilated alveoli. This is generally of no clinical consequence, especially if the patient is receiving supplemental oxygen.

Structure

Beta agonists consist of a benzene ring joined to an aliphatic structure, ethylamine. Modifications of the ring, the two carbons, or the terminal amine alter drug potency, metabolism, and selectivity for $beta_1$ and $beta_2$ receptors (Fig. 3.2). Catecholamines have hydroxyl groups at position 3 and 4 of the benzene ring. Changes in the position of the OH groups on the benzene ring produce noncatecholamine bronchodilators such as resorcinols and saligenins, which resist breakdown by catechol-o-methyltransferase (COMT) and monoamine oxidase (MAO). The catecholamines include isoproterenol and isoetharine. Resorcinols with OH groups on the 3 and 5 positions include metaproterenol, fenoterol, and terbutaline. Saligenins have an OH at position

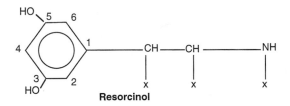

Catecholamine

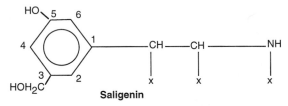

Resorcinol

HO 5 6
4
3 2
HOH₂C
Saligenin

Figure 3.2. Basic structure of common beta agonists.

4 and a CH₂OH at position 5 on the benzene ring. Beta₂ selectivity is increased when OH groups are at position 3 and 5 of the benzene ring. Large amino substitutions also increase beta₂ selectivity and reduce the effect of MAO, prolonging the duration of activity.

Clinical Classification

A useful clinical classification of beta agonists is the duration of action: brief, intermediate, and long (Table 3.1). The equivalent dosages for MDI and SVN delivery are shown in Table 3.2.

BRIEF-DURATION BETA AGONISTS

The short-acting drugs have almost immediate onset of action and reach peak effect in minutes. Bronchodilation, however, generally lasts only approximately 1–1.5 hours. The two drugs in this class are isoproterenol and isoetharine (isoprenaline). Each has important beta₂ activity. The Food and Drug Administration (FDA)-approved doses are 2 puffs 250 μg every 4–6 hours and 2–3 puffs 250–325 μg every 4–6 hours, respectively. *They are not recommended.*

INTERMEDIATE-DURATION BETA$_2$ AGONISTS

Beta$_2$ agonists with an intermediate duration of action are the agents of choice for acute episodes of dyspnea, ranging from the occasional use as a single agent to their

Table 3.1. Commonly Used Beta Agonists Via Metered Dose Inhaler

			Intermediate Duration						
	Onset	Peak	Effective Duration	FDA-Approved Dosage		More Effective Dosage		High Dosage	
Drug	(Minutes)	(Minutes)	(Hours)	Mcg	Puffs	Mcg	Puffs	Mcg	Puffs
Albuterol (U.S.) (Ventolin, Proventil, Airet, Volmax); salbutamol (elsewhere)	<5	15–30	4–6	180	2	360	4	540–1080	6–12
Metaproterenol Orciprenaline	<5	15–30	4–6	130	2	260	4	—	—
Terbutaline (Brethaire, Bricanyl)	<5	15–30	4–6	40	2	8	4	—	—
Pirbuterol (Maxair)	<5	15–30	4–6	4	2	8	4	—	—
Bitolterol (Tornalate)	<5	15–30	4–6	74	2	148	4	—	—
Fenoterol	<5	15–30	4–6	100	2	8	4	—	—
Rimiterol	<5	15–30	4–6	400	2	—	—	—	—
			Long Duration						
Salmeterol (Serevent)	15–30	90–120	~12	84	2	168	4	—	—
Formoterol	<5	60	~12	24	2	96	4	—	—

Table 3.2. Equivalent Dosage Chart for Bronchodilators by Metered Dose Inhaler and Small Volume Nebulizer

Albuterol			Metaproterenol			Terbutaline			Ipratropium		
MDI[a]		SVN[b]	MDI[a]		SVN[b]	MDI[a]		SVN[b]	MDI[a]		SVN[b]
μg	Puffs	Mg	μg	Puffs	Mg	μg	Puffs	Mg	μg	Puffs	Mg
180	2	2.5	130	2	10 (0.2 mL)	40	2	1.0	36	2	500
270	3	3.75	195	3	15 (0.3 mL)	60	3	2.0	54	3	—
390	4	5.0	260	4	20 (0.4 mL)	80	4	3.0	72	4	1000
450	5	6.25				100	5	4.0	90	5	—
540	6	7.5							108	6	1500
630	7	8.75									

[a] MDI = Metered dose inhaler.
[b] SVN = Small volume nebulizer.

addition as rescue therapy to beta$_2$ agonists of long duration and/or corticosteroids. Their onset of action is less than 5 minutes. They reach peak effectiveness in 15 to 30 minutes and provide bronchodilation for 4–6 hours. They include albuterol (Ventolin, Proventil, Airet, Volmax), terbutaline (Brethaire, Bricanyl), pirbuterol (Maxair), bitolterol (Tornalate), fenoterol, and rimiterol.

LONG-DURATION BETA$_2$ AGONISTS

Beta$_2$ agonists with a long duration of action are appropriate for maintenance therapy. Salmeterol (Serevent) is a saligenin with a long lipophilic N-substituent side chain that allows binding with greater affinity at the beta-adenoreceptor site along with persistent binding and prolonged stimulation. Salmeterol's onset of action is approximately 15–30 minutes with peak effectiveness at 60–90 minutes; the clinically effective duration is approximately 12 hours. It is extremely important to emphasize to patients that salmeterol is for maintenance and *should not be used for acute episodes of dyspnea.*

Formoterol is a modification of phenylethanolamine, which is also lipophilic and has a duration of action of approximately 12 or more hours. Its onset, however, is as rapid as the intermediate-duration agents, with peak effectiveness occurring in approximately 60 minutes. Otherwise, salmeterol and formoterol have similar effectiveness.

Long-duration inhaled beta$_2$ agonists are particularly useful for:

• Patients who are awakened from sleep by their asthma;
• Patients who wish to avoid using an inhaler at work or school.

Dosage/Toxicity

One of the most debated issues in the use of bronchodilators is the appropriate dosage; there is concern over the amount per treatment, the frequency of treatment over the day, and the amount over a longer period, such as a month. For 30 years epidemiologic studies of varying quality have reported an association between the use of beta agonists and ''near-fatal'' asthma—arterial hypercarbia ($PaCO_2 > 45$ mm Hg), nonelective intubation during acute asthma, or both—or fatal asthma. Initial concerns were raised over the potential direct arrhythmogenesis of these agents or their excipients. Other investigators speculated that hypokalemia was the mechanism for death in acute severe asthma (so-called ''asphyxic asthma''). A recent large epidemiologic study reported on the association of the use of beta$_2$ agonists, oral corticosteroids, theophylline, and other drugs with ''near-fatal'' or fatal asthma. The authors of this study found crude odds ratios for oral corticosteroids of 5.0, for fenoterol by MDI of 3.7, for albuterol by MDI of 1.5, for albuterol by nebulizer of 3.3, for theophylline of 3.7, and for inhaled corticosteroids or cromolyn of 2.3. Using an ''adjusted'' odds ratio (details not provided but subsequently reported as a multiplicative model), the risk for fenoterol by MDI increased to 6.1 and albuterol by MDI to 4.1. Albuterol by nebulization decreased to 2.5, theophylline to 2.4, oral corticosteroids to 2.5, and inhaled corticosteroids to 1.3. The odds ratio increased from approximately 4 with $\leq$ 1 canister per month to approximately 8 with $>$ 1 to 2 canisters per month to approximately 22 with $>$ 2 canisters per month. These comparisons are with equipotent doses—fenoterol had twice the potency of albuterol per puff at the time of the study. Sixteen percent of the cases versus 10% of the controls, however, were using drugs contraindicated in asthma. Subsequently, these authors have shown that (a) the increased risk was independently associated with increasing use of beta$_2$ agonists over the month before the ''near-fatal'' or fatal event; (b) patients using major psychoactive drugs also had an increased odds ratio 3.2 (95% CI 1.4–2.5); and (c) the odds ratio increased if such drugs had recently been discontinued 6.6 (95% CI 2.5–17.5). The authors cautioned that these findings could reflect the severity of illness rather than the use of the drugs. In a subsequent paper, the authors stated that this was likely the case. In contrast to these epidemiologic reports on patients with asthma, a relationship between the use of beta$_2$ agonists and arrhythmias or sudden death has not been reported in patients with COPD.

In a report on 10 patients with respiratory arrest in ''near-fatal'' (asphyxic) asthma, arrhythmias were not found (heart rate 134 $\pm$ 35 BPM and hypokalemia serum K 3.4 $\pm$ .3 (3.0–3.9)). The respiratory arrests were attributed to asphyxia (pCO$_2$ 97 $\pm$ 31 mm Hg pH 7.01 $\pm$ 11).

These associations are *markers* of risk rather than *determinants* of risk. They indicate that *the greater the severity of illness, the greater the use of medications.* A patient's increasing severity of illness warrants prompt reassessment of current therapy and identification of complicating factors. Assess the following:

• Requirement for inhaled corticosteroids, increase in the dosage of inhaled steroids, a course of oral corticosteroids;
• Need for hospitalization;
• Concurrent infection requiring treatment;
• Changes in medications for asthma or addition of beta blockers or discontinuation of a major psychoactive drug.

In a prospective, double-blind study of patients with chronic airflow obstruction given albuterol as a dry powder in increasing doses of 400 μg (2 capsules, or ~2 puffs, the FDA-approved dose), 1,000 μg, and 2,000 μg, the most effective dose was 1,000 μg (5 capsules or ~11 puffs) as measured by the increase in FEV$_1$ versus side effects. At this dose, there was no increase in heart rate or frequency of ectopic beats.

In a multicenter, randomized, double-blind, parallel group trial of 257 patients with acute severe asthma (FEV$_1$ < 50% of predicted) seen in the emergency department, each patient received either 4 puffs of fenoterol 2,000 μg/puff, or albuterol 1,000 μg/puff, 1 puff every 30 seconds via an MDI attached to a holding chamber. An additional 2 puffs were given every 10 minutes to a maximum of 16 puffs—3,200 μg of fenoterol or 1,600 μg of albuterol. The electrocardiogram and pulse oximetry were recorded continuously. O$_2$ was given to maintain a saturation of $\geq$ 90%. Additional doses were halted if (a) side effects were intolerable to the patient; (b) the FEV$_1$ showed < 10% improvement for 2 doses; (c) cardiac arrhythmias occurred (repetitive ventricular arrhythmias, atrial fibrillation, atrial flutter, or paroxysmal atrial tachycardia); or (d) there was an increase in heart rate of 20 BPM sustained for 1 minute. The most common total dose was 8 puffs, the median 10 puffs, and 32 patients (12.5%) received 16 puffs. Dose increases were stopped in 62% of patients because of a plateau in FEV_1, in 27% of patients because of a decrease in FEV_1 of $> 10\%$, and in 56% with fenoterol and in 45% with albuterol because of tremor; 84% of the side effects occurred with doses greater than 8 puffs. The FEV_1 increased from baseline with increasing doses from 4 to 12 puffs, with extremely small increases above that for fenoterol and a plateau for albuterol. The serum K decreased 0.23 ± 0.04 with albuterol and 0.06 ± 0.03 with fenoterol. There was a slight increase in Q-Tc interval of 0.011 ± 0.003 seconds with fenoterol and 0.003 ± 0.003 seconds with albuterol. Most important, there were no episodes of sustained ventricular tachycardia, ventricular couplets, atrial fibrillation, atrial flutter, or paroxysmal atrial tachycardia. There was a slight decrease in heart rate and blood pressure. The respiratory rate decreased approximately five breaths per minute. In adequately oxygenated patients, doses up to 1,600 μg of albuterol and 3,200 μg of fenoterol by MDI with a holding chamber can be administered with cardiovascular safety.

Table 3.1 lists the commonly used inhaled beta$_2$ agonists with a recommended dose by MDI in three categories: the FDA-approved dose, a more effective dose, and a high dose. The FDA-approved dose is a reasonable starting dose for stable patients and for those with mild exacerbations. The more effective dose is appropriate for use in patients not responding satisfactorily to the FDA-approved dose, either for mild exacerbations or for extended periods. Patients using salmeterol for maintenance do better with four puffs twice daily. The high dose is recommended only for patients with acute exacerbations and adequate oxygenation (e.g., pulse oximetry of 90% or greater) and who are under direct medical supervision. The recommendations for more effective and high doses are based on published prospective, randomized, double-blind studies. The approximately equivalent dose for commonly used beta$_2$ agonists and ipratropium (Atrovent) by MDI and SVN are given in Table 3.2. These bronchodilators are of benefit in patients with asthma, COPD, bronchiectasis, cystic fibrosis, and other diseases characterized by airways obstruction.

ANTICHOLINERGIC (ANTIMUSCARINIC) AGENTS

Natural belladonna alkaloids and atropine were used in the Western world for treating asthma from the 1800s to the early 1900s, when beta agonists, initially epinephrine, became available.

Mechanism of Action

Vagus nerve efferents and afferents supply parasympathomimetic cholinergic innervation to the airways. They are primarily in the larger airways. Their postganglionic fibers are on smooth muscle, cells, pulmonary arterioles, and mucous glands. They release acetylcholine, which results in smooth muscle contraction, increased mucous release, and, possibly, faster ciliary beating. Normal bronchomotor tone is caused by baseline vagal activity. Reflex-mediated bronchoconstriction can originate from the upper and lower airways, esophagus, and the carotid bodies. A variety of nonspecific stimulants such as cold-dry air, irritant gases such as SO_2, mechanical irritation such as bronchoscopy, and various aerosols not containing a bronchodilator may stimulate bronchoconstriction.

Anticholinergic, antimuscarinic agents function as specific antagonists of acetylcholine at the muscarinic receptor, blocking cholinergically mediated bronchoconstriction. They can reduce the baseline bronchomotor tone in normal individuals and reverse or mitigate reflex bronchoconstriction initiated by external mechanisms or associated with asthma and COPD.

Structure

The naturally occurring anticholinergic, antimuscarinic alkaloids are tertiary ammonium compounds; the nitrogen on the tropine ring is trivalent (Fig. 3.3). These compounds are readily absorbed from mucosal surfaces and can be given orally.

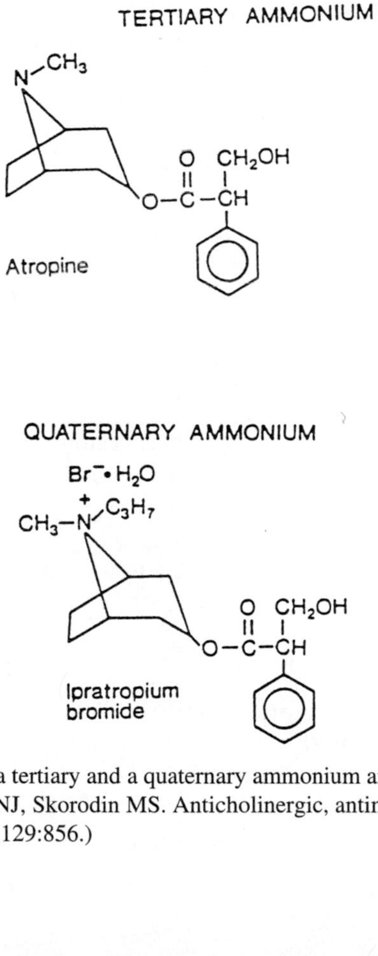

Figure 3.3. Structures of a tertiary and a quaternary ammonium anticholinergic bronchodilator. (Adapted from Gross NJ, Skorodin MS. Anticholinergic, antimuscarinic bronchodilators. Am Rev Respir Dis 1984;129:856.)

Because they are widely distributed, they affect multiple organs: at low doses (0.5 mg), dryness of the mouth and bradycardia may occur; at higher doses (1.0 mg), thirst, pupillary dilation, and tachycardia; at 2 mg, vision may blur and at 5 mg, altered speech, difficulty in swallowing and micturition, dry, red skin, and central nervous system effects such as fatigue, restlessness, and headache. The latter appear because atropine crosses the blood-brain barrier.

Quaternary ammonium compounds have been synthesized. These compounds have a pentavalent nitrogen atom with a charge on the tropine ring (Fig. 3.3). They are not absorbed; thus, systemic effects are essentially nonexistent. They are highly effective locally, however. The prototype is ipratropium bromide (Atrovent). Other quaternary agents include oxitropium, atropine methonitrate, glycopyrrolate, and tiotropium.

Asthma Versus COPD

The response to ipratropium bromide among asthmatics has been variable. The drug reverses or ameliorates reflex bronchoconstriction that occurs with exposure to irritants, dust, inhaled gases, and cold-dry air. Ipratropium decreases elevated baseline bronchomotor tone in stable asthma and COPD. When ipratropium bromide is compared with albuterol, the peak FEV_1 response has been reported to be somewhat less (25–35%) and occurred later (90–120 minutes versus 15–30 minutes). In a long-term study comparing metaproterenol to ipratropium, although the peak response was earlier for metaproterenol, the area under the FEV_1 curves were the same (i.e., ipratropium's duration of action was greater). In acute asthma the *addition* of ipratropium to beta$_2$ agonists has generally resulted in an enhanced response.

In contrast, ipratropium bromide maintenance therapy compared favorably with beta$_2$ agonists in patients with stable COPD. In patients with acute exacerbations of COPD, this agent has usually enhanced the response to inhaled beta$_2$ agonists. Recommendations for the use of ipratropium bromide are:

- Stable asthma: as a possible alternative to chronic beta$_2$ agonist use or the need for increased doses of beta$_2$ agonists;
- Severe stable asthma: as an addition to beta$_2$ agonists and corticosteroids;
- Acute asthma: as an addition to beta$_2$ agonists and corticosteroids;
- Stable COPD: for maintenance (or a long-acting beta$_2$ agonist);
- Stable severe COPD: as an addition to long-acting beta$_2$ agonist;
- Acute exacerbations of COPD: in addition to beta$_2$ agonists and other agents.

Dosage

- Mild asthma: between 2 and 4–5 puffs (36–90 μg); some patients may require doses up to 10 puffs (200 μg);
- Mild, stable COPD: 2 puffs (every 4–6 hours);
- Disease not responding: 4 to 6 puffs every 4–6 hours in combination with other bronchodilators;

- Severe disease or exacerbations that are not responding: 6–10 puffs every 4–6 hours. (See Tables 3.1 and 3.2.)

GLUCOCORTICOIDS

Glucocorticoids are potent antiinflammatory and immunomodulatory agents. They provide the most effective treatment of asthma. Although formidable side effects may accompany the chronic use of oral corticosteroids in high doses, the inhaled corticosteroids currently available minimize or perhaps eliminate clinically important side effects in adults. Glucocorticoids inhibit eosinophils, macrophages, mast cells, T lymphocytes, monocytes, neutrophils, and epithelial cells involved in airway inflammation. They reduce plasma exudation and mucus secretion. They reduce airway hyperresponsiveness to allergens, cold air, irritants, histamine, and cholinergic agonists. Airway narrowing is also reduced.

Mechanism of Action

Glucocorticoids interact with specific intracellular glucocorticoid receptors to regulate the expression of responsive genes (Fig. 3.4). They combine with corticosteroid-binding protein (CBG) entering the cell cytoplasm where they interact with a glucocorticoid receptor (GR). This results in disassociation of the 90-kDa and 70-kDa shock proteins (HSP90 and HSP70) and a 56-kDa immunophilin. The GR-corticosteroid ligand then translocates to the nucleus, where it interacts with specific glucocorticoid-responsive elements (GREs) to induce gene transcription and messenger ribonucleic acid (mRNA) processing. This leads to the binding and inactivation of proinflammatory transcription factors such as activating protein 1 (AP-1) and nuclear factor -κB (NF-κB).

Glucocorticoids affect lymphocytes, macrophages, monocytes, basophils, fibroblasts, eosinophils, neutrophils, and endothelial cells. They inhibit many proinflammatory cytokines, such as the interleukins (IL-1, IL-2, IL-3, and IL-6), tumor necrosis factor α (TNF-α), interferon gamma, and granulocyte-monocyte colony-stimulating factor (GM-CSF). They inhibit arachidonic acid metabolites, prostaglandins and leukotrienes, acute phase reactants (such as the third component of complement), and histamine.

The myriad other physiologic actions of the corticosteroids include their effect on carbohydrate and lipid metabolism, fluid and electrolyte balance, water balance, the kidney, endocrine system, musculoskeletal system, vascular system, and central nervous system.

Structure and Dose

The structures of hydrocortisone and prednisone are shown in Figure 3.5. The 4,5 double bond and the 3-keto group on ring A and an 11-β-hydroxyl group on ring C are required for glucocorticoid activity. A double bond on the 1,2 positions of

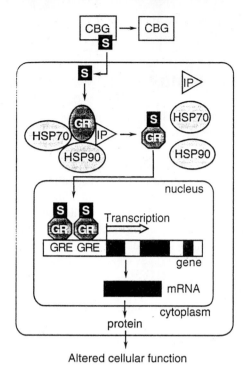

Figure 3.4. Intracellular mechanism of action of the glucocorticoid receptor. (See text for details.) *CBG,* corticosteroid-binding globulin; *S,* steroid hormone; *GR,* glucocorticoid receptor; *HSP90, HSP70,* heat shock proteins 90-kDa and 70-kDa; *IP,* the 56-kDa immunophilin; *GRE,* glucocorticoid response elements in the DNA that recognize and bind GR; *mRNA,* messenger ribonucleic acid; *unshaded,* introns; *shaded,* exons. (From Goodman-Gilman A, et al. The pharmacological basis of therapeutics. New York: McGraw-Hill, 1996. Reprinted with permission.)

ring A, as in prednisone, increases glucocorticoid activity approximately fourfold versus cortisone. A fluoride on the 9α position also increases glucocorticoid activity approximately 10-fold compared with cortisone. The equivalent oral and systemic doses of commonly used glucocorticoids are shown in Table 3.3. In general, the clinically important therapeutic actions and side effects are not different among these agents at equally potent doses.

Inhaled Glucocorticoids

The structures of the commonly used inhaled corticosteroids are shown in Figure 3.6. High topical potency determined by the McKenzie skin blanching test, low systemic bioavailability of the swallowed portion of the dose (80–90%), and rapid metabolic clearance of the amount entering the systemic circulation (high first-pass clearance by the liver) are sought-after properties in these drugs. Budesonide and

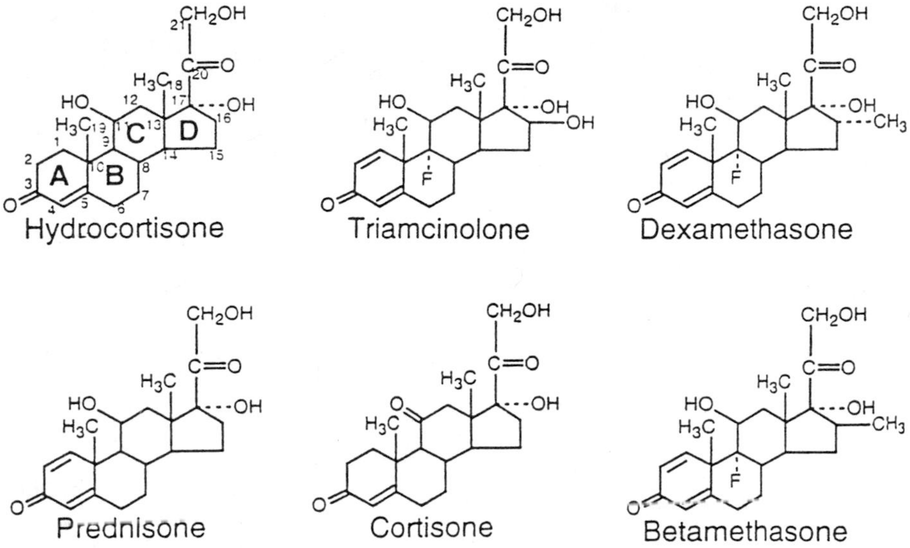

Figure 3.5. Structure and nomenclature of corticosteroid products and selected synthetic derivatives. The structure of hydrocortisone is represented in two dimensions. It should be noted that the steroid ring system is not completely planar and that the orientation of the groups attached to the steroid rings is an important determinant of the biologic activity. The methyl groups at C18 and C19 and the hydroxyl group at C11 project upward (*forward* in the two-dimensional representation and shown by a *solid line* connecting the atoms) and are designated β. The hydroxyl at C17 projects below the plane (*behind* in the two-dimensional representation, and represented by the *dashed line* connecting the atoms) and is designated α. (From Goodman-Gilman A, et al. The pharmacological basis of therapeutics. New York: McGraw-Hill, 1996. Reprinted with permission.)

Table 3.3. Equivalent Doses of the Commonly Used Oral-Systemic Corticosteroids and Relative Duration of Actions

Name	Biologic Half-Life (Hours)	Dose (Mg)
Cortisol (Cortone)	8–12	20
Cortisone (Hydrocortene, Hydrocortone acetate)	8–12	25
Prednisone (Deltasone, Liquid Pred, Prednicen-M, Sterapred)	8–12	5
6-α-methylprednisolone	8–12	4
Triamcinolone (Aristocort, Azmacort)	8–12	4
Betamethasone (Celestone)	36–72	0.75
Dexamethasone (Decadron, Datalone)	36–72	0.75

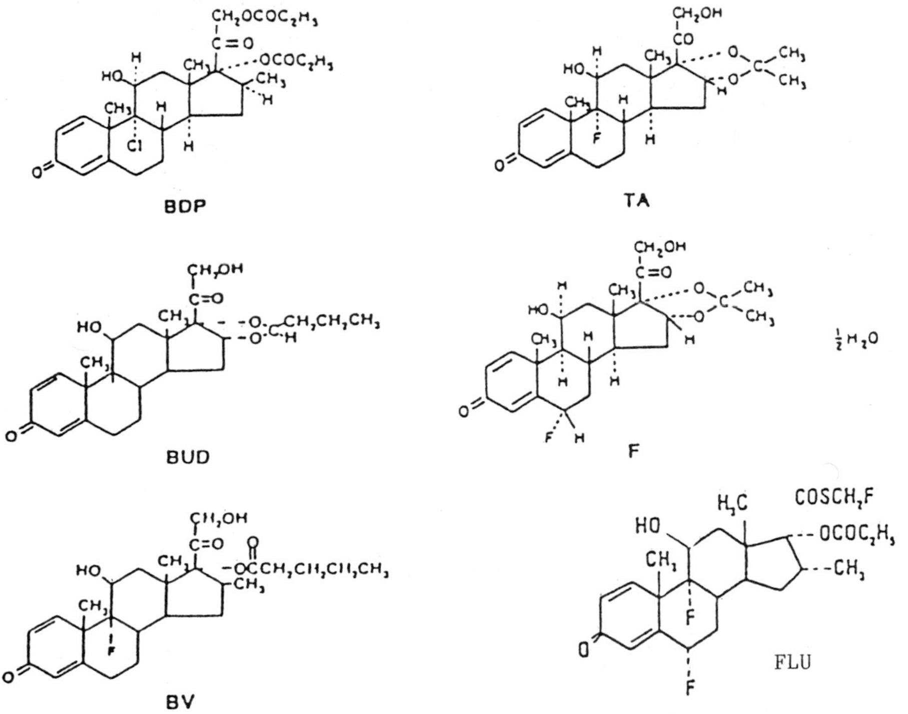

Figure 3.6. Structural formulas for beclomethasone dipropionate (BDP), budesonide (BUD), betamethasone 17-valerate (BV), triamcinolone 16,17-acetonide (TA), flunisolide (F), and fluticasone propionate (FLU). (Adapted from Weiss EB, Stein M. Bronchial asthma: mechanisms and therapeutics. Boston: Little, Brown & Co, 1993.)

flunisolide have extensive first-pass liver metabolism. Beclomethasone dipropionate is metabolized to the monopropionate, which is more active. Although budesonide shows more local potency, clinical trials show equivalence of beclomethasone and budesonide. Fluticasone has low oral bioavailability. Satisfactory comparison trials of betamethasone, triamcinolone, and flunisolide to beclomethasone or budesonide are not available. Clinical trials comparing fluticasone with budesonide show that the former is approximately twice as active by weight. The effect on the hypothalamic-pituitary-adrenal (HPA) axis acceptable to regulatory authorities is that which does not reduce 8:00 AM serum cortisol or the eosinophil count. More sensitive tests of the HPA axis, however, such as the 24-hour urine cortisol, metyrapone stimulation, or cosyntropin stimulation tests show systemic effects with the approved doses. The clinical importance of these findings are unknown. Even higher doses of inhaled glucocorticoids that reduce the plasma cortisol have not been shown to reduce the plasma cortisol response to insulin-induced hypoglycemia, major surgery, or the stress of asthma. The use of a spacer, dry powder inhalers, and rinsing the mouth reduce systemic effects. Studies show that even at a daily dose of 2,000 μg, budesonide or beclomethasone do not affect 24-hour urinary cortisol excretion. Fluticasone

Table 3.4. Relative Potencies of Inhaled Glucocorticoids

Glucocorticoid	Binding Affinity[a,b]	Topical Potency[c]	Systemic Potency[a]	Topical Systemic Potency Ratio[c]	Oral Absorption (Relative Bioavailability)[a]
Beclomethasone dipropionate (Beclovent, Vanceril)	0.4	0.40	3.5	.010	90 (?)
Flunisolide (Aerobid)	1.8	0.70	12.8	0.05	? (21)
Triamcinolone acetonide (Azmacort)	3.6	0.30	5.30	0.05	? (?)
Budesonide	9.4	1.00	1.00	1.00	~100 (11)
Fluticasone propionate (Flovent)	?	1.70	0.07	25.00	80–90 (<1)

[a] Derived from animal models.
[b] Relative to dexamethasone.
[c] Derived from human lung tissue.
Adapted from Kamada AK, et al, and the Asthma Clinical Research Network. Pulmonary perspective: issues in the use of inhaled glucocorticoids. Am J Respir Crit Care Med 1996;153:1739–1748.

Table 3.5. Inhaled Corticosteroid Dosing. Drugs Approved in the U.S. Have μg/Puff at the Mouth Versus Not Approved μg/Puff at the Valve

Drug	μg/Puff	FDA-Approved (Puffs)	High Dose
Beclomethasone (Beclovent, Vanceril)	42[a]	2 QID	10 puffs QID[a,b]
		5 QID	10 puffs QID[a,b]
Beclomethasone dbl strength (Vanceril, dbl strength)	84	2 BID	10 BID
Dexamethasone (Decadron, Datalone)	84	3 QID	?
Triamcinolone (Aristocort, Azmacort)	100	2 QID	?
		4 QID	?
Flunisolide (Aerobid)	250	2 BID	?
		4 BID	?
Fluticasone (Flovent)	44[a]	2 BID	
	110	4 BID	
	220	2 BID	4 BID[a]
Budesonide	50[a]	2 QID	8 QID[a]

[a] Approximate clinical equivalent dose.
[b] Not FDA approved.

appears to have the least effect on the HPA axis, although there are conflicting interpretations of the reported data. The relative potencies are shown in Table 3.4. The recommended and high dosages for the commonly used inhaled glucocorticoids are shown in Table 3.5. The appropriate dose in an individual is best determined by a clinical trial. The full effectiveness of inhaled glucocorticoids on airways hyper-reactivity and the ability to withdraw oral corticosteroids may take months.

Toxicity
Oral

- Edema, hypertension, hypokalemia, metabolic alkalosis, and hyperglycemia;
- Suppression of immunity results in increased susceptibility to infections, particularly to the so-called opportunistic organisms; reactivation of tuberculosis;
- Increased risk of peptic ulcer disease with hemorrhage or perforation, usually when the dose is greater than 25 mg of prednisone daily;
- Proximal limb myopathy is a frequent risk with high doses;
- Mood elevation (most common psychological effect); some patients become extremely hyperactive, anxious, nervous, or have difficulty sleeping; other psychoses may occur; patients may become suicidal or manic;
- Cataracts are a complication of extended use at relatively high doses;
- Osteoporosis; rib and vertebral fractures are the most frequent result of the osteoporosis;
- Osteonecrosis, most frequently of the femoral head, can result from extended use of high-dose corticosteroids in patients with vasculitis or heavy alcohol ingestion; it is not well documented that oral glucocorticosteroids alone can cause osteonecrosis;
- Growth retardation in children.

It is necessary to discuss the benefits and risks of long-term corticosteroids with the patient so that the decision is a participatory one:

- The potential for adrenal insufficiency at the time of withdrawal;
- Withdrawal may cause an exacerbation of asthma;
- Withdrawal of oral corticosteroids or too brief a course after an exacerbation are risk factors for fatal or near-fatal asthma.

Inhaled Corticosteroids

Side effects include:

- Dysphonia (hoarseness) occurs in approximately one-third of patients and is usually well tolerated; it may be caused by laryngeal myopathy;
- Oropharyngeal candidiasis, the incidence of which can be reduced by the use of a spacer and by thoroughly rinsing the mouth after use;
- Rarely, cough and reflex bronchoconstriction; these can be reduced with the use of a spacer or with prior inhalation of a beta$_2$ agonist;
- Osteoporosis has not been observed but a small study has shown decreased bone density in women versus age-matched controls;
- No effect on growth has been shown in children receiving up to 800 μg/day;
- Cataracts or altered glucose metabolism have not been reported;
- Psychiatric symptoms have been reported in an extremely small number of patients;
- There is no evidence of deleterious effects in pregnancy.

The current high cost of inhaled corticosteroids compared with oral prednisone is cause for concern. Most authorities, however, recommend the use of inhaled corticosteroids over oral agents.

Dosage: Acute Asthma

Intravenous methylprednisolone in a loading dose of 60 to 125 mg is recommended for acute exacerbations of asthma. Subsequent doses of 60 to 125 mg every 6 hours are most commonly prescribed, although many patients do well on 15 mg IV every 6 hours. If IV drug is used, change to prednisone when the patient has stabilized—usually in 24–48 hours. In addition, oral prednisone has been shown to be equivalent to IV corticosteroids. It is important that the dose be tapered slowly, over 8–10 days or longer, to avoid re-exacerbations. The effect of corticosteroids takes approximately 4–6 hours to become evident.

Dosage: Chronic Asthma

The use of inhaled corticosteroids is recommended in patients with asthma who have:

- Exacerbations more than 1–2 times/week;
- Exacerbations that affect activity or sleep;
- Nocturnal asthma more than 2 times/month;
- Chronic symptoms requiring intermediate-acting beta$_2$ agonists almost daily;
- A peak expiratory flow rate (PEFR) or FEV$_1$ less than 80% predicted or variability in these measurements of 20 to 30% or more.

The above are the recommendations of the consensus reports of the National Heart, Lung, and Blood Institute Expert Panel on Guidelines for the Diagnosis and Management of Asthma and the International Consensus Report on the diagnosis and treatment of asthma. These are guidelines, not rigid standard of care criteria.

Dosage: COPD

Intravenous corticosteroids cause a modest improvement in FEV$_1$ over the first 24 hours in patients with exacerbations of COPD. They are frequently used for short periods in such exacerbations. Oral corticosteroids may improve FEV$_1$ by 16 to 40% in 15 to 30% of patients (reports vary greatly). A meta-analysis using an improvement in FEV$_1$ of 20% as the criterion found improvement in approximately 10% of patients with COPD receiving corticosteroids for several weeks. There is no convincing evidence at present that inhaled corticosteroids are of benefit in COPD; a long-term trial is in progress.

THEOPHYLLINE AND OTHER METHYLXANTHINES

The role of theophylline in the treatment of airways obstruction is in transition. In the 1970s it was routinely prescribed for acute exacerbations and as chronic maintenance

Table 3.6. Theophylline Drug Interactions

Drugs that Increase Theophylline Levels; May Require Decrease in Theophylline Dose	
Alcohol (0.99 per kg)	Methotrexate
Allopurinol	Mexiletine
Azithromycin	Nicardipine
Cimetidine	Nifedipine
Ciprofloxacin	Norfloxacin
Clarithromycin and other macrolides	Pentoxifylline
Diltiazem	Propafenone
Disulfiram	Propranolol
Enoxacin	Sucralfate
Erythromycin	Tacrine
Estrogen (oral contraceptives)	Thiabendazole
Fluoxamine	Ticlopidine
Influenza vaccine	Troleandomycin
Interferon	Verapamil
Isradipine	Zileuton (lipoxygenase inhibitors ?)
Drugs that Decrease Theophylline Levels; May Require Increase in Theophylline Dose	
Aminoglutethimide	Phenobarbital
Carbamazepine	Phenytoin
Isoproterenol (IV)	Rifampin
Lithium	Sulfinpyrazone
Moricizine	Tobacco smoking

therapy for both asthma and COPD. Most prospective randomized studies that used systemic corticosteroid and beta$_2$ agonists show that IV aminophylline does not provide additional benefit in acute episodes of asthma. One study showed a greater increase in FEV$_1$ in hospitalized patients; another showed a decreased need for hospitalization. In the maintenance therapy of asthma, the role of theophylline has been reduced because of:

- Beneficial effects of inhaled corticosteroids and/or long-acting beta$_2$ agonists;
- Complexities of dosing because of its variable clearance in healthy individuals (a half-life ($t\frac{1}{2}$) in adults of 3 to 16 hours) and a decrease in clearance with liver dysfunction (e.g., cirrhosis, congestive heart failure, hepatitis, cholestasis, septic shock);
- Multiplicity of drug interactions (Table 3.6);
- A relatively narrow therapeutic range (10–20 μg/mL; 10–20 mg/L; 55–110 μmol/L).

Structure

The methylxanthines are methylated forms of xanthine, a dioxypurine. They are found in commonly consumed beverages such as tea (theophylline), coffee, cocoa, and many soft drinks (caffeine); cocoa also contains theobromine. Theophylline is a 1,3-dimethylxanthine and dyphylline is 1,3-dimethyl-7-(2,3–dihydroxypropyl) xanthine.

Mechanism of Action as a Bronchodilator

The mechanism(s) of action of theophylline has not been clearly established. Initially it was thought that its effects were caused by inhibition of phosphodiesterase causing an increase in cAMP. Toxic theophylline levels, however, are required to increase cAMP, and lower theophylline levels result in tracheal smooth muscle relaxation in isolated tracheal muscle. Papaverine and dipyridamole inhibit phosphodiesterase but do not cause relaxation of airway smooth muscle. A second potential mechanism is as an adenosine receptor antagonist. In support of this, theophylline binds to adenosine receptors, protects asthmatic (but not normal) individuals against broncho-constriction from inhaled adenosine, and prevents mediator release in asthmatics. Enprofylline is a more potent bronchodilator, however, and does not antagonize adenosine receptors; 8-phenyltheophylline is a potent adenosine receptor antagonist that does not relax bronchial smooth muscle in vivo. Theophylline releases endoge-nous catecholamines, serum epinephrine and norepinephrine, but there is no parallel increase in bronchodilation. Prostaglandin inhibition also occurs with theophylline administration. Theophylline affects intracellular calcium, which may result in smooth muscle relaxation. Thus, although there is data to support a variety of poten-tial mechanisms of action for bronchodilation, each has confounding data that require further studies to resolve the apparent anomalies.

Pharmacologic Actions

In addition to its action as a modestly effective bronchodilator, theophylline has been shown to have a host of other effects (usually shown in animals or in vitro) that may contribute to its clinical effectiveness and relate to some of the postulates regarding its mechanisms of action. These effects include immunomodulation; down-regulation of inflammatory cells in the presence of airway inflammation; inhibition of cytokine synthesis and release; inhibition of microvascular leakage; attenuation of the late phase response to histamine; decreased response to methacholine, histamine, allergens, irritants; and exercise. These antiinflammatory effects occur at low plasma concentrations (e.g., 5–10 mg/L). Theophylline also increases mucociliary clearance.

Its widespread extrapulmonary effects have some positive aspects but also reflect its side effects. Theophylline stimulates all levels of the central nervous system. Cortical stimulation can result in wakefulness and a decrease in fatigue. Stimulation of the medulla may increase ventilation and increase sensitivity to hypoxia and hypercarbia. Medullary stimulation is the likely mechanism for nausea and vomiting and for reversal of Cheyne-Stokes breathing in patients with congestive heart failure. Theophylline is also a mild diuretic. It may slightly increase cardiac rate and force of contraction while slightly reducing peripheral vascular resistance. It increases diaphragmatic and other striated muscle contraction and reduces muscle fatigue. Theophylline relaxes the lower esophageal sphincter, which may exacerbate gastro-esophageal reflux and thereby asthma. These diverse, positive effects of theophylline generally are modest, and their clinical utility, especially with other more potent medications, is unclear.

Dosing

Both the effectiveness as a bronchodilator and the side effects of theophylline are directly related to serum levels. Because its primary current use is in maintenance therapy, oral long-acting drugs taken every 12 hours are recommended:

- An approximate loading dose of 200 mg/day and increase 200 mg every three days to a maximum dose of 600 mg per day or unless side effects intervene (check serum theophylline concentration (STC) at this point);
- An approximate loading dose of 10 mg/kg of ideal body weight, not to exceed 300 mg/day, with an increase in three days of approximately 13 mg/kg unless side effects intervene—not to exceed 450 mg/day, and a second increase of approximately 16 mg/kg unless side effects intervene—not to exceed 600 mg/day (check STC);
- Adjust the dose to achieve a level within the therapeutic range of 10–20 μg/mL (or mg/L) using the following simple relationship:

$$\frac{\text{Current dose (mg/24 hr)}}{\text{Current STC (mg/L)}} = \frac{\text{New dose (mg/24 hr)}}{\text{Desired STC (mg/L)}}$$

There is little difference, if any, between the two schemes, especially with a person of approximately 70 kg. The second scheme appears to suggest an accuracy that is unlikely to be achieved because of the very variable $t\frac{1}{2}$. Many clinicians recommend seeking theophylline levels of 10 to 12 μg/mL because approximately 75% of improvement in FEV_1 occurs in this range.

The following long-acting preparations have been reported to be completely and consistently absorbed with a peak STC in 3 to 7 hours: Theo-Dur and Slo-bid Gyrocap; and the following, although marketed for once-daily use, when given every 12 hours: Theo-24, Uniphyl, and Uni-Dur. Theophylline is rated as category C by the FDA for pregnant women, although ill effects on the fetus have not been reported. It appears in breast milk and may cause irritability or other side effects in nursing infants.

TOXICITY

The earliest signs of toxicity are nausea, vomiting, abdominal pain, nervousness, tremor, and tachycardia. They almost without exception antedate more serious side effects such as lethargy, disorientation, and supraventricular tachycardia. Seizures, status epilepticus, sustained ventricular tachycardia, and ventricular fibrillation occur rarely and almost without exception at STCs of 40 μg/mL or greater. Underlying central nervous system diseases (vasculitis, seizure disorders, and alcoholism) and rapid IV infusion may precipitate serious complications at lower STCs.

Recommended Indications

In asthmatic patients requiring maintenance therapy:

- As primary therapy in very young children who are unable to effectively use inhalers;

- As primary therapy if compliance with oral therapy is more likely;
- As additional therapy if adequate control, particularly at night, is not achieved with inhaled corticosteroids and long-acting beta$_2$ agonists or as an alternative to the long-acting beta$_2$ agonists;
- As maintenance therapy in COPD if there is evidence of improvement either clinically or by laboratory studies.

The role of theophylline in COPD is unclear because of conflicting reports for and against its use.

MEDIATOR MODULATORS

Chromone Derivatives

Disodium chromoglycate (DSCG), a bischromone drug, was synthesized as an outcome of studies on the naturally occurring smooth muscle relaxant khellin. Khellin is not useful clinically because of its side effects (such as nausea and vomiting). DSCG is not a bronchodilator; rather, it prevents bronchoconstriction resulting from a variety of stimuli.

Mechanism of Action

DSCG has a multitude of inhibitory actions that are varied in different animals, organs, and systems. There are data to support inhibition of:

- Neutrophilic-chemotactic factor release;
- Inflammatory cell activation—eosinophils, neutrophils, and monocytes;
- Bronchial hyperreactivity;
- Early and later asthmatic reactions;
- Reflex bronchoconstriction (via vagus);
- Down-regulation of beta$_2$ receptors;
- Stabilization of mast cells;
- Preservation of mucociliary action after an asthmatic attack.

None of these effects alone is sufficient to satisfactorily explain the mechanism of action of DSCG. There also is considerable conflicting evidence regarding the role of each in human asthma because of differences in study design and the animal, organ, or system studied.

Indications

DSCG is effective in reducing airway hyperreactivity in asthmatics. It can block early and late reactions to antigen challenge. It can prevent exercise-induced asthma. It has been most effective in children and young adults with mild to moderate asthma. Studies have shown a decrease in symptom scores, an improvement in peak expiratory flow and forced expired volume at 1 second, and decreased use of beta agonists, theophylline, and corticosteroids. DSCG has been effective in individuals with occupational asthma resulting from a variety of exposures, such as animals, toluene di-isocyanate, baker's flour, western red cedar, and enzymes. It is not recommended, however, because the primary treatment of individuals with occupational asthma is to terminate exposure. Its effectiveness is said to approximate that of theophylline.

Dose

DSCG is available as 20 mg capsules for inhalation, as 20 mg ampules for nebulization, and in a metered dose device containing 800 μg/puff. The recommended dose is 1 capsule, 1 ampule, or 2 puffs four times a day.

Side Effects

DSCG may cause cough and bronchospasm, which can be ameliorated by the prior inhalation of a beta$_2$ agonist. It may also cause hoarseness and dry mouth. Other side effects that have occurred less commonly include rash, hives, nausea, vomiting, nasal congestion, and dysuria. Rare cases of eosinophilic pulmonary infiltrates and anaphylaxis have occurred.

Recommendations

Because the response to DSCG usually does not appear for several weeks, it is not recommended for acute exacerbations. It is recommended for:

- Children and teenagers with atopic mild to moderate asthma to prevent bronchospasm (as prophylactic);
- As an alternative to a beta agonist to prevent exercise-induced asthma;
- As a possible beta$_2$ agonist or steroid-sparing agent.

Nedocromil

Nedocromil is a pyranoquinolone dicarboxylic acid structurally different from DSCG. In many experimental models, it has been shown to have remarkably similar mechanisms of action as DSCG. In some studies it was more effective. In clinical trials it has been effective in reducing symptom scores, inhaled beta agonists, theophylline, inhaled corticosteroids, and bronchial hyperactivity. It has also been shown to prevent exercise-induced asthma and early and late asthmatic responses. In some studies, PEFR and FEV$_1$ have increased. Most of these studies have been performed in adults. The clinical effectiveness of nedocromil sodium in asthma appears to be similar to that of DSCG. Its side effects are infrequent: bad taste, bronchospasm, headaches, nausea, vomiting, and dizziness. The recommended dose is 3.5 mg, 2 puffs, by MDI four times a day; lower doses may be effective in mild asthmatics. As with DSCG, its action may not be evident for weeks. It is not recommended for acute asthma.

LEUKOTRIENE (5-LIPOXYGENASE INHIBITORS)

Leukotrienes (LT) result from the actions of 5-lipoxygenase and 5-lipoxygenase-activating protein (FLAP) on arachidonic acid, which is released from cell membrane phospholipid by phospholipase A2. As the leukotriene cascade evolves, LTB4 and LTC4 are formed intracellularly. LTC4 is actively transported out of the cell, where it is metabolized to LTD4 and then LTE4. LTB4 is chemoattractant for eosinophils and neutrophils. LTC4, LTD4, and LTE4 (the "cysteinyl leukotrienes" or "sulphidopeptide leukotrienes") are responsible for the development of increased vascular permeability and edema, bronchoconstriction, increased mucus, and cellular infiltrates—the cardinal features of the inflammatory response in asthma. Intense research activity has led to the development of antileukotriene agents of two basic types: receptor, competitive, antagonists of 5-lipoxygenase; and 5-lipoxygenase inhibitors. Agents of both types have been shown to be effective in blocking LTD4-induced bronchospasm, early and late response to allergens, exercise- and cold-induced bronchospasm, bronchial hyperreactivity, and aspirin and nonsteroidal anti-inflammatory drug-induced asthma. They have also been effective in initial trials in chronic asthma. They are given by mouth, which may improve patient compliance.

Lipoxygenase Receptor Antagonists

Zafirlukast (ICI 204,219, Accolate) is a selective peptide leukotriene antagonist. It has been shown to be effective in blocking an LTD4 challenge in a dose-response manner and causing a 90-fold increase in the dose of LTD4 required to produce a 20% reduction in FEV_1; it has blocked allergen challenges. It inhibits exercise-induced bronchoconstriction and has a slight bronchodilator effect. In a prospective, randomized, double-blind study of 266 patients with mild to moderate asthma, FEV_1 40–75% of predicted, approximately 25% each received 10 mg, 20 mg, 40 mg, or a placebo. Improvement was obtained in symptoms; need for albuterol by MDI; and pulmonary function—PEFR, morning and evening, and FEV_1. The 40-mg dose was more effective than 10 or 20 mg; the latter two were similar. Dosage: 20 mg by mouth twice a day.

Lipoxygenase Inhibitors

Zileuton (Zyflo) is one of the direct inhibitors of 5-lipoxygenase with the chemical formula of (N-1-[benzo[b]thien-2-ylethyl]-N-hydroxyurea). It has been shown to be effective in inhibiting postexercise bronchospasm, in reducing airway inflammation after antigen challenge, and in treating patients with mild to moderate asthma. Eight of 266 patients, however, developed clinically silent liver enzyme elevations greater than three times the upper limit of normal; all returned to less than two times normal or below the baseline value over a period of approximately 60 days.

The dose is 600 mg Q.I.D. by mouth. Baseline liver function tests and an alanine aminotransferase (ALT) monthly for 3 months and then every 2 months are recommended. This drug increases serum theophylline levels.

COMBINATION THERAPY

Various combinations of intermediate-acting beta$_2$ agonists, long-duration beta$_2$ agonists, anticholinergic agents, theophylline, corticosteroids (both inhaled and oral-systemic), and antileukotrienes have been shown to be effective. The combination of oral or intravenous corticosteroids with beta$_2$ agonists is the standard therapy for acute exacerbations of asthma. The addition of an inhaled anticholinergic, particularly in difficult cases, is recommended. The value of other agents in episodes of acute asthma has not been well substantiated.

The combination of inhaled glucocorticoids with a long-acting beta$_2$ agonist is useful in the maintenance care of asthma; the long-acting beta$_2$ agonist may obviate the need to use high-dose inhaled corticosteroids. The intermediate beta$_2$ agonists are used for "rescue" therapy. Some patients will benefit from the addition of an anticholinergic to maintenance therapy. An antileukotriene will likely serve as an additional maintenance drug.

In chronic COPD, the addition of a long-acting beta$_2$ agonist to an anticholinergic (or vice versa) improves the outcome. In acute exacerbations of COPD, the use of an intermediate-duration beta$_2$ agonist and an anticholinergic is recommended.

BIBLIOGRAPHY

Hardman JG, Limbird LE, Molinoff PB, Ruddon RW, Goodman Gilman A, eds. Goodman and Gilman's pharmacological basis of therapeutics. 9th ed. New York: McGraw Hill, Health Professions Division, 1996.

Weiss EB, Stein M. Bronchial asthma: mechanisms and therapeutics. 3rd ed. Boston: Little, Brown & Co, 1993.

Wingard LB, Brody TM, Larner J, Schwartz A, eds. Human pharmacology: molecular to clinical. St. Louis: Mosby Year Book, 1991.

Bronchodilators: Effectiveness and Delivery

American Association for Respiratory Care: aerosol consensus statement—1991. Respiratory Care 1991;36:916–921.

Berger R, Smith D. Effect of inhaled metaproterenol on exercise performance in patients with stable "fixed" airway obstruction. Am Rev Respir Dis 1988;138:624–629.

Berry RB, Shinto RA, Wong FH, Despars JA, Light RW. Nebulizer vs. spacer for bronchodilator delivery in patients hospitalized for acute exacerbations of COPD. Chest 1989;96:1241–1246.

Blake KV, Hoppe M, Harman E, Hendeles L. Relative amount of albuterol delivered to lung receptors from a metered-dose inhaler and nebulizer solution. Chest 1992;101:309–315.

Colacone A, Afilalo M, Wolkove N, Kreisman H. A comparison of albuterol administered by metered dose inhaler (and holding chamber) or wet nebulizer in acute asthma. Chest 1993;104:835–841.

Dhand R, Guarte AG, Jubran A, Jenne JW, Fink JB, Fahey PJ, Tobin MJ. Dose-response to bronchodilator delivered by metered-dose inhaler in ventilator-supported patients. Am J Respir Crit Care Med 1996;154:388–393.

Fink JB, Dhand R, Duarte AG, Jenne JW, Tobin MJ. Aerosol delivery from a metered-dose inhaler during mechanical ventilation: an in vitro model. Am J Respir Crit Care Med 1996; 154:382–387.

Fuller HD, Dolovich MB, Posmituck G, Pack WW, Newhouse MT. Pressurized aerosol versus jet aerosol delivery to mechanically ventilated patients: comparison of dose to the lungs. Am Rev Respir Dis 1990;141:440–444.

Fuller HD, Dolovich MB, Turpie FH, Newhouse MT. Efficiency of bronchodilator aerosol delivery to the lungs from the metered dose inhaler in mechanically ventilated patients: a study comparing four different actuator devices. Chest 1994;105:214–218.

Guyatt GH, Townsend M, Nogradi S, Pugsley SO, Keller JL, Newhouse MT. Acute response to bronchodilator: an imperfect guide for bronchodilator therapy in chronic airflow limitation. Arch Intern Med 1988;148:1949.

Harwood R, Rau JL, Thomas-Goodfellow L. A comparison of three methods of metered dose bronchodilator delivery to a mechanically ventilated adult lung model. Respiratory Care 1994;39:886–891.

Hess D, Fisher D, Williams P, Pooler S, Kacmarek RM. Medication nebulizer performance: effects of diluent volume, nebulizer flow, and nebulizer brand. Chest 1996;110:498–505.

Idris AH, McDermott MF, Raucci JC, Morrabel A, McGorray S, Hendeles L. Emergency department treatment of severe asthma: metered-dose inhaler plus holding chamber is equivalent in effectiveness to nebulizer. Chest 1993;103:665–672.

Macintyre NR, Silver RM, Miller CW, Schuler F, Coleman RE. Aerosol delivery in intubated, mechanically ventilated patients. Crit Care Med 1985;13:81–84.

Mcstitz H, Copland JM, McDonald CF. Comparison of outpatient nebulized vs metered dose inhaler terbutaline in chronic airflow obstruction. Chest 1989;96:1237–1240.

Moler FW, Johnson CE, Van Laanen C, Palmisano JM, Nasr SZ, Akingbola O. Continuous versus intermittent nebulized terbutaline: plasma levels and effects. Am J Respir Crit Care Med 1995;151:602–606.

Papo MC, Frank J, Thompson AE. A prospective, randomized study of continuous versus intermittent nebulized albuterol for severe status asthmaticus in children. Crit Care Med 1993;21:1479–1486.

Shim CS, Williams MH. Effect of bronchodilator therapy administered by canister versus jet nebulizer. J Allergy Clin Immunol 1984;73:387–390.

Turner JR, Corkery KJ, Eckman D, Gelb AM, Lipavsky A, Sheppard D. Equivalence of continuous flow nebulizer and metered-dose inhaler with reservoir bag for treatment of acute airflow obstruction. Chest 1988;93:476–481.

Beta Agonists: Dosing/Risks

Ernst P, Habbick B, Suissa S, Hemmelgarn B, Cockcroft D, Buist AS, Horwitz RI, McNutt M, Spitzer WO. Is the association between inhaled beta-agonist use and life-threatening asthma because of confounding by severity. Am Rev Respir Dis 1993;148:75–79.

Ernst P, Spitzer WO, Suissa S, Cockcroft D, Habbick B, Horwitz RI, Boivin J, McNutt M, Buist AS. Risk of fatal and near-fatal asthma in relation to inhaled corticosteroid use. JAMA 1992;268:3462–3464.

Joseph KS, Blais L, Ernst P, Suissa S. Increased morbidity and mortality related to asthma among asthmatic patients who use major tranquillisers. Br Med J 1996;312:79–83.

Maesen FPV, Costongs R, Smeets JJ, Brombacher PJ, Zweers PGMA. The effects of maximal doses of formoterol and salbutamol from a metered dose inhaler on pulse rates, ECG, and serum potassium concentrations. Chest 1991;99:1367–1373.

Nelson HS. β-adrenergic bronchodilators. N Engl J Med 1995;333:499–506.

Newhouse MT, Chapman KR, McCallum AL, Abboud RT, Bowie DM, Hodder RV, Pare PD, Mesic-Fuchs H, Molfino NA. Cardiovascular safety of high doses of inhaled fenoterol and albuterol in acute severe asthma. Chest 1996;110:595–603.

Seider N, Abinader EG, Oliven A. Cardiac arrhythmias after inhaled bronchodilators in patients with COPD and ischemic heart disease. Chest 1993;104:1070–1074.

Spitzer WO, Suissa S, Ernst P, Horwitz RI, Habbick B, Cockcroft D, Boivin J-F, McNutt M, Buist AS, Rebuck AS. The use of β-agonists and the risk of death and near-death from asthma. N Engl J Med 1992;326:501–506.

Suissa S, Blais L, Ernst P. Pattern of increasing β-agonist use and the risk of fatal to near-fatal asthma. Eur Respir J 1994;7:1602–1609.

Suissa S, Ernst P, Boivin J, Horwitz RI, Habbick B, Cockroft D, Blais L, McNutt M, Buist AS, Spitzer WO. A cohort analysis of excess mortality in asthma and the use of inhaled β-agonist. Am J Respir Crit Care Med 1994;149:604–610.

Tashkin DP. Dosing strategies for bronchodilator aerosol delivery. Respiratory Care 1991; 36:977–988.

Vathenen AS, Britton JR, Ebden P, Cookson JB, Wharrad HJ, Tatterfield AE. High-dose inhaled albuterol in severe chronic airflow limitation. Am Rev Respir Dis 1988;138: 850–855.

Beta$_2$ Agonists: Long-Acting

Anderson GP. Long-acting inhaled beta-adrenoceptor agonists: the comparative pharmacology of formoterol and salmeterol. In: Hansel TT, Morley J, eds. New drugs in allergy and asthma. Basel: Birkhäuser Verlag, 1993.

Britton MG, Earnshaw JS, Palmer JBD. A twelve month comparison of salmeterol with salbutamol in asthmatic patients. Eur Respir J 1992;5:1062–1067.

Castle W, Fuller R, Hall J, Palmer J. Serevent nationwide surveillance study: comparison of salmeterol with salbutamol in asthmatic patients who require regular bronchodilator treatment. Br Med J 1993;306:1034–1037.

Cheung D, Timmers MC, Zwinderman AH, Bel EH, Dijkman JH, Sterk PJ. Long-term effects of a long-acting β2-adrenoceptor agonist, salmeterol, on airway hyperresponsiveness in patients with mild asthma. N Engl J Med 1992;327:1198–1203.

D'Alonzo GE, Nathan RA, Henochowicz S, Morris RJ, Ratner P, Rennard SI. Salmeterol xinafoate as maintenance therapy compared with albuterol in patients with asthma. JAMA 1994;271:1412–1416.

Estelle R, Simons R, Soni NR, Watson WTA, Becker AB. Bronchodilator and bronchoprotective effects of salmeterol in young patients with asthma. J Allergy Clin Immunol 1992;90: 840–845.

Rabe KF, Jörres R, Nowak D, Behr N, Magnussen H. Comparison of the effects of salmeterol and formoterol on airway tone and responsiveness over 24 hours in bronchial asthma. Am Rev Respir Dis 1993;147:1436–1441.

Anticholinergic: Bronchodilators

Barnes PJ. Neural mechanisms in asthma. Br Med Bull 1992;48:149–168.

Braun SR, McKenzie WN, Copeland C, Knight L, Ellersieck M. A comparison of the effect of ipratropium and albuterol in the treatment of chronic obstructive airway disease. Arch Intern Med 1989;149:544–547.

Friedman M. A multicenter study of nebulized bronchodilator solutions in chronic obstructive pulmonary disease. Am J Med 1996;100(suppl 1A):30S–39S.

Grandordy BM, Thomas V, de Lauture D, Marsac J. Cumulative dose-response curves for assessing combined effects of salbutamol and ipratropium bromide in chronic asthma. Eur Respir J 1988;1:531–535.

Gross NJ, Petty TL, Friedman M, Skorodin MS, Silvers GW, Donohue JF. Dose response to ipratropium as a nebulized solution in patients with chronic obstructive pulmonary disease. Am Rev Respir Dis 1989;139:1188–1191.

Ikeda A, Nishimura K, Koyama H, Tsukino M, Mishima M, Izumi T. Dose response study of ipratropium bromide aerosol on maximum exercise performance in stable patients with chronic obstructive pulmonary disease. Thorax 1996;51:48–53.

Ind PW, Dixon CMS, Fuller RW, Barnes PJ. Anticholinergic blockade of beta-blocker-induced bronchoconstriction. Am Rev Respir Dis 1989;139:1390–1394.

Maesen FPV, Smeets JJ, Sledsens TJH, Wald FDM, Cornelissen PJG. Tiotropium bromide, a new long-acting antimuscarinic bronchodilator: a pharmacodynamic study in patients with chronic obstructive pulmonary disease (COPD). Eur Respir J 1995;8:1506–1513.

Millar AB, Bush A, Al-Hillawi H, Goldman J, Denison DM. Ipratropium bromide: are patients treated with optimal therapy? Postgrad Med J 1990;66:1040–1042.

Rebuck AS, Marcus HI. SCH 1000 in psychogenic asthma. Scand J Respir Dis 1979; 103(suppl):186–191.

Storms WW, Bodman SF, Nathan RA, Busse WW, Bush RK, Falliers CJ, O'Hollaren JD, Weg JG. Use of ipratropium bromide in asthma: results of a multi-clinic study. Am J Med 1986;81(suppl 5A):61–66.

Yang SC, Yang SP, Lee TS. Nebulized ipratropium bromide in ventilator-assisted patients with chronic bronchitis. Chest 1994;105:1511–1515.

Glucocorticoids

Baraniuk JN. Molecular actions of glucocorticoids: an introduction. J Allergy Clin Immunol 1996;97(suppl):141–142.

Barnes NC, Marone G, Di Maria GU, Visser S, Utama I, Payne SL. A comparison of fluticasone propionate, 1 mg daily, with beclomethasone dipropionate, 2 mg daily, in the treatment of severe asthma. Eur Respir J 1993;6:877–885.

Barnes PJ. Inhaled glucocorticoids for asthma. N Engl J Med 1995;332:868–875.

Barnes PJ. Molecular mechanisms of steroid action in asthma. J Allergy Clin Immunol 1996; 97:159–168.

Fabbri L, Burge PS, Croonenborgh L, Warlies F, Weeke B, Ciaccia A, Parker C. Comparison of fluticasone propionate with beclomethasone dipropionate in moderate to severe asthma treated for one year. Thorax 1993;48:817–823.

Holliday SM, Faulds D, Sorkin EM. Inhaled fluticasone propionate: a review of its pharmacodynamic and pharmacokinetic properties, and therapeutic use in asthma. Drugs 1994;47(2): 318–331.

International Consensus Report on Diagnosis and Treatment of Asthma. Bethesda, MD: NHLBI, NIH publication no. 92–3091. March, 1992. (Also in Eur Respir J 1992;5:601–641 or Clin Exp Allergy 1992;suppl 1:1–72.)

Kamada AK, Szefler SJ, Martin RJ, Boushey HA, Chinchilli VM, Drazen JM, Fish JE, Israel

E, Lazarus SC, Lemanske RF. Issues in the use of inhaled glucocorticoids. Am J Respir Crit Care Med 1996;153:1739–1748.

Leblanc P, Mink S, Keistinen T, Saarelainen PA, Ringdal N, Payne SL. A comparison of fluticasone propionate 200 μg/day with beclomethasone dipropionate 400 μg/day in adult asthma. Allergy 1994;49:380–385.

Management of Asthma During Pregnancy. Washington, DC: U.S. Department of Health and Human Services: Public Health Service; NIH, NHLBI, NAEP September 1993. NIH publication no. 93–3279.

National Asthma Education Program: Expert Panel Report. Guidelines for the diagnosis for management of asthma. August 1991. Publication no. 91–3042.

Rau JL, Restrepo RD, Deshpande V. Inhalation of single vs multiple metered-dose bronchodilator actuations from reservoir devices: an in vitro study. Chest 1996;109:969–974.

Theophylline

Barnes PJ, Pauwels RA. Theophylline in the management of asthma: time for reappraisal? Eur Respir J 1994;7(3):579–591.

Lam A, Newhouse MT. Management of asthma and chronic airflow limitation: are methylxanthines obsolete? Chest 1990;98:44–52.

Newhouse MT. Is theophylline obsolete? Chest 1990;98(1):1–2.

Niewoehner DE. Theophylline therapy: a continuing dilemma. Chest 1990;98(1):5.

Weinberger M, Hendeles L. Theophylline in asthma. N Engl J Med 1996;334(21):1380–1388.

Mediator Modulators

Bousquet J, Aubert B, Bons J. Comparison of salmeterol with disodium cromoglycate in the treatment of adult asthma. Ann Allergy Asthma Immunol 1996;76(2):189–194.

Cherniack RM, Wasserman SI, Rasdell JW, Selner JC, Koepke JW, Rogers RM, Owens GR, Rubin EM, Wanner A (North American Tilade Study Group). A double-blind multicenter group comparative study of the efficacy and safety of nedocromil sodium in the management of asthma. Chest 1990;97:1299–1306.

de Benedictis FM, Tuter G, Pazzelli P, Bertotto A, Bruni L, Vaccaro R. Cromolyn versus nedocromil: duration of action in exercise-induced asthma in children. J Allergy Clin Immunol 1995;96(4):510–514.

Faurshou P, Bing J, Edman G, Engel AM. Comparison between sodium cromoglycate (MDI: metered-dose inhaler) and beclomethasone dipropionate (MDI) in treatment of adult patients with mild to moderate bronchial asthma: a double-blind, double-dummy randomized, parallel-group study. Allergy 1994;49(8):659–663.

Findlay SR, Barden JM, Easley CB, Glass M. Effect of the oral leukotriene antagonist, ICI 204,219, on antigen-induced bronchoconstriction in subjects with asthma. J Allergy Clin Immunol 1992;89:1040–1045.

Finnerty JP, Wood-Baker R, Thomson H, Holgate ST. Role of leukotrienes in exercise-induced asthma; inhibitory effect of ICI 204219, a potent leukotriene D4 receptor antagonist. Am Rev Respir Dis 1992;145:745–749.

Israel E, Chon J, Dubé L, Drazen JM. Effect of treatment with zileuton, a 5-lipoxygenase inhibitor, in patients with asthma: a randomized controlled trial. JAMA 1996;275:931–936.

Piacentini GL, Kaliner MA. The potential roles of leukotrienes in bronchial asthma. Am Rev Respir Dis 1991;143:S96–S99.

Schwartz HJ, Blumenthal M, Brady R, Braun S, Lockey R, Myers D, Mansfield L, Mullarkey M, Owens G, Ratner P, Repsher L, van As A. A comparative study of the clinical efficacy of nedocromil sodium and placebo: how does cromolyn sodium compare as an active control treatment? Chest 1996;109(4):945–952.

Spector SL. Leukotriene inhibitors and antagonists in asthma. Ann Allergy Asthma Immunol 1995;75:463–471.

Spector SL, Smith LJ, Glass M, the ACCOLATE℠ Asthma Trialists Group. Effects of 6 weeks of therapy with oral doses of ICI 204,219, a leukotriene D4 receptor antagonist, in subjects with bronchial asthma. Am J Respir Crit Care Med 1994;150:618–623.

Combination Therapy

Chapman KR. An international perspective on anticholinergic therapy. Am J Med 1996; 100(suppl 1A):2S–4S.

Colice GL. Nebulized bronchodilators for outpatient management of stable chronic obstructive pulmonary disease. Am J Med 1996;100(suppl 1A):11S–18S.

Friedman M. Changing practices in COPD: a new pharmacologic treatment algorithm. Chest 1995;107(suppl 5):194S–197S.

Gross NJ. Airway inflammation in COPD: reality or myth? Chest 1995;107(suppl 5): 210S–213S.

Levin DC, Little KS, Laughlin KR, Galbraith JM, Gustman PM, Murphy D, Kram JA, Hardie G, Reuter C, Ostransky D, McFarland K, Petty TL, Silvers W, Rennard SI, Mueller M, Repsher LH, Zuwallack RL, Vale R. Addition of anticholinergic solution prolongs broncho- dilator effect of β-2 agonists in patients with chronic obstructive pulmonary disease. Am J Med 1996;100(suppl 1A):40S–48S.

Petty TL. The combination of ipratropium and albuterol is more effective than either agent alone. Chest 1995;107(suppl 5):183S–186S.

Rebuck AS, Chapman KR, Abboud R, Pare PD, Dreisman H, Wolkove N, Vickerson F. Nebulized anticholinergic and sympathomimetic treatment of asthma and chronic obstruc- tive airways disease in the emergency room. Am J Med 1987;82:59–64.

Rennard SI. Combination bronchodilator therapy in COPD. Chest 1995;107(suppl 5): 171S–175S.

Serra C, Giacopelli A, Luciani G. Acute controlled study of the dose-response relationship of fenoterol, ipratropium bromide and their combination. Respiration 1986;50(suppl 2): 144–147.

Siefkin AD. Optimal pharmacologic treatment of the critically ill patient with obstructive airways disease. Am J Med 1996;100(suppl 1A):54S–61S.

Tashkin DP, Bleecker E, Braun S, Campbell S, DeGraff Jr AC, Hudgel DW, Boyars MC, Sahn S. Results of a multicenter study of nebulized inhalant bronchodilator solutions. Am J Med 1996;100(suppl 1A):62S–69S.

4 Asthma

Sidney S. Braman

Asthma is a chronic inflammatory disease of the airways that affects up to 10% of the population. Clinical descriptions of the disease have been available since ancient times. Hippocrates in the 3rd century BC and Galen in the 2nd century AD wrote of asthma, describing it as a condition associated with dyspnea of any cause. The medieval physician Maimonides produced a treatise on asthma in 1190. It was, however, Sir John Floyer who wrote the first clear definition and accurate clinical description, having suffered from asthma himself since childhood. He was the first physician to separate asthma from other pulmonary disorders and the first to recognize that bronchospasm was responsible for the symptoms of asthma. Although the inflammatory nature of asthma was recognized in the latter part of the 19th century by Sir William Osler, it has only been in the last decade or so that the emphasis on reversible bronchospasm in the pathogenesis of asthma has shifted to an emphasis on the inflammatory causes of this airways disease. This shift in emphasis has lead to more effective control of symptoms and, in some instances, disease prevention.

A thorough knowledge of the pathophysiology and treatment options available for asthma is essential for the internist and pulmonologist alike for many reasons:

- A relatively large segment of the population is affected with asthma, and there is evidence that both the prevalence and severity of asthma has been increasing in recent years.
- Accurate and inexpensive means to measure lung function are available, thus providing the physician and patient an effective way to monitor disease severity.
- Effective and safe therapy exists for the treatment and prevention of asthma.
- Effective environmental control measures may avoid or even eliminate factors that provoke asthma attacks.

DEFINITION

For most of this century, asthma has been recognized as a disease caused by hyperreactivity of the airways that is manifested by widespread narrowing of the airways that changes either spontaneously or as the result of specific therapy. It is a disease, therefore, that is characterized by wide variations in resistance to airflow over short periods of time. Although this working or operational description is based on the physiologic consequences of asthma and is helpful in distinguishing asthma from other chronic obstructive lung diseases, such as emphysema and chronic bronchitis, it falls short in that it does not recognize the major pathophysiologic mechanism of

177

asthma-airway inflammation. A more recent definition of asthma proposed by the U.S. National Institutes of Health (NIH) states that:

> Asthma is a chronic inflammatory disorder of the airways in which many cells play a role, in particular mast cells, eosinophils, and T-lymphocytes. In susceptible individuals this inflammation causes recurrent episodes of wheezing, breathlessness, chest tightness, and cough, particularly at night and/or in the early morning. These symptoms are usually associated with widespread but variable airflow limitation that is at least partially reversible either spontaneously or with treatment. The inflammation also causes an associated increase in airway responsiveness to a variety of stimuli.

PATHOGENESIS

Asthma is caused by a complex interaction of cells, mediators, and cytokines that results in inflammatory airway disease. The characteristic cellular changes involve (a) constitutive cells, such as epithelial cells, mucous glands, endothelial cells, and myofibroblasts, (b) resident cells, such as bone marrow-derived mast cells and macrophages, and (c) infiltrating cells, such as eosinophils and CD4 (helper cell) T-lymphocytes. Many typical histopathologic findings can be found in the airways of asthmatics:

- Denudation of the airway epithelium can lead to airway edema and loss of substances in the mucosa that protect the airways. Epithelial damage promotes bronchial hyperresponsiveness because access to irritating substances by sensory nerve endings is increased. Similarly, aeroallergens can more readily penetrate the airways.
- The airway architecture is changed by the deposition of type III and V collagen and fibronectin beneath the basement membrane. Airway remodeling may cause permanent changes and fixed airflow obstruction.
- Infiltration of the airways by inflammatory cells, such as mast cells, eosinophils, activated T-lymphocytes, and neutrophils, can be demonstrated by bronchial biopsies and inferred by demonstrating increased numbers of these cells on bronchoalveolar lavage.
- Specific cytokines, most of which are products of lymphocytes and macrophages, appear to direct the movement of cells to the site of airway inflammation. They also activate the cells, causing them to release their mediators (e.g., interleukin-3 and 5 and granulocyte-macrophage colony-stimulating factor) and induce eosinophils to release a number of mediators from their preformed granules. These mediators are major basic protein, eosinophil cationic protein, eosinophil-derived neurotoxin, and eosinophil peroxidase. All have inflammatory effects that contribute to the pathogenesis of asthma.
- Mast cells, usually as a result of IgE-mediated stimulation, also release preformed mediators (such as histamine and tryptase) and further act as a regulator of inflammation by producing cytokines that promote eosinophil infiltration and activation.

There is growing evidence that the neural control of the airways is abnormal in asthma and that neurogenic mechanisms may augment or modulate the inflammatory response. The autonomic nervous system regulates many aspects of airway function, such as airway tone, airway secretions, blood flow, microvascular permeability, and the release of inflammatory cells. A primary defect in autonomic control—the beta adrenoreceptor theory—has been postulated for asthma. It is more likely, however, that autonomic dysfunction is a secondary defect caused by inflammation or by the effects of treatment. For instance, inflammatory mediators can modulate the release of neurotransmitters from airway nerves, such as irritant receptors and C-fiber endings. They can also directly act on autonomic receptors, such as those that cause reflex bronchoconstriction from gastroesophageal reflux.

There is growing evidence for a role of the nonadrenergic, noncholinergic (NANC) nervous system in the pathogenesis of asthma. As the airway epithelium becomes denuded, sensory nerve endings may become exposed, causing a release of potent neuropeptides, such as substance P, neurokinin A, and calcitonin gene-related protein. These neuromediators can lead to bronchoconstriction, microvascular leakage, and mucus hypersecretion. This neurogenic inflammation of the airways, triggered by sensitized sensory nerve endings, has been postulated to cause airway "hyperalgesia" and result in symptoms such as cough and chest tightness. Nitric oxide also appears to be one of the neurotransmitters of the NANC system and is an important braking mechanism that can initiate bronchodilatation.

Airway inflammation is thought to be a key factor in producing a cardinal feature of asthma-bronchial hyperreactivity. This can be described as an exaggerated bronchoconstrictive response of the airways to a variety of stimuli, such as aeroallergens, histamine, methacholine, cold air, and environmental irritants. It is unclear whether bronchial hyperreactivity is entirely acquired or is present at birth and genetically determined to appear with the appropriate stimulus. It is thought that airway inflammation is the stimulus that causes bronchial hyperresponsiveness, whether it is induced by a viral respiratory infection, an allergic IgE-mediated response, or the inhalation of a noxious agent such as ozone or sulfur dioxide. Treatment with antiinflammatory agents, such as inhaled corticosteroids, is effective in reducing bronchial hyperreactivity.

The degree of bronchial hyperreactivity can be determined in the pulmonary function laboratory by standard inhalation challenge testing. The methacholine and histamine inhalation challenges are the most frequently used clinical tools to determine the presence and degree of bronchial hyperreactivity. Cold air and hypotonic saline challenges are also done. Although the result of this testing—airway narrowing—is the same for these provocative agents, the mechanisms that cause the airways to constrict vary. Methacholine and histamine act directly on airway smooth muscle. Exercise and hyperosmolar or hypo-osmolar solutions act indirectly by releasing pharmacologically active substances from mediator-secreting cells, such as mast cells. Sulfur dioxide and bradykinin act by directly stimulating airway sensory nerve endings. The degree of bronchial hyperreactivity usually correlates with the clinical severity of asthma and the medication need of the individual. In addition, fluctuations of diurnal peak flow measurements correlate with the degree of airway reactivity.

Table 4.1. Causes of Airflow Limitation in Asthma

Acute bronchoconstriction
Bronchial wall edema
Inflammatory cell infiltration
Airway wall remodeling (fibrosis)
Smooth muscle hypertrophy
Loss of elastic recoil pressure
Chronic mucus plugging of airway lumen

Airflow obstruction is another cardinal feature of asthma. The causes of airflow limitation in asthma are listed in Table 4.1. In most asthmatics airflow obstruction is completely reversible. Antiinflammatory drugs are used to reduce bronchial hyper-reactivity and reverse other inflammatory sequelae, such as hypersecretion of mucus. In some asthmatics, particularly those with long-standing and severe asthma, airflow obstruction is only partially reversible despite maximal antiinflammatory therapy with large doses of oral corticosteroids. The reasons for these permanent physiologic changes remain obscure, and it is suspected that airway remodeling, at least in part, is responsible.

NATURAL HISTORY

The most reliable information on the natural history of asthma comes from large community surveys. Comparisons from country to country and even within the same country are difficult to make because of varying criteria used to make the diagnosis and the inclusion of cigarette smokers who might also have underlying chronic obstructive pulmonary disease (COPD). The peak prevalence of asthma in all studies is in childhood, affecting approximately 10% of that population. This declines to approximately 5–6% in adolescence and early adulthood, when remission rates are high. The prevalence rises again during later adulthood to 7–9%.

The relationship of atopy and asthma has been carefully studied. In both children and adults, the presence of bronchial hyperreactivity correlates with the presence and number of positive immediate hypersensitivity skin tests to inhalant allergens. The presence of positive skin tests in infants of allergic parents correlates with the onset of asthma in later childhood, and the number of positive skin tests shows a correlation with the severity of asthma in childhood and early adulthood. Studies correlating skin test reactivity to house dust mite and asthma also strongly implicate atopy in the pathogenesis of asthma. One alternative theory is that there is one common mechanism involved in the development of both IgE-mediated hypersensitivity and bronchial hyperreactivity or that the two may be related by genetic linkage. This would suggest that there is not a causal relationship between atopy and asthma and would explain why many asthmatics, especially adults, are skin-test negative and appear to have no allergic basis for their asthma. Although most asthmatics who develop their disease in early childhood will outgrow their asthma by early adult-hood, those with more severe atopy by skin testing, those with a greater degree of bronchial reactivity, and those with more difficult to control asthma are more likely to persist with asthma into adulthood. This is particularly true for young girls.

In adulthood, there is a steady incidence of new-onset asthma through all ages, even in the elderly. Many patients begin with recurrent wheezing following respira-tory viral infections. This pattern may gradually or abruptly develop into persistent wheezing and often severe, poorly responsive disease. At other times asthma devel-ops explosively, with no previous respiratory symptoms, immediately following the onset of a typical viral respiratory infection. In adulthood, asthma may also result from exposure to occupational hazards and may not remit when the patient is re-moved from the offending environment. Not infrequently, heavy cigarette smokers with COPD and predominantly fixed airflow obstruction develop acute broncho-spasm, responsive to inhaled bronchodilators, in a pattern similar to asthma. Because of the underlying chronic bronchitis, these patients are often labeled as asthmatic bronchitis to distinguish them from pure asthma and identify the irreversible compo-

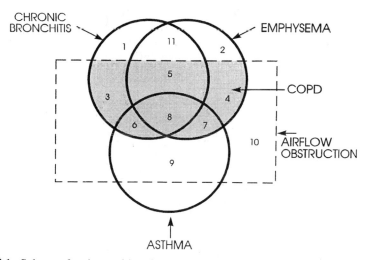

Figure 4.1. Subsets of patients with asthma, bronchitis, and emphysema. Those with chronic irreversible airflow obstruction (COPD) are in the shaded area. Patients with asthma whose airflow obstruction is completely reversible (subset 9) are not considered to have COPD. Patients with asthma who have persistent airflow obstruction are classified as having COPD (subsets 6, 7, and 8). Such patients, when smokers, are often referred to as having asthmatic bronchitis. Chronic bronchitis and emphysema with airflow obstruction usually occur together (subset 5) but may occur independently (subsets 3 and 4). Patients with chronic bronchitis and/or emphysema who do not have airflow obstruction are in subsets 1, 2, and 11. Patients with airflow obstruction caused by other diseases, such as bronchiectasis and cystic fibrosis, are in subset 10. (From Standards for the Diagnosis and Care of Patients with Chronic Obstruc-tive Pulmonary Disease. Am J Respir Crit Care Med 1995;152:S77. Reprinted with permis-sion.)

nent of their disease. Unlike some adult asthmatics, those with asthmatic bronchitis will never have a complete remission of their disease. The relationship among asthma, chronic bronchitis, and emphysema is presented in Figure 4.1.

CLINICAL FEATURES

Symptoms

The typical triad of symptoms of asthma are wheezing, shortness of breath, and cough with or without sputum production. These symptoms are not specific for asthma and can be seen in other acute and chronic airways diseases. The differential diagnosis of asthma is listed in Table 4.2. An acute viral tracheobronchitis associated with or following a typical viral upper respiratory infection (URI), for example, can cause the asthma triad of symptoms and can be associated with bronchial hyperresponsiveness for up to 6 weeks. Unlike asthma, these symptoms usually resolve completely over time.

COPD caused by emphysema and chronic bronchitis can also cause typical asthma symptoms, and the distinction between these conditions can become difficult, especially when COPD is complicated by acute viral or irritant-induced bronchospasm. In general, the symptoms of asthma are considerably more episodic and of sudden onset than those of COPD, and periods of prolonged remission are typical.

Attacks of asthma are likely to be provoked by known aeroallergens, especially in the younger atopic population. It is not unusual for an asthmatic to give a history of wheezing and shortness of breath following exposure to household pets, such as cats and dogs. Animal handlers and laboratory workers may similarly develop sensitivity to rats, guinea pigs, and other small animals. Asthma may occur seasonally, such as during ragweed season in the fall or during flower and tree blooming in the spring. It is believed that exposure to household mites that live in bedding, in floor rugs, and on other fabrics found in the house is also a major cause of asthma symptoms, especially in warmer climates that favor their growth. Similarly, in areas of the inner city, especially where poverty is found, cockroach exposure is an important inciting agent of atopic asthma.

The immediate hypersensitivity reaction (atopic reaction) has two phases, an immediate bronchospastic reaction that causes symptoms within minutes after exposure and a delayed reaction that occurs 6 or more hours after exposure. When there is exposure to an aeroallergen that results in a predominantly delayed allergic bronchospastic reaction, the patient may not realize that the offending agent is the cause because the exposure has occurred many hours before.

Typically the triad of symptoms of asthma present simultaneously, but this is not always the case. There is evidence that some patients with asthma perceive their symptoms poorly. In studies of acutely ill asthmatics, up to 10% of patients have no shortness of breath and only complain of wheezing and cough.

The reasons for the lack of dyspnea remain obscure but several observations are relevant:

- Asthmatic subjects have a higher threshold for tolerating resistive loads than do normal subjects.

Table 4.2. Differential Diagnosis of Asthma

Disease	Distinguishing Features
COPD (emphysema/bronchitis)	Smoking history; irreversible airflow obstruction underlies the reversible bronchospastic component.
Bronchogenic carcinoma	Wheezing often unilateral and accompanied by other symptoms, such as hemoptysis and weight loss; chest roentgenogram shows mass lesion.
Lymphangitic carcinomatosis	This advanced stage of cancer can cause severe dyspnea and wheezing; the chest roentgenogram shows diffuse interstitial infiltrates.
Upper airway obstruction	Wheezing or stridor may occur; flow volume loop shows reduced inspiratory flow with variable extrathoracic obstruction and flattening of the inspiratory and expiratory flow curves with fixed obstruction.
Chronic gastric aspiration	Reflux of gastric acid into the trachea can acutely worsen asthma; chronic aspiration of gastric contents results in aspiration pneumonitis that causes cough and wheezing.
Foreign body aspiration	Foreign bodies may lodge in intrathoracic or extrathoracic airways and cause stridor or wheezing; diagnosis is based on history and chest roentgenogram when the object is opaque.
Pulmonary edema	Cardiac asthma has been recognized for more than a century; inspiratory crackles, gallop rhythm, murmurs, and peripheral edema should be looked for; chest roentgenography may show cardiomegaly and Kerley B lines.
Pulmonary embolism (PE)	Wheezing may be a prominent feature; focal monophonic wheezing, a prominent risk factor for PE, and lack of response to bronchodilator therapy should arouse suspicion, and a lung scan should be ordered.
Carcinoid syndrome	Flushing, hypotension, abdominal cramping, diarrhea, and facial edema are associated with wheezing; confirmation by measurement of 5-hydroxyindoleacetic acid in urine.
Cystic fibrosis	Young patients with long-standing cough and sputum production; evidence of bronchiectasis on chest roentgenogram; sweat chloride test characteristically low.
Vocal cord dysfunction	Caused by adduction of the vocal cords resulting in wheezing or stridor; laryngoscopy shows paradoxical vocal cord motion; most patients have major psychiatric disorders and have been inappropriately treated for asthma.

- Asthmatics with greater resting baseline airflow obstruction are less likely to perceive worsening lung function after an inhalation cholinergic challenge.
- Symptoms caused by a precipitous drop in lung function as a result of the immediate hypersensitivity reaction are better perceived than those that may occur as a result of a slower equal decline in lung function caused by the late onset reaction.

- Abnormalities in the perception of asthma symptoms have important therapeutic implications. An asthmatic who is not able to detect increased airway resistance will not reach for appropriate medication when necessary.
- It has been postulated that poor perception of asthma in some patients may be responsible for fatal and near-fatal attacks, especially in the elderly because impaired perception of bronchospasm is also a feature of aging. Objective monitoring of airway function by spirometry and peak flow meters is essential for asthma prevention.

Variant manifestations of asthma occur:

- Patients with asthma may present with only cough or dyspnea as isolated symptoms. A nonproductive cough may be present for years as a sign of asthma before the full triad of symptoms begin.
- Cough is probably caused by stimulation of airway sensory nerves by inflammatory mediators. The asthmatic cough is often provoked by respiratory irritants (such as cigarette smoke), cold air, laughter, and by cough itself. Many times a single cough will begin a series of violent coughing paroxysms that may last for many minutes and lead to exhaustion. Cough also may be provoked by deep inhalation and by forced exhalation. This may be useful as a bedside test because a coughing paroxysm induced by a deep breathing maneuver suggests hyperreactive asthmatic airways.
- Because patients with isolated cough or dyspnea may have normal pulmonary function studies, reversible airflow obstruction may not be possible to document. In such cases, bronchoprovocation testing with histamine or methacholine may be useful in making the proper diagnosis.
- Other symptoms of asthma are chest tightness, substernal pressure, chest pain, and nocturnal awakenings. These symptoms are more likely to be confused with cardiac disease, especially ischemic heart disease, in the older individual.

Physical Signs

The physical findings associated with acute bronchospasm of asthma are the direct result of:

- Diffuse airway narrowing and hypersecretion of mucus;
- The indirect result of reflex influences from an increase in the work of breathing, increased metabolic demands on the body, and diffuse sympathetic nervous discharge.

Physical signs include:

- Tachypnea and tachycardia are universal features of acute asthma. The average respiratory rate is between 25 and 28 breaths per minute, and average pulse rate is 100 beats per minute. Respiratory rates greater than 30 and heart rates greater than 120 are not uncommon and may be seen in as many as 25 to 30% of patients.
- Diffuse musical wheezes are characteristic of asthma, but their presence or intensity do not reliably predict the severity of asthma. By the time wheezing can be

detected by the stethoscope, peak flow rates may be decreased by as much as 25% or more. In general, wheezing during inspiration and expiration, loud wheezing, and high-pitched wheezing are associated with greater airway obstruction.

- In extremely severe cases wheezing may be absent, suggesting extremely poor air movement and impending respiratory failure.
- A prolonged phase of exhalation is typically seen, as is chest hyperinflation. They are the result of airflow obstruction and air trapping, respectively.
- Accessory muscle use, pulsus paradoxus, and diaphoresis are associated with severe airflow obstruction although their absence does not rule out a severe attack. Accessory muscle use and pulsus paradoxus are caused by large negative swings in intrapleural pressure, and they may not be manifest in the patient with rapid shallow breathing. They are reported to be present in 30 to 40% of patients with acute asthma.
- Cyanosis and signs of acute hypercarbic acidosis, such as mental obtundation, are absent in all but extreme cases.

Objective Measures of Asthma Severity

Objective measurements of pulmonary function are important in asthma because the perception of asthma symptoms is often poor and the physician's findings on physical examination may either overestimate or underestimate the severity of airflow obstruction.

Four tests of pulmonary function are extremely useful for establishing the diagnosis of asthma and for following the clinical course of the patient once the diagnosis has been made:

- Office spirometry;
- Peak expiratory flow rate (PEFR) measurements by a peak flow meter;
- Arterial blood gas analysis;
- Bronchoprovocation testing.

Spirometry can be used to measure maximal inspiratory and expiratory flow rates and lung volumes (see Chapter 2). The timed vital capacity (VC) and flow-volume loop offer similar information, and either technique can be used to measure airway function. During an asthma attack, lung function is characterized by hyperinflation, a prolonged expiratory time, and decreased expiratory flow rates. The PEFR can be measured and requires maximum effort for accuracy. The forced vital capacity (FVC) is the total volume of air that can be expelled rapidly and is usually the best preserved index. The forced expiratory volume in one second (FEV_1) is the volume of air expelled in one second from maximal inspiration, and the maximal midexpiratory flow rate (MMEFR) is the slope of the line between 25 and 50% of the forced expiratory volume. This flow rate is also known as the FEF_{25-50}, the forced expiratory flow between 25 and 50% of the VC. An additional measurement derived from the flow-volume loop, which records instantaneous flow and volume during the forced expiratory maneuver, is the forced expiratory flow at 50 and 75% of the VC (FEF_{50} and FEF_{75}). Computerized analysis of the flow-volume curve routinely derives the FEV_1 and PEFR. The flow-volume loop is especially helpful in distinguishing obstructive disorders of the upper airways (larynx and trachea) from lower airway disorders (such as asthma). This is important because malignant and benign tumors, infections, and inflammatory diseases of the upper airways can masquerade as asthma for months and even years. In such instances, patients may receive unnecessary and, at times, harmful medication such as corticosteroids to alleviate asthma-like symptoms that are caused by obstruction to the upper airway.

- A reduction in the FEV_1 (less than 80% predicted) and MMEFR (less than 70%) with a normal VC indicates obstructive lung disease. The FEV_1/FVC ratio, expressed as a percentage ($FEV_1\%$), is reduced below normal to less than 75% (in children, less than 85%). When the FEV_1 is severely reduced, the FVC can also be reduced as a result of obstruction alone.
- During an acute attack of asthma, on average the FEV_1 is reduced to approximately 30–35% of predicted and the FVC to approximately 50% of predicted. The FEV_1 in absolute terms is reduced to approximately 1 liter. The peak flow (PEFR) is reduced to approximately 150 L/min.
- Reversible airflow obstruction is characteristic of asthma and can be demonstrated by spirometry (Fig. 4.2); a greater than 15% improvement in the FEV_1 (when the absolute value is more than 1 liter) 5 to 10 minutes following treatment with a short-acting inhaled beta$_2$ agonist is generally accepted as diagnostic for asthma. Alternatively, following outpatient treatment, a 15% or greater improvement in the FEV_1 between office visits proves reversible airway disease and a diagnosis of asthma.

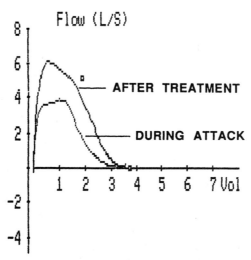

Figure 4.2. A typical flow-volume curve of a patient during an attack of asthma. Peak flow is reduced to less than 4 L/sec with marked improvement to more than 6 L/sec after bronchodilator treatment. The small square above the curve signals a time of 1 second for calculation of the FEV_1.

- When the FVC is reduced and the flow rates are normal, restrictive lung disease should be considered as a cause of the patient's symptoms (see Chapter 6). Lung volume determinations should be measured by helium dilution or other measurements. The total lung capacity (TLC), functional residual capacity (FRC), and residual volume (RV) are all reduced to below normal (less than 80% of predicted).

PEFR measurements can be determined from measurements during office spirometry or with the use of inexpensive portable peak flow meters that can be used by the patient in the home or by emergency room personnel to assess the response to treatment. When done properly, with good effort, the PEFR done by these lightweight plastic devices correlates well with the FEV_1 measurement done by spirometry.

- Short-term home monitoring with the PEFR meter can be useful in diagnosing asthma, in identifying environmental triggers of asthma, and can detect early signs of deterioration when symptoms change. Long-term monitoring is useful for those individuals with severe brittle asthma and for those who have a poor perception of asthma symptoms.
- Peak flow measurements ideally should be done early in the morning (when measurements tend to be lowest) and in the evening (when measurements should be highest), 5 to 10 minutes after inhaling a beta agonist. Each patient should establish a personal best PEFR after a period of maximal therapy.
- The severity of asthma is reflected not only by the level of baseline obstruction but also by its variability over a 24-hour period. A zone system has been devised for patient ease: Green is 80–100% of the personal best and shows good control; yellow is 50–80% of personal best and signals caution that asthma is not under sufficient control; red is below 50% of personal best and signifies danger and need for immediate physician intervention.
- A diurnal variation of PEFR of 20% is diagnostic of asthma. The magnitude of peak flow variability is in general proportional to the severity of the disease. A high degree of variability signals unstable asthma that demands increased medication.

Analysis of arterial blood gases is not necessary in asymptomatic or stable asthma. During an acute attack, an assessment of oxygen saturation by transcutaneous oximetry is helpful to ensure adequate oxygenation. The mechanism of arterial hypoxemia is ventilation/perfusion mismatch. Areas with low ventilation to perfusion ratios cause hypoxemia and are caused by bronchospasm, mucous plugging, and mucosal swelling from inflammation. Virtually all asthmatics have hypoxemia during an acute exacerbation; the more severe the attack the lower the arterial oxygen tension. Arterial blood gas analysis is indicated during a severe attack. Associated with hypoxemia and present in approximately 75% of patients are hypocarbia and respiratory alkalosis. When the obstruction worsens and the FEV_1 approaches approximately 15–20% of predicted, the PCO_2 normalizes. Carbon dioxide retention occurs when the FEV_1 reaches less than 15% of predicted and the absolute FEV_1 is severely reduced to less than 0.5 L. Acute respiratory acidosis results. This occurs in approximately 10% of asthmatics who seek emergency care and often but not invariably requires orotracheal intubation and mechanical ventilation. The mechanism of carbon dioxide retention in severe asthma is severe ventilation/perfusion mismatch. High ventilation to perfusion ratios cause dead space or wasted ventilation. As the work of breathing increases and carbon dioxide production rises, the lungs become incapable of removing the carbon dioxide that is produced and respiratory acidosis occurs. It is believed that respiratory muscle fatigue also contributes to respiratory failure, and in extreme cases, sudden respiratory muscle failure can result in acute cardiopulmonary arrest. Superimposed metabolic acidosis is seen on blood gas analysis in severe cases. This may be the result of lactic acidosis caused by vigorous muscle contraction, inadequate cardiac output, and is possibly a complication of excessive sympathomimetic use.

Sinus tachycardia is also a known complication of sympathomimetic use. Most patients with acute asthma have a sinus tachycardia. It is interesting that as airway function improves with sympathomimetic treatment, sinus tachycardia actually improves rather than worsens. In acute asthma, premature ventricular contractions occasionally occur, while atrial arrhythmias are extremely uncommon. Other electrocardiographic abnormalities seen in acute severe asthma include p-pulmonale, right axis shift, right bundle branch block, and right ventricular strain.

Inhalation challenge testing is useful in some patients when the diagnosis of asthma is not clear. For example, a diagnosis of asthma cannot be proven when the patient has normal peak flow rates and spirometry even when there are typical asthma symptoms. In such cases, an FEV_1 response to bronchodilators or fluctuation in diurnal PEFR cannot be used as criteria for asthma. In such instances, methacholine or histamine bronchoprovocation testing can be useful. Low concentrations of the agonist are inhaled after baseline spirometry ensures normal or near normal airway function. Gradually increasing doses are given, either by tidal volume breathing or

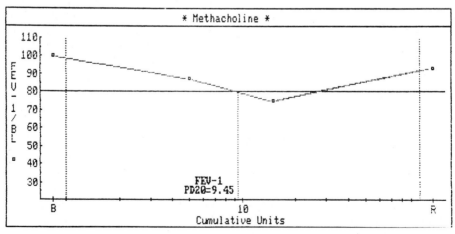

Figure 4.3A. The dose response curve of an asthmatic with a positive methacholine inhalation challenge. A drop in the FEV_1 (vertical axis) of 20% is shown to occur with less than 10 cumulative dose units (horizontal axis). The provocative dose to cause a 20% drop in the FEV_1 (PD_{20}) is shown to be 9.45.

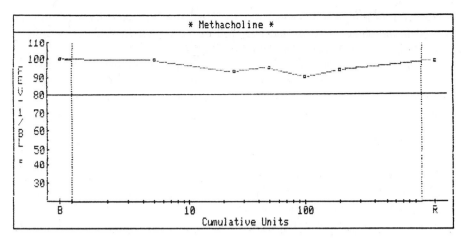

Figure 4.3B. This negative methacholine challenge rules out a diagnosis of asthma. The maximum decrease in FEV_1 of less than 10% seen during the challenge is less than the 20% drop needed for a positive challenge.

by single deep breaths from a dosimeter, and the forced spirogram is repeated after each dose. A calculation of the FEV_1 at each dose produces a dose response curve. If the FEV_1 drops 20% below baseline at any standard dose, the test is positive. An inhaled beta agonist is given that promptly returns lung function to baseline. By a linear interpolation of the dose response curve, the dose of methacholine or histamine that causes a 20% drop in the FEV_1 is calculated (Fig. 4.3). This is called the PD_{20}—the provocative dose that causes a 20% reduction of the FEV_1, or the PC_{20}—the provocative concentration that causes a 20% reduction of the FEV_1. A low PD_{20} is typical of asthma but not specific for asthma because it can be seen in a number of other inflammatory airway diseases. A normal response to methacholine or histamine is incompatible with asthma, and an alternative diagnosis should be considered.

TREATMENT

There are both short-term and long-term therapeutic objectives for every asthmatic patient. Short-term objectives are the control of immediate symptoms and the response to falling peak flow rate measurements. Long-term objectives are those directed to disease prevention because there are now well-proven strategies to avoid serious exacerbations of acute bronchospasm, which often lead to emergency room visits or hospitalization. To meet these therapeutic objectives, four components of asthma care should be addressed:

• Optimal treatment of asthma depends on a careful assessment of the patient's symptoms as well as objective monitoring by office spirometry and home PEFR measurements.

- Treatment of asthma with bronchodilator and antiinflammatory medication is tailored to the patient's needs and relies on a staging system that is based on the symptoms and objective measures of lung function.
- Measures should be taken to avoid respiratory allergens and irritants that can cause worsening of symptoms. These measures include avoidance of outdoor allergens (such as ragweed, grass, pollens, and molds) and indoor allergens (such as animal dander, house dust mites and cockroach antigen). When exposure cannot be avoided, allergen immunotherapy should be considered. Indoor irritants, such as smoke from cigarettes and wood-burning stoves, strong odors, and cleaning solutions, are particularly troublesome.
- Patient education can be a powerful tool in asthma control. Family members also can be helpful, especially with children and elderly adults. Active participation by a patient in monitoring lung function, avoidance of provocative agents, and decisions regarding medications provide asthma management skills that give the patient the confidence to control his or her own disease.

Medications

Antiinflammatory Agents

- Antiinflammatory agents are capable of reducing airway inflammation and thereby improving lung function, decreasing bronchial hyperreactivity, reducing symptoms, and improving the overall quality of life.
- Corticosteroids are the most useful antiinflammatory agents. They act by preventing migration and activation of inflammatory cells, interfering with the production of prostaglandins and leukotrienes, reducing microvascular leakage, and enhancing the action of beta adrenergic receptors on airway smooth muscle.
- Corticosteroids are available for oral, parenteral, and inhaled use. Oral preparations, such as prednisone, are useful for acute exacerbations of asthma unresponsive to bronchodilator therapy. Doses of 40–60 mg/day are given until the patient responds, and then the dosage can be slowly tapered. Often, poorly controlled asthma requires daily or every other day maintenance with prednisone in doses of 10–15 mg. Intravenous corticosteroids, usually given as methylprednisolone, 60–80 mg every 6 to 8 hours for 1 or 2 days, are effective within 4 to 6 hours of administration in preventing further progression of the severe asthma exacerbation that requires hospitalization.
- Inhaled corticosteroids are safe and effective treatment for moderate to severe asthma and have been in use for more than 20 years. Formulations of beclomethasone, triamcinolone, flunisolide, fluticasone, and budesonide can reduce airway inflammation with one to several months of treatment (see Chapter 3).
- Long-term use of inhaled corticosteroids has been associated with a good safety profile. High doses of inhaled steroids (e.g., greater than 1 mg/day of beclomethasone) are capable of causing hypophyseal-pituitary-adrenal (HPA) axis suppression. Local adverse effects, such as hoarseness, dysphonia, cough, and oral candidiasis, do occur but can usually be avoided by using a spacer or holding chamber

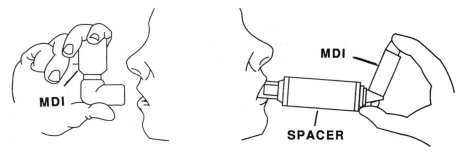

Figure 4.4. A metered dose inhaler (MDI) technique without a spacer is shown in the patient on the left. The inhaler should be shaken before use. The patient breathes out gently, puts the mouthpiece in the mouth or just outside of the mouth, and then starts inspiration. At this point, the cannister is pressed down and the patient inhales slowly and deeply. The breath is then held for approximately 10 seconds. The patient on the right is using a spacer as a holding chamber for the inhaled medication. The patient depresses the cannister into the spacer and breathes in slowly and deeply, holding the breath for 10 seconds.

(Fig. 4.4) and by rinsing the mouth after each use. Oral and parental corticosteroids are associated with many side effects, such as the risk of osteoporosis, cataracts, diabetes mellitus, and, rarely, depression of immunity to infection. Attempts to reduce dependence on oral corticosteroids should be made, especially by the use of inhaled agents.

- Cromolyn sodium and nedocromil sodium are two antiinflammatory agents that are available in inhaled form and that have an extremely good safety profile. A 4–6 week trial may be useful to determine their effectiveness in the prevention of asthma symptoms. These agents are capable of preventing allergen-induced bronchospasm.

Bronchodilators

- Inhaled short-acting beta$_2$ adrenergic agonists are the treatment of choice for the acute exacerbation of asthma symptoms. Inhaled agents can be delivered by metered dose inhaler (Fig. 4.4), dry-powder capsules, and compressor-driven nebulizers. Long-acting beta$_2$ agonists may be helpful for long-term maintenance therapy and to control nocturnal symptoms (see Chapter 3).
- The use of regularly scheduled as opposed to "as needed" (PRN) dosing of beta$_2$ agonists has been associated with diminished control of asthma and heightened bronchial reactivity. In addition, epidemiologic evidence has linked excessive beta$_2$ agonist use to increased mortality. Ideally, short-acting beta$_2$ adrenergic agonists should be prescribed for acute symptom relief on an as-needed basis. The need for regularly scheduled doses should alert the physician to the need for more intense antiinflammatory medication.
- Theophylline is an effective bronchodilator and has antiinflammatory properties. It is available as a sustained release preparation and can be taken once or twice

daily. Monitoring of theophylline blood levels is important to avoid toxicity, especially in the elderly, who are more prone to adverse effects. Gastrointestinal side effects are seen with mild toxicity and blood levels in the range of 20 to 30 $\mu g/$mL. Serious cardiac arrhythmias and seizures may occur with blood levels in excess of this range. A range of 8 to 15 $\mu g/mL$ is generally considered therapeutic.

- Inhaled anticholinergic agents, such as ipratropium, produce bronchodilatation by reducing vagal tone and are widely used in patients with COPD. They may be useful in combination with beta$_2$ agonists for a severe acute exacerbation of asthma. Their role in long-term maintenance in asthma has not been established. They may be tried as a substitute bronchodilator when side effects preclude the use of beta$_2$ agonists, although it must be remembered that they have a slower onset of action of 30–60 minutes until maximal effect.

Treatment Protocols for Asthma

- A global strategy for asthma management and prevention has been proposed through the efforts of the NIH and the World Health Organization (WHO). Treatment protocols use step-care pharmacologic therapy based on the intensity of asthma symptoms and the clinical response to these interventions.
- Mild asthma characterized by intermittent, brief (less than 1 hour) symptoms occurring no more than two times a week can be treated with PRN beta$_2$ agonists.
- Moderate asthma characterized by frequent (more than twice a week) attacks of asthma symptoms or diminished pulmonary function (FEV$_1$ or PEFR 60–80% predicted) requires regularly administered antiinflammatory agents, such as inhaled corticosteroids or cromolyn. Beta$_2$ agonists can be used for rescue therapy. If symptoms persist despite optimal doses of inhaled corticosteroids, several options are available. Sustained-release oral theophylline preparations may be useful, especially in the patient with nocturnal awakenings. Long-acting inhaled beta agonists are also useful when used on a regular daily basis. Alternatively, higher doses or more potent preparations of inhaled corticosteroids can be used, with the knowledge that there is a potential for HPA axis suppression.
- Patients with severe asthma have continuous symptoms, frequent exacerbations, and limited level of activity. Pulmonary function testing shows an FEV$_1$ that is less than 60% predicted and reduced peak flow rates that may show marked diurnal variations. These patients should be evaluated by an asthma expert. It is usually necessary in such patients to treat continuously with inhaled corticosteroids and long-acting bronchodilators, and the patient frequently relies on 2–3 puffs of a short-acting beta$_2$ agonist for rescue therapy. Oral corticosteroids are also useful for exacerbations of severe symptoms and avoidance of hospitalization. Doses of 40–60 mg of prednisone are given and repeated daily until the attack breaks. Rapid tapering can then be accomplished. Some severe asthmatics require daily or alternate-day corticosteroids to control their symptoms. When corticosteroids fail or cause disabling complications or when higher doses must be used over a long period of time, alternate therapies can be considered. These include treatment with methotrexate, cyclosporin A, and intravenous immunoglobulin. Conclusive proof that these agents are useful requires future study.

ASTHMA SYNDROMES
Exercise-induced Asthma (EIA)

Nearly all asthmatics experience increased bronchospasm following vigorous exercise at some point in time in their history. If tested in the pulmonary function laboratory off medication, 70–80% of patients will show a characteristic drop in peak flow or FEV_1 immediately after a 6–8 minute exercise challenge (Fig. 4.5). During exercise patients seem to be protected, as the airways actually dilate, possibly as a result of circulating catecholamines. Symptoms of cough and shortness of breath parallel the drop in lung function, which usually reaches its peak response 5–10 minutes postexercise. Often patients hear no wheezing during the attack, and in some patients, atypical presentations of chest tightness or chest pain alone will occur. A cardiac workup may often precede pulmonary testing in such patients. The symptoms usually abate without treatment, although a short-acting beta agonist immediately returns lung function to normal. Occasionally the attack following exercise can be severe and may require emergency treatment.

The mechanisms that cause exercise-induced bronchospasm in susceptible patients, such as asthmatics, some patients with allergic rhinitis, and patients with cystic fibrosis, have been intensely studied. As ventilation increases with exercise, cooler, dryer air is drawn into the airways in greater quantities, causing heat and water loss from the airways into the airstream. Airway cooling and mucosal drying are thought to trigger mast cells to release their mediators. The greater the heat and water loss, the greater the degree of bronchospasm.

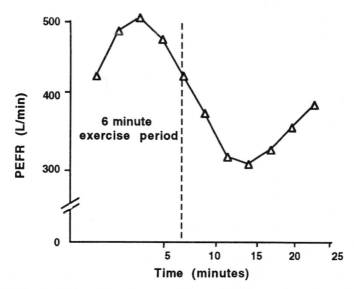

Figure 4.5. Exercise-induced bronchospasm. The peak expiratory flow (PEFR) initially increases during exercise and promptly falls 5–10 minutes after the challenge is completed. Spontaneous resolution without therapy begins in 15–20 minutes.

Many factors may enhance or reduce the risk of exercise-induced bronchospasm:

- Patients with poorly controlled asthma are more likely to have EIA.
- Exercise in cold dry air is more likely to cause EIA.
- Running, especially outdoors, is more likely to cause EIA than are other activities (such as swimming).
- The greater the intensity of the exercise, the more likely the bronchospasm.
- Bronchoconstriction becomes less intense during a second challenge if performed an hour or so after the first. An intense warm-up period 30–60 minutes before competitive sports can be helpful.
- Pretreatment can effectively block EIA in more than 90% of patients. Beta$_2$ agonists are the first choice, and cromolyn is a good alternative. They can be used together if needed.

Nocturnal Asthma

Exacerbations of wheezing and shortness of breath are a common cause of sleep deprivation in asthma and tend to be underreported by patients and overlooked by physicians. Even in patients whose disease is mild and apparently controlled by medication, as many as 25% of patients will awake at least once during the night because of their asthma. Deaths from asthma have been rising in many countries over the past few decades and most of these deaths from asthma occur at night, between midnight and 8 AM. The mechanisms of nocturnal asthma are not completely understood, but it has been observed that lung function has a definite circadian rhythm and that peak expiratory flow rates are highest at 4 PM and lowest at 4 AM. Normal individuals show only an approximate 8% fluctuation, while many asthmatics during periods of unstable symptoms can show as much as a 50% variation in peak expiratory rates in a 24-hour period. This can result in frequent nocturnal awakenings and the need for frequent rescue therapy.

Sustained release theophylline has proven to be a valuable tool in the control of nocturnal asthma. Long-acting beta agonists, such as oral extended-release albuterol and inhaled salmeterol, are also helpful. Because research with bronchoalveolar lavage has shown that levels of inflammatory cells and epithelial sloughing is highest at 4 AM, the keystone to controlling nocturnal asthma is control of the inflammatory response with inhaled or, if necessary, oral corticosteroids.

Aspirin-induced Asthma

Acute idiosyncratic reactions to aspirin may result in either acute bronchospasm or urticaria-angioedema, rarely both together. Aspirin-induced asthma is a syndrome that affects predominantly adults rather than children and nonatopics. One-third of patients, however, may manifest positive immediate skin test hypersensitivity to inhaled aeroallergens. The disease usually evolves over decades and first begins as chronic nonallergic perennial rhinitis, often complicated by nasal polyposis and recurrent bacterial sinusitis. Asthma then appears and is often severe and unremitting, requiring treatment with systemic steroids. Although aspirin may have been tolerated previously, suddenly the patient develops acute bronchospasm thirty minutes to several hours after ingesting a standard dose of oral aspirin. This may also be associated with flushing of the face and ocular and nasal congestion. Cross-sensitivity occurs with other nonsteroidal antiinflammatory drugs, such as indomethacin, naproxen, ibuprofen, sulindac, and piroxicam—all inhibitors of prostaglandin synthesis from the cyclooxygenase pathway of arachidonic acid metabolism. Noninhibitors, such as sodium salicylate, salicylamide, propoxyphene, and acetaminophen, do not cause the reaction. It is believed that by blocking the cyclooxygenase pathway, arachidonic acid metabolism is preferentially shifted to the 5-lipoxygenase pathway to produce leukotrienes, potent bronchoconstrictors. There is a fourfold increase in urinary leukotriene E_4 (LTE_4) after aspirin provocation in the aspirin-sensitive patient.

The prevalence of aspirin-induced bronchospasm in the population of asthmatics depends on the population studied. Approximately 3–5% of hospitalized asthmatics have a history of a reaction to aspirin. This number is higher at highly specialized referral centers where the most severe asthmatics are cared for. Treatment is, of course, avoidance of aspirin and nonsteroidal antiinflammatory agents with known cross-reactivity. For the occasional patient who needs these drugs, oral desensitization protocols using gradually increasing doses of aspirin are effective. Using aspirin desensitization, approximately two-thirds of the patients report significant improvement in their rhinosinusitis and approximately one-half have improvement in their asthma. The recent addition of 5-lipoxygenase inhibitors as therapeutic options for asthma is important because the agents have been shown to block aspirin-induced bronchospasm in sensitive patients.

Occupational Asthma

Asthma that is precipitated by a particular occupational environment and not to stimuli outside of the workplace is called occupational asthma. Two types have been described: (a) asthma that follows a latent period of exposure to either a high or low molecular weight "sensitizing" antigen and (b) asthma that follows exposure to workplace irritants. One form of irritant-induced asthma is called RADS (reactive airways dysfunction syndrome), a condition that usually results from the sudden inhalation of a large dose of a highly irritating substance. Exposure to six major categories of agents can result in occupational asthma:

- Exposure to animals, shellfish, fish, and arthropods can cause asthma in farmers, laboratory workers, grain handlers, and poultry workers.
- Exposure to wood, plants, and vegetables can cause asthma in woodworkers, carpenters, grain handlers, bakers, and tobacco workers.
- Enzymes and pharmaceuticals are known to cause asthma in pharmaceutical workers, pharmacists, and detergent industry workers.
- Low molecular weight chemicals cause asthma in solderers, spray painters, chemical manufacturers, polyurethane manufacturers, and electronics workers.

- Metals and metal salts, such as aluminum, chromium, cobalt, nickel, and platinum fumes, can cause asthma in electroplaters, hard metal workers, polishers, and solderers.
- Dusts, fumes, and gases may cause asthma from a sudden high concentration exposure, usually caused by an accident in the workplace or by less severe repetitive exposures.

Estimates on the prevalence of occupational asthma vary, but it is estimated that 2–15% of all adult-onset asthma is the result of workplace exposure. Seeking occupational causes of asthma in the patient's history can be rewarding and can lead to primary prevention by avoidance of the offending environment.

Cough-variant Asthma

At times, cough may be the sole presenting manifestation of asthma, and the characteristic findings of variable airflow obstruction may not be present. As a result, cough-variant asthma is significantly underdiagnosed. There is evidence that cough receptors in the airways are separate from bronchoconstrictive receptors, and this may explain why such patients do not wheeze. In addition, cough receptors are more abundant in more central airways and uncommon in peripheral airways. The cough receptors are presumably stimulated by the inflammatory cell mediators that are released in the asthmatic process. Inflammation that preferentially involves the central airways could also explain this syndrome.

The diagnosis of cough-variant asthma should be suspected in a patient with a chronic cough that has been present for months and even years and no obvious cause seen on the chest roentgenogram. The history is often suggestive in that the patient coughs vigorously after exposure to fumes, cigarette smoke, and other irritants, and often after laughter and exercise. The diagnosis depends on a positive bronchial inhalation challenge with methacholine, histamine, or exercise, and a clinical response to bronchodilators and/or antiinflammatory agents.

Fatal and Near-fatal Asthma

Despite our better understanding of the pathogenesis of asthma and more effective treatment programs, morbidity and mortality associated with this condition still remain a problem in most countries in the industrialized world. Many factors have been proposed to explain this dilemma. These factors include:

- Poor compliance with medication and asthma monitoring;
- An underestimation by the patient and physician alike of the severity of the asthma;
- Poor long-term access to medical care (especially for the poor);
- Over-reliance on inhaled beta agonist therapy.

Near-fatal attacks of asthma are the result of acute hypercarbic respiratory acidosis and are not associated with serious cardiac arrhythmias. Despite severe degrees of acidosis, even to pH levels below 7.0, recovery can be rapid and complete. In fact,

Table 4.3. Causes Identified with a Near-fatal Asthma Attack

Environmental allergen exposure
Upper respiratory viral infection
Profound emotional upsets
Beta blocker drugs
Air pollution following a thermal inversion
Aspirin and NSAID ingestion in those sensitive

there is evidence that when the asthma attack is sudden, only a few hours of duration before respiratory failure ensues, recovery too is rapid, often more rapid than slowly progressive asthma. The term sudden asphyxic asthma has been given to such attacks. Evidence suggests that such patients are immunohistologically different, in that their airways are characterized by a relative paucity of eosinophils and a large number of neutrophils compared with the classic asthma picture.

The most commonly identified causes of near-fatal asthma are found in Table 4.3. Risk factors for fatal or near-fatal asthma are:

- High medication use (three or more medications);
- Overuse of inhaled beta agonists;
- A history of recurrent hospitalizations;
- Previous occurrences of life-threatening attacks;
- Marked fluctuations in AM and PM peak flow rate measurements.

In addition, recent investigations have shown that patients with near-fatal attacks have abnormal respiratory control mechanisms, such as a blunted perception of dyspnea and a reduced hypoxic ventilatory response to hypoxia.

BIBLIOGRAPHY

Barnes PJ. Mechanisms of action of glucocorticoids in asthma. Am J Respir Crit Care Med 1996;154:S21.

Barnes PJ, Holgate ST, Laitinen LA, Pauwels R. Asthma mechanisms, determinants of severity and treatment: the role of nedocromil sodium. Clin Exp Allergy 1995;25:771.

Bone RC. Goals of asthma management. A step-care approach. Chest 1996;109:1056.

Boulet LP, Cournoyer I, Deschesnes F, et al. Perception of airflow obstruction and associated breathlessness in normal and asthmatic subjects: correlation with anxiety and bronchodilator needs. Thorax 1994;49:965.

Braman SS. Drug treatment of asthma in the elderly. Drugs 1996;51:415.

Busse WW, McGill K, Jarjour NN. Current management of asthma patients with corticosteroid resistance. Am J Respir Crit Care Med 1996;154:570.

Campbell DA, Yellowlees PM, McLennan G, et al. Psychiatric and medical features of near-fatal asthma. Thorax 1995;50:254.

Chan-Yeung M (chair). Assessment of asthma in the workplace (ACCP consensus statement). Chest 1995;108:1084.

Corbridge TC, Hall JB. The assessment and management of adults with status asthmaticus. Am J Respir Crit Care Med 1995;151:1296.

Creer TL, Levstek D. Medication compliance and asthma: overlooking the trees because of the forest. J Asthma 1996;33:203.

Creticos PS, Reed CE, Norman PS, et al. Ragweed immunotherapy in adult asthma. N Engl J Med 1996;334:501.

Devoy MAB, Fuller RW, Palmer JBD. Are there any detrimental effects of the use of inhaled long-acting β2-agonists in the treatment of asthma? Chest 1995;107:1116.

Goldstein RA (moderator), Paul WE, Metcalfe DD, Busse WW, Reece ER (discussants). Asthma (NIH Conference). Ann Intern Med 1994;121:698.

Jarjour NN, Busse WW. Understanding and identifying nocturnal asthma. J Respir Dis 1994; 15:S19.

Johnson M. Pharmacodynamics and pharmacokinetics of inhaled glucocorticoids. J Allergy Clin Immunol 1996;97:169.

Kay AB. Pathology of mild, severe, and fatal asthma. Am J Respir Crit Care Med 1996;154: 566.

Kikuchi Y, Okabe S, Tamura G, et al. Chemosensitivity and perception of dyspnea in patients with a history of near-fatal asthma. N Engl J Med 1994;330:1329.

Lock SH, Kay AB, Barnes NC. Double-blind, placebo-controlled study of cyclosporin A as a corticosteroid-sparing agent in corticosteroid-dependent asthma. Am J Respir Crit Care Med 1996;153:509.

McFadden ER Jr. Exercise-induced airway obstruction. Clin Chest Med 1995;16:671.

Moss RB. Alternative pharmacotherapies for steroid-dependent asthma. Chest 1995;107:817.

National Institutes of Health. Global initiative for asthma. Global strategy for asthma management and prevention. NHLBI/WHO Workshop Report, March 1993. NHLBI Publication #95–3659, January 1995.

Newman KB, Mason UG, Schmaling KB. Clinical features of vocal cord dysfunction. Am J Respir Crit Care Med 1995;152:1382.

O'Byrne PM. The natural history of asthma. Eur Respir Rev 1996;6:23.

Pauwels RA, Joos GF, Kips JC. Leukotrienes as therapeutic target in asthma. Allergy 1995; 50:615.

Peat JK. Prevention of asthma. Eur Respir J 1996;9:1545.

Pedersen S. Important issues in childhood asthma. Eur Respir Rev 1996;6:192.

Robinson DS, Geddes DM. Inhaled corticosteroids: benefits and risks. J Asthma 1996;33:5.

Sears MR. What role for β-agonists in managing asthma today? J Respir Dis 1994;15:S29.

Simpson WG. Gastroesophageal reflux disease and asthma: diagnosis and management. Arch Intern Med 1995;155:798.

Suissa S, Ernst P, Boivin JF, et al. A cohort analysis of excess mortality in asthma and the use of inhaled β-agonists. Am J Respir Crit Care Med 1994;149:604.

Wood AJJ. β-adrenergic bronchodilators. N Engl J Med 1995;333:499.

5 Chronic Obstructive Pulmonary Disease

Bartolome R. Celli

Chronic obstructive pulmonary disease (COPD) has been recently defined by the American Thoracic Society (ATS) as a disease state characterized by the presence of airflow obstruction caused by chronic bronchitis (airways disease) or emphysema (parenchymal destruction with airspace enlargement). The airflow obstruction is generally progressive, may be accompanied by hyperactivity, and may be potentially reversible. This definition is similar to that expressed by other international respiratory societies in similar statements. Inherent to the definition is the acknowledgment that many patients with COPD may show a significant reversible component in their airflow obstruction and that patients with asthma may go on to develop irreversible airflow obstruction indistinguishable from COPD.

Chronic bronchitis is defined in clinical terms as presence of chronic cough with phlegm production for 3 months in each of 2 consecutive years, without other specific causes of cough (e.g., asthma, bronchiectasis, cystic fibrosis). Emphysema is defined pathologically as abnormal airspace enlargement. Figure 5.1 graphically represents the interrelation of the different nosologic components that lead to COPD and helps the reader better understand the concepts. Most patients with asthma have significant reversible airways constriction and respond well to inhaled and systemic antiinflammatory therapy and therefore do not have COPD. As stated before, a minority of asthmatics go on to develop minimally reversible airflow limitation indistinguishable from COPD. This group of patients does have COPD and are treated as such.

EPIDEMIOLOGY AND RISK FACTORS

It is estimated that close to 14 million people in the United States suffer from COPD. This number has increased 42% since 1982. Although between 1979 and 1986 the prevalence varied from 4 to 6% in adult men and from 1 to 3% in adult women, the increase was more prevalent in women than in men. There were 85,544 deaths from COPD in 1991 (death rate of 18 per 100,000 persons). COPD ranks as the fourth leading cause of death, but it was the fastest rising cause (33%) between 1979 and 1991. When adjusted by age, the death rate from COPD rose 72% between 1966 and 1986. This is particularly important because the death rate for all causes decreased 22%, and the death rate from heart and cerebrovascular disease declined 45 and 58%, respectively. Fortunately, there has been a progressive decline in the

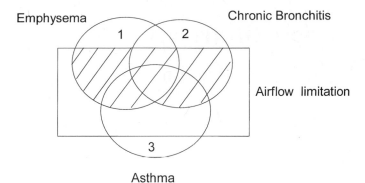

Figure 5.1. Nonproportional Venn diagram. Each circle represents a nosologic entity. The rectangle represents airflow limitation as documented in a forced spirometry. The shaded area corresponds to patients diagnosed as having COPD. Notice that a patient (subset 1) may present with emphysema without COPD (patient with bullae on chest roentgenogram without airflow limitation). Similarly, he or she may present with sputum production and normal spirometry (subset 2, with simple bronchitis). Finally, an asthmatic may present without airflow limitation (subset 3) and will only be diagnosed after a bronchoprovocation test (subset 3).

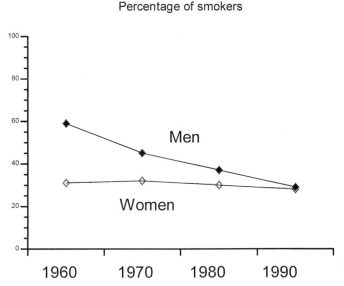

Figure 5.2. Prevalence by decade of smoking habit in the general population of the United States.

percentage of the population who smoke (Fig. 5.2). This should result in decreased mortality from COPD in the near future. Interestingly, most of the decrease is attributable to smoking cessation in men and not in women. Even greater efforts must be devoted to smoking cessation because the habit is still practiced by 75 million citizens in the United States alone. Assuming the same prevalence around the world, there is an astonishing total of 1.2 billion human beings exposed to the ravages of cigarettes.

As shown in Table 5.1, the most important cause of COPD is cigarette smoking. Other possible causes may act as independent risk factors in its genesis, but their importance dwarfs in comparison with the role of cigarette smoking. The only other risk factor comparable to the importance of smoking is α_1-antitrypsin (AAT) deficiency, but AAT accounts for less than 1% of COPD cases.

Children exposed to cigarette smoke manifest a higher prevalence of respiratory symptoms and diseases compared with children of nonsmokers. They also show a measurable decrease in pulmonary function tests. Whether this leads to COPD remains unclear. Air pollution is harmful to patients with heart and lung disease and may be an important factor in certain geographic areas. Studies in nonsmoking persons who use solid fuels for indoor cooling and without adequate ventilation have revealed the presence of COPD in some of the patients. This evidence does support some role for pollutants in the genesis of COPD, but it would be small by comparison with cigarette smoking in countries with better pollution control. Exposure to polluting agents in the environment may operate in the same way and may certainly worsen the function of patients with airflow obstruction. Morbidity and mortality rates from COPD are higher for whites than for nonwhites and are higher in blue-collar versus white-collar workers. COPD also aggregates in families independent of AAT deficiency.

Atopy, hyperresponsive airways, and asthma may play a role in the genesis of COPD. Since it was first proposed by researchers in the Netherlands, the "Dutch Hypothesis" has been the subject of interesting analyses. It has been shown that airway hyperactivity is inversely related to FEV_1 and that it is predictive of an accelerated rate of decline of lung function in smokers. In the Lung Health Study of COPD, a significant proportion of men (59%) and even more women (81%) manifested airways hyperactivity. This suggests that hyperactive airways may be an

Table 5.1. Risk Factors for the Development of COPD

Established	Probable	Possible
Cigarette smoking	Air pollution	Low birth weight
Occupational exposure (work smoke)	Poverty	Childhood respiratory infections
α_1-antitrypsin	Childhood exposure to smoke	Family history
	Alcohol	Atopy
	Hyperreactive airways	IgA nonsecretor
		Blood group A

important factor contributing to FEV_1 decline in some patients with COPD, but its true importance remains undetermined.

The only host factor proven to lead to COPD is deficiency of AAT. This serum protein is made by the liver and its main role is the inhibition of neutrophil elastase. It is a glycoprotein coded for by a single gene on chromosome 14. The normal value of AAT is 150–350 mg/dL (commercial standard) or 20–48 mg/dL (laboratory standard). There are rare instances of patients with normal levels of dysfunctional AAT. Most individuals with severe deficiency are homozygous for the Z allele (PiZZ) and have extremely low levels of AAT (mean 18% of the value seen in normals). The threshold protective level of AAT is approximately 80 mg/dL (35% normal) because heterozygous persons (PiSZ) with these levels rarely develop emphysema. Severe AAT deficiency leads to premature emphysema, often with chronic bronchitis, nonspecific airway hyperactivity, and, occasionally, bronchiectasis. The onset of disease is accelerated by smoking, and dyspnea begins at the median age of 40 in smokers and at 50 in nonsmokers. Not all patients with AAT will develop emphysema, especially if not exposed to cigarettes or pollution. Patients should be screened for AAT if they present with premature onset of COPD (before age 50), predominance of basilar emphysema (by x-ray), presence of nonremitting asthma in a young person, and liver cirrhosis without apparent risk factors.

Natural History

The decline in lung function with time is shown in Figure 5.3. Normal nonsmokers lose between 25 to 35 mL yearly. The rate of decline is steeper for smokers than for nonsmokers. The heavier the smoking, the steeper the decline; likewise, the lower the initial FEV_1, the faster FEV_1 will drop. The FEV_1 of patients with COPD decreases around 90 mL a year. The Lung Health Study showed that patients who stopped smoking had a mean postbronchodilator FEV_1 increase of 57 mL at the first annual visit, compared with a mean FEV_1 decline of 38 mL for those that continued to smoke. This indicates not only will the decline decrease but also that lung function may actually improve after smoking cessation. The natural rate of decline accelerates dramatically in susceptible smokers. The rate of decline returns toward normal soon after smoking cessation in most patients, whereas the development of symptoms with minimal activities will occur much earlier in current smokers than in ex-smokers.

CLINICAL FEATURES

History

The typical patient with COPD has smoked more than 20 pack/years before symptoms develop. He or she commonly presents with productive cough or an acute chest illness at around the 5th decade. Dyspnea usually begins around the 6th or 7th decade but it may become the dominant feature. Dyspnea may become crippling and lead to deconditioning as ever less intense exercise precipitates worsening of the symptom. This vicious cycle is one of the most important problems in patients with

Forced expiratory volume in 1 second (liters)

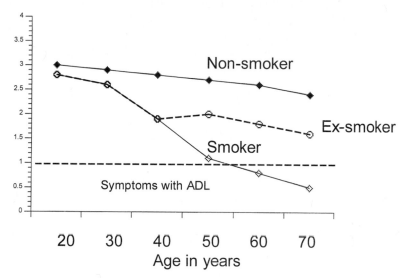

Figure 5.3. Rate of decline of lung function according to smoking habit. Notice that the rate of decline is steeper for current smokers and tends to return to the normal rate after smoking cessation. The onset of symptoms related to COPD will be delayed whenever smoking stops. *ADL,* activity of daily living.

advanced COPD. Breaking the cycle leads to improvement in the functional status of the patient.

Sputum initially occurs only in the morning and is usually mucoid. During exacerbations, it may become purulent. Acute chest illnesses characterized by increased cough, purulent sputum, wheezing, dyspnea, and occasionally fever may occur intermittently. The history of wheezing and dyspnea may lead to the erroneous diagnosis of asthma. As the disease progresses, the intervals between exacerbations shorten. Late in the course, the patient may develop hypoxemia that if severe enough may result in clinical cyanosis, which is accentuated by erythrocytosis. Development of morning headache suggests hypercapnia. Weight loss occurs in some patients, and cor pulmonale with right heart failure and edema may develop in patients with hypoxemia and hypercapnia. Most episodes of hemoptysis are caused by mucosal erosion, not carcinoma. Because bronchogenic carcinoma occurs with increased frequency in smokers with COPD, however, an episode of hemoptysis raises the possibility that a carcinoma has developed. It should prompt an evaluation to rule out this possibility.

Physical Examination

Initially, the chest examination may only show wheezes on forced expiration. As obstruction progresses, hyperinflation becomes evident and the anteroposterior diameter of the chest increases. The diaphragm is depressed and limited in its motion. Breath sounds are decreased at this stage and heart sounds often become distant. Coarse crackles are often heard at the lung bases. An excessively prolonged forced expiratory time (more than 4 seconds with the stethoscope over the trachea) may be seen in patients with a significant degree of airflow limitation. The patient with end-stage COPD may adopt positions that relieve dyspnea, such as leaning forward and supporting weight on the arms. The accessory respiratory muscles of the neck and shoulder girdle are in full use. Expiration often takes place through pursed lips and with forced contractions of the abdominal muscles. Paradoxical drawing in of the lower costal interspace with inspiration is a classic finding, first described by William Stokes in 1837. An enlarged tender liver indicates heart failure. Neck vein distension, especially during expiration, may be observed in the absence of heart failure because of increased intrathoracic pressure. Cyanosis may be present, and asterixis may be seen with severe hypoxemia and hypercapnia.

LABORATORY FINDINGS
Chest Radiography

Because emphysema is defined in anatomic terms, posteroanterior and lateral chest roentgenograms provide evidence of its presence. Hyperinflation is indicated by a low flat diaphragm, an increased retrosternal airspace, and a long narrow heart shadow (see Chapter 1). Rapid tapering of the vascular shadows accompanied by hypertransparency of the lungs is a sign of emphysema; bullae, presenting as radiolucent areas larger than 1 cm in diameter and surrounded by arcuate hairline shadows, suggest its presence. Bullae reflect only locally severe disease, however, and are not necessarily indicative of widespread emphysema. Studies correlating lung structure and the chest radiograph show that emphysema is consistently diagnosed when the disease is severe but is not that accurate when the disease is mild or even moderate. Right ventricular hypertrophy does not result in cardiomegaly in COPD. Comparison with previous chest radiographs may show the enlargement. The hilar vascular shadows are prominent and the heart shadow encroaches on the retrosternal space as the right ventricle enlarges anteriorly. Lung cancer and heart disease are associated with the same risk factor as COPD; namely, smoking. Therefore, a chest roentgenogram is indicated not only to find evidence of emphysema but also to rule out the presence of any of the diseases that may present with similar symptoms.

Computed Tomography

Computed tomography (CT), especially high-resolution CT scans (collimation of 1 to 2 mm), has much greater sensitivity and specificity than does standard chest radiography. Because it rarely alters therapy, however, CT has no place in the routine care of patients with COPD. It is the main imaging tool for evaluating the benefit of pulmonary resection for giant bullous disease and for diagnosing bronchiectasis. It also is gaining ground as a good tool for evaluating potential candidates for lung volume reduction surgery.

Pulmonary Function Tests

Determination of a forced vital capacity is necessary for the diagnosis and assessment of the severity of disease and is helpful in following its progress. The FEV_1 is easily measurable, has less variability than other measurements of airways dynamics, and is more accurately predictable from age, race, gender, and height (see Chapter 2). Roughly comparable information can be obtained from the peak flow measurement or from the forced expiratory flow volume curve. None of these tests can distinguish between chronic bronchitis and emphysema. The FEV_1 and the FEV_1/FVC ratio fall progressively as the severity of COPD increases. In the laboratory, approximately 30% of patients have an increase of 20% or greater in their FEV_1 following a $beta_2$ agonist or ipratropium bromide treatment.

Lung volume measurements show an increase in total lung capacity, functional residual capacity, and residual volume. The vital capacity may be decreased. The single-breath carbon monoxide diffusing capacity (D_{LCO}^{SB}) is decreased in proportion to the severity of emphysema because of the loss of alveolar-capillary bed. The test is not specific, nor can it detect mild emphysema. If the D_{LCO}^{SB} is disproportionally low in comparison with changes in other function tests, emphysema is more likely to be the cause of the obstruction. The presence of a low D_{LCO}^{SB} has correlated with exercise oxygen desaturation in patients with COPD.

Arterial blood gas reveals hypoxemia without hypercapnia in the early stages of the disease. As the disease progresses, hypoxemia becomes more severe and hypercapnia supervenes. Hypercapnia is observed with increasing frequency as the FEV_1 falls below 1 liter. Blood gas abnormalities worsen during acute exacerbations and may worsen during exercise and sleep. Erythrocytosis is infrequently observed in patients living at sea level who have PaO_2 levels greater than 55 mm Hg; the frequency of erythrocytosis increases as PaO_2 levels fall below 55 mm Hg.

Sputum Examination

In stable chronic bronchitis, sputum is mucoid and the predominant cell is the macrophage. With an exacerbation, sputum usually becomes purulent with an influx of neutrophils. Gram's stain usually shows a mixture of organisms. The most frequent pathogens cultured from the sputum are *Streptococcus pneumoniae, Haemophilus influenzae,* and *Moraxella catarrhalis.* Cultures and even Gram's stains, however, are rarely necessary before instituting antimicrobial therapy in the outpatient setting.

Diagnosis and Monitoring

In patients suspected of COPD, a forced spirometry provides the basic physiologic assessment needed to quantify obstruction. Arterial blood gases in patients with severe COPD (stage III) help to identify the presence and severity of hypoxemia and hypercapnia. The effect of inhaling a $beta_2$ agonist or ipratropium on the FEV_1 should be determined. Bronchodilators should not be withheld on the basis of this test. Measurements of lung volumes, diffusing capacity, or physiologic responses to exercise usually add little unless the diagnosis is in doubt or an assessment of operative risk is being made. Arterial blood gas measurements are not needed with mild or moderate disease unless symptoms or specific clinical findings suggest a need for them. With severe disease ($FEV_1 < 1$ liter), serial measurements of FEV_1 become relatively unimportant because of the difficulty of interpreting small changes. Serial blood gas measurements become the major test for monitoring the course of the disease.

Staging

There is no well-accepted staging or severity scoring system for patients with COPD. An ideal system would allow categorization of patients with COPD for epidemiologic and clinical studies, health resource planning, and prognosis. It would also facilitate communication between professionals. The strongest prognostic indicators for mortality are:

• The age of the patient;
• FEV_1;
• The presence of hypoxemia and hypercapnia.

We are limited to grading the disease based on some objective physiologic measure of pulmonary function, usually the FEV_1. The impact of COPD on the ability of patients to perform the normal activities of daily living, however, are incompletely described by the FEV_1. The cardinal symptom of COPD is dyspnea, which often limits functional activity, results in an inability to exercise, and frequently causes the patient to seek medical attention. Because COPD is a chronic disorder that limits the patient's ability to work and, in severe cases, impairs the activities of daily living, a staging system that includes some attribute of this limitation is highly desirable. An ideal classification should include elements of all three factors (FEV_1, capacity to perform activities of daily living (ADL) or to exercise, and dyspnea), but unfortunately this tool has yet to be developed. The current staging system as suggested by the ATS attempts to classify patients according to the degree of FEV_1 value (Table 5.2). This staging system is designed to help the clinician and health care provider identify the possible level of care and the complexity of the patient's illness.

Quality of Life

Not all of the problems associated with the development of COPD are described by physiologic variables (FEV_1 or arterial blood gases). Only weak associations have been described for FEV_1 and quality of life, or FEV_1 and dyspnea. Because of the capacity of certain questionnaires to provide an accurate estimation of a patient's quality of life in chronic diseases, there has been a recent interest to add this dimension to the evaluation of patients with COPD. These tools acquire particular importance in the comprehensive evaluation of different forms of treatment because there need not be an association between physiologic results and how patients perceive

Table 5.2. Staging of COPD

	Stage I	Stage II	Stage III
FEV$_1$ (predicted)	≥ 50%	36–49%	≤ 35%
Usual findings	Most of the patients; may be symptomatic; small impact on health-related quality of life issues; usually managed by primary care physicians	Minority of patients; symptomatic; moderate impact on health-related quality of life issues; may be hypoxemic; may be helped by evaluation from specialist	Small minority of patients; severe symptoms; large impact on health-related quality of life; hypoxemic, may show hypercapnia; best managed by professionals familiar with COPD

Table 5.3. Tools to Assess Outcomes

Quality of Life Assessment Tools
General
Quality of Well-Being Scale
Sickness Impact Profile
Nottingham Health Profile
Medical Outcomes Study Short Form
  (MOS SF-36)

Disease-Specific (Pulmonary)
The St. George's Respiratory Questionnaire
  (SGRQ)
Chronic Respiratory Disease Questionnaire
  (CRQ)
Pulmonary Functional Status and Dyspnea
  Questionnaire (PFSDQ)

Dyspnea Assessment Tools
Functional
Baseline Dyspnea Index (BDI)
Transitional Dyspnea Index (TDI)

Exercise-Related
Borg Scale
Visual Analog Scale (VAS)

Physiologic Tools
Complex
Cardiopulmonary Exercise Test
Pulmonary Function Testing
Graded Exercise Test

Simple
6- and 12-minute walk test
Walk up stairs

the effect of the intervention. A typical example is that of pulmonary rehabilitation. Several controlled trials have shown significant improvement in patients' perceived quality of life without demonstrable evidence of changes in lung function. Table 5.3 shows different quality of life questionnaires that have been validated and that are widely used. Some are generic in nature and are applicable to all forms of chronic diseases. They may not be sensitive enough to detect changes that may arise from improvement secondary to benefits in the respiratory domain. For this reason, there has been recent interest in the development of disease-specific quality of life questionnaires. In particular, the ones shown in Table 5.3 have been validated and proven

Table 5.4. Therapy of Patients with Symptomatic COPD

Interventions That Improve Survival	Interventions That Improve Symptoms
Smoking cessation	Pharmacotherapy
Oxygen therapy if hypoxemic	Rehabilitation:
	Education
	Training and exercise
	Psychological support
	Nutrition
	Surgery (pneumoplasty)

useful when evaluating patients with COPD. They have proven useful in research and may find a role in the everyday management of patients.

COMPREHENSIVE MANAGEMENT

The airflow obstruction of COPD is irreversible; this fact has generated an unjustified nihilistic therapeutic attitude in many health care providers. An optimistic attitude toward these patients, however, goes a long way in relieving patients' fears and misconceptions. Some forms of intervention significantly prolong life (Table 5.4); others improve symptoms and the quality of a patient's life once the diagnosis has been established.

The overall goals of treatment are to:

• Prevent further deterioration in lung function;
• Alleviate symptoms;
• Treat complications as they arise.

The patient should be encouraged to actively participate in his or her own health management. This concept of collaborative management may improve self-reliance and esteem. Although not proven, it may also help improve treatment compliance. Preventive care is extremely important and all patients should receive immunizations, including pneumococcal vaccine and yearly influenza vaccines. An algorithm detailing this comprehensive approach is shown in Figure 5.4.

Smoking Cessation

Because smoking is the major cause of COPD, smoking cessation is the most important component of therapy for patients who still smoke. It should become part of counseling in any patient even without COPD who smokes. Because secondary smoking is known to damage lung function, limitation of exposure to involuntary smoke, particularly in children, should be encouraged. Although most patients agree that smoking is risky, they seem unaware of its true significance. Continuous abstinence in pulmonary patients who have participated in smoking cessation programs

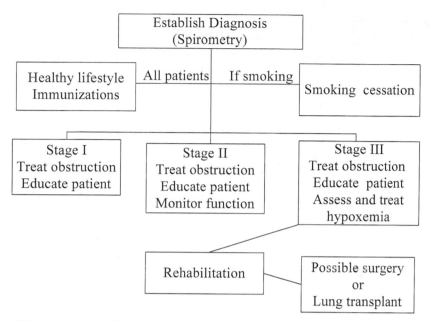

Figure 5.4. Algorithm showing the overall management of patients with COPD.

may be as low as 27% in follow-up periods ranging from 6 months to 7 years. The factors that cause patients to smoke include:

- Addicting potential to nicotine;
- Conditional response to stimuli surrounding smoking;
- Psychosocial problems such as depression, poor education, and low income;
- Forceful advertising campaigns.

Because the causes that drive the patient to smoke are multifactorial, the solutions for smoking cessation should also involve multiple interventions. Elements of successful smoking cessation programs are summarized in Table 5.5.

The clinician should always express strong interest in smoking cessation because a physician's advice to quit smoking discriminates successful from unsuccessful results. A strong social support system including professionals, family, and friends is associated with cessation and long-term abstinence. The smoker should avoid circumstances likely to prompt relapse, including coping with personal and interpersonal stress. It is helpful for the physician to plan a quit date because setting a quit date, to stop "cold turkey," usually holds an advantage over gradual withdrawal. It may be helpful to make a telephone call to the patient at follow-up intervals to encourage cessation of smoking. This call may be made by the physician or a health care worker. Group smoking cessation clinics are offered by many hospitals and in many work sites, as well as by voluntary agencies. They include programs such as the American Lung Association's Freedom from Smoking clinics. Such programs may have an important role in the support of patients who attempt to quit smoking

Table 5.5. Protocol for Smoking Cessation

1. Physician or health care worker should initiate quitting.
   Explain risks of cigarette smoking.
   Offer strong admonition to quit; encourage a quit date; offer referral for self-help or group program.
2. Physician or health care worker may arrange telephone follow-up.
   Call 3–5 days after quit date. Review progress. Counsel regarding quit and recruitment of support individual. Call 1–2 weeks after quit date. Repeat above prn.
3. Physician or health care worker should arrange follow-up. Next regular visit should be < 2 months after initiating quit. May assess the progress with CO and expired air and/or continine in urine, blood, or saliva. If abstinent, should review and reward success. Continue follow-up at increasing intervals for 12 months post-quit.
4. If not abstinent, physician or health care worker should review and emphasize elements of success. Identify circumstances of failure. The physician usually offers nicotine replacement to control the withdrawal symptoms; infrequently other pharmacologic therapy can be considered, such as clonidine or buspirone.

because they effectively integrate behavioral therapy counseling and adjunctive pharmacologic treatment.

Drug Adjuvants

Nicotine is the ingredient in cigarettes that is primarily responsible for smoking addiction. With each cigarette smoked, between 1 and 2 mg of nicotine is delivered to the lungs. Because of rapid absorption into the blood and a half-life of 2 hours, regular daytime smoking can cause nicotine accumulation for an entire 24-hour period. Nicotine is metabolized by the liver. Cotinine, a primary metabolite of nicotine, has a longer half-life and can be searched for in the urine to detect those patients who continue to smoke. Withdrawal from cigarettes causes anxiety, irritability, difficulty concentrating, anger, fatigue, drowsiness, depression, and sleep disruption, especially during the first week of cessation. In a dose-dependent relationship, nicotine replacement following cessation reduces withdrawal symptoms and enhances abstinence. Highly dependent nicotine smokers can be identified as those who smoke more than one pack of cigarettes per day and who require their first cigarette within 30 minutes of arising and who find it difficult to refrain from smoking in places where it is forbidden. Physical dependence can also be assessed by a formal questionnaire, such as the Fagerstrom tolerance questionnaire.

Nicotine polacrilex gum (2 mg per piece) is effective when compared with placebo, especially in self-referred smokers who are highly addicted to cigarettes. Transdermal nicotine patches are more readily available and may be prescribed for the patient who failed smoking cessation efforts in the past or whose smoking cessation has been troubled by withdrawal symptoms. Short-term success rates have varied widely (between 18 and 77%), but in general nicotine patches are approximately two times as effective as placebo. Long-term success rates (6 months and longer) are considerably lower (22–42%) but are consistently better when compared with placebo patch (2–26%).

Adjuvant programs such as individual counseling and group therapy produce a higher success rate when added to pharmacologic intervention. The smoking status (abstinence or continued smoking) during the first two weeks of nicotine patch therapy can serve as a predictor of smoking cessation because smoking during this period is a powerful predictor of failure at the end of a 6-month trial. Patients who fail during the first 2 weeks of therapy should be offered more intense pharmacologic or adjuvant therapy. The ideal time of therapy for each dose has not been established. Recently it has been recommended that nicotine patch therapy beyond 6–8 weeks may not be necessary. Although nicotine patches are well tolerated, mild erythema or other local skin reactions may be seen in up to 50% of patients; however, they can be minimized by rotating the patch to different sites of the skin.

Clonidine, an α-2 adrenergic agonist, may enhance abstinence in the short term but its enduring effects have not been documented. The anxiolytic agent buspirone reduced withdrawal symptoms and may show some benefit on abstinence. Hypnosis may be an effective adjunct but is of little value when offered as a single-session cure. Acupuncture should not be done because there is little evidence that it contributes to smoking cessation beyond its placebo effect.

Pharmacologic Therapy

The pharmacologic therapy of COPD should be organized according to the severity of the disease and the tolerance of the patient for specific drugs. In the outpatient setting, a step-wise approach (Table 5.6) as has been developed for asthma and hypertension is helpful. The most common drugs and dosages that are in current use and the precautions to be taken when indicated are listed in Table 5.6. There is no current evidence that the regular use of any of these drugs alters the progression of COPD. Nevertheless, they alleviate symptoms, improve exercise tolerance, and improve quality of life, all worthwhile goals in COPD. It is important to remember that most COPD patients are older and thereby particularly susceptible to the side effects of medications and that dose adjustments must be made according to each individual circumstance.

Bronchodilators

The bronchodilators used in COPD are similar to those used in asthma, but some differences are noteworthy. Beta$_2$ agonists produce less bronchodilation in COPD and in some patients the spirometric changes may be insignificant, although symptomatic benefit may be experienced perhaps through other mechanisms (such as decreased dynamic hyperinflation) (see Chapter 3). The older age of patients with COPD, however, may result in less tolerance for sympathomimetic-induced tremor, nervousness, and cardiac side effects. Likewise, many older COPD patients cannot effectively activate metered dose inhalers (MDIs), and health providers should recognize this limitation and work with the patient to achieve mastery of the MDI. If this

Table 5.6. Pharmacologic Step-Care of COPD

1. For mild variable symptoms:
   Selective beta$_2$ agonist MDI aerosol 1–2 puffs q 2–6 h prn (not to exceed 8–12 puffs/
   24 h)
   or
   Long-acting beta$_2$ agonist 2 puffs q 12 h
2. For mild to moderate continuing symptoms:
   Ipratropium MDI aerosol 2–6 puffs q 6–8 h (not to be used more frequently)
   plus
   Selective beta$_2$ agonist MDI aerosol 1–4 puffs prn qid (for rapid relief, when needed,
   or as regular supplement)
3. If response to Step 2 is unsatisfactory or for a mild-moderate increase in symptoms, add:
   Sustained release theophylline 200–400 mg bid *or* 400–800 mg h.s. for nocturnal bronchospasm
   and/or
   Consider use of sustained release albuterol 4–8 mg bid, or at night only
   and/or
   Consider use of mucokinetic agent (e.g., organic iodide)
4. If control symptoms is suboptimal:
   Consider a course of oral steroids (e.g., prednisone) up to 40 mg/d for 10–14 days
       if improvement occurs, wean down to low daily or alternate-day dosing (e.g., 7.5
       mg);
       if no improvement occurs, stop abruptly;
       if steroid appears to help, consider possible use of aerosol MDI, particularly if patient
       has evidence of bronchial hyperreactivity
5. For severe exacerbation:
   Increase beta$_2$ agonist dosage (e.g., MDI with spacer 6–8 puffs q ½–2 h) *or* inhalant
       solution, unit dose q ½–2 h *or* subcutaneous administration of epinephrine or terbuta-
       line, 0.1–0.5 mL
   and/or
   Increase ipratropium dosage (e.g., MDI with spacer 6–8 puffs q 3–4 h) *or* inhalant
       solution of ipratropium 0.5 mg q 4–8 h
   and
   Provide theophylline dosage IV with calculated amount to bring serum level to 9–14
       µg/mL (rarely, 12–18 µg/mL)
   Provide methylprednisolone dosage IV giving 50–100 mg stat, then q 6–8 h. Taper as
       soon as possible
   add an antibiotic, if indicated.

is not possible, use of a spacer to facilitate inhalation of the medication will help achieve the desired results. Mucosal deposition in the mouth may result in local side effects (i.e., thrush with inhaled steroids) or general absorption and its consequences (i.e., tremor after beta$_2$ agonists).

Beta$_2$ Agonists

In patients with intermittent symptoms, it is reasonable to initiate drug therapy with an MDI of a beta$_2$ agonist ''as needed'' for relief of symptoms (Table 5.6). Albuterol, pirbuterol, metaproterenol, or terbutaline should be taken up to a maximum of 3 to 4 times a day or as prophylaxis before exercise. The rapid onset of action of $beta_2$ agonist aerosols may lead to dyspneic patients favoring them for regular use. $Beta_2$ agonist therapy decreases dyspnea and improves exercise tolerance in COPD. The potential for arrhythmias necessitates careful dosing in patients with probable or known cardiac disease, although serious cardiac complications are rare with conventional doses.

In more advanced disease, it may be reasonable to use slow-release oral albuterol. Similarly, the new, long-acting aerosol drug salmeterol has been shown to prevent nocturnal bronchospasm. This agent may improve compliance, which can result in an improved outcome in selected patients (see Chapter 3).

Anticholinergics

Once the patient suffers from persistent symptoms, regular use of ipratropium MDI is recommended. The drug has a slower onset and longer action than $beta_2$ agonists such as albuterol and thus is less suitable for "as needed" use. The appropriate dosage is 2–4 puffs three or four times a day, but some patients require and tolerate larger dosages. It has been shown that ipratropium is effective in increasing exercise tolerance and decreasing dyspnea. A recent multicenter, controlled trial of therapy with ipratropium bromide documented a significant bronchodilator effect, but there was no alteration in the rate of decline in lung function in the patients receiving the medication. As is true for $beta_2$ agonists, there is no substantial evidence to suggest that regular use of anticholinergic therapy, with or without a $beta_2$ agonist, leads to a worsening of spirometry. Thus it is appropriate to use regular therapy with ipratropium and to add a $beta_2$ agonist as often as needed for up to four treatments per day.

Theophylline

Theophylline currently represents a third-line agent in the therapy of COPD. The potential for toxicity has led to a decline in its popularity. It is of particular value for less compliant or less capable patients who cannot use aerosol therapy optimally because they can readily take theophylline once or twice a day. Theophylline has been shown to improve the function of the respiratory muscles, stimulate the respiratory center, enhance activities of daily living, and decrease dyspnea. It also improves cardiac output, reduces pulmonary vascular resistance, and improves the perfusion of ischemic myocardial muscle. Recent evidence suggests a modest antiinflammatory role for this drug, thereby expanding its potential indications. It follows that there are several advantages to theophylline therapy in patients with cardiac disease or cor pulmonale, but its use should be carefully followed and intermittent serum levels should be used. The previously recommended therapeutic serum levels of 15 to 20 μg/mL (mg/L) are too close to the toxic range and are frequently associated with side effects. Therefore, a lower target range of 9 to 14 μg/mL (mg/L) is safer and still therapeutic in nature (Table 5.6). The regular use of theophylline has not been shown to have a detrimental effect on the course of COPD. Combination of theophylline, albuterol, and ipratropium can result in maximum benefit in stable COPD.

Antiinflammatory Therapy

In contrast to their value in asthma management, antiinflammatory drugs have not been documented to have a significant role in the routine treatment of COPD. Cromolyn and nedocromil have not been established as useful agents, although they could possibly be helpful if the patient has associated respiratory tract allergy. Corticosteroids may merit more careful evaluation in individual patients on adequate bronchodilator therapy who fail to improve.

In outpatients, exacerbations may necessitate a course of oral steroids, but it is important to wean patients quickly because the older COPD population is susceptible to complications such as skin damage, cataracts, diabetes, osteoporosis, and secondary infection. These risks do not accompany standard doses of steroid aerosols, which may cause thrush but pose a negligible risk for causing pulmonary infection. Most studies suggest that only 10–30% of patients with COPD improve if given chronic oral steroid therapy. The dangers of steroids require the careful documentation of the effectiveness of such therapy before a patient is put on prolonged daily or alternate-day dosing. The latter regimen may be safer, but its effectiveness has not been adequately evaluated in COPD.

Based on preliminary results, two large multicenter trials are being conducted to evaluate the role of inhaled corticosteroids in preventing or slowing the progressive course of patients with symptomatic COPD. Until the results are analyzed, the concurrent use of inhaled steroids with albuterol and ipratropium has to be evaluated on an individual basis.

Mucokinetic Agents

The only controlled study in the United States suggesting a value for mucokinetic agents in the chronic management of bronchitis was a multicenter evaluation of organic iodide. This study demonstrated symptomatic benefits. The values of other agents, including water, have not been clearly demonstrated, although some agents (such as oral acetylcysteine) are favored in Europe for their antioxidant effects in addition to their mucokinetic properties. Genetically engineered ribonuclease may prove to be useful in cystic fibrosis but seems to be of little practical value in COPD.

Antibiotics

Antibiotics are of unproven value in the prevention or treatment of exacerbations of COPD unless there is evidence of infection (such as fever), leukocytosis, and a change in the chest radiograph. If recurrent infections occur, particularly in winter, continuous or intermittent prolonged courses of antibiotics may be useful. When an acute bacterial infection is believed to be present, antibiotic therapy may be justified, but the decision is usually made clinically because culture of sputum is not cost-effective. In prescribing treatment, fiscal concerns should be a consideration because older, less costly agents are often effective (e.g., tetracycline, doxycycline, amoxicillin, erythromycin, or trimethoprim/sulfamethoxazole). The major bacteria to be considered are *Streptococcus pneumoniae, Haemophilus influenzae,* and *Moraxella catarrhalis.* The antibiotic choice will depend on local experience supported by sputum culture and sensitivities if the patient is moderately ill or needs to be admitted to the hospital.

α_1-Antitrypsin

Although replacement with AAT may be indicated in nonsmoking, younger patients with genetically determined emphysema, in practice such therapy is difficult to initiate. There is evidence that the administration of AAT is relatively safe, but the appropriate selection of the candidate for such therapy is not clear. Patients with severe and crippling COPD or those with good lung function are not good candidates for therapy. Likewise, deficient nonsmoker patients are at low risk to develop airflow obstruction. Therefore, the most likely candidates for replacement therapy would be smoking patients with mild COPD. The cost of therapy is such that its use is debatable because its safety and long-term effects remain unknown.

Respiratory Stimulants

Respiratory stimulants are not currently favored, although they are used in some countries. Psychoactive drugs are often sought by older patients to treat depression, anxiety, insomnia, or pain. In general, these agents can be given with appropriate care and with particular awareness of their depressant effect on the respiratory center. Benzodiazepines do not have a marked effect on respiration in mild or moderate COPD but can be suppressive in severe disease, particularly during sleep. The safer hypnotics for use in insomnia include sedating antihistamines, chloral hydrate. Antidepressants may also have the advantage of improving sleep. Concomitant use of cardiovascular drugs may be needed in severe COPD and cor pulmonale. Digoxin is occasionally useful, while beta-adrenergic blockers are generally contraindicated. These drugs must be used cautiously to avoid dehydration, hypotension, myocardial ischemia, and arrhythmias. Because most patients requiring such therapy are elderly or have impaired drug clearance, all potential side effects must be carefully sought and responded to by modifying the drug regimen.

Vaccination

Ideally, infectious complications of the respiratory tract should be prevented in patients with COPD by using effective vaccines. Although the currently available vaccines are not totally effective and are not widely used, there is evidence that COPD patients benefit from their use; thus, routine prophylaxis with pneumococcal and influenza vaccines is recommended.

Management of Acute Exacerbations

In the case of an acute exacerbation, the pharmacologic therapy is initiated with the same therapeutic agents available for its chronic management. As described later in the chapter, care must be taken to rule out heart failure, myocardial infarction, arrhythmias, and pulmonary embolism, all of which may present with clinical signs and symptoms similar to exacerbation of COPD.

The most important components of therapy for acute exacerbation of COPD are anticholinergic and beta$_2$ agonist aerosols. Ipratropium may be administered via an MDI, sometimes with a spacer if the administration is erratic, or as an inhalant solution by nebulization. Although the upper limit of dosage has not been established, the drug is safe, and dosages higher than usual can be given to a poorly responsive patient. The prolonged half-life, however, means that repeat doses should not be given more often than every 4–8 hours. Beta$_2$ agonists should also be administered using the same inhaled techniques. These drugs have a reduced functional half-life in exacerbations of COPD and thus may be given every 30–60 minutes if tolerated. The safety and value of continuous nebulization has not been established but in selected cases may be worth a trial. Subcutaneous or intramuscular dosing are only recommended if aerosol use is not feasible; intravenous administration is not an acceptable practice. Careful administration of theophylline may be useful. The drug can be given as intravenous aminophylline in a severe exacerbation. Serum levels are needed as a guide to avoid toxicity, and in most patients a serum level of 8–12 μg/mL is appropriate. When the patient improves, oral long-acting theophylline can be substituted using 80% of the daily dose of aminophylline.

Combination therapy is often needed, and systemic corticosteroids may then be added to the regimen. Corticosteroids can be effective in patients who demonstrate inadequate responsiveness to beta$_2$ agonist or ipratropium therapy. It is important to avoid prolonged or high-dose therapy in those patients who show little improvement because older patients are susceptible to severe complications such as psychosis, fluid retention, and vascular necrosis of bones. Rapid weaning must be accomplished as soon as possible.

Antibiotics such as amoxicillin, trimethoprim/sulfamethoxazole, doxycycline, or erythromycin have been helpful in exacerbations of COPD. Mucokinetic agents such as iodides given systemically have not been shown to be effective in exacerbations of COPD, although some patients report subjective improvement when given these agents.

HOME OXYGEN THERAPY

Therapeutic oxygen has been used systematically since Barach and then Petty et al. recognized the association between hypoxemia and right heart failure and appreciated the benefit of continuous oxygen delivery to patients with severe COPD. Since then much has been learned about the effects of oxygen and hypoxemia, and progress has been made in the area of mechanical oxygen delivery devices.

The results of the Nocturnal Oxygen Therapy Trial (NOTT) and Medical Research Council (MRC) studies have established that continuous home oxygen improves survival in hypoxemic COPD and that survival is related to the number of hours of supplemental oxygen per day. Other beneficial effects of long-term oxygen include reduction in polycythemia (perhaps related more to lowered carboxyhemoglobin levels than to improved arterial saturation), reduction in pulmonary artery pressures, dyspnea, and rapid eye movement-related hypoxemia during sleep. Oxygen therapy improves sleep and may reduce nocturnal arrhythmias. Oxygen can also improve neuropsychiatric testing and exercise tolerance. Supplemental oxygen increases exercise endurance and has been attributed to central mechanisms causing reduced minute ventilation at the same workload, thereby delaying the time until ventilatory limitations are reached; improved arterial oxygenation, enabling greater oxygen delivery reversal of hypoxemia-induced bronchoconstriction; and the effect of oxygen on respiratory muscle recruitment.

Prescribing Home Oxygen

Patients are evaluated for long-term oxygen therapy (LTOT) by measuring the PaO_2. It is therefore recommended that measurement of PaO_2, not pulse oximetry (SaO_2), be the clinical standard for initiating LTOT, particularly during rest. Oximetry SaO_2 may be used to adjust oxygen flow settings over time. If hypercapnia or acidosis is suspected, an arterial blood gas (ABG) must be performed. Guidelines for long-term oxygen therapy include:

- $PaO_2 \leq 55$ mm Hg at rest breathing room air;
- $PaO_2 < 60$ mm Hg at rest breathing air in patients with either cor pulmonale, pulmonary hypertension, or polycythemia;
- $PaO_2 \leq 55$ mm Hg during exercise or sleep;
- Dose: oxygen flow sufficient to raise PaO_2 to 65 mm Hg or $SaO_2 \geq 90\%$;
- Duration: at least 15 h/day unless only needed during exercise or sleep.

Some COPD patients who were not hypoxemic before the events leading to their exacerbation will eventually recover to the point that they will no longer need oxygen. It is therefore recommended that the need for long-term oxygen be reassessed in 30–90 days, once the patient is clinically stable and receiving adequate medical management. Oxygen therapy can be discontinued if the patient does not meet blood gas criteria. To prescribe LTOT, a certificate of medical necessity (HCFA form 484) must be completed. The HCFA form 484 evolved in an attempt to ensure that the physician, not the home medical equipment (HME) supplier, was in charge of decisions concerning therapy. HCFA requires the physician or an employee of the physician, rather than the HME supplier, to complete form 484.

Like any drug, oxygen has potential deleterious effects that may be particularly relevant to older patients. The hazardous effects of oxygen therapy can be considered under three broad headings:

- Physical risks such as fire hazard or tank explosion, trauma from catheters or masks, and drying of mucous membranes because of high flow rates and inadequate humidification.
- Functional effects related to increased carbon dioxide retention and absorptive atelectasis. Elevated PCO_2 in response to supplemental oxygen is a well-recog-

nized complication in a minority of patients. The mechanism has traditionally been ascribed to reductions in hypoxic ventilatory drive. In many patients, however, the decrease in minute ventilation is minimal. The most consistent finding is a worsening of the pulmonary ventilation to perfusion distribution with an increase in the dead space to tidal volume ratio. This presumably results from oxygen's blockage of local hypoxic vasoconstriction, thereby increasing perfusion of poorly ventilated areas.

• Although possible, cytotoxic and atelectasis effects have not clearly been demonstrated with the low flow rates (1–5 L/min, FIO_2 24–36%) typically used for chronic home oxygen therapy in COPD.

Oxygen Delivery Systems

Long-term home oxygen is available from three different delivery systems: oxygen concentrators, liquid systems, and compressed gas. Each system has advantages and disadvantages, and the correct system for each patient depends on patient limitations and clinical application. Oxygen systems were recently compared on the basis of weight, cost, portability, ease of refilling, and availability. The former three factors may be of particular importance in elderly, often debilitated, patients. Compressed gas is stored in variably sized steel or aluminum cylinders that weight 200, 16, 9, and 4 lbs. and last 2.4 days, 5.2 hours, 2 hours, and 1.2 hours at 2 L/min flow. The advantages of compressed gas oxygen are its low price, availability, and capacity to be stored for long periods. Disadvantages are its weight (with the large cylinders), short oxygen supply time (with the smaller cylinders), potential hazard of a torpedo-like effect if the valve becomes suddenly disconnected from the compressed gas cylinder, and inferior transfilability. Liquid oxygen is stored at very low temperatures that reduce the volume to less than 1% of the room temperature equivalent. Portable containers weigh up to 10 pounds and last 4–8 hours at 2 L/min flow. A wheel-mounted, 140-lb. stationary unit is also available that can last up to 7 days at 1 liter/min. Advantages of this system are its relative portability and ease of transfilability. Disadvantages are its higher cost and requirements for intermittent pressure venting, resulting in oxygen "consumption" even when the system is not being used. Oxygen concentrators are electrical devices that extract oxygen by passing in air through a molecular sieve. The oxygen is delivered to the patient, and the nitrogen is returned to the atmosphere. The devices weigh approximately 35 lbs. and are not portable. They are typically used in a stationary capacity, such as in a car or room, while liquid or gas is used to provide portability. The major advantage of the oxygen concentrator is its relative cost effectiveness; the disadvantages are its need for a power source, regular servicing, and relative lack of portability.

Administration Devices

Oxygen is typically administered with continuous flow by nasal cannula. Because alveolar delivery occurs during a small portion of a spontaneous respiratory cycle (approximately the first one-sixth)—the rest of the cycle being used to fill dead space and for exhalation—the majority of continuously flowing oxygen is not used by the patient and is wasted into the atmosphere. To improve efficiency and increase patient mobility, several devices are available that focus on oxygen conservation and delivery during early inspiration. These devices include reservoir cannulas, demand-type systems, and transtracheal catheters.

Reservoir nasal cannulas and pendants store oxygen during expiration and deliver a 20-mL bolus during early inspiration. Because more alveolar oxygen is delivered, flows may be reduced proportionally. This has been shown to result in a 2 to 4:1 oxygen savings at rest and with exercise. Cosmetic considerations have traditionally limited patient acceptance of these devices.

Demand valve systems have an electronic sensor that delivers oxygen only during early inspiration or provides an additional pulse early in inspiration as an adjuvant to the continuous flow. By restricting or accentuating oxygen during inspiration, wasted delivery into dead space or during exhalation is minimized. This results in a 2 to 7:1 oxygen savings. The effect of mouth breathing on efficacy is not yet clear.

Transtracheal oxygen (TTO) therapy employs a thin flexible catheter placed into the lower trachea for delivery of continuous (or pulsed) oxygen. Because oxygen is delivered directly into the trachea, dead space is reduced and the upper trachea serves as a reservoir of undiluted oxygen. This provides a 2 to 3:1 oxygen savings over nasal cannula. Other benefits of TTO include its relative inconspicuousness; lack of nasal, auricular, or facial skin irritation; stationary position with ambulation or during sleep; and its purported efficacy in providing adequate oxygenation where nasal cannula cannot. TTO therapy has also been reported to reduce minute volume and dyspnea and improve exercise tolerance by mechanisms now owing solely to improvements in oxygenation. TTO appears to reduce dyspnea and improve exercise tolerance through mechanisms that include decreased dead space and decreased minute ventilation.

Complication rates tend to be lower in the larger series and higher in the smaller series. The most frequent complications are dislodged catheters (up to 33%; average 10%), subcutaneous emphysema (up to 10%; average 65%), stomal infection requiring antibiotics (up to 25%; average 6.5%), and the formation of symptomatic mucous balls at the tip of the catheter (up to 25%; average 10%). The latter complication may be potentially serious or even fatal. Other complications of TTO therapy include migration of the catheter into the mediastinum, broken catheter tips in the airways, pneumonia, hemoptysis, keloid formation, hoarseness, cardiac arrhythmias, and tracheal stricture. Overall, the TTO catheter offers several potential advantages over more conventional continuous oxygen administration devices, but it requires a motivated, dexterous patient for routine care and daily cleaning, and it has a modest rate of usually minor but potentially serious complications.

HOSPITALIZATION THERAPY AND DISCHARGE CRITERIA

Although acute exacerbations are difficult to define and its pathogenesis is poorly understood, impaired lung function can lead to respiratory failure requiring intuba-

Table 5.7. Emergency Room Evaluation of Exacerbations of COPD

History	Baseline respiratory status, sputum volume and characteristics, duration and progression of symptoms. Dyspnea severity, exercise limitations, sleep and eating difficulties, home care resources, home therapeutic regimen, symptoms of comorbid acute or chronic conditions.
Physical	Evidence of cor pulmonale, tachypnea, bronchospasm, pneumonia. Hemodynamic instability, altered mentation, respiratory muscle fatigue, excessive work of breathing. Acute comorbid conditions.
Laboratory	ABG, chest radiograph (PA, Lat), ECG, theophylline level (if outpatient theophylline used). Pulse oximetry monitoring ECG monitoring. PostER treatment—spirometry (if FEV_1 changes from baseline to be used as admission criteria), additional studies as clinically indicated.

FEV_1, forced expiratory volume in one second; *ECG,* electrocardiogram; *ER,* emergency room; *ABG,* arterial blood gas; *PA,* posterior-anterior: *Lat,* lateral.

tion and mechanical ventilation. The purpose of acute treatment is to manage the patient's acute decompensation and comorbid conditions to prevent further deterioration and readmission. Table 5.7 lists the components of the history, physical examination, and laboratory evaluation that should be obtained during a moderate to severe acute exacerbation to assist the formulation of therapy and the decision for hospital admission.

Traditionally, the decision to admit derives from subjective interpretation of clinical features, such as the severity of dyspnea, determination of respiratory failure, short-term response to emergency room therapy, degree of cor pulmonale, and the presence of complicating features such as severe bronchitis, pneumonia, or other comorbid conditions. This approach to decision-making is less than ideal because up to 28% of patients with an acute exacerbation of COPD discharged from an ER have recurrent symptoms within 14 days. Additionally, 17% of patients discharged after ER management of COPD will relapse and require hospitalization. Few clinical studies have investigated patient-specific objective clinical and laboratory features that identify patients with COPD who require hospitalization.

General consensus supports the need for hospitalization in patients with:

• Severe acute hypoxemia.
• Acute hypercarbia; less extreme arterial blood gas abnormalities, however, do not assist decision analysis.
• The posttreatment FEV_1 as a percentage of predicted, combined with the clinical assessment, identifies patients in need of admission. Asymptomatic patients with posttreatment FEV_1 less than 40% of predicted were successfully discharged from the ER; patients with a posttreatment FEV_1 less than 40% of predicted accompanied by persistent respiratory symptoms require admission.
• Other factors that identify ''high risk'' patients include a previous emergency room visit within 7 days, the number of doses of nebulized bronchodilators, use of home oxygen, previous relapse rate, administration of aminophylline, and the use of corticosteroids and antibiotics at the time of ER discharge.

The indications for hospital admission are summarized in Table 5.8. Based on expert consensus, they consider the severity of the underlying respiratory dysfunction, progression of symptoms, response to outpatient therapies, existence of comorbid conditions, necessity of surgical interventions that may affect pulmonary function, and the availability of adequate home care. The severity of respiratory dysfunction dictates the need for admission to an ICU (Table 5.9). Depending on the resources available within an institution, admission of patients with severe exacerbations of COPD to intermediate or special respiratory care units may be appropriate if personnel, skills, and equipment exist to identify and manage acute respiratory failure successfully. Limited data support the discharge criteria listed in Table 5.10.

The pharmacologic treatment of acute exacerbations is similar to that available for chronic management. Inhaled administration is preferred, whereas intravenous treatment may be reserved for certain drugs such as corticosteroids and theophylline. Once stable, the patient may be switched to oral and inhaled medications. Once

Table 5.8. Indications for Hospitalization in COPD

The patient has an acute exacerbation of COPD characterized by increased dyspnea, cough, and sputum production with one or more of the following features:
Symptoms that do not adequately respond to outpatient management
Inability of a previously mobile patient to walk between rooms
Inability to eat or sleep because of dyspnea
Family and/or physician assessment that the patient cannot manage at home and supplementary home care resources are not immediately available
Presence of high-risk comorbid pulmonary (e.g., pneumonia) or nonpulmonary conditions
Prolonged, progressive symptoms before emergency room visit
Presence of worsening hypoxemia, new or worsening hypercarbia, or new or worsening cor pulmonale
Acute respiratory failure characterized by severe respiratory distress, uncompensated hypercarbia, or servere hypoxemia
The patient has new or worsening cor pulmonale unresponsive to outpatient management
Invasive surgical or diagnostic procedures are planned requiring analgesics or sedatives that may worsen pulmonary function
Comorbid conditions, such as severe steroid myopathy or acute vertebral compression fractures with severe pain, have worsened pulmonary function

Table 5.9. Indications for ICU Admission of Patients with Acute Exacerbations of COPD

A patient with severe dyspnea does not respond to initial emergency room therapy
A patient demonstrates confusion, lethargy, or respiratory muscle fatigue characterized by paradoxical diaphragmatic motion
Laboratory evidence demonstrates persistent/worsening hypoxemia despite supplemental oxygen or severe/worsening respiratory acidosis (e.g., pH < 7.30)
A patient requires assisted mechanical ventilation by means of an endotracheal tube or noninvasive technique

Table 5.10. Discharge Criteria After Treatment for Acute Exacerbations of COPD

Inhaled beta agonist therapy is required no more frequently than every 4 hours
Previously ambulatory patient is able to walk across the room
The patient is able to sleep without frequent awakening by dyspnea
Any component of reactive airways disease is under stable control
The patient is stable off of parenteral therapy for 12–24 hours
The patient or home care giver is educated as to correct use of medications
Arrangements for follow-up care and home care (e.g., visiting nurse, home oxygen delivery,
    meal provisions) are completed

Note: Patients who do not yet fulfill criteria for discharge to home may be successfully managed at nonacute care placement sites for observation during the final resolution of symptoms.

improved, clinical assessment plans for modifying drug regimens, using home oxygen, or the potential benefits from pulmonary rehabilitation programs should be prepared. Duration of hospitalization in COPD depends at least partially on the existence of a multidisciplinary team that directs respiratory management.

Because of the complex management issues in caring for COPD, patients with impending or frank respiratory failure, physicians with extensive experience in and knowledge of COPD should participate in the care of hospitalized patients who present with severe disease and any of the following:

- Those who require invasive or noninvasive modes of mechanical ventilation;
- Those who develop hypoxemia unresponsive to FIO_2 0.50;
- Those who develop new onset hypercarbia;
- Those who require steroids for more than 48 hours to maintain adequate respiratory function;
- Patients who undergo thoraco-abdominal surgery;
- Those who require specialized techniques to manage copious airway secretions.

Assisted Ventilation

Assisted ventilation should be considered for patients with acute exacerbations of COPD when pharmacologic and other nonventilatory treatments fail to reverse clinically significant respiratory failure.

Progressive airflow obstruction may impair gas exchange to the degree that assisted ventilation will be required. In this clinical context the therapeutic goals are to:

- Support the patient over the short term during the course of acute respiratory failure;
- Enhance gas exchange and functional status in patients with chronically impaired ventilation.

Indications for initiating assisted ventilation during acute COPD exacerbations include:

- Signs of respiratory muscle fatigue;
- Worsening respiratory acidosis;
- Deteriorating mental status.

Although several investigators have reported success with negative pressure ventilation, most studies advocate positive pressure inflation for acute exacerbations of
COPD. Because negative pressure ventilation may cause upper airway obstruction
and arterial oxygen desaturation (when upper airway muscle activation is asynchro-
nous with negative pressure breaths), its role in managing patients with COPD has
been questioned.

The goals of assisted positive pressure ventilation in acute respiratory failure
complicating COPD are:

- Resting of ventilatory muscles and restoration of gas exchange to a stable baseline;
- Avoidance of complications associated with mechanical ventilation;
- Facilitation of weaning and discontinuation of mechanical ventilation as soon as
  possible.

Major complications associated with assisted positive pressure ventilation include
risks of ventilator-associated pneumonia, pulmonary barotrauma, and laryngotracheal complications associated with intubation and/or tracheotomy (see Chapter 12).
In addition to these general hazards, specific pitfalls in ventilating patients with
COPD include:

- Over-ventilation, resulting in acute respiratory alkalemia, especially in patients
  with chronic hypercapnia;
- Creation of auto-PEEP (or intrinsic PEEP), especially when expiratory time is
  inadequate;
- Initiation of complex pulmonary and cardiovascular interactions that result in systemic hypotension.

Auto-PEEP has been reported to occur in up to 39% of mechanically ventilated
patients. Auto-PEEP can best be prevented by carefully instituting ventilatory
changes that decrease hyperinflation, such as decreasing respiratory rate, increasing
inspiratory flow rates to avoid a disadvantageous inspiratory:expiratory (I:E) ratio,
ensuring the use of a large-caliber endotracheal tube, and by reducing compressible
volume in the ventilator circuit.

Modes of Ventilation

Invasive Ventilation

The three ventilatory modes most widely used for managing COPD patients are:

- Assist-control (AC);
- Intermittent mandatory ventilation (IMV);
- Pressure support (PS) ventilation.

Because some clinical reports indicate that PS ventilation provides increased patient comfort, promotes patient synchrony with the ventilator, and may accelerate weaning, it may be a particularly valuable mode of ventilatory support for stabilized patients with COPD and acute respiratory failure who maintain adequate ventilatory drive. No direct evidence exists, however, showing that patient outcome is improved with the use of PS compared with volume-cycled modes of mechanical ventilation in patients with COPD.

Noninvasive Ventilation

Translaryngeal intubation presents risks of nosocomial pneumonia, laryngotracheal injury, and bacterial sinusitis, and also interferes with the patient's capacity for verbal communication. The advent of noninvasive positive pressure-assisted ventilation modes offers an alternative to intubation in some patients with COPD and acute respiratory failure. Noninvasive positive pressure ventilation for acute exacerbations of COPD has been examined in several studies, using both facial and nasal masks in conjunction with volume-cycled ventilation, bilevel positive airway pressure, and pressure support modes. Although available studies suggest a significant success rate in patients with acute respiratory failure complicating COPD, the reported experience is still limited and failure rates up to 40% have been reported in some studies. Primary use of noninvasive techniques for respiratory failure in patients with COPD should be reserved for centers with adequate expertise and supervision to allow safe implementation. Patient features that should discourage considering noninvasive ventilation for acute COPD exacerbations include hemodynamic instability, copious secretions, inability to defend the airways, poor cooperation with the technique, or impaired mental status.

Weaning from Mechanical Ventilation

Many COPD patients who undergo mechanical ventilation for acute bronchospasm, fluid overload, oversedation, or inadvertent hyperoxygenation may experience successful extubation without going through a period of weaning. Some patients with COPD intubated for respiratory failure require graduated weaning. Available techniques for weaning COPD patients from mechanical ventilation include AC ventilation with T-piece trials, IMV, and PS ventilation. Theoretic advantages exist to using IMV and PS modes because they provide partial support when the patient is connected to the ventilator and present less opportunity for barotrauma. Insufficient investigations exist to establish that weaning is accelerated or outcomes improved with any of the available weaning techniques.

Ethical Issues Regarding Initiation and Withdrawing Mechanical Ventilation

Because COPD affects patients at more advanced ages, frequently progresses, and may require highly expensive and prolonged life-saving medical technology, affected patients frequently present ethical dilemmas in their management and care. Deliberations in individual patients require a careful analysis of COPD survival statistics, quality of life, community health care resources, and economic aspects of care. Clinicians commonly attempt to determine the value of mechanical ventilation in individual patients with COPD by subjectively estimating the likelihood of survival after intubation. Unfortunately, subjective bedside assessment is extremely inaccurate in predicting the survival of COPD patients. The predictive accuracy does not correlate with physician experience or level of training.

No correlation exists, for instance, between short-term survival and admission arterial blood gas results, spirometric values, hematocrit, patient age, or number of previous admissions for exacerbations of COPD. Scoring systems such as the Simplified Acute Physiology Score are weak predictors of short-term outcome in patients with COPD and respiratory failure. The presence of nonpulmonary comorbid conditions, such as gastrointestinal hemorrhage, pulmonary embolism, or coronary heart disease, present at the onset of respiratory decompensation contribute to poor patient outcome. Housebound patients with severe, end-stage lung disease and comorbid conditions therefore have a worse short-term prognosis compared with more active patients with less severe underlying pulmonary impairment during episodes of respiratory failure of similar severity. Close to 80% of patients with COPD who require mechanical ventilation for acute respiratory failure survive to hospital discharge. Patients followed from the onset of an episode of acute respiratory failure have a two-year survival rate between 28 to 70%. In contrast to common belief, patients with COPD have the highest survival rate compared with patients with other causes of acute respiratory failure. Finally, the long-term prognosis of patients surviving mechanical ventilation is similar to that of patients with the same degree of underlying respiratory impairment who have not required mechanical ventilation.

Patients with COPD complicated by acute respiratory failure requiring life support measures do not have an overall grim prognosis. Consequently, no fundamental ethical dilemma exists in considering all patients with COPD for intubation and mechanical ventilation. Patients who have poor baseline function, marginal nutritional status, severely restricted activity levels, and inexorable deterioration of their late-stage pulmonary dysfunction, however, may elect to forego intubation when in their and their physician's judgment it will only temporarily interrupt the terminal phase of the disease.

Physicians have an obligation to assist their patients with COPD in formulating advance directives before respiratory decompensation occurs and in counseling patients regarding the value of intubation and mechanical ventilation and the considerations of foregoing life support measures.

The physician has the responsibility to ensure that:

- The patient has decision-making capacity;
- The patient has been informed regarding his or her diagnosis, prognosis, risks, benefits, and consequences for the full range of available medical interventions, including the option of no therapy;
- The patient has received from the physician professional recommendations regard-

ing the medical choices available, including the use of life-sustaining therapy, based on knowledge of both the medical situation and the values and goals of the patient.

Decisions regarding limitations of care are best made during stable periods, before respiratory failure or other life-threatening conditions occur. Patients who choose to forego life support measures should be encouraged to outline their wishes as specifically as possible in an instrument of advance directive, such as a living will. Patients with COPD should specifically define their health care preferences for several clinical situations likely to be encountered, such as intubation, mechanical ventilation, cardiopulmonary resuscitation, tracheotomy, and long-term life support with difficult weaning. The patient should be encouraged to share these preferences with a trusted family member, friend, or other person who can be designated as a surrogate decision maker through a durable power of attorney for health care.

Once these advance directives are properly established or the wishes of an informed patient with decision-making capacity are known, respect for patient autonomy requires physicians in charge of the patient's care to honor the patient's right to forego medical intervention. This is considered distinct from participating in assisted suicide or active euthanasia. Physicians faced with a critically ill patient should determine, however, that requests to forego care are reasonable under the clinical circumstances and derive from deep-seated values and appropriate responses to the severity of underlying disease rather than from endogenous depression or temporary conditions of pain, fear, depression, or anxiety during episodes of acute respiratory failure. Physicians who have personal ethical or religious values that do not allow them to comply with a patient's well-conceived request to forego support should transfer the patient's care to another physician who can honor the patient's directives.

It should be recognized that there is no ethical difference between withholding and withdrawing life support measures in patients with acute respiratory failure. Ethical principles underlying the decision to withhold intubation and mechanical ventilation apply equally when patients or proxies request a discontinuance of care for patients with a terminal disease or a progressive degenerative condition who have no hope for an acceptable and meaningful recovery. Patients electing to have ventilatory support withdrawn may request and receive adequate sedation and analgesia to extinguish all pain and suffering during the dying process even if such treatment accelerates their imminent death.

SURGICAL OPTIONS FOR EMPHYSEMA

In 1959, Otto Brantigan postulated that the tethering force that tends to keep the intrathoracic airways open was lost in emphysema and that by resecting the most affected parts of the lungs in patients with the most severe form of the disease, the force could be partially restored. Indeed, he developed an operation to resect wedges of hyperinflated lungs. In spite of a significant morbidity and mortality (16%), 75%

of his patients manifested clinical improvement for up to five years. Because of a lack of some of the technical material now available (pericardial strips) and the need for bilateral thoracotomy, the procedure was abandoned. Recently, Cooper et al. have reported the results of surgical resection of emphysematous lungs of patients with severe COPD. Using the technique developed by Brantigan but doing both lungs in the same sitting through a median sternotomy, they have reported a 1-year 45% increase in FEV_1, a 25% decrease in total lung capacity, and a significant improvement in exercise performance.

Although the results are preliminary, several groups have shown improvement in lung function, dyspnea, and quality of life. It is difficult to clearly delineate the factors responsible for this improvement, but recent reports indicate a postoperative increase in lung elastic recoil as one likely explanation. The decrease in lung volume lengthens the diaphragm and other respiratory muscles, placing them in a better contractile position of the length-tension curve. This should result in less effort to produce the same ventilatory pressure. Perhaps this decreases respiratory drive and hence reverses some of the factors associated with dyspnea in these patients. More studies are needed to be able to recommend this procedure to most patients with emphysema. Little is known about the factors that help select the best candidates for surgery. More needs to be learned about the best surgical technique and the optimal timing of the surgery. Nevertheless, for a disease with few therapeutic choices when it is advanced, this revival of an old operation seems to offer a possible and reasonable alternative to lung transplant.

Lung transplant, conversely, has become a real option for some patients with advanced COPD. Today it is the most common diagnosis for which lung transplantation has been considered. Close to 40% of all patients undergoing single lung transplant carry the diagnosis of COPD.

The selection of patients to have lung transplant includes:

• Limited life expectancy (less than 3 years);
• Age less than 60 years;
• Failure of maximal medical therapy, and no extrapulmonary organ failure.

Particularly for emphysema, most patients have an FEV_1 lower than 25% predicted, are oxygen dependent, experience limitation of activities of daily living, and are not candidates for lung volume reduction surgery. Patients are not candidates for lung transplants if they continue to smoke, have coronary artery disease, are on long-term corticosteroid therapy, and are either cachectic or obese. Single or bilateral lung transplant can be performed for end-stage emphysema even if pulmonary hypertension is present. Mortality is reduced and improvement in quality of life and exercise capacity is excellent with both procedures. The survival rate at 1 year is close to 75%, with a subsequent yearly mortality of 3 to 6% per year.

SLEEP AND COPD

Patients with COPD seem to have a higher prevalence of insomnia, excessive daytime sleepiness, and nightmares than the general population. This is not caused by the bronchodilators, since studies with these agents have failed to demonstrate any adverse effects on sleep staging or sleep efficiency. Oxygen desaturation during sleep, especially in REM sleep, has been long recognized in patients with COPD. Clinical parameters that have been associated with the presence of nocturnal desaturation include daytime hypoxemia, blunted awake chemosensitivity, severe dysfunction on pulmonary function testing, and chronic CO_2 retention. None of these characteristics have been useful in predicting individual REM desaturators. The mechanisms leading to hypoxemia include ventilation, which is reduced in all stages of sleep—especially in REM sleep. It has also been postulated that hypoxemia may be related to ventilation perfusion imbalance, although this has been difficult to prove. REM-associated falls in SaO_2 are associated with increases in pulmonary artery pressures. It is not clear whether isolated increases in pulmonary artery pressures during sleep can lead to sustained pulmonary hypertension. Recent studies, however, of COPD patients with nocturnal desaturation and daytime PO_2 levels over 60 mm Hg have demonstrated higher daytime resting and exercise-induced pulmonary artery pressures in these patients than in a similar group of patients who did not desaturate at night.

Patients with COPD have increased premature ventricular contractions during sleep, and there is a tendency for these to decrease in frequency when these patients are given supplemental oxygen. The effect of nocturnal oxygen saturation on survival has recently been reported. Both the mean nocturnal SaO_2 and the SaO_2 nadir during sleep were significantly related to survival; however, neither measure improved the prediction of survival over measurements of vital capacity or awake SaO_2. The measurement of nocturnal SaO_2 during sleep therefore cannot be recommended in the routine clinical management of COPD patients. Several studies have demonstrated that COPD and obstructive sleep apnea (OSA) can coexist, but there is no evidence that this coexistence is more common than would be expected from the relative frequencies of these two conditions. The significance of the association seems to be that patients with both disease processes seem more likely to develop pulmonary hypertension and right-sided heart failure than do patients who have either condition alone. Full polysomnography, however, would be beneficial in those COPD patients with symptoms suggestive of coexistent OSA.

AIR TRAVEL

Commercial airline travel exposes passengers to hypobaric hypoxia because aircraft cabins are not routinely pressurized to sea level. In patients who have compensated COPD at sea level, lowering the partial pressure of oxygen in the aircraft cabin can produce severe hypoxemia. Physical exertion during the flight can increase the risk of an exacerbation of symptoms. It is unknown what proportion of patients who suffer cardiac events during air travel have COPD as a comorbid condition. Aircraft are usually pressurized to between 5,000 and 7,000 feet (1,500–2,100 m). For the pre-flight evaluation of most patients, clinicians should consider 8,000 feet (2,438 m) of altitude above sea levels as realistic ''worse case scenarios.''

Pre-flight assessment can be accomplished by estimating the expected degree of hypoxemia at altitude, identifying comorbid disease conditions, and providing an oxygen prescription if necessary. Documentation of the recent clinical condition and laboratory tests—particularly if the patient is traveling abroad—and counseling are also desirable elements of the pre-flight patient care.

The two means of estimating the degree of hypoxia at altitude are:

- The hypoxia inhalation test (HIT);
- The use of regression formulae.

The HIT is not performed in many clinical laboratories in the United States. Regression equations offer the opportunity to compare a patient with a group of patients with similar clinical characteristics who have been previously studied during exposure to hypoxia. Although regression equations may provide a more physiologic basis for the effects of high altitude than the HIT, the regression approach does not assess the individual's susceptibility to the development of symptoms or electrocardiographic changes during hypoxia. The $(A-a)O_2$ gradient generally has no advantages over regression equations. Currently it is recommended that the PaO_2 during air travel be maintained above 50 mm Hg. Although 2–3 liters of oxygen by nasal cannula will replace the inspired oxygen lost at 8,000 feet compared with sea level, lesser increments of oxygen will maintain the PaO_2 above 50 mm Hg in many patients, and a 1–2-liter increment may be sufficient.

COPD patients receiving continuous oxygen at home will require supplementation during air flight. Such patients should receive greater oxygen supplementation during the flight than at sea level. Increments equivalent to 1–2 liters of oxygen by nasal cannula during flight should suffice for most patients. Patients will also require additional oxygen supplementation if the elevation at the destination is significantly greater than at home. The Federal Aviation Administration (FAA) requires a physician's Statement of Oxygen Need for a patient to receive continuous oxygen during flight. Because there is no uniform airline request form, each airline must be contacted by the patient to determine what is required. Because the airlines do not provide oxygen for ground use in the airline terminal, patients who require continuous oxygen should be advised to make plans for such locations. The American Lung Association provides patient education materials for individuals who travel with oxygen entitled "Airline Travel with Oxygen."

NUTRITION

As many as 25% of outpatients with COPD may be malnourished; almost 50% of those patients admitted to the hospital have evidence of malnutrition. Sixty percent of critically ill COPD patients with acute respiratory failure are malnourished. The exact cause is not clear, but factors such as increased work of breathing, decreased food intake because of dyspnea, and secretion of cytokines (such as tumor necrosis factor) may combine to generate the malnutrition state. Malnutrition is associated with wasting of respiratory muscles causing respiratory muscle weakness.

The nutritional assessment of COPD patients includes body weight (loss in excess of 10% ideal body weight), but presence of edema limits the utility of body weight. Hepatic secretory proteins such as albumin, transferrin, retinol binding protein, and prealbumin are markers of visceral protein stores and proposed as methods of nutritional assessment. Unfortunately, all are influenced by numerous factors in addition to the nutritional state. Anthropometry involves application of simple measurements of skin folds and circumferences to divide the body into compartments of fat, muscle tissue, and skeletal mass. This is used with limited success. Depression of cellular immunity is consistently associated with malnutrition and nutritional repletion is associated with improved immunocompetence. The utility of skin testing is limited by multiple factors, which include technical application and interpretation of skin tests. Tests of muscle function are also used as markers of nutritional status. Unfortunately, no simple recommendation can be given regarding the ''best'' test for nutritional assessment. Utilization of any of these methods can be appropriate, provided the limitations are clearly understood.

Nutritional Support

Aggressive oral nutritional supplementation in COPD patients results in improvement of respiratory strength but it is laborious, time-intensive, and often cannot be maintained by the patient. It has been suggested that COPD patients might benefit from a high lipid, low carbohydrate diet because of the reduced respiratory quotient (RQ) when the latter substrates are fed. The clinical benefits of altering fat to carbohydrate ratios in COPD patients when calories supplied are appropriate remains unproven, however. Overfeeding should be avoided. Electrolyte disturbances are common in COPD patients and have the potential for significant adverse outcomes. Hypophosphatemia, hyperkalemia, hypocalcemia, and hypomagnesemia are associated with decreased respiratory muscle function, while repletion of these abnormalities results in improved function. Hypophosphatemia can develop as a consequence of refeeding. Although these complications apply to all patients receiving nutritional support, COPD patients may be at increased risk relative to decreased respiratory muscle function secondary to their prior lung disease. Monitoring electrolyte levels and providing supplemental electrolytes, especially phosphorus in malnourished patients, should be routine in COPD patients with respiratory failure. Patients with COPD should be instructed on good dietary habits. Their weight should approximate ideal body weight. If malnourished, attempts should be made to restore nutritional balance. Several smaller meals a day may help maintain caloric needs but avoid undue dyspnea. Forced nutrition or special diets are not recommended at the present time. The use of hormones to improve muscle functions remains experimental.

CONCLUSION

Over the past two decades, our knowledge about COPD has increased significantly. Smoking cessation campaigns have resulted in a significant decrease in smoking prevalence in the United States. Similar efforts in the rest of the world should have the same impact. The consequence should be a drop in incidence of COPD in the years to come. The widespread application of long-term oxygen therapy for hypoxemic patients has resulted in increased survival. During this time we have expanded our drug therapy armamentarium and have used it to effectively improve dyspnea and quality of life. Noninvasive ventilation has offered new alternatives for the patient with acute failure. The revival of surgery for emphysema, although still experimental, may serve as an alternative to lung transplant for those patients with severe COPD who are still symptomatic on maximal medical therapy. Given all these options, a nihilistic attitude toward these patients is not justified.

BIBLIOGRAPHY

Albert R, Martin T, Lewis S. Controlled clinical trial of methylprednisolone in patients with chronic bronchitis and acute respiratory insufficiency. Ann Intern Med 1980;92:753–758.

AMA Commission on Emergency Medical Services. Medical aspects of transportation aboard commercial aircraft. JAMA 1982;247:1007–1011.

American Thoracic Society. Chronic bronchitis, asthma, and pulmonary emphysema. A statement by the Committee on Diagnostic Standards for Nontuberculous Respiratory Diseases. Am Rev Respir Dis 1962;85:762–768.

American Thoracic Society: Position paper. Withholding and withdrawing life-sustaining therapy. Am Rev Respir Dis 1991;144:726–731.

American Thoracic Society. Standards for the diagnosis and care of patients with chronic obstructive pulmonary disease. Am J Respir Crit Care Medicine 1995;152:78–121.

Anthonisen NR, Connett JE, Kiley JP, Altose MD, Bailey WC, Buist AS, Conway WA, Enright PL, Kanner RE, O'Hara P, Scanlon PO, Tashkin DP, Wise RA. The effects of smoking intervention and the use of an inhaled anticholinergic bronchodilator on the rate of decline of FEV_1: the lung health study. JAMA 1994;272:1497–1505.

Anthonisen NR, Manfreda J, Warren CPW, Hershfield ES, Harding GKM, Nelson NA. Antibiotic therapy in exacerbations of chronic obstructive pulmonary disease. Ann Intern Med 1987;106:196–204.

Aubier M, Murciano D, Milic-Emili M, et al. Effects of the administration of oxygen therapy on ventilation and blood gases in patients with chronic obstructive pulmonary disease during acute respiratory failure. Am Rev Respir Dis 1980;122:747–754.

Aubier M, Murciano D, Lecoguic Y, et al. Effect of hypophosphatemia on diaphragmatic contractility in patients with acute respiratory failure. N Engl J Med 1985;313:420–424.

Bates DV. Respiratory function in disease. 3rd ed. New York: WB Saunders Co, 1989: 172–187.

Belman MJ, Botnick WC, Shin JW. Inhaled bronchodilators reduce dynamic hyperinflation during exercise in patients with chronic obstructive pulmonary disease. Am J Respir Crit Care Med 1996;153:967–975.

Belman MJ, Soo Hoo GW, Kuei JH, Shadonehr R. Efficacy of positive vs. negative pressure ventilation in unloading the respiratory muscles. Chest 1990;98:850–856.

Benditt J, Pollock M, Celli B. Transtracheal delivery of gas decreases the oxygen cost of breathing. Am Rev Respir Dis 1993;147:1207–1210.

Bott J, Carroll MP, Conway JH, et al. Randomised controlled trial of nasal ventilation in acute ventilatory failure due to chronic obstructive airways disease. Lancet 1993;341:1555–1557.

Brantigan O, Mueller E, Kress MB. A surgical approach to pulmonary emphysema. Am Rev Respir Dis 1959;80:194–202.

Brantly M, Nukiwa T, Crystal RG. Molecular basis of alpha-1-antitrypsin deficiency. Am J Med 1988;84:13–31.

Braun SR, Keim NL, Dixon RM, et al. The prevalence and determinants of nutritional changes in chronic obstructive pulmonary disease. Chest 1984;86:558–563.

Brochard L, Isabey D, Piquet J, Amaro P, Mancebo J, Messadi A, Brun-Buisson C, Rauss A, Lemaire F, Harf A. Reversal of acute exacerbations of chronic obstructive lung disease by inspiratory assistance with a face mask. N Engl J Med 1990;323:1523–1530.

Brown DG, Pierson DJ. Auto-PEEP is common in mechanically ventilated patients: a study of incidence, severity, and detection. Respir Care 1986;31:1069–1074.

Buist SA. Smoking and other risk factors. In: Murray JF, Nadel JA, eds. Textbook of respiratory medicine. 2nd ed. Philadelphia: WB Saunders Co, 1994:1259–1287.

Callahan C, Dittus R, Katz BP. Oral corticosteroids therapy for patients with stable chronic obstructive pulmonary disease: a meta-analysis. Ann Intern Med 1991;114:216–223.

Chalker R, Celli B. Special considerations in the elderly. Clin Chest Med 1993;14:437–452.

Chapman KR. Therapeutic algorithm for chronic obstructive pulmonary disease. Am J Med 1991;91(4A):17S–23S.

Chevrolet JC, Jolliet P, Abajo B, Toussi A, Louis M. Nasal positive pressure ventilation in patients with acute ventilatory failure. Chest 1991;100:775–782.

Christopher KL, Spofford BT, Petrun MD, McCarty DC, Goodman JR, Petty TL. A program for transtracheal oxygen delivery: assessment of safety and efficacy. Ann Intern Med 1987; 107:802–808.

Connaughton J, Catteral K, Elton R, Stradling J, Douglas N. Do sleep studies contribute to the management of patients with severe chronic obstructive pulmonary disease? Am Rev Respir Dis 1988;138:341–344.

Cooper J, Trulock E, Triantafillou A, et al. Bilateral pneumectomy (volume reduction) for chronic obstructive pulmonary disease. J Thorac Cardiovasc Surg 1995;109:106–119.

Dardes N, Campo S, Chiappini MG, et al. Prognosis of COPD patients after an episode of acute respiratory failure. Eur J Respir Dis 1986;69(146):377–381.

Dark DS, Pingleton SK, Kerby GR. Hypercapnia during weaning: a complication of nutritional support. Chest 1985;88:141–143.

Dillard TA, Berb BW, Rajagopal KR, Dooley JW, Mehm WJ. Hypoxemia during air travel in patients with chronic obstructive pulmonary disease. Ann Intern Med 1989;111:362–367.

Dillard TA, Beninati WA, Berg BW. Air travel in patients with chronic obstructive pulmonary disease. Arch Intern Med 1991;151:1793–1795.

Dompeling E, van Schayck CP, van Grunsven PM, van Herwaarden CLA, Akkermans R, Molema J, Folgering H, van Weel C. Slowing the deterioration of asthma and chronic obstructive pulmonary disease observed during bronchodilator therapy by adding inhaled corticosteroids: a 4-year prospective study. Ann Intern Med 1993;118:770–778.

Donahue M, Rogers RM, Wilson DO, et al. Oxygen consumption of the respiratory muscles in normal and malnourished patients with chronic obstructive pulmonary disease. Am Rev Respir Dis 1989;140:385–391.

Dunn WF, Nelson SB, Hubmayr RD. Oxygen-induced hypercarbia in obstructive pulmonary disease. Am Rev Respir Dis 1991;144:526–530.

Emerman CL, Effron D, Lukens TW. Spirometric criteria for hospital admission of patients with acute exacerbation of COPD. Chest 1991;99:595–599.

Emerman CL, Connors AF, Lukens TW, Effron D, May ME. Relationship between arterial blood gases and spirometry in acute exacerbations of chronic obstructive pulmonary disease. Ann Emerg Med 1989;18:523–527.

Feinlieb M, Rosenberg HM, Collins JG, Delozier JE, Pokras R, Chevarley FM. Trends in COPD morbidity and mortality in the United States. Am Rev Respir Dis 1989;140:S9–S18.

Ferguson GT, Cherniack RM. Management of chronic obstructive pulmonary disease. N Engl J Med 1993;328:1017–1022.

Fiore MC, Jorenby DE, Baker TB, Kenford SL. Tobacco dependence and the nicotine patch: clinical guidelines for effective use. JAMA 1992;268:2687–2694.

Fletcher E, Miller J, Divine G, Fletcher J, Miller T. Nocturnal oxyhemoglobin desaturation in COPD patients with arterial oxygen tensions above 60 mm Hg. Chest 1987;92:604–608.

Fletcher E, Luckett R, Miller T, Fletcher J. Exercise hemodynamics and gas exchange in patients with chronic obstructive pulmonary disease, sleep desaturation, and a daytime PCO_2 above 60 mm Hg. Am Rev Respir Dis 1989;140:1237–1245.

Fletcher E, Donner C, Midgren B, et al. Survival in COPD patients with a daytime PaO_2 > 60 mm Hg with and without nocturnal oxyhemoglobin desaturation. Chest 1992;101: 649–655.

Gelb AF, Zamel N, Colchen A, et al. Physiologic studies of tracheobronchial stents in airway obstruction. Am Rev Respir Dis 1992;146:1088–1090.

Gift AG. Validation of a vertical visual analogue scale as a measure of clinical dyspnea. Rehab Nurse 1989;14:323–325.

Gong H, Tashkin DP, Simmons MS. Hypoxia-altitude simulation test. Am Rev Respir Dis 1984;130:980–986.

Guyatt GH, Berman LB, Townsend M, et al. A measure of quality of life for clinical trials in chronic lung disease. Thorax 1987;42:773–778.

Higgins MW, Thom T. Incidence, prevalence, and mortality: intra- and Intercountry differences. In: Hensley MJ, Saunders NA, eds. Clinical epidemiology of chronic obstructive pulmonary disease. New York: Marcel Dekker Inc, 1990.

Hill NS. Noninvasive ventilation: does it work, for whom, and how? Am Rev Respir Dis 1993;147:1050–1055.

Hockley B, Johnson NM. A comparison of three high doses of ipratropium bromide in chronic asthma. Br J Dis Chest 1985;79:379–384.

Hodgkin JE. Prognosis in chronic obstructive pulmonary disease. Clin Chest Med 1990;11: 555–569.

Hoffman LA, Wesmiller SW, Sciurba FC, Johnson JT, Ferson PF, Dauber JH. Nasal cannula and transtracheal oxygen delivery: comparison of patient response after six months use of each technique. Am Rev Respir Dis 1992;145:827–831.

Hudson LD. Survival data in patients with acute and chronic lung disease requiring mechanical ventilation. Am Rev Respir Dis 1989;140:S19–S24.

Hudson LD, Monti CM. Rationale and use of corticosteroids in chronic obstructive pulmonary disease. Med Clin North Am 1990;74:661–690.

Jackson RM. Pulmonary oxygen toxicity. Chest 1985;88:900–905.

Jones PW, Quirk FH, Baveystock CM, Littlejohn P. A self-complete measure of health status for chronic airflow limitation. Am Rev Respir Dis 1992;145:1321–1327.

Kaelin RM, Assimacopoulos A, Chevrolet JC. Failure to predict six-month survival of patients with COPD requiring mechanical ventilation by analysis of simple indices. Chest 1987; 92:971–978.

Kanford SL, Fiore MC, Jorenby DE, Smith SS, Wetter D, Baker TB. Predicting smoking cessation: who will quit with and without the nicotine patch. JAMA 1994;271:589–594.

Karpel JP. Bronchodilator responses to anticholinergic and beta-adrenergic agents in acute and stable COPD. Chest 1991;99:871–876.

Karpel JP, Kotch A, Zinny M, Pesin J, Alleyne W. A comparison of inhaled ipratropium, oral theophylline plus inhaled β-agonist, and the combination of all three in patients with COPD. Chest 1994;105:1089–1094.

Keenan R, Landremeau R, Sciurba F, et al. Unilateral thoracoscopic surgical approach for diffuse emphysema. J Thorac Cardiovasc Surg 1996;111:308–316.

Klein JS, Gamsu G, Webb WR, Golden JA, Müller NL. High-resolution CT diagnosis of emphysema in symptomatic patients with normal chest radiographs and isolated low diffusing capacity. Radiology 1992;182:817–821.

Kottke TE, Battista RN, DeFriese GH. Attributes of successful smoking cessation interventions in medical practice: a meta-analysis of 39 controlled trials. JAMA 1988;259: 2882–2889.

Krop AD, Block AJ, Cohen E. Neuropsychiatric effects of continuous oxygen therapy in chronic obstructive pulmonary disease. Chest 1973;64:317–322.

Levi-Valensi P, Weitzenblum E, Rida A, et al. Sleep-related oxygen desaturation and daytime pulmonary hemodynamics in COPD patients. Eur Respir J 1992;5:301–307.

Liebman J, Lucas R, Moss A, Cotton E, Rosenthal A, Ruttenberg H. Airline travel for children with chronic pulmonary disease. Pediatrics 1976;57:408–410.

Lopez-Majano V, Dutton RE. Regulation of respiratory drive during oxygen breathing in chronic obstructive lung disease. Am Rev Respir Dis 1973;108:232–240.

MacIntyre NR. Respiratory function during pressure support ventilation. Chest 1986;89: 677–683.

Mahler DA, Weinburg DH, Wells CK, Feinstein AR. The measurement of dyspnea: contents, interobserver agreement, and physiologic correlates of two new clinical indexes. Chest 1984;85:751–758.

Martin TR, Lewis SW, Albert RK. The prognosis of patients with chronic obstructive pulmonary disease after hospitalization for acute respiratory failure. Chest 1982;82:310–314.

Martinez F, Montes de Oca M, Whyte R, Stetz J, Gay S, Celli B. Lung volume reduction improves dyspnea, dynamic hyperinflation, and respiratory muscle function. Am J Respir Crit Care Med. In press.

McGavin CR, Gupta SP, McHardy GJ. Twelve-minute walking test for assessing disability in chronic bronchitis. Br Med J 1976;1:822–823.

McKay SE, Howie CA, Thomson AH, Whiting B, Addis GJ. Value of theophylline treatment in patients handicapped by chronic obstructive lung disease. Thorax 1993;48:227–232.

McKenna R, Brenner M, Gelb A, et al. A randomized prospective trial of stapled lung reduction versus laser bullectomy for diffuse emphysema. J Thorac Cardiovasc Surg 1996;111: 317–322.

Murata GH, Gorby MS, Chick TW, Halperin AK. Use of emergency medical services by patients with decompensated obstructive lung disease. Ann Emerg Med 1989;18:501–506.

Murata GH, Gorby MS, Kapsner CO, Chick TW, Halperin AK. A multivariate model for the prediction of relapse after outpatient treatment of decompensated chronic obstructive pulmonary disease. Arch Intern Med 1992;152:73–77.

Mushlin AI, Black ER, Connolly CA, Buonaccorso KM, Eberly SW. The necessary length of hospital stay for chronic pulmonary disease. JAMA 1991;266:80–83.

Nisar M, Earis JE, Pearson MG, Calverley PMA. Acute bronchodilator trials in chronic obstructive pulmonary disease. Am Rev Respir Dis 1992;146:555–559.

Nocturnal Oxygen Therapy Trial Group. Continuous or nocturnal oxygen therapy in hypoxemic chronic obstructive lung disease. Ann Intern Med 1980;93:391–398.

O'Donnell DE, Webb KA, Bertley JC, Chau K, Conlan AA. Mechanisms of relief of exertional breathlessness following unilateral bullectomy and lung volume reduction surgery in emphysema. Chest 1996;110:18–27.

O'Donohue WJ. Effect of oxygen therapy on increasing arterial oxygen tension in hypoxemia patients with stable chronic obstructive pulmonary disease while breathing ambient air. Chest 1991;100:968–972.

Pearlman RA. Variability in physician estimates of survival for acute respiratory failure in chronic obstructive pulmonary disease. Chest 1987;91:515–521.

Pepe PE, Marini JJ. Occult positive end-expiratory pressure in mechanically ventilated patients with airflow obstruction: the auto-PEEP effect. Am Rev Respir Dis 1982;126:166–170.

Petty TL. The National Mucolytic Study: results of a randomized, double-blind, placebo-controlled study of iodinated glycerol in chronic obstructive bronchitis. Chest 1990;97: 75–83.

Postma DS. Inhaled therapy in COPD: what are the benefits. Respir Med 1991;85:447–449.

Postma DS, Sluiter HJ. Prognosis of chronic obstructive pulmonary disease: the Dutch experience. Am Rev Respir Dis 1989;140:S100–S105.

President's Commission for the Study of Ethical Problems in Medicine and Biomedical and Behavioral Research. Making health care decisions: the ethical and legal implications of informed consent in the patient-practitioner relationship. Vol 1. Washington, DC: US Government Printing Office, 1982.

Prochaska JO, Goldstein MG. Process of smoking cessation. Clin Chest Med 1991;12: 727–735.

Redline S, Weiss ST. Genetic and perinatal risk factors for the development of chronic obstructive pulmonary disease. In: Hensley MJ, Saunders NA, eds. Clinical epidemiology of chronic obstructive pulmonary disease. New York: Marcel Dekker, 1989:139–168.

Rennard SI, Serby CW, Ghafouri M, Johnson PA, Friedman M. Extended therapy with ipratropium is associated with improved lung function in patients with COPD. Chest 1996; 110:62–70.

Report of the Medical Research Council Working Party. Long-term domiciliary oxygen therapy in chronic hypoxic cor pulmonale complicating chronic bronchitis and emphysema. Lancet 1981;1:681–685.

Rodnick JE, Gude JK. The use of antibiotics in acute bronchitis and acute exacerbations of chronic bronchitis. West J Med 1988;149:347–351.

Salzman GA, Steele MT, Pribble JP, Elenbaas RM, Pyszczynski DR. Aerosolized metaproterenol in the treatment of asthmatics with severe airflow obstruction. Comparison of two delivery methods. Chest 1989;96:1017–1020.

Sanders C. The radiographic diagnosis of emphysema. Radiol Clin North Am 1991;29: 1019–1030.

Schlick W. Selective indications for use of antibiotics: when and what. Eur Respir Rev 1992; 2:9, 187–192.

Schwartz JL. Methods for smoking cessation. Clin Chest Med 1991;12:737–753.

Sciurba F, Rogers R, Keenan R, et al. Improvement in pulmonary function and elastic recoil after lung reduction surgery for diffuse emphysema. N Engl J Med 1996;334:1095–1099.

Skorodin MS. Pharmacotherapy for asthma and chronic obstructive pulmonary disease. Arch Intern Med 1993;153:814–828.

Snider GL. Pulmonary disease in alpha-1-antitrypsin deficiency. Ann Intern Med 1989;111: 957–959.

Snider GL, Kleinerman J, Thurlbeck WM, Bengali ZK. The definition of emphysema: report of a National Heart, Lung and Blood Institute, Division of Lung Diseases, Workshop. Am Rev Respir Dis 1985;132:182–185.

Sweer L, Zwillich CW. Dyspnea in the patient with chronic obstructive pulmonary disease. Clin Chest Med 1990;11(3):417–445.

Tarpy S, Celli B. Long-term oxygen therapy. N Engl J Med 1995;333:710–719.

Thomas P, Pugsley JA, Stewart JH. Theophylline and salbutamol improve pulmonary function in patients with irreversible chronic obstructive pulmonary disease. Chest 1992;101: 160–165.

Tiep BL. Medicare regulations for oxygen reimbursement. In: Tiep BL, ed. Portable oxygen therapy: including oxygen conserving methodology. Mt. Kisco, NY: Futura Publishing Co, 1991;15.

Tiep BL, Christopher KL, Spofford BT, Goodman J, Worley PD, Macey SL. Pulsed nasal and transtracheal oxygen delivery. Chest 1990;97:364–368.

Travis J. Alpha-1-proteinase inhibitor deficiency. In: Massaro M, ed. Lung cell biology. New York: Marcel Dekker, 1989:1227–1246.

Weitzenblum E, Sautegeau A, Ehrhart M, Mammosser M, Pelletier A. Long-term oxygen therapy can reverse the progression of pulmonary hypertension in patients with chronic obstructive pulmonary disease. Am Rev Respir Dis 1985;131:493–498.

West GA, Primeau P. Nonmedical hazards of long-term oxygen therapy. Respir Care 1983; 28:906–912.

Ziment I. Pharmacologic therapy of obstructive airway disease. Clin Chest Med 1990;11: 461–486.

6 Restrictive Lung Disease

David R. Moller, Joseph P. Lynch, III

The term "restrictive lung disease" encompasses a large, diverse group of diffuse lung diseases characterized by filling of the alveoli and/or infiltration of the pulmonary interstitium, which results in a characteristic pattern of restrictive lung impairment with reduction in lung volumes and decrease in the compliance of the lung. A classification based on the known cause or symptom complex of this group of disorders is given in Table 6.1.

PATHOPHYSIOLOGY

Disorders involving the pulmonary interstitium are associated with inflammation and/or fibrosis of the alveolar structures. The inflammatory component may be dominated by mononuclear cells, neutrophils, eosinophils, or lymphocytes and is termed an alveolitis. The inflammatory process may be associated with various degrees of fibrosis. Both processes result in restrictive physiologic disturbances.

- Forced vital capacity (FVC) and forced expiratory volume in one second (FEV_1) are reduced proportionately in the absence of associated obstructive airways disease. Thus, the FEV_1/FVC is commonly normal or supranormal.
- Lung volumes (total lung capacity (TLC), vital capacity (VC), and residual volume (RV)) are reduced.
- Lung compliance is reduced.
- Diffusing capacity for carbon monoxide (DL_{CO}) is reduced and the difference between the alveolar and arterial oxygen tensions ((A-a)O_2 gradient) is widened.
- Hypoxemia results from mismatching of ventilation and perfusion. Chronic respiratory alkalosis occurs, and respiratory acidosis may supervene with advanced disease.
- Gas exchange is typically disturbed during exercise and often correlates with the severity of the disease.
- Similar physiologic changes are noted with airspace involvement, except that hypoxemia may be more severe because of greater shunt fractions compared with disorders with predominant interstitial involvement.

APPROACH TO THE DIAGNOSIS

Management of patients with restrictive lung disease begins by establishing a definitive diagnosis whenever possible. Most patients have progressive dyspnea and/or

237

Table 6.1. Classification of Restrictive Lung Disease

Familial or congenital	Physical reagents
Familial pulmonary fibrosis	Radiation lung disease
Gaucher's disease	Rejection-associated pulmonary fibrosis
Niemann-Pick disease	Primary eosinophilic pneumonias
Hermansky-Pudlak syndrome	Löffler's syndrome
Familial hypercalciuric hypercalcemia	Chronic eosinophilic pneumonia
and interstitial lung disease	Allergic bronchopulmonary aspergillosis
Neurofibromatosis and tuberous sclerosis	Tropical pulmonary eosinophilia
Environmental lung disease	Pulmonary vasculitis—Churg-Strauss
Inorganic dust diseases	syndrome
(pneumoconiosis)	Hypereosinophilic syndromes
Asbestosis	Disorders of unknown cause
Silicosis	Sarcoidosis
Coal workers' pneumoconiosis	Idiopathic pulmonary fibrosis (IPF)
Siderosis	Collagen vascular lung disease
Talcosis	Bronchiolitis obliterans–organizing
Hard metal disease	pneumonia (BOOP)
Hypersensitivity pneumonitis	Eosinophilic granuloma (EG)
Organic dusts	Pulmonary vasculitis
Chemicals	Wegener's granulomatosis
Granulomatous diseases	Goodpasture's syndrome
Beryllium disease	Systemic necrotizing vasculitis
Diffuse lung injury	Hypersensitivity vasculitis
NO_2 (silo-filler's disease)	Lymphomatoid granulomatosis
Irritant chemicals	Lymphocytic infiltrative disorders
Infections	Idiopathic pulmonary hemosiderosis
Viral	Lymphangioleiomyomatosis
Bacterial	Amyloidosis
Mycobacterial	Pulmonary alveolar proteinosis (PAP)
Fungal	Pulmonary alveolar microlithiasis
Parasitic	Lipoid pneumonia
Drug reactions	
Chemotherapeutic agents	
Antiarrhythmic agents	
Antibiotics	
Illicit drugs	
Miscellaneous	

diffuse pulmonary infiltration on chest x-ray. Review of the clinical history, physical examination, and all previous and current chest radiographs give important clues to the diagnosis and chronicity of the disease.

The initial diagnostic sequence starts by excluding multiple other possible causes of progressive dyspnea and/or diffuse pulmonary infiltration. Left ventricular failure, primary pulmonary hypertension, and pulmonary embolism must be considered. Patients should be evaluated for known causes of interstitial lung disease, such as occupational and environmental agents, drugs, connective tissue diseases, and infectious pneumonias, by performing a detailed history and physical examination and, where appropriate, serum studies.

History

- Rapid changes in symptoms and radiologic pattern are unusual except in pulmonary edema, hemorrhage, or pneumonia.
- Careful occupational, environmental, and drug histories are critical and can lead to specific diagnoses.
- Fever suggests an infectious process, a collagen vascular disorder, malignancy, hypersensitivity pneumonitis (HP), sarcoidosis, or drug reaction.
- Hemoptysis is commonly seen in advanced fibrocystic sarcoidosis, pulmonary vasculitis (e.g., Wegener's granulomatosis, Goodpasture's syndrome), blood dyscrasias, or infections.

Physical Examination

- Interstitial pulmonary fibrosis is frequently associated with end-inspiratory, "Velcro" crepitations (crackles).
- Bronchiolitis obliterans–organizing pneumonia (BOOP), HP, or idiopathic pulmonary fibrosis (IPF) may demonstrate high-pitched, musical, mid-inspiratory squeaks.
- Digital clubbing is found in up to 25% of patients with pulmonary fibrosis, usually as a late manifestation.

Chest X-ray

Chest x-rays may narrow the differential diagnosis when combined with the history and physical examination (see Chapter 1). Traditionally, diseases causing diffuse infiltration on chest x-ray are divided into interstitial or alveolar disorders based on radiographic features (Table 6.2). Alveolar-filling diseases are associated with small, nodular, ill-defined infiltrates reflecting material in the distal airspaces. Confluence of these opacities may lead to large areas of consolidation with air bronchograms and silhouetting of normal structures. Interstitial processes are associated with reticular, reticulonodular, or nodular patterns or a ground glass appearance.

- Many restrictive diseases involve both alveolar and interstitial components, and the radiographic pattern is mixed.
- Four to ten percent of symptomatic individuals with diffuse lung disease initially have normal chest x-rays.
- Mediastinal adenopathy is common in sarcoidosis, lymphoma, granulomatous infections, lymphangitic carcinomatosis, silicosis, berylliosis, and amyloidosis, and is uncommon in Wegener's granulomatosis (WG) or IPF.
- Pleural effusions associated with interstitial lung disease are commonly seen with

Table 6.2. Radiographic Features of Restrictive Lung Disease

Predominantly Alveolar Pattern	*Predominantly Interstitial Pattern*
Diffuse pulmonary hemorrhage	Inflammatory disorders
Goodpasture's syndrome	Sarcoidosis
Idiopathic pulmonary hemosiderosis	Pneumoconiosis
Vasculitis	Eosinophilic granuloma (EG)
Bleeding diathesis	Hypersensitivity pneumonitis (HP)
Drugs	Idiopathic pulmonary fibrosis (IPF)
Pulmonary exudates	Interstitial pneumonitis associated with
Infectious pneumonias	collagen vascular disorders
Eosinophilic pneumonias	Familial pulmonary fibrosis
Pulmonary alveolar proteinosis (PAP)	Bronchiolitis obliterans–organizing
Lipoid pneumonia	pneumonia (BOOP) (mixed pattern)
Sarcoidosis	Infections
Idiopathic pulmonary fibrosis (IPF)	Neoplasms
(desquamative phase)	Lymphangitic carcinomatosis
Neoplasms	Metastatic carcinoma
Bronchoalveolar cell carcinoma	Lymphoma
Lymphoma	
Metastatic carcinoma	

tuberculosis and other infections, collagen vascular diseases, asbestos-related diseases, and lymphangitic carcinomatosis, and are uncommon in lymphangioleiomyomatosis (chylous effusions) and drug reactions (e.g., nitrofurantoin).

- Diffuse pulmonary infiltration in immunocompromised patients suggests opportunistic infections, diffuse pulmonary hemorrhage or edema, malignancy, or drug reactions.

High-Resolution Computed Tomography (HRCT)

Computed tomography of the lungs is an important advance in the evaluation of patients with restrictive lung diseases and is best performed using high-resolution, thin-section (1- to 2-mm-thick slices) techniques (HRCT). HRCT does not require contrast and is superior to conventional chest radiographs in delineating parenchymal details and lung architecture. Specific patterns of aberrations on HRCT are characteristic of specific diseases and may narrow the differential diagnosis. Findings on HRCT are discussed in greater detail in the sections on individual diseases later in this chapter.

Laboratory Studies

A specific diagnosis can sometimes be confirmed by noninvasive tests. Sputum cultures and cytologies are generally of low yield. Serologies (e.g., antinuclear antibody (ANA), rheumatoid factor, antineutrophil cytoplasmic antibody, angiotensin-converting enzyme, complement fixation antibodies for fungi) are helpful in selected patients but are usually nonspecific. Biopsies of extrapulmonary sites (e.g., skin, superficial lymph nodes) are appropriate in selected patients with malignancy, sarcoidosis, or granulomatous infections. Lung biopsy (transbronchial or thoracoscopic) is usually required, however, to substantiate a specific etiologic diagnosis.

Fiberoptic Bronchoscopy

When noninvasive studies are nondiagnostic, fiberoptic bronchoscopy with transbronchial lung biopsies is warranted to evaluate diffuse pulmonary infiltrates (unless specific contraindications exist). Multiple transbronchial biopsies (TBBs) obtained from upper and lower lobe sites are sent for histologic analysis. Bronchoalveolar lavage (BAL) fluid may be sent for cytologies (to look for malignant cells or fungi) and cultures (usually fungal, mycobacterial, or viral). When enlarged paratracheal, subcarinal, or hilar nodes are present, Wang needle aspiration biopsy may confirm granulomatous or neoplastic processes.

- Bronchoscopic biopsy is effective in diagnosing infectious diseases (tuberculosis, fungal infection, *Pneumocystis carinii*), sarcoidosis, lymphangitic carcinomatosis, eosinophilic granuloma (EG), pulmonary alveolar proteinosis (PAP), and eosinophilic pneumonia. In contrast, the yield of bronchoscopy in pulmonary WG is less than 10%.
- BAL may provide diagnostic information with appropriate microbiologic and cytologic analysis of the fluid. Although the role of BAL in the diagnosis and staging of noninfectious, nonmalignant interstitial diseases is unproven, differential cell counts show characteristic profiles in many interstitial lung diseases. The risk of transbronchial lung biopsies is small, with a less than 1% incidence of pneumothorax in experienced hands. Serious bleeding is rare, but biopsies should not be performed if bleeding diathesis, coagulopathy, or thrombocytopenia are present.

Surgical (Open or Thoracoscopic) Lung Biopsy

Surgical (open or thoracoscopic) lung biopsies may be necessary when prior investigations (including transbronchial lung biopsies) are nondiagnostic. Thoracoscopic lung biopsy is less invasive than open biopsy, reduces the duration of hospitalization, and is preferred in most cases.

- Thoracoscopic (or open) lung biopsy should only be performed if the findings will alter the approach to treatment.

THERAPY

Management involves specific therapy for treatable diseases (Table 6.3) and general supportive care for all patients. Supportive care includes:

Table 6.3. Therapy of Some Treatable Restrictive Lung Diseases

Disorder	Primary Therapy	Secondary Therapy
Known etiology		
Infections	Antimicrobials	
Pneumoconiosis	Removal from exposure	
Hypersensitivity pneumonitis (HP)	Removal from exposure	Corticosteroids
Drug reactions	Discontinue drugs	Corticosteroids
Unknown etiology		
Sarcoidosis	Corticosteroids	
Idiopathic pulmonary fibrosis (IPF)	Corticosteroids	Cytotoxic agents[a]
Interstitial pneumonitis associated with collagen vascular disorders	Corticosteroids	Cytotoxic agents[a]
Bronchiolitis obliterans organizing pneumonia (BOOP)	Corticosteroids	
Wegener's granulomatosis	Cytotoxic agents[a] plus corticosteroids	?Co-trimoxazole
Goodpasture's syndrome	Plasmapheresis, corticosteroids	Cytotoxic agents[a]
Pulmonary vasculitis	Corticosteroids	Cytotoxic agents[a]
Eosinophilic granuloma (histiocytosis X) (EG)	Quit smoking	Corticosteroids
Chronic eosinophilic pneumonia	Corticosteroids	
Tropical pulmonary eosinophilia	Diethylcarbamazine citrate	
Pulmonary alveolar proteinosis (PAP)	Lung lavage	

[a] Cyclophosphamide, azathioprine are most commonly used.

- Supplemental oxygen for exercise-associated or resting hypoxemia;
- Bronchodilators for bronchial hyperresponsiveness or endobronchial involvement;
- Infection prophylaxis with influenza and pneumococcal vaccines;
- Antibiotic therapy begun promptly at the first sign of an upper respiratory tract infection or exacerbation of cough and sputum production;
- Diuretic therapy with the appearance of cor pulmonale.

In the sections that follow, individual diseases will be discussed in depth, with an emphasis on clinical, radiographic, and histopathologic features, and an approach to management.

IDIOPATHIC PULMONARY FIBROSIS

Idiopathic pulmonary fibrosis, also known as cryptogenic fibrosing alveolitis, is a disease of unknown cause that produces diffuse inflammation and fibrosis of the alveolar interstitium, resulting in cough, dyspnea, and respiratory insufficiency. The clinical course is highly variable, but progression to severe respiratory failure and death within 2–10 years is characteristic. Five-year mortality exceeds 40%. Spontaneous resolution occurs in fewer than 1% of cases. Progressive respiratory failure is the leading cause of death, but lung cancer complicates IPF in 9–11% of patients.

Clinical Features

- Onset is usually after age 40, with a peak incidence in the 7th and 8th decades of life.
- Prevalence (per 100,000) is less than 3 for adults between the ages of 35–44 years but exceeds 175 for adults older than 75 years. IPF is rare in children.
- Gradual, progressive dyspnea on exertion and nonproductive cough are characteristic.
- Extrapulmonary involvement does not occur.
- Chest auscultation reveals bibasilar, late inspiratory, Velcro crackles in more than 80% of patients.
- Clubbing of the fingers is found in 25% or more of patients.
- Cardiac examination is normal except in advanced stages when signs of pulmonary hypertension (cor pulmonale) develop.
- Blood or serologic studies are of no value in the diagnosis or follow-up of IPF.
- Nonspecific elevations in the erythrocyte sedimentation rate (ESR) are noted in 60–94% of patients with IPF; circulating antinuclear antibodies or rheumatoid factor, in 10–20%. These serologic studies do not correlate with extent or activity of the disease and do not predict therapeutic responsiveness.

Chest Radiographs

- Conventional chest radiographs are abnormal in 95% of patients with IPF (see Chapter 1). Typical features include diffuse reticular (linear) or reticulonodular interstitial infiltrates, with a basilar predominance, and small lung volumes. The disease is usually bilateral and symmetric; strictly unilateral disease is rare. With disease progression, infiltrates may extend to the apices, and lung volumes shrink. Alveolar or ground glass patterns are occasionally observed and reflect a more cellular and earlier phase of the disease. Small cystic radiolucencies 3 to 15 mm in diameter (termed honeycomb cysts) indicate end-stage, irreversible fibrosis and poor responsiveness to therapy. Chest radiographs are normal in 5–10% of patients with IPF at the time of presentation. Pleural effusions or intrathoracic lymphadenopathy are not features of IPF.

High-Resolution Computed Tomographic Scans (HRCT)

High-resolution, thin-section CT scans (HRCT) (using 1- to 2-mm slices) are more sensitive than conventional chest radiographs in evaluating the extent and nature of the parenchymal abnormalities. Characteristic HRCT findings in IPF include patchy interstitial infiltrates (reticulation), focal ground glass opacities, air bronchograms, cystic radiolucencies (honeycomb cysts), ragged pleural surfaces, irregular or thickened bronchial walls, and traction bronchiectasis. A striking and highly characteristic feature is the heterogeneity of the process. The involvement is patchy, with a striking proclivity for the peripheral (subpleural) and basilar regions of the lungs. This anatomic distribution, with a basilar predominance, distinguishes IPF from other disorders that exhibit a propensity for upper lobe involvement (e.g., pulmonary EG, sarcoidosis, silicosis, chronic eosinophilic pneumonia). HRCT features that may be observed with far advanced IPF include traction bronchiectasis, distortion of alveolar structures, severe volume loss, and dilated pulmonary arteries. The predominant pattern on HRCT may have prognostic value. Foci of alveolar (ground glass) opacities correlate with a more cellular biopsy (i.e., active alveolitis) and greater response to corticosteroid therapy. Reticular or interstitial patterns can be seen with either inflammation or fibrosis but usually do not improve with therapy. Honeycomb cysts indicate end-stage fibrosis and destroyed lung parenchyma. The prognostic significance of HRCT is influenced by the underlying histopathologic pattern observed on open lung biopsy. In patients with usual interstitial pneumonitis, ground glass attenuation usually increases in extent (worsens) or progresses to fibrosis in spite of therapy. In contrast, in patients with desquamative interstitial pneumonitis (DIP), areas of ground glass opacities usually improve or stabilize with therapy. Although HRCT is undoubtedly superior to conventional chest radiographs in assessing the extent and nature of pulmonary parenchymal involvement, HRCT is expensive, and its role in the diagnosis or follow-up evaluation of IPF is controversial.

Radionuclide Imaging

Radionuclide imaging with gallium-67 citrate or positron emission tomographs (PET scans) have been used as adjunctive measures of alveolitis. These studies are expensive, logistically difficult, and do not predict clinical course or therapeutic responsiveness. We see no current role for radionuclide studies in the diagnosis or follow-up of IPF.

Physiologic Aberrations

- Pulmonary function tests (PFTs) typically demonstrate reduced lung volumes (FVC, TLC), impaired diffusing capacity(DL_{CO}), and impaired oxygenation (either at rest or with exercise). Expiratory flow rates and FEV_1 are usually preserved. DL_{CO} is the most sensitive of the static parameters and is disproportionately reduced compared with lung volumes. In smokers, lung volumes may be higher and gas exchange worse compared with nonsmokers. Severe derangements in PFTs (e.g., VC or TLC less than 60% predicted or DL_{CO} less than 40% predicted) are associated with 2-year mortality rates exceeding 50%.
- Exercise studies are highly sensitive, even to mild cases of IPF. The alveolar-arterial oxygen gradient $(A-a)O_2$ is widened in more than 85% of patients with IPF, and invariably worsens with exercise. Other characteristic aberrations in IPF

include markedly limited exercise tolerance, respiratory alkalosis, reduced oxygen consumption, increased dead space ($V_D V_T$), and reduced compliance. Formalized exercise tests with arterial cannulation are expensive and may be difficult in elderly or debilitated patients. Less formalized tests (i.e., finger oximetry and distance walked in 6 minutes) may be adequate to quantify or follow the course of the disease.

- PFTs quantitate the extent of impairment but cannot discriminate alveolitis from fibrosis. Serial PFTs are necessary to determine response (or lack of response) to therapy. In this context, spirometry (with VC) and oximetry are adequate for most patients. More sophisticated and expensive studies, although more sensitive, can be reserved for specific indications.

Lung Biopsies

Clinical, radiographic, and physiologic studies overlap with myriad other interstitial lung disorders that may mimic IPF. In addition, these studies cannot reliably discriminate alveolitis (which may be amenable to therapy) from fibrosis (which would not be influenced by therapy). Given the potential for serious toxicities with corticosteroids or with immunosuppressive or cytotoxic agents, lung biopsy is required to exclude alternative etiologies.

Histopathologic Features

Cardinal features of IPF on lung biopsies are focal areas of alveolar septal (interstitial) and intraalveolar inflammation (alveolitis) and fibrosis. Mononuclear cells (lymphocytes, plasma cells, monocytes) infiltrate the alveolar spaces and interstitium; scattered neutrophils and eosinophils may also be present. The disease is patchy and heterogeneous, with preferential involvement of the basilar and peripheral (subpleural) regions of the lung. As the disease progresses, the inflammatory infiltrates regress, but the alveolar spaces are replaced and distorted by dense collagen, extracellular matrix, and fibrosis. Destruction of the lung architecture leads to dilated cystic airspaces (honeycombing). Granulomas or vasculitis are absent. In far advanced cases, end-stage honeycomb lung, marked smooth muscle hyperplasia, secondary pulmonary hypertension, and traction bronchiectasis may be prominent. The constellation of features of disruption of the alveolar architecture, significant interstitial fibrosis or inflammation, heterogeneous involvement, and a minimal or absent intraalveolar component is termed usual interstitial pneumonitis (UIP). This histologic variant typifies most cases of IPF and is associated with patchy peripheral (subpleural) distribution, reticular shadows, and honeycomb cysts on HRCT. In contrast, DIP is a histologic variant characterized by homogeneous filling of the alveolar spaces with macrophages, preservation of the lung architecture, and limited or no fibrosis. DIP is associated with a more favorable prognosis and responsiveness to therapy and is considered by most experts to be a disease distinct from UIP. While the relationship of UIP and DIP is controversial, these histologic patterns may reflect stereotypical responses to lung injuries of various etiologies.

Fiberoptic Bronchoscopy

Fiberoptic bronchoscopy with TBBs and BAL can be performed in the ambulatory setting with minimal morbidity and is the preferred *initial* biopsy technique in patients with chronic interstitial lung disease (CILD). A specific histologic diagnosis can be established by TBBs or BAL in several CILDs that mimic IPF, including: sarcoidosis, lymphangitic carcinomatosis, PAP, granulomatous infections, EG, and HP. Because of small sample size, TBBs cannot be considered specific for IPF, however, even if histopathologic features of interstitial inflammation or fibrosis are observed.

- The presence of patchy fibrosis or interstitial pneumonitis in TBBs may, however, *support* the diagnosis of IPF in patients with classical historic, clinical, physiologic, and radiographic (particularly HRCT) features.
- BAL demonstrates increases in BAL neutrophils or eosinophils (or both) in 67–90% of patients with IPF. Increases in BAL lymphocytes are present in up to 15% of patients. BAL lymphocytosis has been associated with a more cellular biopsy, less honeycombing, and a higher rate of response to corticosteroids. In contrast, BAL neutrophilia has no prognostic value. In some studies, BAL eosinophils have been associated with a poor therapeutic response. Despite these clinical caveats, BAL has marginal clinical value in staging or monitoring IPF and should be considered investigational.

Surgical (Open or Thoracoscopic) Lung Biopsy

Thoracoscopic or open lung biopsies are required to establish the diagnosis of IPF with certainty and to more objectively ascertain the extent of inflammatory or fibrotic components, respectively. Biopsies should be obtained from at least two sites (typically upper and lower lobes from one side).

- Histopathologic features associated with an improved prognosis include DIP, cellular inflammation, preservation of the alveolar architecture, minimal or absent honeycombing or fibrosis.
- Adverse prognostic factors include extensive disruption or destruction of the alveolar architecture, fibrosis, and honeycomb cysts.
- Because of the patchy and heterogeneous nature of the disease, the prognostic value of even surgical lung biopsies is controversial.
- In experienced hands, the yield of thoracoscopic biopsies is excellent and comparable to open lung biopsies. Thoracoscopy has lower morbidity than open lung biopsy and is preferred.
- The risk of surgical lung biopsies may be excessive in debilitated or elderly patients. In this context, the constellation of clinical, radiographic, physiologic, and transbronchial lung biopsies may be sufficient to determine a course of therapy.

Pathophysiology

- A chronic active immunologic and inflammatory reaction of the lung interstitium leads to destruction and distortion of alveoli, with fibrosis and progressive disorganization of pulmonary architecture. The physiologic consequences are stiff, non-compliant lungs that increase the work of breathing and impair gas exchange.

- Although inciting causes have not been elucidated, IPF likely represents an exuberant host response to lung injury, possibly resulting from inhaled antigen(s). Injury to lung epithelial and endothelial cells are uniformly present. Activated macrophages, neutrophils, lymphocytes, and eosinophils are present in increased numbers in the lower respiratory tract and contribute to parenchymal injury. Cytokines and inflammatory mediators enhance fibroblast recruitment and proliferation, leading to increased deposition of lung collagen and extracellular matrix, distorting and destroying the alveolar architecture.
- Cigarette smoking or occupations resulting in inhalation of hazardous dusts, metals, or chemicals may increase the risk.
- No clear genetic basis or predisposition has been found, but rare cases of IPF within families have been cited. The presence of specific genes on chromosome 14 may be associated with an increased risk of IPF.

Therapy

Corticosteroids or immunosuppressive or cytotoxic agents are the mainstay of therapy for IPF, but fewer than 30% of patients respond to therapy. Responses are usually partial and often transient; complete, sustained remissions are rare (less than 3% of patients). Optimal therapy for IPF is controversial because accurate predictors of the eventual course of IPF or responsiveness to therapy are lacking, and toxicities of the therapeutic agents may be considerable. The decision to treat must be individualized, based on the severity and acuity of the disease and on the presence of risk factors or toxicities associated with corticosteroids or immunosuppressive agents.

- Important factors to consider in determining appropriate therapy include patient age, duration of disease, rate of progression, degree of respiratory impairment, and the presence of comorbidities that may increase the toxicities of therapy.
- Individuals with severe pulmonary impairment or incapacitating complicating diseases may not be candidates for aggressive diagnostic studies (e.g., lung biopsy).
- Factors associated with a favorable response to therapy include younger age at presentation, mild pulmonary function abnormalities, a cellular lung biopsy, and elevated proportion of lymphocytes in BAL fluid. Unfavorable prognostic factors include advanced age at presentation, severe pulmonary impairment, widespread honeycomb pattern on chest x-ray, and extensive fibrosis on lung biopsy.
- Response to therapy cannot be accurately predicted by any combination of factors. Therapy should not be withheld because of unfavorable prognostic factors, but the aggressiveness of therapy may be modified.
- Determining response to therapy may be difficult because up to 20% of patients with IPF stabilize without specific therapy. While stability is considered a response by some investigators, lack of progression even for several months in some patients may simply reflect the natural history of the disease. Spontaneous remissions rarely occur in IPF, but a subset of patients have minimal symptoms or physiologic

aberrations and may remain stable for years after an initial downhill course. Discriminating these patients *a priori* from patients with a progressive deteriorating course is not possible. Because the majority of patients with IPF deteriorate, treatment of IPF is usually indicated unless stability has been assured over prolonged follow-up (two or more years). Even in this cohort, follow-up examinations at 4–6-month intervals are necessary to assess stability of the disease.

- Serial evaluations should be done to evaluate the response to therapy (or natural history of the disease). Clinical assessment, chest radiographs, and PFTs (FVC, FEV_1, DL_{CO}) are most useful in this regard. HRCT provides useful adjunctive information but is expensive, and its prognostic value requires further study. Radionuclide scans (e.g., gallium-67) and BAL have no clinical value in monitoring the disease and should be reserved for research studies.

Corticosteroids

Corticosteroids have been the cornerstone of therapy for more than four decades. Many investigators advocate doses of 1.0 mg/kg/day for up to 3 months. Some employ doses as high as 1.5 mg/kg/day for 6 weeks, tapered to 1.0 mg/kg/day for an additional 6 weeks. Others have used doses of 30–40 mg/day for 1 month, with a gradual taper. Optimal dose or duration of therapy have not been determined because studies comparing specific dosage regimens or duration of therapy have not been performed. Toxicity is invariable at high-dose regimens.

- Improvement or stabilization with corticosteroids occurs in only 10–30% of patients.
- We advise initial therapy with prednisone (40–60 mg/day or equivalent) for 3 months, at which time objective parameters (e.g., PFTs, chest radiographs, or HRCT) should be obtained to assess the presence or absence of response.
- If a favorable response is to occur, objective improvement should be noted within 3 months. Patients failing to respond by this time should be considered nonresponders. In this context, the steroid should be tapered and discontinued over the next few weeks.
- Patients responding to initial therapy should be maintained on prednisone for a minimum of 1–2 years, albeit at lower maintenance doses. The dose of prednisone can usually be tapered to 30 mg/day by 4 months and to 15–20 mg/day by 6 months. An equivalent alternate dose regimen may be substituted.
- The dose and rate of corticosteroid taper must be individualized according to objective parameters of response and toxicities.
- Progression or relapses of disease with corticosteroid taper may necessitate escalation of the dose or addition of an immunosuppressive agent.
- Patients exhibiting multiple relapses require long-term therapy (indefinite) with low-dose alternate-day corticosteroids.

Adverse Effects (Table 6.4): Adverse effects are nearly universal with high-dose corticosteroids used for IPF. Neuropsychiatric effects, bloating, weight gain, glucose intolerance, osteoporosis, peptic ulcer disease, and heightened susceptibili-

Table 6.4. Complications of Corticosteroid Therapy

Adverse Effects	Surveillance/Intervention
Endocrine: Increased appetite, weight gain, cushingoid habitus, hyperglycemia, adrenal axis suppression	Monitor weight, blood, urine, sugar; diet and insulin if needed; steroid replacement during stress
Neurologic: Emotional lability, depression, psychosis, pseudotumor cerebri	Mental status examination; use lowest possible dose
Cardiac: Sodium and fluid retention, hypertension	Monitor weight and blood pressure; 4 gm sodium restriction; treat sustained hypertension
Ocular: Glaucoma, cataracts	Ophthalmologic examination
Musculoskeletal: Osteopenia, osteoporosis, aseptic necrosis of bone, compression fractures, myopathy	Exercise program; possibly supplemental calcium and vitamin D for women
Gastrointestinal: Peptic ulcer, pancreatitis	Antacids or sucralfate for history of peptic ulcers
Cutaneous: Striae, ecchymosis, easy bruisability, acne	

ties to infection are common. Because of potential toxicities, alternative agents (e.g., azathioprine or cyclophosphamide) may be considered in lieu of corticosteroids in patients with specific risk factors for corticosteroid adverse effects (e.g., osteoporosis, advanced age (age more than 70 years), for insulin-dependent diabetes mellitus, extreme obesity, and poorly controlled hypertension).

Alternative Agents

CYCLOPHOSPHAMIDE (CYTOXAN)

Cyclophosphamide, an alkylating agent with potent inhibitory effects on diverse arms of the immune response (Table 6.5), has been reserved primarily as therapy for IPF patients failing corticosteroids. Data are limited to a few retrospective series and two prospective studies. A 6-month trial at the National Institutes of Health randomized 28 patients with midcourse IPF to prednisone alone, prednisone plus oral cyclophosphamide (1.5 mg/day), or oral cyclophosphamide alone. Compared with prednisone, cyclophosphamide reduced BAL neutrophil counts at 3 and 6 months, but PFTs did not change in any group. Johnson and colleagues randomized 43 patients with untreated IPF to either oral cyclophosphamide (1–2 mg/kg/day) *plus* alternate day prednisolone (20 mg every other day) or high-dose prednisone *alone.* Mortality at 3 years was lower in the cyclophosphamide group (3 of 21 deaths) than in the prednisolone-only group (10 of 22 deaths), but the difference may have reflected a bias in favor of cyclophosphamide at the time of randomization. Patients failing either arm of therapy were allowed to crossover to the alternative regimen. Only 3 of 16 patients who failed prednisolone responded to cyclophosphamide.

Table 6.5. Pharmacology of Cytotoxic Agents Used in the Treatment of Interstitial Lung Disease

	Cyclophosphamide	*Azathioprine*
Trade name	Cytoxan	Imuran
Oral form	25 and 50 mg tablets	25 and 50 mg tablets
Route of administration	Oral, IV	Oral
Mechanism of action	Cytotoxicity; immunosuppression	Immunosuppression; cytotoxicity
Active metabolites	Phosphoramide mustard, acrolein	6-mercaptopurine
Metabolism	Hepatic, renal	Hepatic, renal
Dosage range	1–2 mg/kg/day	2–3 mg/kg/day
Approved indications	Many neoplastic disorders	Adjunctive therapy in transplant rejection; severe rheumatoid arthritis
Complications	Leukopenia	Leukopenia
	Hemorrhagic cystitis	Toxic hepatitis (rare)
	Anorexia, nausea, vomiting[a]	Dermatitis (rare)
	Alopecia[a,b]	Anorexia, nausea, vomiting[a]
	Gonadal dysfunction (common)	Gonadal dysfunction (uncommon)
	Pulmonary fibrosis (rare)	Pulmonary fibrosis (rare)
	Bladder fibrosis	Potential carcinogenesis
	Potential carcinogenesis	
Interactions	—	Allopurinol (inhibits metabolism of 6-mercaptopurine; reduce to 25% of usual dose)

[a] Uncommon with doses usually employed for IPF.
[b] Reversible with discontinuing drug.

Among patients failing cyclophosphamide, 1 of 8 responded to high-dose prednisolone. Despite these sobering statistics, favorable responses have been noted following introduction of cyclophosphamide even in corticosteroid-recalcitrant patients. A trial of cyclophosphamide can be offered to patients failing corticosteroids or experiencing steroid side effects, but patients should be informed about potential toxicities and the relatively low rate of anticipated response.

Dosage: 1.5–2.0 mg/kg/day in a single morning oral dose. An initial daily dose of 75–100 mg is reasonable, with increments by 25–50 mg every 2 weeks as needed (maximal dose 200 mg/day). Dose reductions are required if toxicity or cytopenias develop. Intermittent, intravenous pulse (once monthly) cyclophosphamide has been used, but no studies have compared oral with pulse cyclophosphamide for IPF.

Adverse Effects (Table 6.5): Toxicities of cyclophosphamide include stomatitis, bone marrow suppression, opportunistic infections, alopecia, gastrointestinal irritation, infertility, hemorrhagic cystitis, and neoplasms. Hemorrhagic cystitis occurs in up to one-third of patients. Patients should be instructed to force fluids and void frequently to minimize the local bladder toxicity. Hematologic malignancies develop in 1–2% of patients receiving long-term cyclophosphamide; bladder carcinomas, in 3–10% of patients.

Monitoring: Bone marrow suppressant effects of cyclophosphamide lag 1–weeks. Complete blood counts and differential and platelet counts should be measured at 2 weeks, 4 weeks, and once monthly while on therapy. The dose of cyclophosphamide should be reduced when leukocyte or platelet counts fall below 3,000 (absolute neutrophil count more than 1,000) or 100,000 cells/mm^3, respectively. Urinalyses should be done every 3 to 6 months. The development of microscopic hematuria warrants cystoscopy to exclude hemorrhagic cystitis. Hemorrhagic cystitis mandates discontinuation of therapy. With careful monitoring, cyclophosphamide is often better tolerated than are high doses of corticosteroids.

Duration of Therapy

Because responses to cyclophosphamide may be delayed for 3–6 months, an empiric trial for 6 months is warranted. Clinical and physiologic parameters should be assessed at 3 and 6 months. At this point, a decision should be made to either continue or discontinue therapy. Because of its potential toxicity, cyclophosphamide should be stopped after 6 months in patients failing to demonstrate objective improvement. Among responders, cyclophosphamide should be continued for a minimum of 12–18 months. At this point, the drug should be gradually tapered because long-term toxicity (including neoplasms) is substantial with chronic therapy.

AZATHIOPRINE (IMURAN)

Azathioprine has a role in patients failing corticosteroids or experiencing steroid side effects. Data evaluating azathioprine as therapy for IPF are limited to anecdotal reports and two prospective trials (only one of which was randomized). In both prospective studies, azathioprine was *added* to conventional doses of corticosteroids. In the first study, 20 patients with progressive IPF were initially treated with high-dose prednisone for 3 months. At that point, azathioprine (3 mg/kg/day) was added and the combination of azathioprine and low-dose prednisone was continued for 9 months. Favorable responses were noted in 12 of 20 (60%) with this regimen. In 1991, Raghu and colleagues reported results of a randomized, double-blind trial comparing azathioprine plus prednisone with prednisone alone for previously untreated IPF. At the end of 1 year, mortality and PFTs were similar in both groups. Late mortality was lower in patients receiving prednisone/azathioprine (43%) compared with those receiving prednisone/placebo (77%), but this was not statistically significant. No studies have directly compared azathioprine with cyclophosphamide as therapy for IPF. Azathioprine is less potent than cyclophosphamide but has fewer side effects. Because of its lower toxicity, azathioprine may be considered as initial therapy for IPF in patients with specific contraindications to corticosteroids (e.g., osteoporosis, insulin-dependent diabetes mellitus, advanced age, massive obesity) or in patients experiencing corticosteroid side effects. Patients who have failed treatment with both corticosteroids and cyclophosphamide are unlikely to respond to azathioprine.

Dosage: 2–3 mg/kg/day orally (not to exceed 250 mg/day).

Adverse Effects: Principal toxicities of azathioprine include bone marrow suppression, opportunistic infections, and gastrointestinal irritation. Azathioprine does not cause bladder toxicity and has no direct oncogenic effects.

Duration: An empiric trial for 6 months is warranted. Prolonged therapy should be reserved for patients exhibiting unequivocal responses to therapy.

COLCHICINE

Colchicine inhibits collagen formation in animal models, inhibits neutrophil function, and in one study suppressed the release of fibroblast growth factors in vitro from alveolar macrophages obtained by BAL from patients with IPF and sarcoidosis. Oral colchicine 0.6 mg once or twice daily has been used to treat IPF, but data are limited to anecdotal, nonrandomized trials. Colchicine is rarely associated with serious adverse effects; principal toxicities are nausea or diarrhea. The role of colchicine is controversial. We have not observed favorable responses to colchicine and are skeptical that this approach has merit, particularly in patients who have previously failed therapy with corticosteroids or immunosuppressive agents. Advocates of colchicine recommend an empiric trial (0.6 mg b.i.d for 6 months) in deteriorating patients who have failed or who are not candidates for treatment with corticosteroids or immunosuppressive agents.

Dosage: 0.6 mg orally once or twice day.

Lung Transplantation

Single lung transplantation has been successfully accomplished for end-stage restrictive lung disease (including IPF). Three-year survival approximates 70%. Recurrent IPF following lung transplantation has not been described. Long-term survival is limited by chronic allograft rejection (obliterative bronchiolitis), which occurs in 30–60% of patients by 5 years. Because the waiting time for a donor organ may exceed 18 months, patients with severe, progressive IPF unresponsive to medical therapy should be referred to transplant centers if no specific contraindications exist. Contraindications to transplantation include age more than 60 years (some centers accept patients up to age 65 years), significant extrapulmonary disorders that independently affect survival, and unstable or inadequate psychosocial profile.

COLLAGEN VASCULAR LUNG DISEASE

The collagen vascular disorders are systemic, multi-organ diseases that are grouped together because of their common association with inflammation of blood vessels,

Table 6.6. Pulmonary Manifestations of Some Collagen Vascular Diseases

Rheumatoid arthritis
  Pleural disease (effusions)
  Diffuse interstitial pneumonitis
  Necrobiotic nodules
  Caplan's syndrome
  Pulmonary hypertension (arteritis)
  Apical fibrobullous disease
  Bronchiolitis obliterans with and without
    organizing pneumonia
  Cricoarytenoid arthritis
Systemic lupus erythematosus
  Pleural disease (pleuritis, effusions)
  Atelectasis
  Acute lupus pneumonitis
  Diffuse interstitial lung disease
  Pulmonary hemorrhage
  Respiratory muscle dysfunction
Progressive systemic sclerosis
  Diffuse interstitial fibrosis
  Pulmonary vascular disease
  Respiration pneumonia
  Chest wall restriction secondary to
    thoracic skin sclerosis
  Pleural disease

Polymyositis—Dermatomyositis
  Interstitial pneumonitis
  Aspiration pneumonia
  Respiratory myositis
  Pulmonary hypertension
  BOOP
Mixed connective tissue disease
  Diffuse interstitial lung disease
  Pulmonary hypertension (vasculitis)
  Pleural disease
  Diaphragmatic muscle dysfunction
Sjögren's syndrome
  Respiratory mucosal dryness
  Pleurisy
  Chronic airway disease
  Lymphocytic interstitial pneumonia
  Pseudolymphoma
  Lymphoma
  Amyloid
  Pulmonary hypertension (vasculitis)

connective tissues, and serosal surfaces. Each disorder is associated with a spectrum of lung diseases (Table 6.6).

Chronic Interstitial Lung Disease

Chronic interstitial lung disease may complicate each of the collagen vascular disorders but is most prevalent in rheumatoid arthritis (RA) and PSS. Clinical, physiologic, radiographic, and histopathologic features are similar to IPF, but the course of collagen vascular disease-associated pulmonary fibrosis (CVD-PF) is more indolent. An alveolitis characterizes the early phases of CILD. Persistent alveolitis may cause injury, disruption of the normal alveolar architecture, and progressive pulmonary fibrosis. Historically, the approach to CVD-PF has been nihilistic, owing to the chronicity of the process and low rate of responsiveness to therapy. Recent studies have shown that subsets of patients with CVD-PF and active alveolitis benefit from aggressive therapy with corticosteroids and/or immunosuppressive or cytotoxic agents.

• Dyspnea and cough are the cardinal symptoms with moderate or advanced disease.
• Patients with early or minimal disease may be asymptomatic.

- Bibasilar end-inspiratory Velcro rales are characteristic.
- Chest x-rays are similar to IPF, with bibasilar interstitial infiltrates, honeycombing, and small lung volumes. Foci of ground glass (alveolar) opacities are occasionally seen.
- HRCT scans demonstrate varying degrees of honeycombing, ground glass opacities, reticular infiltrates, and a predilection for the peripheral (subpleural) and basilar regions of the lung. These features are indistinguishable from IPF.
- PFTs typically reveal reduced lung volumes, low diffusing capacity, and hypoxemia at rest or with exercise.
- BAL may demonstrate increases in neutrophils, eosinophils, or lymphocytes in patients with active alveolitis. Persistent elevations in neutrophils or eosinophils may be associated with a deteriorating course.
- The activity or course of CVD-PF may not correlate with extrapulmonary or systemic manifestations of the collagen vascular disorder. The lung lesion may progress even when articular or systemic components are quiescent.
- Other causes of interstitial lung disease may complicate CVD and need to be excluded (e.g., infection, neoplasm, drug-induced pulmonary toxicity).

Histopathologic Features

- Histopathologic features of CVD-PF are indistinguishable from IPF; however, in addition to classical features of IPF, some patients with CVD-PF manifest prominent lymphoid follicles or foci of BOOP.
- Fiberoptic bronchoscopy with TBBs and BAL can often corroborate the diagnosis of CVD-PF and exclude other causes.
- Findings of interstitial pneumonitis or fibrosis on TBBs are nonspecific, but in the context of characteristic clinical and HRCT findings are sufficient to support the diagnosis of CVD-PF.
- Open lung biopsy is rarely necessary because the diagnosis of CVD-PF can be presumed in patients with known CVD, typical clinical and HRCT features of pulmonary fibrosis, negative BAL, and ''consistent'' TBBs.

Therapy

- Empiric therapy with corticosteroids or immunosuppressive/cytotoxic agents should be considered in patients with CVD-PF and severe functional impairment or deteriorating clinical course.
- The decision to treat is difficult because complications associated with corticosteroids or cytotoxic agents may be substantial, particularly when therapy is prolonged.
- Because of the oncogenic risk with cyclophosphamide, azathioprine is often preferred as a steroid-sparing agent or in corticosteroid-refractory cases.

Rheumatoid Lung

- CILD in RA, termed rheumatoid lung, occurs in 10–50% of patients with RA but is severe and disabling in fewer than 5% of patients.

- Other pleuropulmonary manifestations of RA include pleural effusions, pulmonary vasculitis, bronchiolitis obliterans, necrobiotic (rheumatoid) nodules, and Caplan's syndrome.
- Risk factors associated with a higher prevalence of CILD in RA include male gender, age older than 60 years, history of smoking, α_1-antitrypsin variant phenotype, high levels of circulating rheumatoid factor, and prominent extra-articular manifestations.
- The presence of CILD does not correlate with the extent or duration of RA or with the presence of articular or systemic symptoms or sedimentation rate.
- Radiographic features are similar to IPF except for a higher prevalence of pleural thickening in rheumatoid CILD.
- The course of the rheumatoid CILD varies greatly but is usually less aggressive than IPF.
- BAL may reveal increases in neutrophils, lymphocytes, or eosinophils consistent with an inflammatory alveolitis.

Therapy

Although randomized, controlled therapeutic trials have not been performed, anecdotal successes have been noted with corticosteroids and immunosuppressive or cytotoxic agents as therapy for severe rheumatoid CILD. Unless specific contraindications exist, corticosteroids are considered as first-line therapy. Initial therapy with prednisone (40–60 mg/day or equivalent) for 3 months is recommended. If no improvement has occurred within this time frame, the corticosteroid should be tapered and discontinued. Corticosteroids should be continued, in a taper schedule, among patients exhibiting *objective* and unequivocal responses to therapy. The dose and rate of taper must be individualized but are similar to that for IPF. Cyclophosphamide or azathioprine can be considered in patients failing corticosteroids or experiencing serious adverse effects from corticosteroids (dose and schedule similar to that outlined for IPF).

Progressive Systemic Sclerosis

Pulmonary complications (principally CILD and pulmonary hypertension) occur in more than 90% of patients with PSS. Aspiration pneumonitis is a well-recognized complication in patients with esophageal disease. Clinical, radiographic, physiologic, and histopathologic features of CILD complicating PSS are similar to those features of IPF but the course is more indolent in PSS. Cough, dyspnea, or interstitial infiltrates on chest radiographs have been noted in 30–60% of patients with PSS. PFTs in CILD complicating PSS demonstrate reductions in lung volumes or DL_{CO}. A concomitant obstructive defect may reflect peribronchiolar fibrosis. Raynaud's phenomenon, digital pitting or ulceration, history of smoking, and peripheral vascular involvement have been associated with a more rapid decline of DL_{CO} and a higher likelihood of developing pulmonary hypertension. The presence of pulmonary hypertension or DL_{CO} less than 40% predicted is associated with striking increases in mortality. Open lung biopsies are rarely performed in CILD complicating PSS, but histopathologic features are similar to those of IPF.

Therapy

Because the course is indolent and chronic, therapy for PSS-associated CILD has usually been withheld. A subset of patients, however, exhibit acute alveolitis, associated with increased intrapulmonary uptake of gallium-67, increased neutrophils or neutrophil products on BAL, and ground glass opacities on HRCT. Patients with acute alveolitis are more likely to benefit from aggressive therapy with corticosteroids or immunosuppressive or cytotoxic agents. While controlled, randomized trials are lacking, favorable responses have been noted with corticosteroids or cyclophosphamide. No data are available regarding azathioprine. Given the chronicity of PSS and the likely need for prolonged therapy, we favor a trial of corticosteroids in patients with progressive, symptomatic CILD. The dose and rate of taper is similar to that for IPF and other CVD-PF. Cyclophosphamide is reserved for steroid-recalcitrant patients with severe and progressive disease.

Polymyositis/Dermatomyositis

CILD complicates polymyositis or dermatomyositis in 3–10% of patients. The course and prognosis are heterogeneous, but severe and fatal respiratory insufficiency may occur. Features of CILD complicating polymyositis or dermatomyositis include:

- Circulating autoantibodies to the enzyme histidyl-tRNA-synthetase (anti-Jo-1, anti-PL7, anti-PL-12, KJ) are noted in at least 50–70% of patients.
- Histopathologic features are similar to IPF but also include BOOP, cellular interstitial pneumonitis, and diffuse alveolar damage.
- The severity or clinical course of CILD does not correlate with the extent or activity of the muscle disease or systemic features.

Therapy

A trial of corticosteroids or immunosuppressive/cytotoxic agents is warranted in patients with severe or progressive CILD. The dose and duration are similar to treatment for IPF or other forms of CVD-PF.

Mixed Connective Tissue Disease

Mixed connective tissue disease (MCTD) combines clinical features that overlap with two or more collagen vascular disorders (e.g., RA, PSS, polymyositis/dermatomyositis, systemic lupus erythematosus). Patients with MCTD exhibit high titers of serum antibodies to extractable nuclear antigen (ENA) and to ribonucleoprotein (anti-RNP). Extrapulmonary features (e.g., sclerodactyly, polyarthritis, myositis, Raynaud's phenomenon) occur in 70–90% of patients and often dominate. CILD complicates MCTD in 30–85% of patients; pulmonary hypertension, in 15–30% of patients. The course of CILD is variable, but progressive fatal respiratory insufficiency may occur. Corticosteroids and/or immunosuppressive or cytotoxic agents are reserved for patients with severe or progressively worsening disease.

Sjögren's Syndrome

Sjögren's syndrome, characterized by xerostomia, xerophthalmia (sicca syndrome), and lymphocytic infiltration of exocrine glands, may occur as a primary disorder or as a complication of collagen vascular disease. Clinically significant pulmonary complications occur in at least 10% of patients with Sjögren's syndrome; asymptomatic involvement is considerably higher. Salient pulmonary complications include:

• Lymphocytic interstitial pneumonitis (LIP) or pseudolymphoma;
• Lymphoproliferative disorders (including lymphoma);
• CILD (pneumonitis or fibrosis);
• BOOP.

As with other CVD-associated CILD, increases in lymphocytes or neutrophils or both have been observed on BAL.

Therapy

Although controlled studies have not been performed, corticosteroids are recommended in patients with symptomatic or progressive CILD, BOOP, or lymphoid interstitial pneumonia. Cytotoxic agents are reserved for patients with severe disease refractory to corticosteroids.

Systemic Lupus Erythematosus (SLE)

Pleuropulmonary manifestations of systemic lupus erythematosus are protean and include pleuritis, acute lupus pneumonitis, alveolar hemorrhage, pulmonary vasculitis, pulmonary embolism (resulting from circulating anticardiolipin antibodies), and CILD. Chronic interstitial pneumonitis or fibrosis occurs in fewer than 5% of patients with SLE and is rarely severe. As with other CILD complicating CVD, corticosteroids or cytotoxic agents may be considered for patients with severe or progressive disease.

DRUG-INDUCED INTERSTITIAL LUNG DISEASE

Many drugs can induce pathophysiologic reactions that can be classified into one of the following syndromes:

• Chronic interstitial pneumonitis and fibrosis;
• Hypersensitivity reactions;

- Pulmonary infiltrates with eosinophilia;
- Drug-induced lupus syndrome;
- Diffuse alveolar hemorrhage.

Chronic Interstitial Pneumonitis and Fibrosis

Patients with drug-induced CILD typically develop cough, dyspnea, bibasilar crackles, interstitial bibasilar pulmonary infiltrates, restrictive lung impairment, and hypoxemia. The most commonly implicated drugs include bleomycin, busulfan, cyclophosphamide, nitrosourea compounds, amiodarone, nitrofurantoin, and hexamethonium. A dose-dependent relationship exists for some agents (e.g., bleomycin, busulfan, the nitrosoureas, and amiodarone). The pathogenesis is thought to result from both direct toxic effects of the implicated drug and indirect toxicity from the associated inflammatory and reparative responses. Toxic oxygen-derived radicals likely mediate the lung toxicity in bleomycin, busulfan, and nitrofurantoin drug reactions.

Therapy

- The prognosis is variable even when the drug is discontinued. Improvement, stabilization, or progressive fibrosis may occur.
- An empiric trial of corticosteroids is warranted in severe or progressive cases.

Hypersensitivity Drug Reactions

HP may occur as a response to numerous drugs (e.g., nitrofurantoin, sulfonamides, amiodarone, methotrexate, gold salts, salicylates, and nonsteroidal antiinflammatory agents). Clinical features include acute onset of cough, dyspnea, fever, myalgias, and arthralgias; urticaria, pleuritis, and peripheral blood eosinophilia are occasionally noted. Chest radiographs typically demonstrate alveolar and/or interstitial infiltrates; pleural effusions or intrathoracic adenopathy may also occur.

- BAL frequently demonstrates increased numbers and proportions of lymphocytes and CD8 + T-cytotoxic cells. Similar findings are seen in classic HP (to be discussed in detail later), suggesting similar immunopathogenic mechanisms.
- Complete resolution usually ensues following discontinuation of the implicated drug. For fulminant or protracted cases, a short course of corticosteroids is indicated.

Miscellaneous Drug Reactions

Intrapulmonary hemorrhage has been described as a rare complication of D-penicillamine, occupational exposure to trimellitic anhydride, and cocaine. Acute eosinophilic pneumonia may complicate use of various pharmacologic agents including methotrexate, salicylates, nitrofurantoin, sulfa drugs, penicillins, amiodarone, gold compounds, and procarbazine. The process is self-limiting following discontinuation of the drug. Corticosteroids are reserved for severe or protracted cases. A lupus-like syndrome, with fever, pleuritis, arthralgias, and pulmonary infiltrates, has been described in association with procainamide, hydralazine, diphenylhydantoin, and isoniazid. Renal or neurologic involvement is not a feature of this syndrome.

- Antinuclear antibody and antihistone antibody are positive, but anti-double-stranded DNA antibody (anti-dsDNA) is negative.
- Prompt resolution usually occurs following discontinuation of the offending agent.
- Corticosteroids may hasten recovery.

HYPERSENSITIVITY PNEUMONITIS (EXTRINSIC ALLERGIC ALVEOLITIS)

HP (also termed extrinsic allergic alveolitis) is characterized by a cell-mediated immunologic reaction to a variety of inhaled organic dusts or inorganic chemicals (Table 6.7). The occupational origin of many of these agents has led to descriptive names for each clinical syndrome. The prototype of HP is farmer's lung, which is caused by inhalation of thermophilic actinomycetes spores from moldy hay. In Mexico, domestic exposure to pigeon antigens (pigeon-breeder's lung) is the most common cause of HP. Although the agents differ widely, the clinical presentations are similar.

Clinical Features

Clinical presentations may be acute, subacute, or chronic.

- Acute form: Fever, chills, dyspnea, cough, and fine crackles with transient leukocytosis, pulmonary infiltrates, and restrictive impairment noted 4–12 hours following

Table 6.7. Etiologic Agents in Hypersensitivity Pneumonitis

Occupation	Dust Exposure	Antigen
Farmer	Moldy compost (hay, sugar cane, mushrooms)	Thermophilic actinomycetes
Home/office worker	Contaminated ventilation system	Thermophilic actinomycetes, amebae
Bird breeder	Avian dust	Avian proteins
Animal handler	Rodent dander	Rodent proteins
Detergent worker	Bacterial enzymes	Bacillus subtilis proteins
Woodworker	Moldy wood dust	Fungi—*Aspergillus, Alternaria, Pullularia* spp.
Malt/cheese worker	Malt or cheese mold	Fungi—*Penicillium* spp.
Wheat worker	Infested wheat	Wheat weevil protein
Plastics worker	Plastic components	Isocyanates, anhydrides
Painters	Paint hardeners	Isocyanates

exposure. Recovery occurs in 24–48 hours with no further exposure. With repeated acute exposures, the relationship between symptoms and exposure may not be obvious. (Example—cleaning bird cages by sensitized individuals.)

- Chronic form: Insidious progression of dyspnea, cough, anorexia, weight loss, and progressive interstitial lung disease. Hypoxemia, a restrictive ventilatory defect on PFTs, and diffuse reticulonodular infiltrates on chest radiographs are typical. (Example—farmer with chronic low-level exposure to moldy hay or women with chronic exposure to domestic pigeons.)
- Airways obstruction is uncommon but may reflect nonspecific bronchial hyperresponsiveness. The presence of significant airways obstruction raises the possibility of occupational asthma, because many occupations involve exposures to dusts known to elicit IgE-mediated and non–IgE-mediated asthma.

Radiographic Features

Conventional chest radiographs typically demonstrate bilateral mixed interstitial and alveolar infiltrates that may be patchy or diffuse. In chronic forms of HP, honeycombing, small lung volumes, and reticular or reticulonodular infiltrates are similar to IPF. High-resolution, thin-section CT scans reveal areas of ground glass opacities, hyperlucency, and foci of fibrosis and honeycombing. Centrilobular, peribronchiolar, indistinct nodules are characteristic features on HRCT. These nodules represent intraluminal granulation tissue within bronchioles or an active inflammatory process in the surrounding peribronchiolar regions. Bronchial obstruction may cause patchy areas of hyperlucency in a lobular distribution. With end-stage disease, fibrosis and areas of emphysema may be observed.

Diagnosis

A careful occupational and environmental history is the key to a diagnosis. In the acute form, correlation of symptoms to exposure is highly suggestive of HP. The diagnosis may not be suspected in chronic forms and relies heavily on identifying exposure to putative disease-causing agents.

- Positive serum precipitating antibodies to the organic dust (or avian antigen, etc.) are virtually always present in patients with HP. Circulating antibodies are not diagnostic of disease but may be seen in asymptomatic, exposed individuals without disease.
- Inhalation challenge testing under controlled conditions can establish a diagnosis in acute or subacute disease but entails risk in patients with significant respiratory impairment.

Histopathologic Features

Lung biopsies reveal intense mononuclear cell infiltration (lymphocytes, plasma cells, foamy macrophages) within the alveolar interstitium and bronchioles, scattered poorly formed granulomas and multinucleated giant cells, areas of fibrosis, and lymphoid follicles. The process is bronchocentric in distribution. Foci of proliferative bronchiolitis obliterans were noted in 50% of open lung biopsies in patients with farmer's lung but were not observed in a recent study of open lung biopsies in patients with chronic pigeon-breeder's HP. With chronic continuous exposure, severe, end-stage honeycomb lung (indistinguishable from IPF) may be observed.

- Bronchoscopy with BAL and transbronchial lung biopsies may establish the diagnosis of HP, particularly if the clinical history and features are consistent. Striking increases in BAL lymphocytes (40–80% of cells), predominantly expressing CD8 phenotype, are characteristic of HP.
- Thoracoscopic lung biopsies may be needed if bronchoscopy is nondiagnostic.

Pathophysiology

A heightened immunologic response to inhaled antigens results in circulating antibodies and a cellular immune (lymphocytic-mononuclear) response. The prominence of foamy macrophages and CD8 + T-cytotoxic lymphocytes suggests an important role for these cells in the immunopathogenesis of HP. Additional cofactors or genetic susceptibilities may be required to elicit symptomatic disease.

Therapy

Avoidance of the offending agent is the mainstay of treatment.

- Clean humidifiers and change humidifier water frequently.
- Reduce occupational exposure to organic dusts whenever possible by improved industrial hygiene, ventilation, and air purification.
- Discourage dependence on personal dust respirators because they are difficult to use properly and do not exclude all respirable dust. The remaining fraction can cause new attacks in a sensitized person.
- Avoid workplace or a vocational exposure if environmental control measures are ineffective in preventing disease. Unfortunately, many individuals refuse to restrict exposures and return to work (e.g., farmers) or a vocation (e.g., bird breeders). Patients should be advised of the risk for progressive interstitial fibrosis with continued exposure.

Corticosteroids

Corticosteroids are effective in alleviating acute symptoms and improving chest radiographs and should be used for severe cases.

ACUTE DISEASE

- Respiratory symptoms are self-limiting, and treatment may not be necessary.
- For acutely ill patients with significant radiographic infiltration and hypoxemia, corticosteroids are indicated.

Dosage: Prednisone 40–60 mg/day in divided doses for 1–2 weeks or until significant clinical, radiologic, and physiologic improvement occurs. Taper over 4–6 weeks.

SUBACUTE DISEASE (REPEATED ACUTE EXPOSURES)

- Reduce exposure;
- Long-term corticosteroid therapy.

Dosage: Prednisone 40–60 mg/day for 2 weeks. Taper slowly over 3–4 months until a dose of 15–30 mg/day is reached. Slowly taper to lowest effective dose. Alternate-day therapy may minimize long-term complications.

CHRONIC DISEASE

- Decrease exposure;
- Trial of corticosteroids as outlined for subacute disease. Evaluate response at 6 months using clinical, radiologic, and PFTs. Continue therapy only if an objective response can be documented.

SARCOIDOSIS

Sarcoidosis is a multisystemic disorder of unknown cause characterized by noncaseating granulomata in affected organs. Pulmonary manifestations typically dominate, but virtually any organ can be affected. The clinical course is heterogeneous. Spontaneous remissions occur in nearly two-thirds of patients. Progressive destruction of involved organs may result in irreversible fibrosis and sequelae. Fatalities occur in 1–4% of patients. The disease is found worldwide, but geographic and racial differences in the prevalence are striking. In North America, the prevalence approximates 10–20 cases per 100,000. Sarcoidosis is eight times more common in blacks and slightly more common in women.

Clinical Features

- More than 80% present between age 20 and 40; sarcoidosis is rare at extremes of age.
- The lungs are affected in more than 90% of patients but virtually any organ can be involved.
- Pulmonary manifestations usually dominate, but clinical manifestations are protean and reflect the specific organ(s) involved.
- Forty to sixty percent of patients with sarcoidosis are asymptomatic.
- Skin, eye, and peripheral lymph nodes are each involved in 20–30% of patients.
- Symptomatic involvement of heart, central nervous system, bone, kidney, liver, or spleen occurs in 2–6% of patients.
- Asymptomatic involvement of extrapulmonary organs is common. Noncaseating

granulomas have been detected in 40–70% of sarcoid patients by percutaneous liver biopsy, even in the absence of specific signs or symptoms.
- Chest radiographs are abnormal in more than 90% of patients and are often the sentinel reason for suspecting the diagnosis. Bilateral hilar lymphadenopathy (BHL) (with or without right paratracheal adenopathy) is most common.
- Cough, dyspnea, or chest discomfort may reflect endobronchial or pulmonary parenchymal involvement. Sputum production and hemoptysis may be seen in advanced fibrotic disease.
- The course of sarcoidosis is markedly heterogeneous.
- The constellation of erythema nodosum, fever, BHL, and arthritis (often associated with uveitis), is termed Löfgren's syndrome and reflects an early inflammatory phase. Spontaneous remissions occur in more than 85% of patients with Löfgren's syndrome.
- Factors associated with a poor prognosis include black race, lupus pernio (disfiguring nasolabial cutaneous lesions), chronic hypercalcemia, bone lesions, and chronic pulmonary sarcoidosis.
- Fatalities occur in 1–4% of patients, usually as a result of pulmonary insufficiency or cardiac involvement.

Laboratory Features

- Hypercalcemia is present in 2–5% of patients with sarcoidosis. Chronic hypercalcemia or hypercalciuria may cause nephrolithiasis or nephrocalcinosis.
- Anemia occurs in fewer than 6% of sarcoid patients and warrants investigation for alternative causes.
- Increased transaminases are noted in 10–20% of patients.
- Hypergammaglobulinemia occurs in more than 25% of patients with chronic progressive sarcoidosis but is nonspecific.
- Serum angiotensin-converting enzyme (SACE) is elevated in 30–80% of sarcoid patients and may be a surrogate measure of granuloma burden.
- Cutaneous anergy to recall antigens, such as tuberculin, *Candida,* mumps, and *Trichophyton,* is characteristic.

Chest Radiographs

- Chest radiographs are abnormal in more than 90% of patients (see Chapter 1). BHL is the classical and predominant feature, noted in 50–85% of patients. Enlargement of other lymph nodes in the paratracheal, pretracheal, para-aortic, and subcarinal areas is common but may not be obvious by conventional radiographs. Parenchymal infiltrates are present in 25–50% of patients. These infiltrates have a predilection for the upper and posterior lung zones and may mimic tuberculosis.
- Other disorders that may cause upper lobe parenchymal infiltrates include granulomatous infections, silicosis, EG, ankylosing spondylitis, and chronic eosinophilic pneumonia.

- In severe cases, marked destruction of lung parenchyma result in bullae, cysts, pneumothorax, and upward retraction of hilae.
- Pleural effusions occur in only 1–3% of patients with sarcoidosis and should prompt evaluation for other causes, such as tuberculosis, congestive heart failure, or pulmonary embolism.
- Chest x-rays are classified by international convention as stage I (BHL only), stage II (BHL and pulmonary infiltrates), and stage III (parenchymal infiltrates without BHL). Some advocate stage IV to refer to extensive fibrosis, cystic changes, and distortion, but this is not uniform.
- Although exceptions exist, prognosis is related to radiographic stage. Spontaneous remissions occur in more than 80% of patients with stage I disease but in only 30–60% with stage II and less than 20% with stage III disease.

High-Resolution, Thin-Section CT Scans (HRCT)

- High-resolution, thin-section CT scans (HRCT) typically demonstrate micronodules (1–3 mm in size) along bronchovascular bundles and conglomerate alveolar infiltrates (sometimes with air bronchograms). Other abnormalities include ground glass opacities, traction bronchiectasis, honeycomb cysts, linear bands, and distortion or displacement of vessels or bronchi. Parenchymal abnormalities have a distinct predilection for upper lung zones with relative sparing of the bases. Enlarged lymph nodes in pretracheal, paratracheal, para-aortic, and subcarinal regions may be apparent. Despite the increased sensitivity of HRCT as compared with conventional chest x-rays, CT scans are expensive and have limited prognostic value. Thus, routine CT scans are not necessary or cost-effective in managing sarcoidosis.

Pulmonary Function Tests

- PFTs are normal in more than 80% of patients with stage I disease, but abnormalities are present in 40–70% of patients with stage II or III disease. A restrictive defect is characteristic, but concomitant airways obstruction is present in one-third or more of patients. The diffusing capacity may be reduced in patients with stage II or III disease and may be associated with impaired oxygenation.
- Hypoxemia is rare at presentation but may be observed in patients with chronic, severe pulmonary parenchymal involvement.
- Exercise tests may detect mild abnormalities (e.g., excessive ventilation, increased dead space) even in asymptomatic patients with normal spirometry and DL_{CO}.
- Neither PFTs nor exercise tests can distinguish alveolitis (which may be amenable to therapy) from fibrosis.
- Serial PFTs are useful to quantitate the degree of pulmonary impairment and follow the course of the disease (or response to therapeutic interventions).
- Spirometry (FVC, FEV_1) is usually adequate to follow the disease longitudinally. More expensive tests, such as DL_{CO}, lung volumes, or exercise tests, can be reserved for specific indications.

Histopathologic Features

- The hallmark of sarcoidosis is multiple, confluent noncaseating (nonnecrotizing) granulomata. These granulomata are composed of epithelioid cells, multinucleated giant cells, and a cuff of lymphocytes and plasma cells in the periphery. Varying degrees of fibrosis and distortion or destruction of parenchymal architecture may be noted.
- Because noncaseating granulomas may be found in infectious granulomas, special stains for acid-fast bacilli (AFB) and fungi (and often cultures) should be done before the diagnosis of sarcoidosis can be assumed.
- In the lung, the granulomas are preferentially located along bronchovascular bundles and in the bronchial submucosa, which explains the high yield of fiberoptic bronchoscopy.

Diagnosis

A diagnosis of sarcoidosis is based on a compatible clinical picture, histologic confirmation of noncaseating granulomas, and absence of other known causes of granulomas. Tuberculosis, fungal diseases, lymphoma, beryllium disease, drug reactions, and local sarcoid reactions must be excluded. Tuberculin skin tests (PPD) should be performed because clinical and radiographic features of granulomatous infections may be indistinguishable from sarcoidosis. In endemic areas, serum complement fixation tests for *Histoplasma capsulatum* or *Coccidioides immitis* are advised.

Biopsies

- Fiberoptic bronchoscopy with transbronchial lung biopsies is the procedure of choice for stage I, II, or III disease (diagnostic yields of 60–90%).
- Mediastinoscopy should be reserved for when bronchoscopy is nondiagnostic or when malignancy is suspected (e.g., extensive mediastinal or asymmetric hilar adenopathy).
- Symmetric BHL is rarely a presenting feature of malignancy. When malignancy is present, symptoms or abnormalities on routine physical examination are virtually always present.
- Thoracoscopic or open lung biopsies are rarely warranted because the diagnosis of sarcoidosis can almost always be established by bronchoscopy or mediastinoscopy.
- Biopsies of skin, palpable lymph nodes, lip, or conjunctivae may be diagnostic provided these sites are involved clinically.

Prognosis

Spontaneous remissions occur in more than 80% of patients with stage I sarcoidosis (i.e., BHL alone). Unless specific complications develop, patients with stage I sarcoidosis rarely require specific therapy. In contrast, most patients with stage III disease require therapy because spontaneous remissions occur in fewer than 20%

of patients in this context. The prognosis for stage II disease is intermediate (spontaneous remission rate of 30–60%). Treatment is warranted in patients with severe or progressive symptoms (irrespective of radiographic stage) or with persistent radiographic infiltrates. By the time symptoms of cough or dyspnea develop, irreversible damage may have occurred. Patients with stage II or III disease and mild or no symptoms may be observed without specific therapy for 6–12 months to determine if remission will occur spontaneously. More than 80% of spontaneous remissions occur within 2 years of onset. Persistent or progressive infiltrates warrant treatment.

Pathophysiology

Although the inciting stimulus is unknown, sarcoidosis is characterized by a heightened immune response with increased numbers of activated T helper-inducer (CD4+) lymphocytes and macrophages at sites of active disease. Interactions between these activated immune effector cells induce granulomas; progression of the inflammatory process may injure and distort parenchymal architecture and result in tissue destruction and fibrosis.

Therapy

Baseline chest radiographs, PFTs (FVC, FEV_1, diffusing capacity), liver function tests (alkaline phosphatase, aspartate aminotransferase (AST), alanine aminotransferase (ALT)), serum calcium, complete blood count, and complete ophthalmologic examinations should be performed. The role of SACE is controversial. Additional studies may be required when specific extrapulmonary features are present.

- Serial clinical evaluations, chest x-rays, PFTs, or abnormal serologic studies suffice to monitor patients and determine the need for treatment. Radionuclide studies (e.g., gallium scans) and BAL are expensive and nonspecific and have no role in monitoring.

  Indications for treatment are listed below:

- Asymptomatic individuals with stage I or II disease and normal lung function should be observed and do not require specific therapy.
- Acute inflammatory manifestations (e.g., fever, polyarthritis, erythema nodosum) should initially be treated with nonsteroidal antiinflammatory agents (NSAIDs). Corticosteroids are indicated for symptomatic patients failing NSAIDs and are virtually always efficacious.
- Corticosteroids are the mainstay of treatment for sarcoidosis with serious or progressive pulmonary or extrapulmonary disease.
- The antimalarials (i.e., chloroquine or hydroxychloroquine) may be used for skin involvement, but data are limited.
- Methotrexate or azathioprine may be used in patients with progressive or severe disease refractory to corticosteroids, provided appropriate guidelines and monitoring are followed.

- Although anecdotal successes have been noted with the alkylating agents (cyclo-phosphamide and chlorambucil), these agents are potentially oncogenic and should generally be avoided.

Corticosteroids

Corticosteroids are the drugs of choice for symptomatic or progressive pulmonary or extrapulmonary sarcoidosis. Favorable responses have been noted in 60–90% of patients treated with corticosteroids, but relapses occur in 20–50% of patients as the dose is reduced or the drug withdrawn.

INDICATIONS FOR CORTICOSTEROID THERAPY

- Corticosteroids are recommended for the following indications: ocular, myocardial, or neurologic involvement; hypercalcemia; significant or progressive hepatic, renal, or muscle involvement; persistent or progressive symptomatic pulmonary or extrapulmonary sarcoidosis.
- Minimally symptomatic patients with near normal lung function and stable pulmonary infiltrates that have persisted for 1–2 years should be given a trial of corticosteroids (20–30 mg daily of prednisone or equivalent for 3–4 months) to determine potential for improvement.
- Topical corticosteroids are adequate for anterior uveitis; systemic steroids are indicated for posterior eye disease.

Although the optimal dose and duration of therapy in patients with sarcoidosis has not been elucidated, modest doses are usually adequate to control the disease. The role of alternate day versus daily dosing of prednisone is controversial. As initial therapy in patients with mild to moderate disease, daily prednisone (20–30 mg daily or equivalent) for 3–4 months is often adequate. In patients with more extensive or acute disease, higher doses are warranted (40 mg daily or equivalent, with a gradual taper once clinical improvement has occurred). Initial doses as high as 60 mg daily are reserved for specific complications (e.g., myocardial, neurologic, or severe pulmonary involvement). The dose and rate of taper of corticosteroid must be individualized, depending on the acuity and severity of the disease and the presence or absence of side effects. In most patients exhibiting complete and sustained remissions, the prednisone dose can be reduced to 15 mg daily (or 30 mg every other day) within 4–6 months. A minimum of 12–18 months of therapy is warranted for patients with chronic or severe sarcoidosis. Patients exhibiting a propensity for repetitive relapses may require indefinite chronic suppressive therapy. For long-term maintenance, doses of 5–10 mg of prednisone daily (or 10–20 mg alternate day) may be adequate. Intensification of the corticosteroid dose is required for recrudescent disease. Inhaled steroids may ameliorate symptoms in patients with endobronchial involvement but have limited benefit for pulmonary sarcoidosis. Immunosuppressive or cytotoxic agents are reserved for patients failing or experiencing severe side effects from corticosteroids.

Adverse Effects (Table 6.4): Low-dose daily or alternate-day corticosteroids as maintenance therapy for sarcoidosis are usually well tolerated. Weight gain, neuropsychiatric effects, hypertension, osteoporosis, cataracts, and diabetes (in susceptible individuals) are the most common adverse effects.

Chloroquine and Hydroxychloroquine

- These antimalarial drugs have been used as first-line therapy for skin and mucosal sarcoidosis but are of doubtful efficacy for pulmonary or systemic sarcoidosis.
- May be useful in severe nasal, sinus, and laryngeal sarcoidosis refractory to corticosteroids alone.

CHLOROQUINE PHOSPHATE (ARALEN)

Dosage: 500 mg daily for 2 weeks, then 250 mg daily for 5½ months. Use no longer than 6 months at a time, followed by a 6-month rest period. This regimen may be repeated as needed. A major concern is ocular toxicity with long-term administration. Ophthalmologic examinations should be performed prior to administration and at 3- and 6-month intervals.

ADVERSE EFFECTS

- Retinopathy;
- Gastrointestinal upset (mild); transient headache;
- Discoloration of nail beds and mucous membranes;
- Dermatitis, reversible.

Caution: High daily doses of chloroquine (more than 250 mg) may cause retinopathy, toxic cardiomyopathy, and neuropathy. Do not exceed 250 mg daily after first 2 weeks.

HYDROXYCHLOROQUINE SULFATE (PLAQUENIL)

Hydroxychloroquine may be less effective than chloroquine to treat mucocutaneous sarcoidosis but it is less toxic. Serious ocular toxicity is rare with hydroxychloroquine at doses of 400 mg/day or less, even when administered for prolonged periods.

Dosage: 200 mg once or twice daily for a minimum of 6 months.

Management Problems in Pulmonary Sarcoidosis

Hemoptysis

Hemoptysis may complicate advanced fibrocystic sarcoidosis and may reflect underlying bronchiectasis, bronchopulmonary suppurative infections, or mycetomas. Broad-spectrum antibiotics should be administered. For severe hemoptysis, hospitalization is indicated. Elective arteriography and embolotherapy can be considered for massive hemoptysis following localization of the bleeding site by bronchoscopic examination.

Mycetomas (Fungus Balls)

Mycetomas are a complication of advanced fibrocystic sarcoidosis. The most frequent causative organism is *Aspergillus fumigatus,* which may colonize preexisting cavities or bullae. Invasive *Aspergillus* infection is rare, even in the presence of low-dose corticosteroids. Bacterial infection of the surrounding bronchitic and bronchiectatic areas is common and leads to chronic sputum production and hemoptysis. Treatment should be conservative with broad-spectrum antibiotics. Some patients benefit from daily antibiotics, rotated at 2- to 4-week intervals, to suppress recurrent infections and hemoptysis.

- Antifungal agents have been used but do not penetrate the fungus ball and are likely of limited efficacy.
- Surgical resection is rarely feasible because of severe restrictive lung disease superimposed on fibrocystic disease.

PRIMARY EOSINOPHILIC PNEUMONIAS

The primary eosinophilic pneumonias are characterized by pulmonary infiltration by eosinophils with or without peripheral blood eosinophilia (Table 6.1). Eosinophils possess a wide array of proinflammatory substances, such as major basic protein, lysosomal hydrolases, cytokines, and arachidonic acid metabolites, which may cause direct tissue injury, as well as mediating antiparasitic and antimicrobial effects. Persistent eosinophilic lung inflammation may be associated with fibrosis and restrictive impairment.

Löffler's Syndrome

Acute eosinophilic pneumonia (Löffler's syndrome) is a self-limited illness characterized by migratory pulmonary infiltrates, blood eosinophilia, and mild pulmonary symptoms. Many cases are probably caused by unrecognized drug reactions, parasitic infestations, or allergic bronchopulmonary aspergillosis. Cough, malaise, fever, and fluffy alveolar infiltrates on chest radiographs are characteristic. Extrapulmonary involvement does not occur. Histopathologic features are indistinguishable from chronic eosinophilic pneumonia (discussed below). BAL typically demonstrates marked increases in eosinophils (often more than 40% on differential count). TBBs and BAL are usually adequate to support the diagnosis provided clinical and radiographic features are consistent. Open or thoracoscopic lung biopsies are rarely necessary. Because the disease resolves spontaneously within 2–6 weeks, no specific therapy is required. If a drug or parasite is implicated, removal or treatment directed against the offending agent is curative. A careful history for infectious etiologies is important, particularly in patients residing in endemic areas or with relevant exposures.

Tropical Pulmonary Eosinophilia

Tropical pulmonary eosinophilia is caused by a local hypersensitivity response to helminths (e.g., *Wuchereria bancrofti, Brugia malayi,* or *Dirofilaria immitis*) introduced by mosquito bites as the microfilaria lodge in pulmonary vessels.

- Suspect in individuals from endemic areas (India, Sri Lanka, Southeast Asia, Pakistan, or Indonesia).

Clinical Features

- New onset asthma, severe cough, chest pain, and hemoptysis are characteristically worse at night; fevers, fatigue, and weight loss are common.
- Wheezing and/or crackles may be present.
- Extrapulmonary manifestations may occur (e.g., hepatosplenomegaly, lymphadenopathy, gastrointestinal symptoms, muscle tenderness, skin lesions).
- Restrictive lung impairment more common than airways obstruction.
- Chest x-ray may be normal or show mixed alveolar and reticulonodular infiltrates; cavitation or pleural effusions are rare.
- Marked peripheral eosinophilia (more than 2,000/mm^3), elevated IgE levels, and high titers of antifilarial antibodies are present.

Therapy

- The antifilarial drug diethylcarbamazine citrate.

Dosage: 5 mg/kg/day for 7–10 days. Treatment causes a rapid disappearance of symptoms (usually within 2 weeks). Relapses usually respond to retreatment, but longstanding disease may lead to irreversible pulmonary fibrosis and a protracted course.

Chronic Eosinophilic Pneumonia

Chronic eosinophilic pneumonia, originally described in 1969, is characterized by transient alveolar infiltrates, pulmonary and constitutional symptoms, and blood eosinophilia. The cause is unknown, but the course is protracted (over years) in the absence of treatment.

Clinical Features

- It is most common in middle-aged women.
- Dyspnea, productive cough, fevers, night sweats, weight loss, and wheezing are predominant symptoms.
- Chest x-rays typically show dense peripheral (subpleural) alveolar infiltrates, with central clearing. This pattern has been termed the "photographic negative of pulmonary edema." These infiltrates exhibit a distinct predilection for the upper lobes.
- Peripheral blood eosinophilia is found in 80% of patients.
- Elevations in blood eosinophils and ESR usually correlate with activity of the disease.
- Increases in serum IgE are common.

- BAL findings of more than 40% eosinophils (normal less than 1%) are highly suggestive of eosinophilic pneumonia in the proper clinical and radiologic context.
- Restrictive lung impairment, often with superimposed airflow limitation, low DL_{CO}, and hypoxemia, is characteristic.
- The course is subacute or chronic, with symptoms developing over weeks or months.
- An acute form, progressing to severe respiratory failure, has been described.

Histopathologic Features

- Lung biopsies demonstrate dense aggregates of eosinophils within the alveolar spaces, interstitium, and bronchioles. Multinucleated giant cells and histiocytes are prominent, with scattered lymphocytes and plasma cells. Other features include degenerating eosinophils, Charcot-Leyden crystals, and alveolar macrophages containing eosinophilic fragments. Extensive fibrosis or necrosis does not occur.
- Surgical (open or thoracoscopic) lung biopsy is rarely necessary. The diagnosis can usually be made on the basis of symptoms, a characteristic radiographic pattern, BAL and transbronchial lung biopsies, and the exclusion of other causes of pulmonary eosinophilia.

Therapy

Corticosteroids are the treatment of choice. Response to steroids is usually dramatic. Symptoms improve within hours or days; partial radiographic clearing is evident within 2–3 days. Chest radiographs usually normalize within 2–3 weeks.

Dosage: Prednisone 40–60 mg/day for 2 weeks, with a taper to 40 mg alternate day by 6–12 weeks. The rate of taper can be guided by clinical and radiographic criteria and peripheral eosinophil counts. Prednisone can usually be tapered to 30 mg every other day within 6 months, but the dose should be very gradually tapered beyond that point. Some patients relapse each time the corticosteroid dose is reduced below a certain threshold. Low-dose prednisone (10–20 mg alternate day) is often sufficient to prevent relapse. Treatment should be continued for a minimum of 12–18 months. Following discontinuation of corticosteroids, relapses occur in 80% of patients. Patients exhibiting a propensity to relapse may require prolonged therapy for years (sometimes indefinite). In this context, the lowest dose prednisone necessary to maintain remissions should be used.

BRONCHIOLITIS OBLITERANS–ORGANIZING PNEUMONIA

Bronchiolitis obliterans–organizing pneumonia (also termed cryptogenic organizing pneumonia) usually presents as a poorly resolving pneumonia (mimicking community-acquired pneumonia). In up to one-third of patients, diffuse reticulonodular infiltrates (similar to IPF) may be evident. BOOP may complicate collagen vascular disease, toxic fume exposures, organ transplantation, pharmacologic agents, or specific pulmonary infections (e.g., viruses, *Mycoplasma, Legionella*). When no cause is identified, the term idiopathic BOOP is applied. The prevalence of BOOP is uncertain, but the diagnosis is substantiated in only 2–4 patients annually in most medical centers. This may in part reflect underrecognition because of the overlap of symptoms with community-acquired pneumonia and other diagnoses.

Clinical Features

- Most patients are 40–60 years old, but all ages may be affected.
- Persistent nonproductive cough, dyspnea, and malaise are typical presenting features.
- The course is subacute, with symptoms developing over 2 weeks to 6 months.
- A respiratory tract infection or flulike illness antedates the onset of symptoms by 1–3 months in 40–60% of patients.
- Despite pronounced constitutional symptoms in some patients, extrapulmonary involvement does not occur.
- Physical examination reveals crackles in 60% of patients; mid-inspiratory "squeaks" are noted in 40–70% of patients. Overt wheezing is rare.
- Chest x-rays demonstrate bilateral, patchy, ground glass opacities in more than two-thirds of patients; a bibasilar predominance is common, but any lobe may be affected.
- Diffuse reticulonodular infiltrates, indistinguishable from IPF or other CILDs, are noted in 20–40% of patients. Chest radiographs are normal or exhibit only hyperinflation in 4–10% of patients.
- Dense alveolar infiltrates are associated with a more acute course and greater responsiveness to corticosteroids. In contrast, a reticulonodular or interstitial pattern is associated with a more chronic course and lower rate of response to therapy.
- PFTs characteristically show a restrictive defect (e.g., reduced lung volumes), low diffusing capacity, and hypoxemia. A pure obstructive defect is rare. These defects usually normalize or improve following corticosteroid therapy.
- HRCT scans demonstrate distinctive focal alveolar infiltrates with ground glass opacities and consolidation juxtaposed to normal or hyperlucent areas. Honeycombing does not occur.
- BAL demonstrates increases in neutrophils or lymphocytes; eosinophils may also be present.

Histopathologic Features

The histologic hallmark of BOOP is polypoid masses of granulation tissue filling and obstructing terminal and respiratory bronchioles. The inflammatory cellular infiltrate is composed of lymphocytes, foamy macrophages, plasma cells, polymorphonuclear leukocytes, and scattered eosinophils and multinucleated giant cells. Extension of the inflammatory process to contiguous alveolar ducts and alveolar spaces results in the "organizing pneumonia" component. Other distinct features include broncho-centricity, patchy involvement, preservation of the alveolar architecture, and lack of significant fibrosis or honeycombing.

- The diagnosis of BOOP can be confirmed by TBBs, provided the key histologic and clinical features are present. Given the patchy nature of BOOP and the small sample size of TBB, thoracoscopic lung biopsy should be performed in equivocal or nondiagnostic cases.

Pathophysiology

BOOP likely represents a stereotypic host response to diverse injurious or inflamma-tory stimuli. Injury to the bronchioles leads to an inflammatory and reparative re-sponse involving neutrophils, lymphocytes, macrophages, fibroblasts, and possibly other cells. The inciting stimuli are likely diverse, and elicit immune complexes in response to inhaled antigen(s).

Therapy

Corticosteroids are the cornerstone of therapy for BOOP. An initial dose of 40–60 mg prednisone (or equivalent) daily for 2–4 weeks is adequate. Favorable responses are achieved in 60–80% of patients. Responses are often dramatic, with marked clinical improvement within days of institution of therapy. Radiographic improve-ment ensues within 1–4 weeks. The dose is gradually tapered according to clinical symptoms, chest radiographs, and PFTs. Pulmonary fibrosis develops in fewer than 20% of patients. Fatality rates range from 3 to 10%. A subset of patients manifest a more fulminant course, leading to severe fibrosis and even death. Immunosuppres-sive or cytotoxic agents should be given for corticosteroid-recalcitrant cases, but data are limited to anecdotal cases.

Dosage: Prednisone (40–60 mg/day) for 2–4 weeks; gradually taper to 40 mg alternate day by 3–4 months. The rate of taper should be individualized and guided by clinical, radiographic, and physiologic parameters. In patients exhibiting complete and sustained remissions, the dose can be reduced to 20 mg every other day within 6–9 months. Therapy should be continued for a minimum of 12–18 months because relapse is common with early cessation of treatment.

RESPIRATORY BRONCHIOLITIS

Respiratory bronchiolitis is a rare disorder in cigarette smokers with features that overlap with BOOP and CILDs.

Clinical Features

- Most patients are asymptomatic but mild cough, dyspnea, or sputum production may be present.

- In contrast to BOOP, fever, constitutional symptoms, or dense alveolar infiltrate do not occur with respiratory bronchiolitis.
- Basilar rales are noted in 40% of patients; clubbing does not occur.
- Chest radiographs reveal fine reticulonodular interstitial infiltrates or accentuated bronchopulmonary markers ("dirty lungs") in 70–80% of patients. Chest radiographs are normal in the remaining patients.
- HRCT demonstrates finely irregular bronchiolar and peribronchiolar nodules and foci of patchy ground glass opacities. Honeycombing is absent.
- PFTs usually reveal reduced DL_{CO} and mild airways obstruction with preserved lung volumes.
- BAL findings are similar to those of normal smokers and do not reveal the striking neutrophilia characteristic of BOOP.

Histopathologic Features

The salient finding is dense aggregates of pigmented, golden-brown macrophages in respiratory and terminal bronchioles and adjacent airspaces. This may mimic DIP. Peribronchiolar fibrosis may be present but is rarely severe.

Therapy

- Smoking cessation is the mainstay of therapy.
- Following cessation of smoking, symptoms resolve in 80% of patients, and serious sequelae are rare.
- Corticosteroids should be reserved for patients with persistent or progressive symptoms despite cessation of smoking.

PULMONARY VASCULITIS

Systemic necrotizing vasculitis involves the lung primarily in the context of granulomatous vasculitic syndromes (e.g., WG, Churg-Strauss angiitis) or pulmonary renal syndromes (e.g., microscopic polyangiitis, pauci-immune glomerulonephritis). Classical (macroscopic) polyarteritis rarely involves the lung. Pulmonary arterial aneurysms or hemorrhage are rare complications of Takayasu's disease or Behçet's disease. Lymphomatoid granulomatosis, initially grouped among the pulmonary vasculitides, represents a spectrum of lymphoproliferative syndromes and will not be further discussed.

Wegener's Granulomatosis

Wegener's granulomatosis is the most common of the pulmonary vasculitides. In its classical form, WG involves the upper respiratory tract (e.g., ears, sinuses, oropharynx, nasopharynx), lower respiratory tract (e.g., bronchi, lung), and kidney, with varying degrees of disseminating vasculitis. The prevalence is between 1.3 to 3 cases per 100,000 persons per 5-year period. In the absence of therapy, mortality rates for generalized WG exceeds 80% within 3 years. Limited forms of the disease (affecting only one or two organs) have a much better prognosis.

Clinical Features

- Clinical features are protean; virtually any organ can be involved.
- Upper respiratory tract symptoms are present in more than 90% of patients and often are the dominant manifestations.
- Sinus pain, otitis media, hearing loss, epistaxis, saddle nose deformity, nasal or oropharyngeal ulcers are typical complaints.
- Sinusitis is noted on radiographs or CT in more than 80% of patients.
- Lung involvement occurs in 60–80% of patients.
- Tracheal or bronchostenosis occurs in 10–20% of patients.
- Cough, dyspnea, or hemoptysis are present in one-third of patients.
- Abnormalities on chest radiographs are present in more than 80% of patients at some point in the course of the disease.
- Severe alveolar hemorrhage (as a result of capillaritis) occurs in fewer than 5% of patients but may be lethal.
- Glomerulonephritis occurs in 70–85% of patients at some point in the course of the disease (often manifests initially by proteinuria or microscopic hematuria).
- Severe renal failure is noted at the onset of disease in fewer than 20% of patients.
- Chronic renal failure requiring dialysis occurs in 10–30% of patients with WG.
- Ocular involvement occurs in 20–50% of patients. Findings range from superficial conjunctivitis or scleritis to sight-threatening complications of uveitis, vasculitis, or compression of the optic nerve. Blindness occurs in 2–9% of patients.
- Systemic vasculitis frequently involves several organ systems (e.g., the joints, eyes, skin, central nervous system, heart).

Laboratory Investigations

- Chest radiographs: focal nodular or alveolar infiltrates are most common and may be asymptomatic; cavitation occurs in one quarter of patients. Simultaneous clearing and worsening in different areas of the lung may be seen. Pleural effusions occur in 20% of patients. Mediastinal adenopathy is rare.
- PFTs: Reduced lung volumes and diffusing capacity are characteristic. Airways obstruction may reflect granulomatous involvement or stenosis of the trachea or bronchi.
- Serum studies: The ESR and C-reactive protein are elevated in more than 90% of patients with active disease and are invaluable in monitoring the course of the disease.
- Antineutrophil cytoplasmic antibodies (ANCA): Elevated titers of ANCA (typically c-ANCA) are present in more than 90% of patients with disseminated WG but are present in only two-thirds of patients with limited disease.

Histopathologic Features

The salient histopathologic features of WG in involved organs include:

- A necrotizing vasculitis involving capillaries, venules, and arterioles;
- Mixed inflammatory cellular infiltrate (composed of lymphocytes, plasma cells, histiocytes, and scattered neutrophils and eosinophils);
- Geographic necrosis;
- A granulomatous component.

The renal lesion is different and manifests nonspecific features of a segmental, pauci-immune glomerulonephritis. With fulminant disease, a necrotizing, crescentic glomerulonephritis may be seen. Granulomatous vasculitis is noted in fewer than 10% of renal biopsies.

Biopsy Confirmation

A diagnosis of WG requires biopsy confirmation. The triad of granulomas, small vessel vasculitis, and necrosis is the cardinal histologic criteria. Biopsies of sinuses, nasopharynx, or oropharynx typically demonstrate nonspecific inflammation or necrosis but demonstrate vasculitis in fewer than 20% of cases. Even in patients with radiographic evidence for lung involvement, bronchoscopic biopsies (transbronchial or bronchial) are diagnostic in fewer than 10%. Surgical (open or thoracoscopic) lung biopsies are usually required to establish a definitive diagnosis of pulmonary WG. Percutaneous renal biopsies demonstrate focal, segmental glomerulonephritis, but rarely reveal vasculitis.

Pathophysiology

The pathogenesis likely involves a hypersensitivity response by T cells to unknown antigen(s) with the development of necrotizing granulomas and vasculitis and subsequent tissue injury. Antineutrophil cytoplasmic antibodies (c-ANCA) directed against myeloid lysosomal enzymes are markers for the disease and may play pathogenic roles.

Therapy

Oral cyclophosphamide (2 mg/kg/day) combined with corticosteroids (prednisone 1 mg/kg/day, with gradual taper) is the treatment of choice for WG. Oral trimethoprim/sulfamethoxazole (TMP/SMX) (one double-strength tablet twice daily) should be added as adjunctive therapy. TMP/SMX has been shown to reduce the rate of relapses and intercurrent infections.

Cyclophosphamide Dosage: 2 mg/kg/day as a single morning oral dose. Adjust the dosage to keep peripheral blood leukocyte count more than 3,000 and platelet count more than 100,000 mm^3. Cyclophosphamide should be continued for a minimum of 1 year after complete clinical and biochemical remission has been achieved.

At that point, cyclophosphamide can be tapered by 25-mg increments every 2–3 months. Intravenous "pulse" cyclophosphamide has been tried as therapy for WG but appears to be less effective than daily oral cyclophosphamide.

- Expect 2–6 weeks for maximal response to cyclophosphamide.

Corticosteroid Dosage: Prednisone (1 mg/kg/day) for 2 weeks, then taper (if clinical remission has occurred) to 60 mg alternate day within 2 months. The rate of taper must be individualized according to the severity of the disease and treatment response. Prednisone can usually be tapered to 40 mg alternate day by 6 months and to 20 mg alternate day by 12 months. For adverse effects, refer to Tables 6.4 and 6.5.

TMP/SMX (BACTRIM, SEPTRA)

Anecdotal successes have been noted with TMP/SMX as primary therapy in patients with mild, indolent disease or in patients with progressive, active disease refractory to conventional therapy with cyclophosphamide and prednisone. Although its role as primary therapy is highly controversial, the addition of TMP/SMX to cyclophosphamide and prednisone was recently shown to reduce the rate of relapses and secondary infections in a multicenter randomized placebo controlled trial. Thus, TMP/SMX should be given as adjunctive therapy in patients with WG, not only for its efficacy in preventing opportunistic infections (e.g., *Pneumocystis carinii, Nocardia*) but also to reduce the rate of relapses of vasculitis. We do not believe TMP/SMX has a role as primary therapy for WG.

Alternative Therapies

- Methotrexate (in combination with prednisone) may be given in patients experiencing serious adverse effects from cyclophosphamide or in lieu of cyclophosphamide in patients with mild disease. Although randomized trials have not been done, a recent study at the National Institutes of Health of patients with non–life-threatening WG cited favorable responses to once-weekly methotrexate (mean dose 20 mg/week) in 30 of 42 patients (71%). Toxicity was generally mild, but four patients developed *Pneumocystis carinii* pneumonia (two of whom died). This complication can be averted by concomitant use of TMP/SMX.
- Azathioprine and chlorambucil have each been used, with anecdotal successes, in patients with WG. Although controlled studies have not been performed, azathioprine is less effective than cyclophosphamide and data affirming its efficacy are limited. Chlorambucil is potentially leukemogenic. We believe methotrexate is preferred among patients unable to tolerate or failing cyclophosphamide.

THERAPIES FOR SPECIFIC COMPLICATIONS OF WG

- Pyogenic infections of the sinuses or lower respiratory tract are common and warrant aggressive antibiotic therapy. Surgical drainage of the sinuses may be needed for persistent sinusitis refractory to medical therapy.

- Upper airways obstruction secondary to tracheal stenosis may require surgical dilatation or tracheostomy.
- Renal transplantation has been successful in patients with end-stage renal failure as long as the systemic vasculitis is in remission.

ALVEOLAR HEMORRHAGE COMPLICATING WEGENER'S GRANULOMATOSIS

Severe alveolar hemorrhage, associated with rapidly progressive glomerulonephritis and respiratory failure, may be a catastrophic complication of WG. Early mortality exceeds 35%, even with aggressive therapy. In this context, intravenous pulse methylprednisolone, followed by oral (or intravenous) cyclophosphamide should be given.

Therapy

- Intravenous methylprednisolone (1 gm daily for 3 days), followed by a corticosteroid taper *plus* cyclophosphamide (2 mg/kg/day orally or intravenously).

Churg-Strauss Syndrome

Churg-Strauss syndrome, also known as allergic angiitis and granulomatosis, is a rare necrotizing granulomatous vasculitis associated with asthma, allergic rhinitis, fever, and eosinophilia (in peripheral blood and tissue). The annual incidence has been estimated at 2.4 cases per million. Asthma or allergic rhinitis symptoms may antedate the diagnosis for years. Chest x-rays demonstrate focal alveolar infiltrates in 30–70% of patients. A diagnosis of acute or chronic eosinophilic pneumonia commonly precedes the diagnosis of Churg-Strauss syndrome. Allergic rhinitis, nasal polyposis, and sinusitis are noted in more than two-thirds of patients. Fever, weight loss, and malaise occur in more than 90% of patients. Neurologic involvement (particularly mononeuritis multiplex) occurs in up to two-thirds of patients and may presage disseminated vasculitis. Cutaneous involvement occurs in two-thirds of patients; skin biopsies demonstrate eosinophilic or leukocytoclastic vasculitis. The heart is involved in 30–50% of patients; the gastrointestinal tract, in one-third of patients. Renal failure is rare, but hypertension develops in nearly 50% of patients. During the active vasculitis phase, striking increases in blood eosinophil counts and ESR are evident. Both ESR and blood eosinophil counts usually correlate with activity of disease. Circulating ANCA (either c-ANCA or p-ANCA) have been noted in Churg-Strauss syndrome.

Histopathologic Features

Histopathologic features of Churg-Strauss syndrome are characterized by a necrotizing vasculitis affecting arterioles, venules, and capillaries, with granulomatous and eosinophilic components. Eosinophilic infiltration of vascular walls is usually striking. Granulomas, eosinophils, multinucleated giant cells, and palisading histiocytes in extravascular tissues are characteristic.

Treatment

Corticosteroids are the mainstay of treatment for mild to moderate cases. Prednisone (1 mg/kg/day for 4 weeks, followed by a gradual taper) achieves remissions in more than 80% of patients. For severe disease or when unfavorable prognostic features are present (e.g., renal failure, gastrointestinal, cardiac, or CNS involvement), oral cyclophosphamide should be added (similar to the regimen used for WG). The prognosis is usually favorable with both treatment regimens (3-year survival rates of 80–90%; 10-year survival, 70–80%). For fulminant cases, pulse methylprednisolone (1 gm daily for 3 days) followed by oral cyclophosphamide (2 mg/kg/day) and prednisone is advised.

EOSINOPHILIC GRANULOMA OF THE LUNG

Pulmonary EG (also called histiocytosis X or Langerhans' cell granulomatosis) is a rare granulomatous disorder usually seen in smokers that may present with cough, dyspnea, and interstitial, nodular, or cystic infiltrates on chest radiographs. Like Letterer-Siwe disease and Hand-Schüller-Christian disease in children, EG shares in common an abnormal accumulation of atypical histiocytes and stellate-shaped granulomatous inflammatory lesions in affected tissues.

Clinical Features

- More than 90% of patients with pulmonary EG are smokers.
- Pulmonary EG is almost exclusively seen in Caucasians.
- Adults (age 20–50 years) are usually affected; pulmonary EG is rare in children.
- Cough or dyspnea are the most common symptoms (noted in 60–75% of patients).
- Low grade fever, malaise, or anorexia occur in 15–30% of patients.
- Extrapulmonary involvement (e.g., osteolytic bone lesions or diabetes insipidus) occurs in 15–20% of patients.
- Ten to twenty-five percent of patients are asymptomatic.
- Pneumothorax, resulting from rupture of subpleural cysts, occurs in 6–20% of patients.
- PFTs are abnormal in 80–85% of patients with pulmonary EG. Pure restrictive or mixed restrictive/obstructive defects may be observed. Diffusing capacity, VC, and/or TLC are reduced in 50–80% of patients. FEV_1 is often reduced, but FEV_1/FVC ratio is normal or increased. Hypoxemia is common, particularly with exercise.
- The incidence of bronchogenic carcinoma is increased in smokers with pulmonary EG.

Radiographic Features

- Chest x-rays show nodular or reticulonodular infiltrates with a predilection for the mid and upper lung zones; costophrenic angles are spared. Extensive honeycombing, fibrocystic changes, and pneumothorax are seen in more advanced disease. Pleural effusions or intrathoracic lymphadenopathy are not features of pulmonary EG.

- HRCT is highly distinctive. Numerous thin-walled cysts are evident in more than 90% of patients. Peribronchiolar nodules (typically 1–4 mm in diameter) are present concomitantly in 60–78% of patients. Coalescence of cysts may result in bullous lesions exceeding 2–3 cm in diameter. Ground glass opacities are rarely prominent. The combination of numerous cysts and nodules involving the upper lobes strongly suggests the diagnosis of pulmonary EG.

Histopathologic Features

- Pulmonary EG is characterized by inflammatory, cystic, nodular, and fibrotic lesions involving the bronchioles and pulmonary interstitium.
- Destruction of bronchioles and lung parenchyma leads to numerous peribronchiolar nodules and cysts.
- The lesions are distributed around bronchioles (bronchocentric).
- A ''stellate'' or star-shaped pattern of fibrosis can be identified in up to 80% of cases under low power light microscopy.
- Eosinophils are not a constant feature of the inflammatory lesions.
- The inflammatory process can lead to fibrocystic changes and end-stage honeycomb lung.
- Atypical histiocytes (Langerhans' cells (LCs)) are the cornerstone of the diagnosis. These large ovoid histiocytes, with pale eosinophilic cytoplasm, an indented nucleus, and inconspicuous nucleoli, may comprise up to 30–50% of cells in the dense inflammatory lesions.
- LCs can be recognized by conventional hematoxylin-eosin stains in most cases. When light microscopic features are not definitive, positive immunohistochemical stains may substantiate their identity (i.e., S-100 protein or common thymocyte antigen (OKT6)).
- With far advanced disease, the distinctive LCs may no longer be present and changes of honeycomb lung may be indistinguishable from other CILDs.
- Transbronchial lung biopsies should be done in suspected cases but are often nondiagnostic because of the small amount of tissue sampled.
- BAL typically shows a marked increase (more than 10%; normal less than 1%) in the proportions of OKT6-staining mononuclear cells. This finding may not be seen in more advanced disease.
- If the diagnosis is uncertain, thoracoscopic lung biopsy of the inflammatory lesions, in addition to S-100 and OKT6 staining, may be required. Electron microscopy is used primarily for research purposes.

Pathophysiology

- Although the cause is unknown, pulmonary EG likely represents an uncontrolled immune response initiated or controlled by LCs. Components in tobacco smoke may be implicated, as more than 90% of cases occur in smokers. Cigarette smoke may stimulate and recruit LCs and other immune effector cells to the lung. Replication of LCs and release of cytokines in the alveolar structures may recruit other inflammatory cells and perpetuate the alveolitis.

Therapy

Management is tempered by the fact that the course of the disease is unpredictable and may be self-limiting. In more than two-thirds of patients the disease stabilizes or improves, often within 6–24 months of onset of symptoms. Pulmonary EG progresses in 15–31% of patients. Severe late sequelae include pulmonary fibrosis, cor pulmonale, or respiratory failure. Fatality rates range from 6–25%. Multisystemic disease, multiple pneumothoraces, or severe honeycombing on chest radiographs have been associated with a worse prognosis.

- Primary therapy begins by counseling the patient to quit smoking.
- Anecdotal responses have been noted with corticosteroids, but their efficacy remains unproven. Corticosteroids should be reserved for selected patients with severe or progressive disease despite smoking cessation. In such cases, a 3- to 6-month trial is reasonable. A prolonged course should be continued only in patients exhibiting unequivocal responses.
- Isolated, symptomatic bony lesions can be treated with curettage or local radiotherapy.
- For progressive, widespread disease unresponsive to corticosteroids, vinblastine (a vinca alkaloid) or a cytotoxic agent may be considered, but data affirming their efficacy are lacking.
- Single lung transplantation has been successfully accomplished in patients with EG and end-stage pulmonary fibrosis.

PULMONARY ALVEOLAR PROTEINOSIS

Pulmonary alveolar proteinosis, also termed alveolar phospholipidosis, is a rare disorder of unknown cause described in 1958 and characterized by accumulation of lipoprotein-rich, surfactant-like material within the alveolar spaces. Massive intrapulmonary shunting results in progressive hypoxemia, cough, dyspnea, and respiratory insufficiency. PAP is exceptionally rare, with an estimated prevalence of one case per million adults. The disease is two to three times more common in males and usually occurs between age 20–50 years, but all ages can be affected.

Clinical Features

- Usually presents insidiously with dyspnea, cough, and occasional sputum production.

- Crackles are often present on chest auscultation.
- Serum lactate dehydrogenase is elevated in 80% of patients.
- Chest x-ray demonstrates diffuse, bilateral alveolar infiltrates, often in a perihilar distribution; pleural effusion and hilar adenopathy are not features of PAP.
- Often a marked disparity exists between mild clinical symptoms and extensive radiographic infiltrates.
- The characteristic physiologic abnormality is severe hypoxemia, resulting from intrapulmonary shunting.
- PFTs demonstrate mild reductions in VC or diffusing capacity; expiratory flow rates are usually preserved.
- Infections caused by intracellular pathogens (e.g., *Nocardia, Staphylococci, Mycobacteria*) may complicate PAP as a result of an acquired defect in alveolar macrophages.

Histopathologic Features

Alveolar spaces are filled with dense surfactant-like material that stains bright pink with periodic acid-Schiff (PAS) reagent and negative with alcian blue. This foamy intraalveolar exudate resembles pneumonia caused by *Pneumocystis carinii* but lacks the interstitial inflammatory component or damage seen in that condition. In PAP, the alveolar septae are normal and interstitial inflammation or fibrosis are not found. The intraalveolar material contains many lamellar bodies, similar to inclusions within type II pneumocytes.

- Fiberoptic bronchoscopy with TBBs and BAL is often definitive. The gross and microscopic appearance of BAL fluid is distinctive. Lavage effluent reveals thick, opaque, yellowish-white milky fluid, which sediments into multiple layers on standing. Positive PAS and negative alcian blue stains of BAL fluid may corroborate the diagnosis.
- TBBs may demonstrate the characteristic histopathologic features of PAP, but because of sampling error, the diagnosis may be missed.
- When bronchoscopy is nondiagnostic, thoracoscopic lung biopsy should be done.

Pathophysiology

The pathogenesis of PAP is unknown. The massive accumulation of surfactant-like material in alveolar spaces suggests defects in surfactant homeostasis (i.e., impaired clearance or excessive production). The inciting signals or stimuli for PAP have not been identified, but a history of exposure to chemicals, solvents, hydrocarbons, minerals, or hard metals has been elicited in 50% or more of cases. Diverse animals models resembling PAP have been produced by inhalation of fine dust particles (e.g., volcanic ash, titanium, silica) or ingestion of specific drugs (e.g., amiodarone, chlorphentermine). PAP has rarely been described in families and in association with hematologic malignancies.

Therapy

- Whole lung lavage is the treatment of choice. The procedure requires general anesthesia and involves placing a double lumen tube. The most severely affected lung is deflated and lavaged with 20–30 liters of saline (warmed to body temperature) while the contralateral lung is continuously ventilated. With progressive lavage, the viscid fluid is removed and the effluent clears. Whole lung lavage requires 3–5 hours to complete and has significant potential morbidity. This procedure should be performed by experienced medical teams. Following lavage, gradual improvement in chest radiographs, symptoms, and blood gases ensues. Maximal improvement may take up to 6 weeks. We often wait a few weeks before lavaging the contralateral lung, but immediate lavage can be performed in fulminant or severe cases. Improvement occurs in 75–95% of patients following whole lung lavage. Relapses occur in up to one-third of patients but usually respond to repeat lavage. Serial chest radiographs, PFTs, and serum lactate dehydrogenase may be useful to monitor patients.

BIBLIOGRAPHY

Overview of Interstitial Lung Disease

Lynch JP, Chavis A. Chronic interstitial pulmonary disorders. In: Victor L, ed. Clinical pulmonary medicine. Boston: Little, Brown, 1992:193–264.

High-Resolution Lung Computed Tomography

Colby TV, Swensen SJ. Anatomic distribution and histopathologic patterns in diffuse lung disease: correlation with HRCT. J Thorac Imaging 1996;11:1–26.

Grenier P, Chevret S, Beigelman C, et al. Chronic diffuse infiltrative lung disease: determination of the diagnostic value of clinical data, chest radiography, and CT with Bayesian analysis. Radiology 1994;191:383–390.

Primack S, Hartman T, Hansell D, et al. End-stage lung disease: CT findings in 61 patients. Radiology 1993;189:681–686.

Raghu G. Interstitial lung disease: a diagnostic approach: are CT scan and lung biopsy indicated in every patient? Am J Respir Crit Care Med 1995;151:909–914.

Idiopathic Pulmonary Fibrosis

Clinical Series and Reviews

Agusti C, Xaubet A, Agusti AGN, Roca J, Ramirez J, Rodriquez-Roisin R. Clinical and functional assessment of patients with idiopathic pulmonary fibrosis: results of a 3-year follow-up. Eur Respir J 1994;7:643–650.

Johnston ID, Gomm SA, Kalra A, et al. The management of cryptogenic fibrosing alveolitis in three regions of the United Kingdom. Eur Respir J 1993;6:891–893.

Meier-Sydow J, Weiss SM, Buhl R, Rust M, Raghu G. Idiopathic pulmonary fibrosis: current concepts and challenges in management. Semin Respir Crit Care Med 1994;15:77–96.

Panos RJ, Mortenson RL, Niccoli SA, King GE Jr. Clinical deterioration in patients with idiopathic pulmonary fibrosis: causes and assessment. Am J Med 1990;88:396–404.

Schwartz DA, Van Fossen DS, Davis CS, Helmers RA, Dayton CS, Burmeister LF, Hunninghake GW. Determinants of progression in idiopathic pulmonary fibrosis. Am J Respir Crit Care Med 1994;149:444–449.

Schwartz DA, Helmers RA, Galvin JR, Van Fossen DS, et al. Determinants of progression in idiopathic pulmonary fibrosis. Am J Respir Crit Care Med 1994;149:450–454.

Wells AU, Cullinan P, Hansell DM, Rubens MB, et al. Fibrosing alveolitis associated with systemic sclerosis has a better prognosis than lone cryptogenic fibrosing alveolitis. Am J Respir Crit Care Med 1994;149:1583–1589.

Epidemiology

Coultas DB, Zumwalt RE, Black WC, Sobonya RE. The epidemiology of interstitial lung diseases. Am J Respir Crit Care Med 1994;150:967–972.

Hubbard R, Johnston I, Coultas DB, Britton J. Mortality rates from cryptogenic fibrosing alveolitis in seven countries. Thorax 1996;51:711–716.

Iawai K, Mori T, Yamada N, Yamaguchi M, Hosoda Y. Idiopathic pulmonary fibrosis: epidemiologic approaches to occupational exposure. Am J Respir Crit Care Med 1994;150: 670–675.

Raghu G, Hert R. Interstitial lung diseases: genetic predisposition and inherited interstitial lung diseases. Semin Respir Med 1993;14:323–332.

Schwartz DA, Merchant RK, Helmers RA, Gilbert SR, Dayton CS, Hunninghake GW. The influence of smoking on lung function in patients with idiopathic pulmonary fibrosis. Am J Rev Respir Dis 1991;144:504–506.

Computed Tomographic Scans

Agusti C, Xaubet A, Luburich P, Ayuso MC, Roca J, Rodriguez-Roisin R. Computed tomographic-guided bronchoalveolar lavage in idiopathic pulmonary fibrosis. Thorax 1996;51: 841–845.

Akira M, Sakatani M, Ueda E. Idiopathic pulmonary fibrosis: progression of honeycombing at thin-section CT. Radiology 1993;189:687–691.

Hartman TE, Primack SL, Swensen SJ, Hansell D, et al. Desquamative interstitial pneumonia: thin-section CT findings in 22 patients. Radiology 1993;187:787–790.

Hartman TE, Primack SL, Kang EY, Swensen SJ, Hansell D, et al. Disease progression in usual interstitial pneumonia compared with desquamative interstitial pneumonia. Chest 1996;110:378–382.

Lee JS, IM JG, Ahn JM, Kim YM, Han MC. Fibrosing alveolitis: prognostic implication of ground-glass attenuation at high-resolution CT. Radiology 1992;184:451–454.

Nishimura K, Kitaichi M, Izumi T, Nagai S, Kanaoka M, Itoh H. Usual interstitial pneumonia: histologic correlation with high-resolution CT. Radiology 1992;182:337–342.

Remy-Jardin M, Giraud F, Remy J, et al. Importance of ground-glass attenuation in chronic diffuse infiltrative lung disease: pathologic-CT correlation. Radiology 1993;189:693–698.

Wells AU, Rubens MB, du Bois RM, Hansell DM. Serial CT in fibrosing alveolitis: prognostic significance of the initial pattern. AJR 1993;161:1159–1165.

Wells AU, Hansell DM, Rubens MB, Cullinan P, Black CM, du Bois RM. The predictive value of appearances on thin-section computed tomography in fibrosing alveolitis. Am Rev Respir Dis 1993;148:1076–1082.

Pulmonary Function Tests/Exercise Tests

Dunn TL, Watters LC, Hendrix C, Cherniak RM, Schwarz MI, King TE Jr. Gas exchange at a given degree of volume restriction is different in sarcoidosis and idiopathic pulmonary fibrosis. Am J Med 1988;85:221–224.

Harris Eze AO, Sridhar G, Clemens RE, Gallagher CG, Marciniuk DD. Oxygen improves maximal exercise performance in interstitial lung disease. Am J Respir Crit Care Med 1994;150:1616–1622.

Robertson HT. Clinical application of pulmonary function and exercise tests in the management of patients with interstitial lung disease. Semin Respir Crit Care Med 1994;15:1–9.

Lung Biopsy

Bernsard DD, McIntyre RC, Simon JS, et al. Comparison of video thoracoscopic lung biopsy to open lung biopsy in the diagnosis of interstitial lung disease. Chest 1993;103:765–770.

Cherniack RM, Colby TV, Flint A, Thurlbeck WM, Waldron JA Jr, Ackerson L, et al. Correlation of structure and function in idiopathic pulmonary fibrosis. Am J Respir Crit Care Med 1995,151:1180–1188.

Corrin B. Pathology of interstitial lung disease. Semin Respir Crit Care Med 1994;15:61–76.

Katzenstein AA, Fiorelli RF. Nonspecific interstitial pneumonia/fibrosis. Histopathologic features and clinical significance. Am J Surg Pathol 1994;18:136–147.

Bronchoalveolar Lavage

Boomars KA, Wagenaar SS, Mulder PG, van Velzen-Blad H, van den Bosch JM. Relationship between cells obtained by bronchoalveolar lavage and survival in idiopathic pulmonary fibrosis. Thorax 1995;50;1087–1092.

Turner-Warwick M, Haslam PL. The value of serial bronchoalveolar lavages in assessing the clinical progress of patients with cryptogenic fibrosing alveolitis. Am Rev Respir Dis 1987; 135:26–34.

Watters LC, Schwarz MI, Cherniak RM, et al. Idiopathic pulmonary fibrosis. Pretreatment bronchoalveolar lavage cellular constituents and their relationships to lung histopathology and clinical response to therapy. Am Rev Respir Dis 1987;135:696–704.

Treatment of IPF

Hosenpud JD, Novick RJ, Bennett LE, Keck BM, Fiol B, Daily OP. The Registry of the International Society for Heart and Lung Transplantation: Thirteenth Official Report—1996. J Heart Lung Transplant 1996;15:655–674.

Hunninghake GW, Kalica AR. Approaches to the treatment of pulmonary fibrosis. Am J Respir Crit Care Med 1995;151:915–918.

Johnson MA, Kwan S, Snell NJC, Nunn AJ, Darbyshire JH, Turner-Warwick M. Randomized controlled trial comparing prednisolone alone with cyclophosphamide and low dose prednisolone in combination with cryptogenic fibrosing alveolitis. Thorax 1989;44:280–288.

Peters SG, McDougall JC, Douglas WW, Coles DT, DeRemee RA. Colchicine in the treatment of pulmonary fibrosis. Chest 1993;103:101–104.

Raghu G, DePaso WJ, Cain K, Hammar SP, et al. Azathioprine combined with prednisone in the treatment of idiopathic pulmonary fibrosis: a prospective, double-blind, randomized, placebo-controlled trial. Am Rev Respir Dis 1991;144:291–296.

van Oortegem K, Wallaert B, Marquette CH, Ramon P, et al. Determinants of response to immunosuppressive therapy in idiopathic pulmonary fibrosis. Eur Respir J 1994;7: 1950–1957.

Collagen Vascular Disease-associated Interstitial Lung Disease

Agusti C, Xaubet A, Roca J, Agusti AGN, Rodriguez-Roisin R. Interstitial pulmonary fibrosis with and without associated collagen vascular disease: results of a two-year follow-up. Thorax 1992;47:1035–1040.

Lynch JP III, Hunninghake GW. Pulmonary complications of collagen vascular disease. In: Creger WP, ed. Annual review of medicine. Vol. 42. Palo Alto, CA: Annual Reviews, Inc., 1992;43:17–35.

Martinez FM, Lynch JP III. Collagen vascular disease-associated bronchiolitis obliterans–organizing pneumonia. In: Epler GR, ed. Diseases of the bronchioles. New York: Raven Press, 1994:347–366.

McCune WJ, Vallance D, Lynch JP III. Immunosuppressive drug therapy for rheumatic disease. Current Opin Rheumatol 1994;6(3):262–272.

Toews GB, Lynch JP III. Pathogenesis and clinical features of pulmonary infections in patients with rheumatic disease. In: Cannon GW, Zimmerman GA, eds. The lung in rheumatic diseases. Lung biology in health and disease. New York: Marcel Dekker, Inc., 1990;45: 179–226.

Vallance D, Lynch JP III, McCune WJ. Immunosuppressive treatment of the pulmonary manifestations of progressive systemic sclerosis. Curr Opin Rheum 1995;7:174–182.

Rheumatoid Arthritis

McDonagh J, Greaves M, Wright AR, Heycock C, Owen JP, Kelly C. High-resolution computed tomography of the lungs in patients with rheumatoid arthritis and interstitial lung disease. Br J Rheumatol 1994;33:118–122.

Remy-Jardin M, Remy J, Cortet B, Mauri F, Delcambre B. Lung changes in rheumatoid arthritis: CT findings. Radiology 1994;193:375–382.

Yousem SA, Colby TV, Carrington CB. Lung biopsy in rheumatoid arthritis. Am Rev Respir Dis 1985;131:770–777.

Progressive Systemic Sclerosis (Scleroderma)

Akesson A, Scheja A, Lundin A, Wollheim FA. Improved pulmonary function in systemic sclerosis after treatment with cyclophosphamide. Arthritis Rheum 1994;37:729–735.

Behr J, Vogelmeier C, Beinert T, Meurer M, Krombach F, Konig G, Fruhmann G. Bronchoalveolar lavage for evaluation and management of scleroderma disease of the lung. Am J Respir Crit Care Med 1996;154:400–406.

Johkoh T, Ikezoe J, Kohno N, et al. High-resolution CT and pulmonary function tests in collagen vascular disease: comparison with idiopathic pulmonary fibrosis. Eur J Radiol 1994;18:113–121.

Remy-Jardin M, Remy J, Wallaert B, Bataille D, Hatron PY. Pulmonary involvement in progressive systemic sclerosis: sequential evaluation with CT, pulmonary function tests, and bronchoalveolar lavage. Radiology 1993;188:499–506.

Sato S, Ihn H, Kikuchi K, Takehara K. Antihistone antibodies in systemic sclerosis: association with pulmonary fibrosis. Arthritis Rheum 1994;37:391–394.

Silver RM, Warrick JH, Kinsella MB, Staudt LS, Baumann MH, Strange C. Cyclophosphamide and low-dose prednisone therapy in patients with systemic sclerosis (scleroderma) with interstitial lung disease. J Rheumatol 1993;20:838–844.

Steen VD, Lanz JK Jr, Conte C, Owens GR, Medsger TA Jr. Therapy for severe interstitial lung disease in systemic sclerosis. A retrospective study. Arthritis Rheum 1994;37:1290–1296.

Wells AU, Hansell DH, Rubens MB, Cullinan P, Haslam PL, Black CM, Du Bois RM. Fibrosing alveolitis in systemic sclerosis: bronchoalveolar lavage findings in relation to computed tomographic appearance. Am J Respir Crit Care Med 1994;150:462–468.

Polymyositis and Dermatomyositis

Marguerie C, Bunn CC, Beynon H, Bernstein RM, Hughes JM, et al. Polymyositis, pulmonary fibrosis, and autoantibodies to aminoacyl-tRNA synthetase enzymes. Q J Med 1990;77:1019–1038.

Targoff IN, Arnett FA, Berman L, O'Brien C, Reichlin M. Anti-KJ: a new antibody associated with the syndrome of polymyositis and interstitial lung disease. J Clin Invest 1989;84:162–172.

Tazelaar H, Viggiano R, Pickersgill J, Colby T. Interstitial lung disease in polymyositis and dermatomyositis. Clinical features and prognosis as correlated with histologic findings. Am Rev Respir Dis 1990;141:727–733.

Mixed Connective Tissue Disease

Lazaro M, Maldonado, Cocco J, Catoggio L, Babini S, et al. Clinical and serologic characteristics of patients with overlap syndrome: is mixed connective tissue disease a distinct clinical entity? Medicine (Baltimore) 1989;68:58–65.

Prakash UB. Lungs in mixed connective tissue disease. J Thorac Imaging 1992;7:55–61.

Sullivan WD, Hurst DJ, Harmon CE, Esther JH, et al. A prospective evaluation emphasizing pulmonary involvement in patients with mixed connective tissue disease. Medicine (Baltimore) 1984;63:92–104.

Sjögren's Syndrome

Alkhayer M, McCann BG, Harrison BD. Lymphocytic interstitial pneumonitis in association with Sjögren's syndrome. Br J Dis Chest 1988;82:305–309.

Dalavanga YA, Constantopoulos SH, Galanopoulou V, Zerva L, Moutsopoulos HM. Alveolitis correlates with clinical pulmonary involvement in primary Sjögren's syndrome. Chest 1991;99:1394–1397.

Hansen LA, Prakash UBS, Colby RV. Pulmonary lymphoma in Sjögren's syndrome. Mayo Clin Proc 1989;64:920–931.

Systemic Lupus Erythematosus

Andronopoulos AP, Costantopoulos SH, Galanopoulou V, Drosos AA, et al. Pulmonary function in non-smoking patients with systemic lupus erythematosus. Chest 1992;92:312–315.

Fenlon HM, Doran M, Sant SM, Breatnach E. High-resolution chest CT in systemic lupus erythematosus. AJR 1996;166:301–307.

Orens J, Martinez F, Lynch JP III. Pleuropulmonary manifestations of systemic lupus erythematosus. Rheum Clin N Am 1994;20:159–193.

Drug-induced Pneumonitis

Overview

Barry SG, Wesslius LJ. Drug-induced lung disease: keys to diagnosis and management. Clin Pulmonary Med 1996;3:157–163.

Benson MK, Bentley AM. Lung disease induced by drug addiction. Thorax 1995;50:125–127.

Reed CR, Glauser FL. Drug-induced non-cardiogenic pulmonary edema. Chest 1991;100: 1120–1124.

Rosenow EC III, Limper AH. Drug-induced pulmonary disease. Semin Respir Infect 1995; 10:86–95.

Zitnik RJ, Cooper JA Jr. Pulmonary disease due to antirheumatic agents. Clin Chest Med 1990;11:139–154.

Chemotherapy or Radiation-induced Pneumonitis

Anderson BS, Lunga MA, Yee C, Hiu KK, et al. Fatal pulmonary failure complicating high dose cytosine arabinoside therapy in acute leukemia. Cancer 1990;65:1079–1084.

Comis RL. Bleomycin pulmonary toxicity: current status and future directions. Semin Oncol 1992;19:64–70.

Kalaycioglu M, Kavaru M, Tuason L, Bolwell B. Empiric prednisone therapy for pulmonary toxic reaction after high dose chemotherapy containing carmustine (BCNU). Chest 1995; 107:482–487.

Kreisman H, Wolkove N. Pulmonary toxicity of anti-neoplastic therapy. Semin Oncol 1992; 19:508–520.

Salinas FV, Winterbauer RH. Radiation pneumonitis: a mimic of infectious pneumonitis. Semin Respir Infect 1995;10:143–153.

Twohig KJ, Matthay RA. Pulmonary effects of cytotoxic agents other than bleomycin. Clin Chest Med 1990;11:31–54.

Specific Drugs

Coudert B, Bailly F, Lombard JN, et al. Amiodarone pneumonitis: bronchoalveolar lavage findings in 15 patients and review of the literature. Chest 1992;102:1005–1112.

Klinger JR, Bensadown E, Carrao WM. Pulmonary complications from alveolar accumulation of carbonaceous material in a cocaine smoker. Chest 1992;101:1171–1173.

Tashkin DP, Khalsa ME, Gorelick D, Chang P, et al. Pulmonary status of habitual cocaine smokers. Am Rev Respir Dis 1992;145:92–100.

van der Veen MJ, Dekker JJ, Dinant HJ, van Soesbergern RM, Bijlsma JW. Fatal pulmonary fibrosis complicating low dose methotrexate therapy for rheumatoid arthritis. J Rheumatol 1995;22:1766–1768.

Hypersensitivity Pneumonitis

Adler BD, Padley SP, Muller NL, Remy-Jardin M, Remy J. Chronic hypersensitivity pneumonitis: high-resolution CT and radiographic features in 16 patients. Radiology 1992;185: 91–95.

Akira M, Kita N, Higashihara T, et al. Summer-type hypersensitivity pneumonitis. Comparison of high-resolution CT and plain radiographic findings. Am J Roentgenol 1992;158: 1223–1228.

Gurney JW. Hypersensitivity pneumonitis. Radiol Clin North Am 1992;30:1219–1230.

Kokkarinen J, Tukiainen H, Terho EO. Mortality due to farmer's lung in Finland. Chest 1994; 106:509–512.

Kokkarinen J, Tukiainen H, Terho EO. Recovery of pulmonary function in farmer's lung—a five-year follow-up study. Am Rev Respir Dis 1993;147:793–796.

Lalancette M, Carrier G, Laviolette M, Ferland S, et al. Farmer's lung: long-term outcome and lack of predictive value of bronchoalveolar lavage fibrosing factors. Am Rev Respir Dis 1993;148:216–221.

Lynch DA, Newell JD, Logan PM, King TE Jr, Muller NL. Can CT distinguish hypersensitivity pneumonitis from idiopathic pulmonary fibrosis? AJR 1995;165:807–811.

Perez-padilla R, Gaxiola M, Salas J, Mejia M, Ramos C, Selman ML. Bronchiolitis in chronic pigeon breeder's disease: morphologic evidence of a spectrum of small airways lesions in hypersensitivity pneumonitis induced by avian antigens. Chest 1996;110:371–377.

Perez-padilla R, Salas J, Chapela R, et al. Mortality in Mexican patients with chronic pigeon breeders lung compared with those with usual interstitial pneumonia. Am Rev Respir Dis 1993;148:49–53.

Sharma OP, Fujimura N. Hypersensitivity pneumonitis: a noninfectious granulomatosis. Semin Respir Infect 1995;10:96–106.

Sarcoidosis

Clinical Series and Reviews

Gideon NM, Mannino DM. Sarcoidosis mortality in the United States, 1979–1981: an analysis of multiple-cause mortality data. Am J Med 1996;100:423–427.

Hillerdal G, Nou E, Osterman K, Schmekel B. Sarcoidosis: epidemiology and prognosis. A 15-year European study. Am Rev Respir Dis 1984;130:29–32.

Neville E, Walker AN, James DG. Prognostic factors predicting the outcome of sarcoidosis: an analysis of 818 patients. Quart J Med 1983;208:525–533.

Reich JM, Johnson RE. Course and prognosis of sarcoidosis in a nonreferral setting: analysis of 86 patients observed for 10 years. Am J Med 1985;89:61.

Romer FK. Presentation of sarcoidosis and outcome of pulmonary changes. A review of 243 patients followed for up to 10 years. Dan Med Bull 1982;29:27–32.

Sharma OP, Badr A. Sarcoidosis: diagnosis, staging, and newer diagnostic modalities. Clin Pulmon Med 1994;1(1):18–26.

Radiographic Manifestations

Brauner MW, Lenoir S, Grenier P, Cluzel P, Battesti JP, Valeyre D. Pulmonary sarcoidosis: CT assessment of reversibility. Radiology 1992;182:345–349.

Chiles C, Putnam CE. Pulmonary sarcoidosis. Semin Respir Med 1992;13:345–357.

Lenique F, Brauner MW, Grenier P, Battesti JP, Loiseau A, Valeyre D. CT assessment of bronchi in sarcoidosis: endoscopic and pathologic correlations. Radiology 1995;194: 419–423.

Mana J, Tierstein AS, Mendelson DS, Padilla ML, DePalo LR. Excessive thoracic computed tomographic scanning in sarcoidosis. Thorax 1995;50:1264–1266.

Murdoch J, Muller NL. Pulmonary sarcoidosis: changes on follow-up CT examination. AJR 1992;159:473–477.

Nishimura K, Itoh H, Kitaichi M, Nagai S, Izumi T. CT and pathological correlation of pulmonary sarcoidosis. Semin Ultrasound CT MR 1995;16:361–370.

Winterbauer RH, Belic N, Moores KD. A clinical interpretation of bilateral hilar adenopathy. Ann Intern Med 1973;78:65–71.

Pulmonary Function Tests

Miller A, Brown LK, Sloane MF, Bhuptani A, Teirstein AS. Cardiorespiratory responses to incremental exercise in sarcoidosis patients with normal spirometry. Chest 1995;107: 323–329.

Angiotensin-Converting Enzyme Activity

Arbustini E, Grasso M, Leo G, Tinelli C, et al. Polymorphism of angiotensin-converting enzyme gene in sarcoidosis. Am J Respir Crit Care Med 1996;153(2):851–854.

Brice EA, Friedlander W, Bateman ED, Kirsch RE. Serum angiotensin-converting enzyme activity, concentrations, and specific activity in granulomatous interstitial lung disease, tuberculosis, and COPD. Chest 1995;107:706–710.

Bronchoalveolar Lavage (BAL)

Laviolette M, LaForge J, Tennina S, Boulet LP. Prognostic value of bronchoalveolar lavage lymphocyte count in recently diagnosed pulmonary sarcoidosis. Chest 1991;100:380–384.

Muller-Quernheim J, Pfeifer S, Strausz J, Ferlinz R. Correlation of clinical and immunologic parameters of the inflammatory activity of pulmonary sarcoidosis. Am Rev Respir Dis 1991;144:1322–1329.

Striz I, Zheng L, Wang YM, Pokorna H, Bauer PC, Costabel U. Soluble CD14 is increased in bronchoalveolar lavage of active sarcoidosis and correlates with alveolar macrophage membrane-bound CD14. Am J Respir Crit Care Med 1996;153(2):544–547.

Gallium Scanning (⁶⁷Ga)

Sulavik SB, Spencer RP, Palestro CJ, Swyer AJ, Teirstein AS, Goldsmith SJ. Specificity and sensitivity of distinctive chest radiographic and/or ⁶⁷Ga images in the noninvasive diagnosis of sarcoidosis. Chest 1993;103:403–409.

Pathogenesis

Girgis RE, Basha MA, Maliarik M, Popovich J Jr, Iannuzzi MC. Cytokines in bronchoalveolar lavage fluid of patients with active pulmonary sarcoidosis. Am J Respir Crit Care Med 1996;152:71–75.
Thomas PD, Hunninghake GW. Current concepts of the pathogenesis of sarcoidosis. Am Rev Respir Dis 1987;135:747–760.

Therapy

Alberts C, van der Mark TW, Jansen HM. Inhaled budesonide in pulmonary sarcoidosis: a double-blind, placebo-controlled study. Dutch Study Group on Pulmonary Sarcoidosis. Eur Respir J 1995;8:682–688.
Baughman RP, Lower EE, Lynch JP III. Treatment modalities for sarcoidosis. Clin Pulmonary Med 1994;1(4):223–231.
Gibson GJ, Prescott RJ, Muers MF, Middleton WG, et al. British Thoracic Society Sarcoidosis study: effects of long-term corticosteroid treatment. Thorax 1996;51:238–247.
Hunninghake GW, Gilbert S, Pueringer R, Dayton C, Floerchinger C, Helmers R, Merchant R, Wilson W, Galvin J, Schwartz D. Outcome of the treatment for sarcoidosis. Am J Respir Crit Care Med 1994;149:893–898.
Lower EE, Baughman RP. Prolonged use of methotrexate for sarcoidosis. Arch Intern Med 1995;155:846–851.
Sharma OP. Pulmonary sarcoidosis and corticosteroids. Am Rev Respir Dis 1993;147:1598–1600.

Eosinophilic Pneumonias

Buchheit J, Rodgers G, Feger T, Yakoub O. Acute eosinophilic pneumonia with respiratory failure: a new syndrome? Am Rev Respir Dis 1992;145:716–718.
Jederlinic PJ, Sicilian L, Gaensler EA. Chronic eosinophilic pneumonia. A report of 19 cases and a review of the literature. Medicine (Baltimore) 1988:154–162.
Naughton M, Fahy J, FitzGerald MX. Chronic eosinophilic pneumonia. A long-term follow-up of 12 patients. Chest 1993;103:162–165.
Rohatgi PK, Smirniotopoulos TT. Tropical eosinophilia. Semin Respir Med 1991;12:98–106.
Shannon J, Lynch JP III. Eosinophilic pulmonary syndromes. Clin Pulmonary Med 1995;2:19–38.

Bronchiolitis Obliterans±Organizing Pneumonia (BOOP)

Alasaly K, Muller N, Ostrow DN, Chamion P, FitzGerald JM. Cryptogenic organizing pneumonia: a report of 25 cases and a review of the literature. Medicine (Baltimore) 1995;74: 201–211.

Bouchardy LM, Kuhlman JE, Ball WC Jr, Hruban RH, Askin FB, Siegelman SS. CT findings in bronchiolitis obliterans–organizing pneumonia (BOOP) with radiographic, clinical, and histologic correlation. J Comput Assist Tomogr 1993;17:352–357.

Colby TV, Myers JL. The clinical and histologic spectrum of bronchiolitis obliterans including bronchiolitis obliterans–organizing pneumonia. Semin Respir Med 1992;13:119–133.

Cordier JF. Cryptogenic organizing pneumonia. Clin Chest Med 1993;14:677–692.

Lee KS, Kullnig P, Hatman TE, Muller NL. Cryptogenic organizing pneumonia: CT findings in 43 patients. AJR 1994;162:543–546.

Nishimura K, Itoh H. High-resolution computed tomographic features of bronchiolitis obliterans–organizing pneumonia. Chest 1992;102:26S–31S.

Miscellaneous Forms of Small Airways Disorders and BOOP

Cohen A, King TE Jr, Downey GP. Rapidly progressive bronchiolitis obliterans with organizing pneumonia. Am J Respir Crit Care Med 1994;149:1670–1675.

Chan CK. Bone marrow transplantation bronchiolitis obliterans. In: Epler GR, ed. Diseases of the bronchioles. New York: Raven Press, Ltd., 1994:247–257.

Fitzgerald JE, King TE Jr, Lynch DA, Tuder RM, Schwarz MI. Diffuse panbronchiolitis in the United States. Am J Respir Crit Care Med 1996;154:497–503.

Iwata M, Sato A, Colvy TV. Diffuse panbronchiolitis. In: Epler GR, ed. Diseases of the bronchioles. New York: Raven Press, Ltd., 1994:153–179.

Paradis I, Yousem S, Griffith B. Airway obstruction and bronchiolitis obliterans after lung transplantation. Clin Chest Med 1993;14:751–764.

Yousem SA, Colby RV, Gaensler EA. Respiratory bronchiolitis-associated interstitial lung disease and its relationship to desquamative interstitial pneumonia. Mayo Clin Proc 1989; 64:1373–1380.

Pulmonary Vasculitis (Overview)

Hammar SP. Granulomatous vasculitis. Semin Respir Infect 1995;10:107–120.

Jaffe E, Travis WD. Lymphomatoid granulomatosis and lymphoproliferative disorders of the lung. In: Lynch JP III, DeRemee RA, eds. Immunologically mediated pulmonary diseases. Philadelphia, PA: Lippincott Co., 1991:274–301.

Jeannette JC, Falk RJ, Andrassy K, Bacon PA, et al. Nomenclature of systemic vasculitides. Proposal of an International Consensus Conference. Arthritis Rheum 1994;37:187–192.

ter Maaten JC, Franssen CF, Gans ROB, Strack van Schjindel RJM, Hoorntje SJ. Respiratory failure in ANCA-associated vasculitis. Chest 1996;110:357–362.

Antineutrophil Cytoplasmic Antibodies (ANCA)

Gaudin PB, Askin FB, Falk RJ, Jennette JC. The pathologic spectrum of pulmonary lesions in patients with anti-neutrophil cytoplasmic autoantibodies specific for anti-proteinase 3 and anti-myeloperoxidase. Am J Clin Pathol 1995;104:7–16.

Kerr G, Fleisher TA, Hallahan CW, et al. Limited prognostic value of changes in anti-neutrophil cytoplasmic antibody titer in patients with Wegener's granulomatosis. Arthritis Rheum 1993;36:365–371.

Rao JK, Weinberger M, Oddone EZ, Allen NB, et al. The role of anti-neutrophil cytoplasmic antibody (c-ANCA) testing in the diagnosis of Wegener's granulomatosis. A literature review and meta-analysis. Ann Intern Med 1995;123:925–932.

Wegener's Granulomatosis

Daum TE, Specks U, Colby TV, Edell ES, et al. Tracheobronchial involvement in Wegener's granulomatosis. Am J Respir Crit Care Med 1995;151:522–526.

DeRemee RA. The treatment of Wegener's granulomatosis with trimethoprim/sulfamethoxazole: illusion or vision? Arthritis Rheum 1988;31:1068–1072.

Devaney KO, Travis WD, Hoffman GS, Leavitt RY, Lebovics R, Fauci AS. Interpretation of head and neck biopsies in Wegener's granulomatosis. A pathologic study of 126 biopsies in 70 patients. Am J Surg Pathol 1990;14:555–564.

Hoffman GS, Kerr GS, Leavitt RY, Hallahan CW, et al. Wegener's granulomatosis: an analysis of 158 patients. Ann Intern Med 1992;116:488–498.

Sneller MC, Hoffman GS, Talar-Williams C, Kerr GS, Hallahan CW, Fauci AS. An analysis of forty-two Wegener's granulomatosis patients treated with methotrexate and prednisone. Arthritis Rheum 1995;38:608–613.

Stegeman CA, Cohen Tervaert JW, de Johng PE, Kallenberg CGM, et al. Trimethoprim/sulfamethoxazole (co-trimoxazole) for the prevention of relapses in Wegener's granulomatosis. N Engl J Med 1996;335:16–20.

Talar-Williams C, Hijazi YM, Walther MM, Linehan WM, et al. Cyclophosphamide-induced cystitis and bladder cancer in patients with Wegener's granulomatosis. Ann Intern Med 1996;124:477–484.

Travis WD, Hoffman GS, Leavitt RY, Pass HI, Fauci AS. Surgical pathology of the lung in Wegener's granulomatosis. Review of 87 open lung biopsies from 67 patients. Am J Surg Pathol 1991;15:315–333.

Churg-Strauss Syndrome and Polyarteritis Nodosa

Calabrese LH, Hoffman GS, Guillevin L. Therapy of resistant systemic necrotizing vasculitis. Polyarteritis, Churg-Strauss syndrome, Wegener's granulomatosis, and hypersensitivity vasculitis group disorders. Rheum Dis Clin North Am 1995;21:41–57.

Churg A, Ballas M, Cronin SR, Churg J. Formes frustes of Churg-Strauss syndrome. Chest 1995;108:320–323.

Fortin PR, Larson MG, Watters AK, Yeadon CA, et al. Prognostic factors in systemic necrotizing vasculitis of the polyarteritis nodosa group—a review of 45 cases. J Rheumatol 1995; 22:78–84.

Guillevin L, Lhote F, Cohen P, Jarrousse B, et al. Corticosteroids plus pulse cyclophosphamide and plasma exchanges versus corticosteroids plus pulse cyclophosphamide alone in the treatment of polyarteritis nodosa and Churg-Strauss syndrome patients with factors predicting poor prognosis. Arthritis Rheum 1995;38:1638–1645.

Guillevin L, Lhote F, Gayraud M, Cohen P, et al. Prognostic factors in polyarteritis nodosa and Churg-Strauss syndrome. Medicine (Baltimore) 1996;75:17–28.

Guillevin L, Visser H, Noel LH, et al. Antineutrophil cytoplasm antibodies in systemic polyarteritis nodosa with and without hepatitis B infection and Churg-Strauss syndrome—62 patients. J Rheumatol 1993;20:1345–1349.

Lanham JG, Elkon KB, Pusey CD, et al. Systemic vasculitis with asthma and eosinophilia: A clinical approach to the Churg-Strauss syndrome. Medicine (Baltimore) 1984;63:65–81.

Lynch JP III, Fantone JC III. Other pulmonary granulomatous vasculitis syndromes. In: Lynch JP III, DeRemee RA, eds. Immunologically mediated pulmonary diseases. Philadelphia, PA: JB Lippincott, 1991:302–319.

Masi AT, Hunder GG, Lie JT, Michel BA, Bloch DA, Arend WP, et al. The American College of Rheumatology 1990 criteria for the classification of Churg-Strauss syndrome (allergic granulomatosis and angiitis). Arthritis Rheum 1990;33:1094–1100.

Sehgal M, Swanson JW, DeRemee RA, Colby TV. Neurologic manifestations of Churg-Strauss syndrome. Mayo Clin Proc 1995;70:337–341.

Watts RA, Carruthers DM, Scott DG. Epidemiology of systemic vasculitis: changing incidence or definition? Semin Arthritis Rheum 1995;25:28–34.

Eosinophilic Granuloma (EG)

Auerswald U, Barth J, Magnussen H. Value of CD-1 positive cells in bronchoalveolar lavage fluid for the diagnosis of pulmonary histiocytosis X. Lung 1991;169:305–309.

Brauner MW, Grenier P, Mouelhi MM, Mompoint D, Lenoir S. Pulmonary histiocytosis X: evaluation with high-resolution CT. Radiology 1989;172:255–258.

Crausman RS, Jennings CA, Tuder RM, Ackerson LM, Irvin CG, King TE, Jr. Pulmonary histiocytosis X: pulmonary function and exercise physiology. Am J Respir Crit Care Med 1996;153:426–435.

Housini I, Tomashefski JF, Cohen A, Crass J, Kleinerman J. Transbronchial biopsy in patients with pulmonary eosinophilic granuloma. Comparison with findings on open lung biopsy. Arch Pathol Lab Med 1994;118:523–530.

Moore ADA, Godwin JD, Muller NL, Naidich DP, et al. Pulmonary histiocytosis X: comparison of radiographic and CT findings. Radiology 1989;172:249–254.

Prakash U. Eosinophilic granuloma. In: Lynch JP III, DeRemee RA, eds. Immunologically mediated pulmonary diseases. Philadelphia, PA: JP Lippincott Co., 1991:432–448.

Selman M, Carillo GH, Gaxiola M, Ramos C. Pulmonary histiocytosis X (eosinophilic granuloma): clinical behavior, pathogenesis, and therapeutic strategies of an unusual interstitial lung disease. Clin Pulmonary Med 1996;3:191–198.

Stern EJ, Webb WR, Golden JA, Gamsu G. Cystic lung disease associated with eosinophilic granuloma and tuberous sclerosis: air trapping at dynamic ultrafast high-resolution CT. Radiology 1992;182:325–329.

Tazi A, Bonay M, Grandsaigne M, Battesti JP, Hance AJ, Soler P. Surface phenotype of Langerhans cells and lymphocytes in granulomatous lesions from patients with histiocytosis X. Am Rev Respir Dis 1993;147:1531–1536.

Tomashefski JF, Khiyami A, Kleinerman J. Neoplasms associated with pulmonary eosinophilic granuloma. Arch Pathol Lab Med 1991;115:499–506.

Travis WD, Borok Z, Roum JH, Zhang J, et al. Pulmonary Langerhans cell granulomatosis (histiocytosis X). A clinicopathologic study of 48 cases. Am J Surg Pathol 1993;17: 971–986.

Pulmonary Alveolar Proteinosis (PAP)

Cordonnier C, Fleury-Feith J, Escudier E, et al. Secondary alveolar proteinosis is a reversible cause of respiratory failure in leukemic patients. Am J Respir Crit Care Med 1994;149: 788–794.

Hoffman R, Rogers R. Pulmonary alveolar proteinosis. In: Lynch JP III, DeRemee RA, eds. Immunologically mediated pulmonary diseases. Philadelphia, PA: JP Lippincott, 1991: 449–472.

Prakash UB, Barham SS, Carpenter HA, et al. Pulmonary alveolar phospholipoproteinosis: experience with 34 cases and a review. Mayo Clin Proc 1987;62:499–518.

7 Bacterial Pneumonia

Joseph P. Lynch, III

Despite the proliferation of an array of potent, broad-spectrum antimicrobials within the past decade, mortality from bacterial pneumonia remains high. Pneumonia is the fourth leading cause of death among elderly patients (sixth overall) and is the leading cause of death resulting from nosocomial infections. The past decade has been marked by increasingly resistant microorganisms capable of generating more sophisticated enzymes that inactivate even the most advanced antimicrobial drugs. This chapter reviews the specific organisms involved in bacterial pneumonia and the appropriate use of antimicrobials for the treatment of this complication in both community and hospital settings. The clinical features, prognosis, relevant pathogens, and therapeutic strategies differ markedly between these disparate patient populations. Certain pathogens, such as *Pseudomonas aeruginosa* and *A. calcoaceticus,* are virtually only seen in nosocomial settings in critically ill, debilitated patients. By contrast, *Streptococcus pneumoniae* and *Mycoplasma pneumoniae,* common pathogens in the community setting, are rarely implicated in nosocomial pneumonias. Recognition of the differences between pneumonias that arise in these settings is critical for arriving at curative yet cost-effective treatment strategies. Community-acquired pneumonia and the salient pathogens involved (some of which overlap with nosocomial pneumonia) are reviewed initially. Nosocomial pneumonia is then covered, with an emphasis on the importance of enteric Gram-negative bacilli (EGNB) and the pathogenic mechanisms responsible for acquisition of EGNB in the lower respiratory tract. We review diagnostic techniques to define the microbiology, the specific pathogens involved in both community and nosocomial pneumonias, and controversies and strategies of antibiotic use.

COMMUNITY-ACQUIRED PNEUMONIA
Epidemiology

Community-acquired pneumonia (CAP) remains an important cause of morbidity and mortality. In the United States, more than 3 million cases of CAP occur annually, resulting in more than 900,000 hospitalizations and more than 60,000 deaths. Only 20 to 30% of cases of CAP occur in young, previously healthy adults. Mortality is low (1–3%) in young adults without comorbidities, and many patients can be treated with oral antibiotics as outpatients. In the remaining cases, a predisposing risk factor can be identified (e.g., old age, a history of cigarette smoking, chronic ethanol abuse, chronic obstructive lung disease, malignancy, cardiac disease, diabetes mellitus, corticosteroid or immunosuppressive therapy, residence in a nursing home, liver disease, renal insufficiency, previous strokes, debilitation, or any serious preexisting disease). Mortality of CAP is increased in the elderly or in patients with significant associated conditions. Several prospective investigations of CAP in adults have cited mortality rates ranging from 5 to 13% among patients requiring hospitalization. Mortality is higher (from 15 to 30%) in the presence of multilobar involvement, bacteremia, tachypnea (more than 30/min), diastolic hypotension, renal failure, or shock. Progression of CAP to respiratory failure requiring mechanical support occurs in 10 to 20% of patients; in this context, *S. pneumoniae* and *Legionella pneumophila* are the most likely pathogens. Broad-spectrum parenteral antimicrobials are appropriate for severe CAP or for patients with comorbidities. Oral agents may be appropriate for mild CAP in adults without serious associated conditions. Antimicrobials must be modified according to clinical and host factors, including age, presence or absence of underlying disease, prior use of antibiotics, extent of radiographic changes, and severity of the pneumonia.

Microbiologic Cause

The most important pathogens implicated in CAP have been well delineated in epidemiologic studies applying both cultural and serologic data. In individual cases, however, a specific microbiologic cause can be demonstrated in only 30 to 60% of patients. An awareness of the likely pathogens (based on epidemiologic studies) may guide therapy even when a precise microbiologic diagnosis is not possible. The prevalence of microorganisms not previously appreciated as community-acquired pathogens, such as *Haemophilus influenzae, Staphylococcus aureus,* and enteric Gram-negative bacteria, has increased during the past two decades. Recent epidemiologic studies have implicated these pathogens in 17 to 30% of CAP requiring hospitalization.

- *Streptococcus pneumonia* (pneumococcus) is the most important pathogen in all age groups, accounting for 30–70% of CAP.
- *Mycoplasma pneumoniae* is the causative agent in 20–30% of adults younger than age 35, but accounts for only 1–9% of CAP in older adults.
- *Legionella* spp. account for only 2–10% of CAP, but are second only to pneumococcus as a cause of death from CAP.
- *Chlamydia pneumoniae* has been implicated in 2–8% of CAP, but severe pneumonias are rare with this pathogen.
- *H. influenzae* accounts for 5–18% of CAP in adults (higher rates in smokers with chronic obstructive pulmonary disease).
- Enteric Gram-negative rods (predominantly Enterobacteriaceae) account for 3–8% of CAP (only in patients with comorbidities).
- *S. aureus* accounts for 3–8% of CAP in adults (only in patients with risk factors such as nursing home residence, advanced age, IV drug abuse, chronic dialysis, or following influenza).
- *Moraxella (Branhamella) catarrhalis* accounts for only 1–2% of CAP (more common in patients with chronic obstructive lung disease).

- Viruses are implicated in 5–15% of CAP (most cases occur during the winter months).

Clinical and Radiographic Features

- Clinical and radiographic features of CAP suggest certain pathogens but are not specific.
- An abrupt onset, high fever, shaking chill, pleuritic chest pain, and lobar consolidation are characteristic of bacteremic infections caused by *S. pneumoniae,* other bacteria, or *Legionella* spp. This presentation is rare with *Mycoplasma* or *Chlamydia.*
- The "classic" features of acute bacillary pneumonia may be absent, particularly in elderly or debilitated patients.
- Nearly 25% of patients older than 65 years of age with CAP are afebrile; leukocytosis is present in only 50–70%. Clinical features of pneumonia in this context may be subtle. Lethargy, fatigue, nausea, anorexia, or deterioration in overall condition may be the predominant features.
- Delay in recognizing and treating pneumonia may be disastrous. Mortality of CAP in the elderly population ranges from 10 to 25%.

Chest radiographic changes in CAP are variable (see Figs. 1.65, 1.67, 1.68).

- Patchy bronchopneumonic infiltrates are most common.
- Lobar consolidation with air bronchograms occurs in less than 33%.
- Pleural effusions complicate CAP in 10–25% of patients (not etiologically specific).
- Cavitation is rare with *S. pneumoniae, Mycoplasma,* or *Chlamydia* (suggests *S. aureus,* EGNB, anaerobes, fungi, mycobacteria, or neoplasm).
- An air-fluid level is characteristic of a lung abscess (usually mixed anaerobic/aerobic).
- Basilar interstitial or reticulonodular infiltrates suggest *Mycoplasma* spp. (but lobar pneumonia may be seen in 20% of CAP caused by *Mycoplasma* spp.).
- Radiographic features favor certain pathogens, but significant overlap exists.
- Smears and cultures of sputum, blood, or pleural fluid (when present) may substantiate a specific microbiologic diagnosis.

Etiologic (Cultural) Diagnosis

Although sensitivity and specificity is low, an initial sputum smear and cultures should be obtained in patients with suspected or proven pneumonia. The sputum Gram's stain is most useful to distinguish Gram-negative from Gram-positive organisms but is not specific for a unique organism.

- Sputa demonstrating numerous leukocytes, rare or absent epithelial cells, uniform morphology and staining, and many intracellular organisms within leukocytes may guide therapy.

- Lancet-shaped diplococci in pairs suggest *S. pneumoniae;* clumps of Gram-positive cocci suggest *S. aureus;* Gram-negative coccobacilli suggest *H. influenzae;* Gram-negative rods are characteristic of *Klebsiella* spp. or other Enterobacteriaceae.
- In most instances, mixed Gram-negative and Gram-positive organisms are observed. Even when a dominant pathogen is noted, the reliability of sputum smears is inexact.
- One should be cautious about basing initial therapy solely on a sputum Gram's stain.
- Sputum cultures yield a pathogen in only 25 to 50% of cases of CAP.
- Even in bacteremic cases of CAP, the pathogen is isolated from sputum in only 40 to 60%.
- Identification of microorganisms in cultures may take 2 to 3 days (antimicrobial susceptibility profiles take even longer).
- The value of sputum cultures is confounded because potential pathogens, such as *S. pneumoniae* and *H. influenzae,* may be part of normal oral flora. Isolation of a potential pathogen from sputum does not prove causation.
- In pneumonias caused by atypical pathogens, *Legionella* spp., or anaerobes, routine sputum cultures may yield only normal oral flora.
- In summary, Gram's stain and cultures of sputum may be helpful in some cases but are often nondiagnostic and can be misleading.

Ancillary Diagnostic Techniques

Fiberoptic bronchoscopy with bronchoalveolar lavage (BAL) and protected brush (PB) for quantitative cultures are more accurate than sputa cultures in establishing the microbiology of pneumonia. Bronchoscopy is invasive and expensive (cost exceeds $500 in most centers), however, and is inappropriate for the *routine* diagnosis of CAP. Blood culture studies should be performed in patients with CAP requiring hospitalization but are positive in only 5–20% of cases. Thoracentesis should be done when a substantial pleural effusion is present, but this occurs in fewer than 15% of patients. Isolation of a pathogen from blood or pleural fluid is highly specific. Routine cultures for viruses or atypical pathogens are not cost-effective, but these studies may be warranted in selected patients. Serologic tests (IgG and IgM antibodies) for *Mycoplasma, Legionella,* or *Chlamydia* spp. are useful in large epidemiologic investigations but are of limited practical value in individual patients.

Specific Pathogens Encountered in CAP

Prior to discussing therapy, the salient features of the most important pathogens involved in CAP will be reviewed.

Typical Pneumonias

STREPTOCOCCUS PNEUMONIAE

Epidemiology

- *S. pneumoniae* (pneumococcus) is a major cause of morbidity and mortality as a result of pneumonia, meningitis, bacteremia, sinusitis, and otitis media, resulting in annual expenditures in the United States exceeding $ 4 billion.

- *S. pneumoniae* accounts for 30–70% of CAPs and has been associated with the most fatalities.
- *S. pneumoniae* has a predilection for the elderly and for patients with preexisting disease (e.g., ethanol abuse, chronic lung disease) but can affect previously healthy individuals.
- Outbreaks of severe, invasive infections caused by *S. pneumoniae* may occur in nursing homes, prisons, and chronic care facilities.
- *S. pneumoniae* is the leading cause of pneumonia in all age groups. Empiric therapy for CAP should always cover *S. pneumoniae*.
- Penicillin-resistant (and often multiply antibiotic-resistant) strains are increasing and threaten the future efficacy of antibiotics.

Clinical Features

- Classic features include a temperature higher than 103° F, drenching sweats, chills, purulent sputum, pleuritic chest pain, and lobar consolidation. These features occur in 50–70% of persons with bacteremic pneumonia caused by *S. pneumoniae* but do not distinguish pneumococcal pneumonia from other causes.
- Bacteremia occurs in 15–30% of patients; the rate is higher in patients with lobar consolidation and rigors.
- These manifestations are often absent in nonbacteremic forms, in the elderly, or in patients with serious associated diseases.
- A single shaking chill, often stated to be a hallmark for pneumococcal pneumonia, occurs in fewer than 10% of patients; recurrent chills are more common.
- Blood-tinged sputum occurs in 15% of patients.
- Myalgias, nausea, vomiting, and prostration may be prominent.
- Headache is a common early feature; stiff neck may reflect meningeal spread.
- Diarrhea occurs in fewer than 10% of cases of pneumococcal pneumonia.

The course of pneumococcal pneumonia is highly variable but may be fulminant. Mortality in bacteremic cases of pneumococcal pneumonia ranges from 15 to 30% and has not changed significantly over the past three decades. Multilobar involvement, respiratory failure requiring mechanical ventilatory support, extrapulmonary spread (endocarditis, meningitis) leukopenia, age older than 60 years, and certain serotypes (e.g., type 3 strains) have been associated with even higher mortality.

Laboratory Studies: Lancet-shaped, Gram-positive diplococci on sputum Gram's stain support the diagnosis, particularly when intracellular forms are present within leukocytes. Sputum cultures are positive in only 40–60% of bacteremic cases. Counterimmunoelectrophoresis (CIE) can be done in cerebrospinal fluid or pleural fluid, but is rarely employed in tracheobronchial secretions. Peripheral blood leukocytosis or left shift on differential occurs in more than 80% of patients. Leukopenia occurs in one-third of alcoholic or debilitated patients and suggests a worse prognosis. Chest x-rays demonstrate lobar consolidation in 30–60% of patients; patchy bronchopneumonic infiltrates occur commonly. Pleural effusions occur in 15–20% of patients; empyema, in less than 5%.

Antimicrobial Resistance: Resistance to penicillin, tetracyclines, macrolides, trimethoprim/sulfamethoxazole (TMP/SMX), cephalosporins, and other antibiotics has increased dramatically over the past two decades, which reflects patterns of antibiotic use. Penicillin resistance is chromosomally mediated and results from alterations in penicillin-binding proteins (PBPs). Resistance of pneumococci to penicillin is defined in terms of the minimal inhibitory concentration (MIC), the lowest concentration of penicillin that inhibits growth. Susceptibilities are characterized as follows: MIC of less than 0.1 μg/mL, fully susceptible; MIC of 0.1–1 μg/mL; intermediate resistance; MIC of 2 μg/mL or greater is considered high-grade or fully resistant. In France, Spain, and Eastern Europe, 15–40% of pneumococci exhibit high-grade resistance to penicillin; 6–49% are also resistant to erythromycin. Penicillin resistance has not yet been noted in Finland and has only recently emerged in North America. A nationwide surveillance program in the United States detected high-grade resistance to penicillin in only 0.02% of pneumococci isolated from 1979 to 1987. By 1992, 1.3% of isolates were resistant. Recent studies cited substantially higher rates of resistance. A 1994 survey in Atlanta noted penicillin resistance in 25% of pneumococci (7% were highly resistant). Rates of resistance in that study to other antibiotics were alarming (26% to TMP/SMX; 15% to erythromycin; 9% to cefotaxime). Risk factors for penicillin resistance include age under 6 years, prior use of β-lactam antibiotics, and nosocomial acquisition. Five serotypes (e.g., 23F, 6, 9, 14, 19) are responsible for most resistant isolates. Virulence of penicillin-resistant pneumococci is similar to penicillin-sensitive strains; however, penicillin-resistant pneumococci are often resistant to tetracyclines, erythromycin, and TMP/SMX as well. Resistance to quinolone antibiotics is unrelated to penicillin susceptibility. Erythromycin-resistant pneumococci are increasing in frequency worldwide. The incidence of erythromycin-resistant strains is less than 3% in South Africa, Israel, the United States, and most European countries, but resistance rates ranging from 15 to 49% have been noted in France, Spain, Uruguay, and Hungary. Only 0.3% of pneumococci isolated in the United States in 1987 were resistant to erythromycin; currently 6–15% of strains are resistant in some areas. Erythromycin-resistant strains are resistant to other macrolides and are usually resistant to penicillin and tetracycline. Most penicillin-resistant or erythromycin-resistant strains remain susceptible to imipenem, cefotaxime, and ceftriaxone. Cephalosporin-resistant strains, however, have also increased. In Spain, cephalosporin resistance increased from 2% of isolates in 1984–1988 to 9% in 1989–1993. In the United States, cephalosporin resistance has been noted in up to 9% of pneumococci in some areas. Resistance to tetracycline antibiotics is variable. In South Africa, 5.2% of pneumococci isolated from 1987–1990 were resistant to tetracyclines. In France, the rate of resistance to tetracycline increased from 14% in 1970 to 47% in 1978, and then decreased to 20% by 1990. In two recent studies in Spain, 45 and 48% of pneumococci were resistant to tetracycline. In the United States, 6 to 30% of pneumococci are resistant to tetracycline. Resistance to TMP/SMX is approximately 5% in Sweden and in the United States, but rates as high as 24–44% have been noted in some European and African countries. In France, 9.5% of pneumococci were resistant to TMP/SMX in 1984; by 1990, 24% were resistant. In Barcelona, Spain, 42% of pneumococci isolated from 1979–1990 were resistant to TMP/SMX. Antibiotic resistance varies considerably among geographic regions, continues to evolve rapidly, and reflects disparate patterns of antibiotic use. Fortunately, all pneumococci are susceptible to vancomycin, irrespective of susceptibilities to other classes of antibiotics.

Preferred Therapy

For susceptible strains or in areas where rates of penicillin-resistant strains are low:

• Penicillin G, 4.8–10 million units IV (until clinical improvement);
• Penicillin VK, 500 mg q.i.d. orally.

As empiric therapy when penicillin resistance is suspected:

• Cefotaxime 1 gm q8h or ceftriaxone 1 gm q24h.

For strains resistant to penicillin and cephalosporins:

• Vancomycin (100% active);
• Imipenem/cilastin (active against more than 90% of isolates).

Alternative Agents

• Macrolide antibiotic (e.g., erythromycin, clarithromycin, or azithromycin);
• β-lactams and clindamycin are usually active;
• Tetracyclines and TMP/SMX inconsistent (6 to 30% are resistant).

Note: Penicillin G is less expensive and less toxic than alternative agents and should be used for susceptible strains.

Pneumococcal Vaccination: The efficacy and indications for pneumococcal vaccine (Pneumovax) remain controversial. Early studies published in the 1970s confirmed that pneumococcal vaccination was effective in reducing pneumococcal infections in closed populations at high risk (e.g., South African gold miners, New Guinea highlanders, immunocompetent Air Force recruits) and in children with sickle cell anemia. Despite the widespread use of the 14-valent vaccine for more than 10 years, its efficacy in preventing pneumococcal infections in high-risk patients was far from clear. Studies assessing the 14-valent vaccine yielded discrepant results; this vaccine failed to influence the rate of pneumococcal infections in a large Veterans Cooperative Study. In some studies, failures were associated with a serotype not encompassed by the vaccine. Because the 14-valent vaccine covered only 75–80% of serotypes, a 23-valent vaccine (currently in clinical use) was developed to cover more than 90% of strains implicated in pneumococcal infections. Efficacy of this 23-valent vaccine has been estimated at 60–70% among targeted patients. Failures are usually the result of an inability of patients with impaired immune defenses to mount an antibody response rather than failure of the vaccine to cover serotypes. Vaccination is recommended for the following groups: adults older than 65 years of age; adults or children older than 2 years of age with chronic pulmonary or cardiovascular diseases, diabetes mellitus, alcoholism, cirrhosis, or CSF leaks; immunocompromised patients; those with sickle cell disease; those with chronic renal failure; those with a prior history of invasive pneumococcal infection. Revaccination is advised every 6 years.

HAEMOPHILUS INFLUENZAE

Epidemiology

- *H. influenzae* is a pleomorphic Gram-negative rod that accounts for 5–18% of pneumonias, both community- and hospital-acquired.
- Both typeable (encapsulated, primarily type B) and nontypeable (nonencapsulated) strains can cause disease.
- *H. influenzae* is a common commensal (colonizes the oropharynx in 20–40% of healthy individuals and in 50–70% of smokers).
- *H. influenzae* pneumonia or bronchitis characteristically affects smokers, the elderly, or debilitated patients but may affect previously healthy individuals.

Clinical Features: Clinical features of *H. influenzae* pneumonia are nonspecific. Mortality with bacteremic pneumonia is 10–20% but may be higher in debilitated individuals.

Diagnosis: Pleomorphic Gram-negative rods are characteristic on Gram's stain. Because *H. influenzae* is often part of normal oral flora, distinguishing infection from colonization is difficult. The diagnosis of lower respiratory tract infection caused by *H. influenzae* may be confounded by the fastidious growth requirements of the organism; other bacteria may overgrow the culture plates. Even in bacteremic cases of *H. influenzae* pneumonia, sputum cultures yield the organism in only 40–60%.

Antimicrobial Susceptibility: Antimicrobial resistance has increased dramatically in the past two decades. In the early 1970s, more than 99% of strains were susceptible to ampicillin. By the early 1980s, β-lactamase-producing (ampicillin-resistant) strains of *H. influenzae* emerged. By 1990, 10–20% of strains were resistant to ampicillin. First-generation cephalosporins or erythromycin are not reliable (only 40–60% of strains are susceptible). The activity of tetracyclines is modest. More than 90% of strains are susceptible to TMP/SMX. Virtually all isolates are susceptible to ampicillin/sulbactam, cefuroxime, third-generation cephalosporins, extended-spectrum penicillins, imipenem, fluoroquinolones, clarithromycin, and azithromycin.

Preferred Therapy

- Ampicillin/sulbactam, cefuroxime, or ceftriaxone;
- Oral agents (amoxicillin/clavulanate, cefuroxime axetil, TMP/SMX) (for mild infections or following initial parenteral therapy).

Alternative Agents

- TMP/SMX, fluoroquinolones, azithromycin, or clarithromycin;
- Ampicillin or amoxicillin (only for β-lactamase-negative strains);
- Activity of erythromycin is inconsistent.

MORAXELLA (BRANHAMELLA) CATARRHALIS

Epidemiology

- *M. catarrhalis* (formerly termed *Neisseria catarrhalis* or *Branhamella catarrhalis*) is part of the normal flora of the upper respiratory tract and is an important pathogen in otitis media, sinusitis, and acute exacerbations of bronchitis;
- *M. catarrhalis* accounts for 1–3% of CAPs (most frequently in the winter months);
- More than 80% of lower respiratory tract infections caused by *M. catarrhalis* occur in patients with COPD or underlying diseases;
- Probably not important as a nosocomial pathogen.

Clinical Features: The virulence of *M. catarrhalis* is low, and respiratory tract infections caused by *M. catarrhalis* typically manifest as exacerbations of chronic bronchitis or tracheobronchitis. Rhinorrhea, headache, and myalgias are rare. Fever occurs in fewer than 50% of patients. Pneumonia occurs in only 5–20% of cases of *M. catarrhalis* infections and is usually mild. Pleuritic chest pain, dense lobar consolidation, and extreme prostration rarely occur. Chest x-rays usually show patchy bronchopneumonic infiltrates. Empyema, necrotizing pneumonia, cavitation, and fatalities have rarely been described.

Diagnosis: Morphologically, *M. catarrhalis* resembles other *Neisseria* species. Kidney bean-shaped Gram-negative diplococci are characteristic.

Antimicrobial Susceptibility: Resistance of *M. catarrhalis* to penicillins increased dramatically in the past two decades. In 1977, the first β-lactamase(penicillinase)-producing strains of *M. catarrhalis* were described. Now, 50–85% of isolates produce β-lactamase and are resistant to penicillins. Penicillins with β-lactamase inhibitors, second- or third-generation cephalosporins, TMP/SMX, tetracycline, macrolides, and the fluoroquinolones are active against β-lactamase-positive or negative strains. β-Lactamase-negative strains are susceptible to penicillin, ampicillin, and most β-lactams. β-Lactamase-producing *M. catarrhalis* may also confer antimicrobial resistance among coinfecting pathogens (a phenomenon termed indirect pathogenicity). Production of β-lactamases by *M. catarrhalis* may result in clinical resistance of β-lactamase-negative strains of organisms primarily responsible for the infections (such as *H. influenzae* or *S. pneumoniae*). In such cases, antibiotics effective against both *M. catarrhalis* and the coinfecting pathogen are required.

Preferred Therapy

- Cefuroxime, ampicillin/sulbactam, or amoxicillin/clavulanate.

Alternative Therapy

- TMP/SMX, macrolide, tetracycline, or fluoroquinolones.

Atypical Pneumonias

Pneumonia caused by *Mycoplasma pneumoniae, C. pneumoniae* (TWAR), and viruses may be grouped under the term "atypical pneumonias." These pathogens are considered atypical because many of the cardinal features of acute bacterial pneumonia, such as leukocytosis, pleuritic chest pain, rigors, and consolidation, are often lacking. Cough is often nonproductive and extrapulmonary features, such as sore throat, arthritis, myalgias, gastrointestinal symptoms, headache, and viral pro-dromal symptoms, may dominate the clinical picture. *Mycoplasma pneumoniae* has a predilection for previously healthy young individuals. *C. pneumoniae* and viruses affect all age groups. Pneumonias caused by *Mycoplasma* or *Chlamydia* are usually mild and self-limited; fatalities are rare. The spectrum of viral pneumonitis is varied and is covered in the next chapter. Bibasilar interstitial infiltrates or small, patchy, subsegmental infiltrates are characteristic findings on chest radiographs. Classic lobar pneumonia indistinguishable from bacillary pneumonias may occur, however, in 10–20% of patients. Clinical and radiographic features do not reliably discriminate between atypical and typical bacterial pathogens.

MYCOPLASMA PNEUMONIAE

Epidemiology

- *Mycoplasma pneumoniae,* a cell wall-deficient microbe within the class Molli-cutes, accounts for 2–14% of CAP.
- *Mycoplasma pneumoniae* has a striking predilection for younger patients and often spares older individuals, suggesting that preexisting antibody or prior exposure confer lasting protection.
- *Mycoplasma pneumoniae* accounts for 20–30% of CAP in adolescents and adults younger than age 35; 2–9% of pneumonias among adults between the ages of 40 and 60; only 1–3% of CAP in adults over age 60.
- Epidemics of *Mycoplasma* may occur in university dormitories, military institu-tions, schools, and families. Prolonged close contact is usually necessary for trans-mission of infection. Pneumonia caused by *Mycoplasma pneumoniae* occurs in only 3–10% of exposed individuals.
- *Mycoplasma* is rarely implicated as a nosocomial pathogen.

Clinical Features

- Pneumonia caused by *Mycoplasma pneumoniae* is usually mild and rarely life-threatening. Bronchitis and upper airway symptoms predominate. Pneumonia oc-curs in only 5–15% of infected individuals and rarely warrants hospitalization.
- The onset of mycoplasmal pneumonia may be insidious, and the course may be protracted. Cough, malaise, and fatigue may persist for 4–6 weeks.
- Typical features include fever, malaise, headache, and an intractable, hacking cough. Pleuritic chest pain, rigors, and lobar consolidation are uncommon. Rhonchi and a few scattered crackles may be detected on auscultation; consolidation find-ings are rare.
- Progression to respiratory failure is rare.
- Rhinorrhea, sore throat, earache, and hoarseness occur in 25–50% of infections. On physical examination, erythema of the oropharynx and tender cervical lym-phadenopathy can be appreciated in 30–50% of patients.

- Bullous myringitis, a frequently emphasized feature of mycoplasmal pneumonia, occurs in 3–7% of patients.
- Nausea, vomiting, diarrhea, myalgias, and arthralgias occur in 20–45% of patients with mycoplasmal pneumonia; skin rashes, in 10–15% of patients.
- Encephalitis, neurologic symptoms, myocarditis, pericarditis, or hemolytic anemia have been noted in 1–3% of patients with mycoplasmal infections.

Ancillary Laboratory Features: Chest x-ray findings are variable. Diffuse or patchy interstitial infiltrates or patchy bronchopneumonia are most common. Lobar consolidation with air bronchograms is evident in fewer than 20% of patients. Cavitation does not occur. Small pleural effusions are noted in 5–15% of patients. Peripheral blood leukocyte counts are usually normal, but neutrophilia or a left shift occurs in 60–80% of patients. Cold agglutinin IgM antibodies are present in 40–70% of patients but may also be detected in 10–15% of viral or bacterial pneumonias and are of limited diagnostic value.

Diagnosis: Diagnosis of *Mycoplasma* is difficult in the early phases of the disease. Cultures of sputum or pharyngeal washings require specialized techniques, and isolation may take 2–3 weeks. cDNA probes specific for *Mycoplasma* spp. have sensitivities and specificities of up to 89%. In most cases, the diagnosis is substantiated by serologic techniques after the disease has run its course. Serum complement fixation (CF) antibodies against *Mycoplasma* spp. are highly specific and sensitive. A fourfold titer rise from acute to convalescent sera or single titers of greater than 1:128 are considered diagnostic of recent or active infection. Indirect fluorescent antibody and enzyme-linked immunosorbent assay (ELISA) methods may detect IgM antibodies but are not superior to CF titers.

Preferred Therapy

- Macrolide antibiotic (erythromycin, azithromycin, or clarithromycin);
- Doxycycline (100 mg b.i.d. orally or IV).

Therapy should be continued for 14–21 days to prevent relapse.

Alternative Agents

- Fluoroquinolones (e.g., ciprofloxacin, ofloxacin).

Note: Because *Mycoplasma* spp. lack a cell wall, β-lactams and other cell wall-active antibiotics have no significant activity.

CHLAMYDIA PNEUMONIAE (TWAR)

Epidemiology: *C. pneumoniae* (strain TWAR), an obligate intracellular bacteria, may cause rhinitis, sinusitis, pharyngitis, tonsillitis, bronchitis, and pneumonia. *C. pneumoniae* (TWAR) is one of three recognized species within the genus *Chlamydia;* the other species are *C. trachomatis* and *C. psittaci.* Grayston and coworkers first described *Chlamydia*-TWAR as a causative agent of pneumonia in 1986, when serologies implicated *Chlamydia*-TWAR in 9 of 76 pneumonias at the Student Health Service at the University of Washington. By 1988, serologic investigations implicated *Chlamydia*-TWAR as the cause of epidemic outbreaks of pneumonia in Finland, Denmark, Norway, and England. Prospective studies demonstrated that *Chlamydia*-TWAR was endemic in the United States, Canada, and Europe, accounting for 2–8% of CAP. *Chlamydia*-TWAR rarely causes nosocomial pneumonia. Worldwide, the prevalence of TWAR antibody in sera ranges from 25 to 86%. Rates of circulating antibody are low in young children, increase from adolescence to middle age, and remain elevated even in the elderly.

Clinical Features

- Clinical features are similar to *Mycoplasma pneumoniae*. Fever and cough occur in 50–80% of patients.
- Severe sore throat, often with hoarseness, occur in more than one-third (may be the presenting feature).
- Chest x-rays typically demonstrate small (2 to 3 cm), patchy bronchopneumonic infiltrates; lobar consolidation is rare. Pleural effusions are rare in young adults but occur in 10–20% of older adults (many of whom may have coexisting organisms).
- Peripheral blood leukocyte and differential counts are usually normal.
- The illness is usually mild (albeit often protracted); hospitalization is rarely necessary.
- Fatalities are rare but may occur in patients with serious, coexisting disease(s).
- Tetracyclines or macrolides may shorten the duration of illness.
- Associations of *Chlamydia* infections and coronary artery disease, asymptomatic carotid atherosclerosis, asthma, and sarcoidosis have been *suggested* based on serologic studies, but the clinical significance of these observations is not known.

Diagnosis: Diagnosis of *Chlamydia*-TWAR pneumonia is difficult. The organism is difficult to culture. Even with specialized culture methods (HeLa 229 or yolk sac of embryonic chicken eggs), sensitivity is low. Direct fluorescent antibody (DFA) stains of sputum or tracheal secretions may demonstrate the organism but data affirming its sensitivity and specificity are limited. Serologies are performed in only a few reference laboratories. The microimmunofluorescence test (micro-IF), which measures both IgM and IgG titers, is the most accurate serologic assay (more than 90% sensitive and more than 95% specific). IgM titers greater than 16 or IgG titers greater than 512 suggest recent or active infection. Antibodies do not appear until 10 or more days after the onset of illness; titers peak at 6–12 weeks. A recent study in Rhode Island, however, noted high titers in 13% of healthy individuals, suggesting that the false–positive rate may be higher than previously suggested. CF titers are less specific than micro-IF titers and are only 70% sensitive. A fourfold rise in CF titer or single titers exceeding 64 are considered evidence of recent infection. Primary infection is associated with a striking rise in IgM titer within the first 3 weeks, followed by a rise in IgG titer at 8 weeks. Reinfection with *Chlamydia*-TWAR may occur, particularly in older adults. In this context, striking increases in IgG titers are observed without elevation in IgM. Because circulating *Chlamydia*-TWAR antibodies require two or more weeks to become detectable, serologies have little practical value in individual patients.

- An aggressive search for *Chlamydia*-TWAR in patients with CAP is not cost-effective.
- Empiric therapy with tetracyclines should be considered for patients with protracted bronchitis or CAP refractory to β-lactam antibiotics, even if a microbiologic diagnosis has not been established.

Preferred Therapy

- Doxycycline or tetracycline orally for 14–21 days.

Alternative Agents

- Oral macrolides;
- Fluoroquinolones (limited data in vivo).

Note: β-Lactams and aminoglycosides have no activity.

LEGIONELLA SPP.

Epidemiology

Pneumonia caused by *L. pneumophila* (Legionnaire's disease), first described in Philadelphia in 1976, may cause pneumonia in both community and nosocomial settings. Several species and strains of *Legionella* exist, but *L. pneumophila* accounts for more than 95% of infections. The prevalence of legionellosis is highly variable and depends on local and geographic factors. Legionellae thrive in warm water, and inhalation or aspiration of contaminated water has been implicated in both community and nosocomial outbreaks.

- *Legionella* spp. are endemic in the community, accounting for 2 to 10% of CAP.
- Nosocomial legionellosis is rare in most hospitals but may occur when the hospital water supplies are contaminated with *L. pneumophila*. Environmental control measures that eradicate *Legionella* spp. from hospital water distribution systems may limit nosocomial legionellosis.
- Risk factors for legionellosis and more severe disease include advanced age, renal failure, cigarette smoking, ethanol abuse, organ transplantation, corticosteroids, and serious underlying disease.

Clinical Features

- Severe respiratory failure occurs in 20–40% of patients with legionellosis; fatality rates range from 10 to 30%.
- Clinically, pneumonia caused by *Legionella* spp. is indistinguishable from other bacterial pneumonias. Pleural effusions occur in fewer than 10%; cavitation is rare.

Features commonly associated with *Legionella* pneumonia include:

- Progression of pneumonia while taking antimicrobials;
- Hyponatremia (20–50%);
- Neurologic symptoms (confusion, lethargy, headache) in 20–30%;

- Gastrointestinal symptoms (principally nausea, vomiting, diarrhea) in 20–40%;
- Elevations in serum transaminases (20–40%).

These features do not distinguish legionellosis from other types of pneumonia.

Diagnosis

- *Legionella* spp. are Gram-negative rods but are difficult to visualize on Gram's stain.
- Legionellae can be identified in tissue or in secretions by DFA stains; sensitivity is only 25–65%.
- Cultures using specialized media are positive in 30–90%; requires 3 to 5 days to grow.
- Urinary antigen assays are sensitive but only detect *L. pneumophila* serotype 1.
- ELISA and gen-probe techniques: their role has not been established.
- Serum antibodies against *Legionella* spp. by indirect fluorescence are useful in epidemiologic surveys but are of limited value in individual patients (results take 2–4 weeks; single titer of 1:256 or a fourfold titer rise suggest acute infection).

Preferred Therapy

- Intravenous erythromycin, 1000 mg q6h IV. Substitute oral erythromycin (500 mg q.i.d.) following clinical improvement and defervescence. A 21-day course is recommended.
- Rifampin may be synergistic in vitro (combine with erythromycin in seriously ill or immunocompromised hosts).

Alternative Therapy

- Clarithromycin (500–1000 mg b.i.d. for 21 days).
- Ciprofloxacin (750 mg b.i.d.) or ofloxacin (400 mg b.i.d.) for 21 days).

Note: β-Lactams and aminoglycosides are not active against Legionellae.

VIRUSES

Pneumonia caused by viruses (e.g., influenza A and B, parainfluenza, respiratory syncytial virus, and adenovirus) account for 5–15% of CAP and may be indistinguishable from bacterial or atypical pneumonias. Viral pneumonias are reviewed in the next chapter.

Empiric (Initial) Therapy for CAP

In most cases of pneumonia, therapy is empiric. Initial treatment for CAP (undertaken while waiting for cultures) should be sufficiently broad to cover most likely pathogens while avoiding polypharmacy or excessively expensive or toxic antimicrobials. Choice of empiric therapy must be modified based on clinical features such as age, the presence or absence of underlying disease, radiographic appearance, prior use of antimicrobials, and severity of the pneumonia. Given the high mortality (8–20%) of CAP in elderly adults or in patients with serious associated diseases, parenteral antibiotics are preferred as initial therapy in these patients. Other factors that warrant parenteral therapy include multilobar pneumonia, hypoxemia, respiratory distress, hypotension, acuity of illness, or noncompliance. With few exceptions, oral therapy should be reserved for patients meeting all the following criteria:

- Age under 60 years;
- No prior underlying disease;
- Pneumonia confined to a segment or lobe;
- No hypoxemia or respiratory distress;
- Clinically not toxic, hypotensive, or severely ill;
- No nausea, vomiting, or gastrointestinal symptoms that preclude predictable oral absorption;
- Reliable patient, committed to taking the antibiotic and assuring outpatient follow-up examination.

Unless all these conditions are met, hospitalization should be considered. Hospitalization ensures adequate administration of antimicrobials and allows closer scrutiny of the patient and prompt response to any complications that may develop (e.g., shock, empyema). The duration of hospitalization must be individualized. Parenteral therapy is advised until clinical improvement and defervescence have been achieved. Oral agents may be substituted within 2–4 days in patients responding promptly to therapy. A total course of 10–14 days (parenteral plus oral) is advised. For less severely ill ambulatory patients but with risk factors for infections with aerobic EGNB, outpatient therapy with intramuscular ceftriaxone (1 gm/day) is a reasonable alternative. The first dose can be given in the outpatient clinic or physician's office, with supplemental doses given daily for 1–2 additional days. Once a favorable response has been documented, an oral agent may be substituted. Therapeutic strategies for CAP are described in detail in the sections that follow.

Previously Healthy Adults (No Coexisting Illnesses)

Pneumonia in previously healthy adults (under age 60) can be successfully treated with relatively narrow-spectrum antibiotics. *S. pneumoniae* and atypical pathogens (including Legionellae) account for more than 85% of CAP in this population. Other pathogens include *H. influenzae* (2–6%); viruses (5–15%); Enterobacteriaceae or *S. aureus,* less than 2%. Oral macrolide antibiotics are usually adequate for mild CAP in patients without comorbidities. Parenteral therapy is advised for patients who are acutely ill, toxic, hypoxemic, or who exhibit multilobar involvement. In this context, we prefer a β-lactam combined with an oral macrolide as initial therapy. An oral agent can be substituted once clinical improvement and defervescence have occurred (choice of antibiotic depends on pathogen and clinical course).

EMPIRIC STRATEGIES FOR CAP IN ADULTS UNDER AGE 60 OR WITH NO COMORBIDITIES

MILD CAP NOT REQUIRING HOSPITALIZATION:

- An oral macrolide antibiotic is preferred (covers atypicals, *S. pneumoniae,* and most strains of *H. influenzae*);

- Penicillin or ampicillin may be adequate when *S. pneumoniae* is strongly suspected (in communities where the rate of penicillin-resistant pneumococci is low);
- Second-generation oral cephalosporin or amoxicillin/clavulanate;
- Tetracyclines inexpensive, but not reliable against *S. pneumoniae* or *H. influenza* (alternative agents are preferred);
- Activity of the fluoroquinolones against *S. pneumoniae* is modest (alternative agents are preferred).

MODERATE CAP REQUIRING HOSPITALIZATION:

- Intravenous ampicillin/sulbactam, cefuroxime, ceftriaxone, or cefotaxime (*plus* an oral macrolide to cover atypicals);
- When penicillin-resistant pneumococci is a possibility, ceftriaxone or cefotaxime are superior to cefuroxime or ampicillin/sulbactam;
- Ofloxacin (for penicillin-allergic patients).

SEVERE, LIFE-THREATENING, OR MULTILOBAR CAP REQUIRING HOSPITALIZATION:

- Ceftriaxone *plus* high-dose IV erythromycin (1 gm q6h);
- Ceftriaxone *plus* IV fluoroquinolone (ofloxacin or ciprofloxacin);
- Piperacillin/tazobactam (3.375 gm q6h) *plus* IV erythromycin (1 gm q6h);
- Piperacillin/tazobactam (3.375 gm q6h) *plus* a fluoroquinolone;
- Fluoroquinolone (ofloxacin or ciprofloxacin) (for penicillin-allergic patients).

Adults Older than 60 Years of Age or with Preexisting Disease (Comorbidity)

Adults older than 60 years of age or with preexisting disease (e.g., ethanol abuse, diabetes mellitus, chronic obstructive lung disease, congestive heart failure, renal failure, malnutrition, residence in chronic care facilities, or any serious underlying disease) are at increased risk for colonization or infection with EGNB, *H. influenzae, M. catarrhalis,* and *S. aureus,* in addition to *S. pneumoniae* and atypical pathogens. In patients with comorbidities, *H. influenzae* accounts for 8–30% of CAP; EGNB, 3–10%; *S. aureus,* 3–9%. Thus, broad-spectrum β-lactams to cover these pathogens are required in this patient population. By contrast, *Mycoplasma pneumoniae,* a frequent pathogen in young adults, accounts for only 1–3% of CAP in adults over age 60 years. Legionellae and *C. pneumoniae* each account for 3–9% of CAP in patients with comorbidities. The decision to add a macrolide antibiotic (to cover atypicals) in older patients should be individualized.

EMPIRIC STRATEGIES FOR CAP IN ADULTS OLDER THAN 60 YEARS OF AGE OR WITH COMORBIDITIES

MILD PNEUMONIA NOT REQUIRING HOSPITALIZATION:

- Second-generation oral cephalosporin or amoxicillin/clavulanate.

Note: Consider adding a macrolide antibiotic if atypical pathogens suspected. Options for penicillin-allergic patients:

- Ciprofloxacin or ofloxacin;
- Oral macrolide (clarithromycin or azithromycin);
- TMP/SMX.

MODERATE PNEUMONIA REQUIRING HOSPITALIZATION:

- Cefuroxime or ceftriaxone *plus* an oral macrolide;
- Ampicillin/sulbactam less active than cephalosporins against EGNB;
- Penicillin G and ampicillin are too narrow-spectrum (not recommended);
- Antipseudomonal penicillins or imipenem are efficacious, but too expensive;
- Ciprofloxacin or ofloxacin may be used, but activity against *S. pneumoniae* and anaerobes is marginal. Avoid fluoroquinolones when these pathogens are likely.

SEVERE, RAPIDLY PROGRESSIVE, OR MULTILOBAR PNEUMONIA REQUIRING HOSPITALIZATION:

- Ceftriaxone *plus* high-dose IV erythromycin (1 gm q6h);
- Piperacillin/tazobactam *plus* high-dose IV erythromycin (1 gm q6h).

 Options for penicillin-allergic patients:

- Fluoroquinolone
- TMP/SMX *plus* erythromycin;
- Combination of clindamycin, aztreonam, and erythromycin.

ANAEROBIC PLEUROPULMONARY INFECTIONS

Epidemiology

Aspiration of oropharyngeal bacilli may lead to a spectrum of pleuropulmonary manifestations, including acute pneumonitis, necrotizing pneumonia with cavitation, lung abscess, and empyema. Anaerobes (often admixed with other pathogens) may have a primary role in all these pleuropulmonary syndromes. Oropharyngeal anaerobes include *Bacteroides melaninogenicus, Fusobacterium nucleatum, Peptococcus, Peptostreptococcus,* and microaerophilic streptococci. *Bacteroides fragilis* and species within the *B. fragilis* group (e.g., *B. ovatus, B. vulgatus,* and *B. thetaiotamicron*) account for 10–15% of isolates. Anaerobes have been implicated as either sole or concomitant pathogens in 60–97% of aspiration pneumonias or primary lung abscess.

Clinical Features

Aspiration pneumonia should be considered in patients with primary neurologic or esophageal disease. Common associated conditions include reduced level of consciousness, alcohol or drug abuse, general anesthesia, previous strokes, seizures, periodontal disease, and the presence of nasogastric, endotracheal, and tracheostomy tubes. Aspiration pneumonia preferentially involves the dependent segments of the lung (posterior segments of the upper lobes and superior segments of the lower lobes) as a result of gravitational forces. Basilar infiltrates may also occur. Community-acquired aspiration pneumonia often is indolent, evolving over 1 to 3 weeks. Cough, sputum production, and low-grade fever are characteristic. The hallmarks of acute bacillary pneumonias, such as chills, rigors, pleuritic chest pain, and consolidation, are usually lacking. Weight loss, anemia, and generalized weakness may be the presenting features. The course of aspiration pneumonitis may be more fulminant, particularly when *S. aureus* or EGNB are present concomitantly. Chest x-rays typically demonstrate patchy infiltrates without consolidation; persistence of the pneumonic infiltrate may lead to necrosis and cavitation. An air-fluid level indicates a lung abscess.

Microbiology

The microbiologic aspects of aspiration pneumonitis or lung abscess differ depending on risk factors for the acquisition of EGNB. Normal oral flora consist largely of anaerobes and aerobic Gram-positive cocci; aerobic EGNB are absent. By contrast, aerobic EGNB frequently colonize the oropharynx and lower respiratory tract of hospitalized patients or patients with comorbidities. When aspiration occurs in the community, streptococci, *H. influenzae,* and anaerobes may be involved. Aspiration pneumonia in patients in hospitals, nursing homes, chronic care facilities, or in patients with comorbidities may include an admixture of anaerobes and aerobic EGNB.

Clarification of the microbiologic cause of aspiration pneumonia (or lung abscess) is difficult. Expectorated sputum cultures often grow only normal oral flora, because concomitant upper respiratory tract flora usually overgrow anaerobes. Foul-smelling, putrid sputum is a clue to the presence of anaerobes but is only present in one-third of patients. Gram's stain of expectorated sputum or empyema fluid may demonstrate a mixture of both Gram-negative (e.g., *Bacteroides* spp., *Fusobacterium nucleatum*) and Gram-positive (e.g., streptococci, peptococci) organisms. Pioneering studies in the early 1970s by Gorbach, Finegold, and Bartlett (using transtracheal aspirates) elegantly delineated the organism(s) responsible for aspiration pneumonia or primary lung abscess in the community. Fifty percent of primary lung abscesses were caused by pure anaerobes; 47% by a mixture of anaerobes and aerobes; only 3% were exclusively aerobic. Percutaneous needle or transtracheal aspirates are reliable sources for anaerobic cultures but are potentially dangerous and are no longer recommended.

Antimicrobial Susceptibility

Virtually all anaerobes (including those of the *B. fragilis* group) are susceptible to imipenem, extended-spectrum penicillins with β-lactamase inhibitors, and metronidazole. Clindamycin is excellent against most anaerobes, but 4–22% of strains of *B. fragilis* (or *B. fragilis* group) are now resistant. Penicillin G and ampicillin have exquisite activity against normal oral anaerobes, but more than 90% of *B. fragilis* spp. are resistant. Anaerobic activity of cephalosporins is modest. The cephamycins (cefoxitin and cefotetan) are the most active cephalosporins, but 5–30% of *B. fragilis* are resistant. Activity of ceftazidime and cefoperazone is poor. Aztreonam, the fluoroquinolones, and TMP/SMX have poor anaerobic activity.

Therapy

Community-acquired aspiration pneumonia or lung abscess in patients without serious associated diseases can be treated with narrow-spectrum agents. Penicillin G (8–12 million U daily) is inexpensive, well-tolerated, and may be adequate for uncomplicated lung abscess. Clindamycin has superior activity against anaerobes (including *B. fragilis*) compared with penicillin G and is preferred by some physicians for treating community-acquired aspiration pneumonia or lung abscess. In one multicenter prospective study of community-acquired lung abscess, patients treated with intravenous clindamycin (600 mg q8h) exhibited more rapid clinical improvement and defervescence and had a lower rate of relapses compared with patients who received penicillin (6 million U daily). Despite these data, many authors still advocate penicillin G as primary therapy for uncomplicated lung abscess or aspiration pneumonia because of its lower cost and historical success over many years. Clindamycin or a penicillin with β-lactamase inhibitor is preferred for complicated lung abscess or for patients failing therapy with penicillin. When aspiration pneumonia occurs in patients with serious associated disease(s), extended-spectrum penicillins with β-lactamase inhibitors or cefotetan (2 gm q12h) are preferred because of their superior activity against EGNB compared with clindamycin or penicillin G. Ciprofloxacin and TMP/SMX lack activity against many anaerobes and are not advised for polymicrobial anaerobic infections. Metronidazole has exquisite activity against anaerobes (including *B. fragilis*) but has been associated with a high failure rate when used as monotherapy for pulmonary anaerobic infections. The poor results achieved with metronidazole may reflect its poor activity against aerobic and micro-aerophilic streptococci, which are often present concomitantly.

Preferred Therapy for Community-acquired Lung Abscess

- Penicillin G for uncomplicated lung abscess in community (because of low cost);
- Clindamycin (for complicated lung abscess or penicillin failure);
- Ampicillin/sulbactam (when concomitant EGNB suspected);
- Oral antibiotics (penicillin VK, clindamycin, or amoxicillin/clavulanate may be substituted following clinical response to parenteral therapy).

Note: Metronidazole has been associated with a high failure rate for anaerobic infections above the diaphragm and is not recommended.

Alternative Agents

- Cefotetan or extended-spectrum penicillins with β-lactamase inhibitors (useful when infection with EGNB coexists).

Clinical Response

Antibiotic therapy is almost always sufficient to treat anaerobic pneumonitis or lung abscess. Drainage of abscess cavities can usually be accomplished by expectoration of sputum and local percussion and drainage. Empyema requires surgical drainage in addition to antibiotics. Acute anaerobic pneumonitis usually responds rapidly to antibiotics, with lysis of fever within 48 hours; more than 80% of patients are afebrile within 5 days. For aspiration pneumonia without lung abscess, a 14-day course of therapy is advised. A more prolonged febrile pattern is typical of lung abscess (cavitation with an air-fluid level). Fever may persist for 5–10 days or longer, despite adequate antimicrobial therapy. For a frank lung abscess, parenteral therapy is initiated until clinical response has occurred, at which time an oral antibiotic can be substituted (e.g., penicillin VK, ampicillin, amoxicillin/clavulanate, or clindamycin). Therapy for a lung abscess should be continued for 2–4 months to prevent recrudescence of infection.

ANTIMICROBIAL RESISTANCE: AN INCREASING PROBLEM IN COMMUNITY AND NOSOCOMIAL SETTINGS

Antimicrobial resistance has increased at an alarming rate in both community and nosocomial settings, primarily as a result of selection pressure from use of antibiotics. Antimicrobial resistance may develop when single classes of antibiotics are used extensively. Bacteria acquire resistance by multiple mechanisms, including:

- Enzymatic inactivation of the antibiotic (β--lactamases, aminoglycoside-modifying enzymes);
- Alteration of target sites (PBPs, DNA gyrases, ribosomes, RNA polymerase);
- Decreased antibiotic permeability through the bacterial cell wall (resistance to imipenem or quinolones);
- Active efflux of antibiotic from the bacteria.

β-Lactamases are the most important causes of resistance to β-lactam antibiotics. β-Lactamases differ in selectivity for the target (e.g., penicillinases, cephalosporinases) and stability. In the 1940s (in the earliest days of penicillin use), most staphylococci were susceptible to penicillin. By the late 1950s, most staphylococci produced penicillinase (a β-lactamase) and were resistant. These isolates remained susceptible to antistaphylococcal penicillins, such as methicillin. Alterations in PBPs led to methicillin-resistant *S. aureus* (MRSA) and penicillin-resistant *S. pneumoniae*. Currently, more than 5% of strains of *S. pneumoniae* in the United States are resistant to penicillin by this mechanism; in some countries, more than 40% of isolates are resistant. Emergence of resistance has been dramatic with other pathogens. β-Lactamase-producing (ampicillin-resistant) strains of *Escherichia coli* were rare in the 1960s. Currently, more than 30% of isolates are resistant to ampicillin. In 1974, the first β-lactamase-producing strain of *H. influenzae* was identified. Within a decade, 15–20% of isolates were resistant to ampicillin. Similarly, β-lactamase-positive strains of *M. catarrhalis* constituted fewer than 1% of isolates in 1977; now, 55–80% of strains produce β-lactamase and are resistant to penicillin. Plasmid- and chromosomally mediated β-lactamases have increased dramatically as a cause of resistance to antibiotics among aerobic EGNB. Within the past decade, a striking increase in plasmid-mediated β-lactamases and extended-spectrum β-lactamases produced by

Enterobacteriaceae has been noted. These newer β-lactamases inactivate third-generation cephalosporins, antipseudomonal penicillins, and aztreonam but do not affect imipenem. Some of these plasmid-mediated β-lactamases confer multiple drug resistance, even to antibiotics of a different class (e.g., gentamicin, tetracycline, chloramphenicol). Outbreaks of nosocomial infection caused by bacteria exhibiting multiple antibiotic resistances have been reported with increasing frequency over the past decade. Resistance to aminoglycosides, carbapenems, fluoroquinolones, and vancomycin has also increased dramatically. Resistance to imipenem may develop via chromosomally mediated β-lactamases, carbapenemases, changes in permeability, or changes in penicillin-binding affinity. Changes in permeability of the bacterial cell wall emerge rapidly in *P. aeruginosa* with the fluoroquinolones or imipenem and may result in cross-resistance to antibiotics of unrelated classes. With liberal use of fluoroquinolones, resistant *P. aeruginosa* Enterobacteriaceae or *S. aureus* may emerge, which are also less susceptible to β-lactams, aminoglycosides, and tetracyclines. Although fewer than 4% of Enterobacteriaceae (and only 1.6% of *E. coli*) are resistant to fluoroquinolones in the United States, prevalence rates exceeding 35% were noted in Europe in a cohort of patients with hematologic malignancies following prolonged use of prophylactic norfloxacin. Liberal use of a single class of antibiotic may promote resistance. MRSA, a rarity only 2 decades ago, now constitutes 15–40% of nosocomial isolates. Vancomycin- and aminoglycoside-resistant enterococci have increased dramatically in nosocomial settings and correlate with prior therapy with these antibiotics. These resistance trends bode poorly for the future. The pharmaceutic industry will have to meet the challenge to keep ahead of these "smart organisms." Antimicrobial susceptibility profiles will undoubtedly change radically in the next decade, and some antibiotics currently in use may become obsolete or distinctly less effective. Antimicrobials that were efficacious only two decades ago for CAP, such as ampicillin, are no longer adequate for empiric treatment of CAP. Since 1983, strains of Enterobacteriaceae producing novel β-lactamases, such as *Klebsiella* spp., *E. coli,* and *Proteus* spp., have markedly reduced the effectiveness of first-generation cephalosporins and penicillins. An awareness of the changing patterns of antimicrobial resistance is critical to develop rational treatment strategies.

NOSOCOMIAL PNEUMONIA
Microbiology and Epidemiology

Pneumonia develops in 0.5–2% of hospitalized patients and has been associated with a mortality rate of 30 to 60%. Nosocomial pneumonia accrues costs in excess of $3 billion in the United States annually. In striking contrast to CAP, aerobic EGNB are responsible for 65–85% of nosocomial pneumonias. Enterobacteriaceae (primarily *Klebsiella* and *Enterobacter* spp.) account for 30–50% of nosocomial pneumonias; 15–20% are caused by *P. aeruginosa*. *H. influenzae* is responsible for 3–8% of nosocomial pneumonias, but the incidence is higher in pneumonias acquired within the first 3 hospital days. *Serratia marcescens, Acinetobacter* spp., *Citrobacter,*

Providencia, Morganella, and a host of highly virulent EGNB may cause nosocomial pneumonia. Staphylococci and streptococci account for 10–25% of cases (usually in the context of polymicrobial pneumonia). Anaerobes have been implicated in only 2–5% of nosocomial pneumonias in most studies, but prevalence rates of 30% have been cited when meticulous culture techniques are used. Anaerobes are probably less important as primary pathogens but may play important contributory roles in polymicrobial infections, which account for 20–40% of nosocomial pneumonias. Sporadic cases and epidemic outbreaks of nosocomial pneumonia caused by *Legionella* spp., viruses, *Mycobacterium tuberculosis, Pneumocystis carinii,* and invasive fungi have been described but are rare. Nonbacterial pathogens are discussed in the next chapter.

Prognostic Factors

Host factors and difference in virulence among infecting organisms influence prognosis and mortality of nosocomial pneumonia. Factors that increase mortality include age greater than 60 years, renal or hepatic failure, coma, multi-organ failure, hypotension, debilitation, malnutrition, prior treatment with corticosteroids or chemotherapy, or any disorder that may impair immune defenses. Mortality rates for aerobic Gram-negative bacillary pneumonia (30–50%) are higher than pneumonia because of Gram-positive bacilli (5–25% mortality). For *P. aeruginosa* or *Acinetobacter* spp., mortality approaches 60–80%. Several factors contribute to this higher mortality:

- *P. aeruginosa* may release virulence factors and exotoxins that inactivate host defenses and cause necrosis of lung parenchyma.
- Nosocomial Gram-negative pathogens are often highly resistant to antibiotics.
- Infected patients are often debilitated with severe comorbidities that independently increase mortality.

Pathogenesis

Both environmental and host factors contribute to the high prevalence of pneumonia. The risk of nosocomial pneumonia is increased in the elderly, in patients with serious associated diseases, and with increasing duration of hospital stay. The incidence is particularly high (10–40%) in critically ill patients requiring mechanical ventilatory support for more than 48 hours. The prevalence is lower in patients not requiring ventilatory support or in coronary care units. Mechanical ventilation is an independent risk factor for pneumonia but also identifies a population of patients who are debilitated and have more serious concurrent illnesses. Invasive devices, such as central venous catheters, arterial lines, indwelling bladder catheters, and endotracheal, nasotracheal, or tracheostomy tubes, have been associated with a higher prevalence of nosocomial infections and pneumonia. Inadequate hand-washing by medical personnel may be a source of spread of potentially pathogenic bacteria, particularly in the intensive care unit (ICU). Bloodborne seeding to the lung from extrapulmonary sites, such as wounds, soft tissue, or urinary tract, may result in pneumonia. The dominant mechanism by which nosocomial pneumonia occurs is via aspiration of endogenous oropharyngeal bacilli into the tracheobronchial tree. Oropharyngeal and tracheal colonization with EGNB is markedly increased in hospitalized patients with underlying diseases and is an important precursor of infection. Once colonization with EGNB has occurred, aspiration may precipitate lower respiratory tract infection in patients with impaired host defenses. The gastrointestinal tract serves as a reservoir for proliferation of EGNB, which may later colonize the lower respiratory tract. Agents that increase gastric pH, such as histamine-2 (H_2) antagonists or antacids, have been associated with higher rates of nosocomial pneumonia in critically ill, mechanically ventilated patients. Prophylactic regimens for stress ulcers that employ sucralfate (an agent that does not affect gastric pH) have been associated with a lower rate of bronchopulmonary colonization and pneumonia in mechanically ventilated patients compared with antacids or H_2 antagonists.

Selective Digestive Tract Decontamination (SDD)

Aggressive prophylactic regimens to reduce gastrointestinal tract colonization and infection with EGNB have been tried in patients at high risk for nosocomial pneumonia in an attempt to reduce nosocomial infections. This concept, known as selective digestive tract decontamination, employs nonabsorbable antibiotics (polymyxin E, tobramycin, and amphotericin B) given orally and as an adhesive paste applied to the oral mucosa every 6 hours. This regimen is often combined with a 4-day course of intravenous cefotaxime. In several studies, SDD prophylaxis reduced tracheal colonization with EGNB and nosocomial pneumonias but failed to influence overall mortality or length of stay. SDD is expensive, logistically difficult, and may increase the risk for antimicrobial resistance. Thus we see no role for SDD as routine prophylaxis for nosocomial settings. Focused use of SDD may be considered in selected high-risk patient populations (e.g., organ transplant recipients, trauma patients, etc.), but additional studies are required to determine its role.

Diagnosis

The diagnosis of nosocomial pneumonia may be difficult, particularly in patients in the ICU or in postsurgical patients. Congestive heart failure, atelectasis, pulmonary embolism, or adult respiratory distress syndrome (ARDS) may produce infiltrates on chest radiographs, mimicking pneumonia. Further, more than one process may be present concomitantly. Pneumonia complicates ARDS in 50–75% of patients. Persistence or progression of respiratory failure in ARDS may reflect concomitant pulmonary suppuration. Critically ill or debilitated patients may not mount an adequate host response to infection. Thus, the usual hallmarks of bacterial infection may be lacking. Pleuritic chest pain, high fever, and chills are usually absent in nosocomial pneumonias. Chest x-rays may demonstrate only minimal, patchy infiltrates that mimic fluid overload or congestive heart failure. Frank consolidation with air bronchograms or cavitation is present in a minority of patients. A high index of suspicion is required to make a diagnosis of lower respiratory tract infection in a timely fashion. Unexplained leukocytosis (or left shift), worsening dyspnea, purulent tracheobronchial secretions, or new infiltrates on chest x-ray warrant an aggressive approach. Gram's stain and cultures of expectorated sputum or tracheal secretions should be done to assess a predominant organism. Only Gram's stains showing greater than 25 leukocytes and fewer than 10 epithelial cells per low power field are acceptable for culture. Unfortunately, these techniques are neither sensitive nor specific. Potential pathogens are found in culture of tracheal aspirates in 60–100% of pneumonias, but specificity is low (less than 20%). Blood cultures should be done, but only 5–10% of cases of nosocomial pneumonias are bacteremic. In many cases of nosocomial pneumonia, a precise microbiologic etiology is never established.

Invasive Techniques

Fiberoptic bronchoscopy using a PB or BAL and quantitative cultures may more accurately define the microbacteriology of nosocomial pneumonia. Thresholds established for quantitative cultures are $>10^3$ organisms/mL in a PB or $>10^4$ by BAL. Using these criteria, sensitivities of PB or BAL range from 70 to 95% in patients with bacterial pneumonia, with false–positive rates of less than 10%. Stains of cytocentrifuged BAL fluid (Gram's stain, Diff-Quik) may more immediately characterize the predominant organism(s). Numerous intracellular organisms with polymorphonuclear leukocytes are highly predictive of infection. Unfortunately, false–negative results are higher in patients already receiving antibiotics. This underscores the importance of performing bronchoscopy prior to initiating antibiotic therapy. Unfortunately, this is often impractical. The routine use of bronchoscopy in suspected nosocomial pneumonia has not been shown to reduce morbidity or mortality. In view of its expense and potential morbidity, we do not recommend bronchoscopy in patients with uncomplicated nosocomial pneumonia. Bronchoscopy may be invaluable, however, in patients with nosocomial pneumonia failing therapy or in immunocompromised patients at risk for nonbacterial opportunistic pathogens. Additional studies are warranted to define the impact of bronchoscopic techniques on prognosis in selected patient populations. Less invasive nonbronchoscopic techniques using plugged or protected catheters and quantitative cultures are promising, but their use is limited to ventilated patients. Quantitative cultures of sputum or endotracheal aspirates (using 10^6 organisms as a threshold) have been as sensitive as PB (55–82%) with specificity exceeding 80%. Quantitative cultures are superior to conventional sputum cultures but are logistically difficult. The role of these techniques needs to be better defined in studies that assess outcome and cost-effectiveness. Because of the high mortality associated with nosocomial pneumonia, we initiate empiric antibiotic therapy for suspected cases, even when the diagnosis has not been substantiated with certainty.

Specific Pathogens

In the following sections, the epidemiologic characteristics, clinical features, and antimicrobial susceptibility of specific pathogens are reviewed.

ACINETOBACTER SPP. (*A. CALCOACETICUS* OR *A. BAUMANNII*)

Epidemiology: *Acinetobacter* spp. are aerobic Gram-negative coccobacilli of relatively low virulence that may emerge by selection pressure in critically ill, debilitated patients. *Acinetobacter* spp. are found in water and soil and are common commensals in humans; colonization rates of 7% for throat and 25% for skin have been reported. The lung is the most common site of primary infection, followed by urinary tract, surgical wounds, and skin. *Acinetobacter* accounts for only 1–3% of nosocomial pneumonias, but the rate is higher (5–15%) in mechanically ventilated ICU patients. Risk factors for acquisition of *Acinetobacter* include tracheostomy or endotracheal intubation, surgery, residence in an ICU, prolonged mechanical ventilatory support, invasive devices, and recent use of antibiotics. Outbreaks of nosocomial pneumonia transmitted by hospital personnel or contaminated environmental sources (e.g., nebulizers, dialysis baths, and hospital equipment) have been described. Mortality rates for *Acinetobacter* pneumonia exceed 50%. *Acinetobacter* rarely causes CAP. The largest series of community-acquired *Acinetobacter* pneumonia included only six patients diagnosed over a 5-year period from three teaching hospitals in the United States.

Antimicrobial Susceptibility: *Acinetobacter* spp. are highly resistant to multiple antibiotics. Most isolates are resistant to ampicillin and first- and second-generation cephalosporins; activity of third-generation cephalosporins is variable. High-grade resistance to aminoglycosides has recently been described. Risk factors for aminoglycoside-resistant *Acinetobacter* spp. include prior therapy with cephalosporins or aminoglycosides, extended ICU care, and prolonged respiratory therapy.

Preferred Therapy

- Choice of agent depends on results of susceptibility testing;
- Ceftazidime, antipseudomonal penicillins, imipenem/cilastatin, aminoglycosides, TMP/SMX, and fluoroquinolones may be active but variable;
- Combine with an aminoglycoside to confer synergy.

ENTEROBACTERIACEAE

Enterobacteriaceae (which include *Enterobacter* spp., *Klebsiella* spp., *E. coli, Proteus, Serratia, Citrobacter*) account for 30–50% of nosocomial pneumonias and may cause CAP in elderly or debilitated patients with risk factors for acquisition of EGNB. Enterobacteriaceae may possess inducible β-lactamases that inactivate cephalosporins, antipseudomonal penicillins, and monobactams. These inducible β-lactamases are common with *Enterobacter* and *Serratia* spp. but are rare with *E. coli* or *Klebsiella pneumoniae*. For most strains of *E. coli* or *K. pneumoniae*, monotherapy with cephalosporins is adequate. Serious infections caused by β-lactamase-producing organisms may warrant combination therapy (e.g., an antipseudomonal penicillin plus an aminoglycoside). Fluoroquinolones (as monotherapy) are usually effective against both β-lactamase ($-$) and ($+$) Enterobacteriaceae.

ENTEROBACTER SPECIES (*E. CLOACAE, E. AEROGENES*)

Epidemiology: Infections caused by *Enterobacter* spp. have increased dramatically in recent years as a cause of nosocomial or community-acquired infections.

Enterobacter spp. are now the third most common cause of nosocomial pneumonia (behind *P. aeruginosa* and *S. aureus*), accounting for 7–12% of nosocomial pneumonias. The emergence of *Enterobacter* spp. reflects selection pressure from the use of antimicrobials to which these organisms are resistant.

Antimicrobial Susceptibility: Virtually all isolates of *Enterobacter* spp. are resistant to penicillin, ampicillin, and first-generation cephalosporins. Fewer than 50% of isolates are susceptible to second-generation cephalosporins. Twenty to forty percent of isolates are resistant to third-generation cephalosporins; 20–30% are resistant to antipseudomonal penicillins. Imipenem is usually active even in strains resistant to other β-lactams. Chromosomally mediated inducible β-lactamases may be triggered on exposure to cephalosporins and may be facilitated by extensive use of monotherapy with third-generation cephalosporins. These β-lactamases confer resistance to multiple β-lactam antibiotics and are not inhibited by clavulanate, sulbactam, or tazobactam. In a multicenter prospective study of *Enterobacter* bacteremia, resistance emerged during therapy in 19% of patients receiving third-generation cephalosporins but in none of 50 patients receiving other β-lactams and in only 1 of 89 receiving aminoglycosides. Because of their potential to induce resistance, cephalosporins should not be used for *Enterobacter* infections, regardless of in vitro susceptibility. Activity of fluoroquinolones, TMP/SMX, and aminoglycosides is excellent, but aminoglycoside resistance is increasing. Amikacin may be active against strains resistant to gentamicin or tobramycin.

Preferred Therapy

- Imipenem (combine with aminoglycoside);
- Antipseudomonal penicillin (combine with aminoglycoside);
- Ciprofloxacin or ofloxacin;
- Cephalosporins should not be used (irrespective of susceptibilities).

Alternative Agents

- TMP/SMX, aztreonam.

Note: Third-generation cephalosporins should not be used; may induce resistance. Sulbactam, clavulanate, or tazobactam do not affect β-lactamases produced by *Enterobacter* spp.

ESCHERICHIA COLI

Epidemiology: *E. coli* remains an important pathogen in both community- and hospital-acquired bacteremias and infections. Urinary tract and gastrointestinal sites are the most common sources of infection. *E. coli* accounts for 6–8% of nosocomial pneumonias, however, and for 1% of CAPs. Mortality from *E. coli* pneumonia has been 20–30%. Most deaths have been in elderly, debilitated patients and may reflect impairments in host defenses rather than failure of antibiotics.

Antimicrobial Susceptibility: In the 1970s, ampicillin was the treatment of choice for infections caused by *E. coli*. β-Lactamase-producing strains have increased dramatically within the past decade. Thirty to fifty percent of *E. coli* are now resistant to ampicillin. Nearly 100% of strains (β-lactamase-positive or negative) are susceptible to ampicillin/sulbactam, cefuroxime, cephamycins (cefoxitin, cefotetan), and third-generation cephalosporins. Eighty-five to ninety-five percent of strains are susceptible to ticarcillin/clavulanate or piperacillin. Imipenem, aztreonam, TMP/SMX, the fluoroquinolones, and aminoglycosides have excellent activity. Pneumonia caused by *E. coli* can usually be treated with ampicillin/sulbactam or a second-generation cephalosporin (e.g., cefuroxime or cefotetan) alone. An aminoglycoside could be added for serious, life-threatening cases.

Preferred Therapy

- Ampicillin/sulbactam, cefuroxime, or cefotetan;
- Ampicillin (only for β-lactamase-negative strains).

Alternative Agents

- TMP/SMX, fluoroquinolones, third-generation cephalosporins, aztreonam, imipenem.

KLEBSIELLA PNEUMONIAE

Epidemiology: *K. pneumoniae,* an aerobic EGNB within the family Enterobacteriaceae, accounts for 5–9% of nosocomial pneumonias and has been implicated in 1–5% of CAPs in debilitated patients with risk factors for acquisition of EGNB or residents of nursing homes or chronic care facilities. Clinical features are indistinguishable from other pneumonias, but a high rate of bacteremia and suppurative complications has been noted.

Antimicrobial Susceptibility: *K. pneumoniae* is resistant to penicillin and ampicillin but is highly susceptible to cefuroxime, third-generation cephalosporins, imipenem, aztreonam, fluoroquinolones, aminoglycosides, and TMP/SMX. Most strains are susceptible to first-generation cephalosporins, but the MIC may be marginal. More than 90% of isolates are susceptible to piperacillin, whereas fewer than 30% are susceptible to ticarcillin or azlocillin. More than 95% of strains are susceptible to ticarcillin/clavulanate or piperacillin/tazobactam. Recently, *K. pneumoniae*-producing plasmid-mediated extended-spectrum β-lactamases that confer resistance to ceftazidime have been isolated in Europe and in the United States. Epidemics of infection caused by β-lactamase-producing *K. pneumoniae* have correlated with extensive use of cephalosporin monotherapy and may be curtailed by switching to extended-spectrum penicillins or imipenem/cilastatin. For susceptible strains, cefuroxime is usually efficacious and less expensive than other extended-spectrum agents. Combination therapy with an aminoglycoside may confer synergy but is usually not necessary except in fulminant or refractory cases. Fluoroquinolones are acceptable alternatives for patients allergic to β-lactams.

Preferred Therapy

- Second- or third-generation cephalosporins (monotherapy is usually adequate);
- Aminoglycosides may be added for synergy in fulminant or refractory cases.

Alternative Agents

- Imipenem, fluoroquinolone, aztreonam, TMP/SMX.

SERRATIA MARCESCENS

Epidemiology: *Serratia* spp. (primarily *S. marcescens*) account for 2–5% of nosocomial pneumonias, with even higher rates in mechanically ventilated patients in ICUs. Rare cases of CAP may occur in patients with risk factors for Gram-negative infections (e.g., ethanol abuse, nursing home residence, diabetes mellitus, and intravenous drug abuse). Clinical features are nonspecific, but a necrotizing pneumonia with cavitation is characteristic. Pseudohemoptysis may result from the red pigment produced by *S. marcescens.* Mortality rates for pneumonia caused by *Serratia* spp. exceed 60% in some studies.

Antimicrobial Susceptibility: *Serratia* spp. are resistant to penicillin, ampicillin, ampicillin/sulbactam, and most first-generation cephalosporins. Most isolates are highly susceptible to third-generation cephalosporins, aztreonam, imipenem, fluoroquinolones, and aminoglycosides. Antipseudomonal penicillins are less consistently effective. In view of the high mortality associated with *Serratia pneumonia,* we recommend combination therapy with a β-lactam plus an aminoglycoside.

Preferred Therapy

- Third-generation cephalosporin (combine with aminoglycoside).

Alternative Agents

- Imipenem, aztreonam, fluoroquinolone, or TMP/SMX.

PSEUDOMONAS AERUGINOSA

Epidemiology: *P. aeruginosa* accounts for 15–20% of nosocomial pneumonias, with even higher rates (20–30%) among mechanically ventilated patients in ICUs. *P. aeruginosa* is ubiquitous in hospital environments and can survive in distilled water, ventilator tubing, sinks, plants, and other environmental sources. Colonization of the respiratory tract is common in mechanically ventilated or intubated patients and is facilitated by prior antibiotic use. In a study by Rello and colleagues of ventilator-associated pneumonias, *P. aeruginosa* was the causative agent in 40% of pneumonias in patients who had received prior antibiotics but in only 5% of antibiotic-naive patients. *P. aeruginosa* is a rare cause of CAP except among patients with specific risk factors, such as bronchiectasis, cystic fibrosis, tracheostomy, immunosuppressive or corticosteroid therapy, intravenous drug abuse, or granulocytopenia. *P. aeruginosa* produces a necrotizing pneumonia, with frequent cavitation and microabscess formation. Mortality from *Pseudomonas* pneumonia is 50–70%, which reflects the debilitated state of patients infected with this pathogen and the high virulence of these organisms. Relapses or antimicrobial resistance develop in 30–50% of patients.

Antimicrobial Susceptibility: *P. aeruginosa* is resistant to most antibiotics. Antipseudomonal penicillins are active against 80–95% of strains. Piperacillin is the most active of the penicillins. Among the cephalosporins, only ceftazidime and cefoperazone can be considered active (80–95% of isolates are susceptible). Other agents with excellent antipseudomonal activity include imipenem, aztreonam, aminoglycosides, and ciprofloxacin. Piperacillin and ceftazidime (in combination with an aminoglycoside) are preferred agents for *P. aeruginosa*. Imipenem/cilastin or ciprofloxacin should be reserved for infections resistant to these β-lactams. Resistance may develop rapidly when imipenem or ciprofloxacin are used as monotherapy. Aminoglycosides are inadequate as single agents but may be important to confer synergistic killing. Provided the isolates are susceptible, gentamicin is preferred because of its lower cost. Tobramycin or amikacin should be reserved for gentamicin-resistant strains (or strains exhibiting a high MIC). For *P. aeruginosa* pneumonia, combination therapy with an aminoglycoside and an antipseudomonal β-lactam (or fluoroquinolone) for 14–21 days is advised. Oral ciprofloxacin may be substituted after 7–10 days of parenteral therapy (provided the isolate is susceptible and patients are responding clinically).

Preferred Therapy

• Piperacillin or ceftazidime (combine with aminoglycoside);
• Imipenem (reserve for resistant strains; combine with aminoglycoside).

Alternative Agents

• Ciprofloxacin or aztreonam (combine with aminoglycoside).

PSEUDOMONAS (BURKHOLDERIA) CEPACIA

Epidemiology: *Pseudomonas (Burkholderia) cepacia,* a member of the *Pseudomallei* group of pseudomonads, is an aerobic Gram-negative rod that is virtually nonpathogenic in normal, healthy individuals. *P. cepacia* is ubiquitous in the environment and can thrive and proliferate in tap water, antiseptic solutions, disinfectants, and medications. *P. cepacia* is of low virulence but is a well-recognized cause of respiratory tract infection and colonization in patients with cystic fibrosis. Lower respiratory tract colonization with *P. cepacia* in patients with cystic fibrosis has been associated with increasing severity of disease, prior use of aminoglycosides, a deteriorating course, and shortened survival. Virtually all cystic fibrosis patients colonized with *P. cepacia* are coinfected with *P. aeruginosa*. *P. cepacia* rarely causes community-acquired infections, but *P. cepacia* endocarditis in intravenous drug abusers and dermatitis in soldiers following prolonged immersion in contaminated water have been described. *P. cepacia* may rarely cause nosocomial pneumonia in patients with specific risk factors (e.g., mechanical ventilation, multiple courses of antimicrobials—particularly imipenem, debilitation, or impaired immune defenses). The mechanism of transmission is poorly understood. Both environmental sources and man-to-man transmission have been cited. Sporadic outbreaks of infection or colonization with *P. cepacia* have been noted in burn units, oncology wards, intensive care units, and in patients with surgical wounds or indwelling catheters. Contaminated nebulizer devices, irrigation or disinfectant solutions, or topical anaesthetics have been associated with nosocomial epidemics of *P. cepacia* pneumonia or bacteremias. Fatalities resulting from *P. cepacia* lung abscess, empyemas, or necrotizing pneumonias in immunocompromised patients have been described.

Antimicrobial Susceptibility: *P. cepacia* is highly resistant to multiple antibiotics. Virtually all isolates are resistant to penicillin, ampicillin, first- and second-generation cephalosporins, imipenem, and aminoglycosides. Susceptibility to antipseudomonal penicillins is variable. TMP/SMX, chloramphenicol, ceftazidime, minocycline, ciprofloxacin, and aztreonam are the most active agents; however, 20–50% of isolates are resistant to these antimicrobials. Imipenem has no activity against *P. cepacia* and may predispose to colonization or superinfection with this organism.

Preferred Therapy

* TMP/SMX, chloramphenicol, and ceftazidime are the most active agents.
* Aztreonam, ciprofloxacin, minocycline may be active (variable).
* Choice depends on in vitro susceptibility (but correlation to in vivo efficacy imperfect).
* Combinations of agents may be optimal (data lacking).
* Aminoglycosides may confer synergy in some strains.

Note: Virtually all isolates are resistant to imipenem.

STENOTROPHOMONAS (XANTHOMONAS) MALTOPHILIA

Epidemiology: *Stenotrophomonas* (formerly *Xanthomonas maltophilia* or *Pseudomonas maltophilia*) is a nonfermenting Gram-negative rod that is a rare opportunist in nosocomial settings. *X. maltophilia* may be isolated from hospital sinks, nebulizers, and environmental sources. *X. maltophilia* may colonize the respiratory tract in patients who have received repeated courses of antimicrobials (particularly imipenem). Other predisposing factors for nosocomial colonization or infections caused by *X. maltophilia* include residence in an ICU, indwelling central venous or arterial lines, tracheostomies, neutropenia, diabetes mellitus, malignant neoplasms, and intravenous drug abuse. Septicemias, wound infections, soft tissue infections, catheter infections, and pneumonias caused by *X. maltophilia* may occur in immunocompromised or debilitated hosts. Prognosis for catheter-induced bacteremias has been excellent following removal of the catheter and appropriate antibiotics. Mortality associated with *X. maltophilia* nosocomial pneumonia exceeds 50%. This high mortality likely reflects the debilitated state of patients who acquire this organism and the high-grade resistance to most antibiotics. *Stenotrophomonas maltophilia* is not a cause of CAP but may colonize or infect the lower respiratory tract in patients with cystic fibrosis. In this setting, *P. aeruginosa* is virtually always present concomitantly. Endocarditis in intravenous drug abusers has rarely been described.

Antimicrobial Susceptibility: *Stenotrophomonas maltophilia* is highly resistant to most β-lactams. Isolates are uniformly resistant to ampicillin, first- and second-generation cephalosporins, aztreonam, and imipenem. Fewer than 40% of isolates are susceptible to the antipseudomonal penicillins or aminoglycosides; 30–70% are susceptible to ceftazidime or cefoperazone. Most strains are sensitive to TMP/SMX, chloramphenicol, fluoroquinolones, and minocycline. Antibiotic combinations should be used in severe or refractory cases. Synergy has been achieved with TMP/SMX plus antipseudomonal penicillins or rifampin. The combination of ciprofloxacin and ceftazidime or antipseudomonal penicillins may also be synergistic.

Preferred Therapy

- Intravenous TMP/SMX (pending susceptibility);
- Ciprofloxacin, chloramphenicol, or minocycline more active than β-lactams;
- Ceftazidime or antipseudomonal penicillins with β-lactamase inhibitors (variable activity);
- Combinations of agents may be synergistic;
- Addition of aminoglycosides does not confer synergy.

Gram-positive Cocci

STREPTOCOCCI

Epidemiology: *Streptococcus* spp. other than *S. pneumoniae* (e.g., hemolytic and viridans streptococci) account for 1–4% of CAPs and play contributory roles in community-acquired lung abscess. Streptococci have been isolated in 1–8% of nosocomial pneumonias, usually as part of mixed (polymicrobial) infections. Because streptococci are part of normal oral flora, isolation of streptococci from tracheobronchial secretions must be interpreted with caution. Severe pneumonia caused by streptococci may occur even in previously healthy young adults, but most infections occur in patients with serious underlying disease(s). Dementia, esophageal disease, prior strokes, old age, and neurologic impairment are predisposing factors. Streptococci exhibit a striking proclivity for necrosis, abscess formation, and empyema. Aspiration pneumonitis progressing to a necrotizing pneumonitis is characteristic. Coinfection with other pathogens is common.

Antimicrobial Susceptibility: Penicillin G and ampicillin are highly active and are the preferred agents. Activity of antipseudomonal penicillins is no greater than penicillin G or ampicillin. Cephalosporins have excellent activity against streptococci; activity of imipenem is outstanding. Aztreonam is inactive. Activity of fluoroquinolones is modest: ofloxacin is superior to ciprofloxacin. Erythromycin, clindamycin, and vancomycin may be used in patients allergic to β-lactams. Aminoglycosides may confer synergistic activity and may be combined with penicillin for fulminant, life-threatening infections.

Preferred Therapy

- Penicillin G or ampicillin;
- Combine with aminoglycosides for life-threatening infections.

Alternative Agents

- Third-generation cephalosporins, imipenem, antipseudomonal penicillins;
- Erythromycin, clindamycin, vancomycin for patients allergic to penicillin.

GROUP D STREPTOCOCCI (ENTEROCOCCI)

Epidemiology: Group D streptococci (enterococci) include *S. faecalis* (85–90%), *S. faecium* (5–15%), and *S. durans* (less than 1%). Enterococci frequently cause urinary tract, pelvic, and intraabdominal infections but only rarely cause pneumonia. Enterococci are isolated frequently in sputum or tracheal secretions, particularly in patients previously treated with cephalosporins, but account for no more than 1–2% of nosocomial pneumonias. Risk factors for acquisition of enterococci include instrumentation of the gastrointestinal or genitourinary tract, immunosuppression, diabetes, cancer, debilitation, prolonged hospitalization, and prior cephalosporin use.

Antimicrobial Susceptibility: Enterococci are uniformly susceptible to vancomycin and ampicillin, but these agents are bacteriostatic. Thus, an aminoglycoside (typically gentamicin) should be added to confer synergy. Unfortunately, plasmids conferring vancomycin resistance have recently emerged among enterococci in some hospitals and chronic care facilities, and pose a serious threat to the future usefulness of vancomycin. Penicillin is slightly less active than ampicillin. Susceptibility to erythromycin is variable. Enterococci are resistant to all cephalosporins because of altered penicillin binding proteins. β-Lactamases are rare. Plasmid-mediated, aminoglycoside-modifying enzymes may confer high-grade resistance to aminoglycosides.

Preferred Therapy

• Ampicillin (or vancomycin) combined with an aminoglycoside.

Note: Enterococci are uniformly resistant to cephalosporins.

STAPHYLOCOCCUS AUREUS

Epidemiology: Coagulase-positive *S. aureus* may cause both community- and hospital-acquired pneumonia. Staphylococci have been implicated in 2–8% of CAP, almost exclusively in patients with specific risk factors (e.g., nursing home residence, diabetes mellitus, postinfluenza, intravenous drug abuse, debilitation, intravenous lines, Hickman catheters, hematologic malignancy). Staphylococci rarely cause CAP in previously healthy hosts. In nosocomial settings, *S. aureus* accounts for 15–30% of pneumonias, but these infections are usually polymicrobial. Risk factors for colonization or infection with *S. aureus* include recent neurosurgery, head trauma, diabetes mellitus, renal failure, burns, and corticosteroids. Fifteen to forty percent of nosocomial isolates are methicillin resistant (MRSA). Prior antibiotic use, prior nasal carriage, or transmission from medical personnel are risk factors for acquisition of MRSA. Staphylococci may cause a necrotizing pneumonia, lung abscess, or empyema. Multiple nodular or fluffy infiltrates suggest hematogenous spread, a pattern often observed in drug addicts or in endocarditis. Staphylococci should be considered when sputum or tracheal secretions demonstrate Gram-positive cocci in clusters. Prognosis for pneumonia depends on the severity and extent of comorbidities. Mortality rates for pneumonia caused by methicillin-sensitive *S. aureus* range from 5 to 21% but may exceed 40% in patients with serious coexisting illness or MRSA.

Antimicrobial Susceptibility: Most isolates of *S. aureus* are resistant to penicillin G and ampicillin but are susceptible to the antistaphylococcal penicillins (oxacillin, nafcillin, and cloxacillin) or cefazolin. Ceftazidime has only modest activity against staphylococci. The antipseudomonal penicillins and imipenem/cilastin are active against methicillin-sensitive strains. MRSA is resistant to all β-lactams. Clindamycin, fluoroquinolones, or TMP/SMX may be active against methicillin-susceptible or methicillin-resistant strains, but this is variable.

Preferred Therapy

- Oxacillin or cloxacillin (only for monomicrobial infections caused by methicillin-susceptible strains);
- Vancomycin (uniformly active for both methicillin-susceptible and methicillin-resistant strains).

Alternative Agents

- Cefazolin, clindamycin, or imipenem.

METHICILLIN-RESISTANT *STAPHYLOCOCCUS AUREUS* (MRSA)

Epidemiology: Within the past two decades, MRSA has emerged as an important problem in hospitalized patients, intravenous drug users, nursing homes, and chronic care facilities. Fifteen to forty percent of *S. aureus* in nosocomial settings are methicillin resistant. Concomitant infections with *P. aeruginosa* or aerobic EGNB are common. Mortality rates for pneumonia caused by MRSA may exceed 40% in debilitated patients with serious comorbidities.

Antimicrobial Susceptibility: Methicillin resistance results from alterations of PBPs, which also confer resistance to cephalosporins. Resistance to other classes of antibiotics (e.g., erythromycin, aminoglycosides, tetracycline, clindamycin) is common among MRSA strains. Patterns of resistance differ among geographic regions. Vancomycin is highly active against even these resistant strains and is the drug of choice. Clindamycin, TMP/SMX, or the quinolones may be used to treat some strains of MRSA but are less consistently active. Teicoplanin, a novel glycopeptide antibiotic related to vancomycin with less toxicity and a longer half-life, is not yet available in the United States.

Preferred Therapy

- Vancomycin (for monomicrobial infections);
- Additional antibiotics (to cover EGNB) may be required for polymicrobial infections.

Alternative Agents

- TMP/SMX, clindamycin, imipenem (for patients intolerant of vancomycin).

COAGULASE-NEGATIVE STAPHYLOCOCCI (*STAPHYLOCOCCUS EPIDERMIDIS*)

Epidemiology: Coagulase-negative staphylococci (*Staphylococcus epidermidis*) may cause bacteremia in granulocytopenic patients, infected Hickman or central venous catheters, neurosurgical and arterio-venous shunts, and prosthetic heart valves. *S. epidermidis* has been implicated in fewer than 3% of nosocomial pneumonias and is often mixed with other pathogens. Because most nosocomial pneumonias are polymicrobial, specific therapy against *S. epidermidis* may not be necessary.

Antimicrobial Susceptibility: By the late 1980s, 35–70% of coagulase-negative staphylococci were resistant to methicillin. Most hospital isolates of *S. epidermidis* are resistant to all β-lactams; virtually all isolates are susceptible to vancomycin. Many community-acquired strains of *S. epidermidis* are inhibited by β-lactams.

Preferred Therapy

• Vancomycin;
• Nafcillin (only for susceptible strains).

Empiric Therapy of Nosocomial Pneumonia

Because the diagnostic techniques used to ascertain the microbiologic cause of pneumonia remain inexact, treatment of nosocomial pneumonia often remains empiric. In view of the potential lethality of nosocomial pneumonia, we initiate therapy with broad-spectrum parenteral antibiotics pending clarification of the etiology. Selection of antibiotics should take into account host and environmental factors, findings on sputum Gram's stain, the known frequency of specific isolates in the hospital or ICU setting, and antimicrobial susceptibility patterns within institutions (and individual ICUs). Antimicrobial therapy can be switched to a narrower-spectrum agent once a definitive microbiologic diagnosis has been established. Patients who have recently received antibiotics are at risk of acquiring highly resistant organisms, such as *P. aeruginosa, Acinetobacter, Serratia* spp., and MRSA. Antibiotic resistance patterns vary widely within hospitals or even within ICUs within hospitals, and reflect previous trends of antibiotic use. At the University of Michigan, sweeping changes in antimicrobial resistance have been noted over the past decade. In 1981, fewer than 1% of *S. aureus* isolates were resistant to methicillin; by 1989 and 1994, 17% and 38% of strains were methicillin resistant, respectively. The prevalence of gentamicin-resistant *P. aeruginosa* increased from 3% in 1982 to 12% in 1989, and to 33% by 1994. High-level gentamicin-resistant enterococci climbed from fewer than 1% of isolates in 1982 to 20% in 1989, and to 22% in 1994. During that same time frame, *E. cloacae* isolates resistant to cefotaxime increased from 7% to 24% to 33%. Similar disturbing trends have been noted in other institutions. An awareness of existing (or recent) antimicrobial susceptibility data within institutions (or individual ICUs) may guide therapy. Selection pressure from prior antimicrobials administered for prophylaxis or treatment of infections in individual patients may predispose to highly resistant pathogens (e.g., *Enterobacter* spp. among patients receiving third-generation cephalosporins; *P. cepacia* following the use of imipenem). When nosocomial pneumonia develops (or progresses) in a patient receiving antibiotics, we usually switch to a different class of antimicrobials or to agents with a differing spectrum.

Treatment Regimens for Serious Nosocomial Pneumonia

Optimal antibiotic strategies for empiric therapy of nosocomial pneumonia are controversial. Several strategies have been advocated, including monotherapy with a broad-spectrum β-lactam or fluoroquinolone; combinations of a β-lactam or fluoroquinolone with an aminoglycoside; other antibiotic combinations (e.g., fluoroquinolones plus penicillins, clindamycin, or metronidazole); aztreonam plus vancomycin or clindamycin; TMP/SMX (alone or combined with an aminoglycoside). Prospective randomized trials assessing these options are limited.

MONOTHERAPY WITH BROAD-SPECTRUM β-LACTAMS

Monotherapy with a broad-spectrum β-lactam (e.g., third-generation cephalosporin, antipseudomonal penicillin/β-lactamase inhibitor, or imipenem/cilastin) is an attractive concept because the toxicities and expense of aminoglycosides (or additional agents) are avoided. Monotherapy with ceftazidime, cefoperazone, or imipenem/cilastin has been associated with favorable responses in 65–88% of cases of nosocomial pneumonia. A high rate of clinical and bacteriologic failures and relapses has been noted with monotherapy, however, when *P. aeruginosa* has been implicated. Less data are available regarding monotherapy with antipseudomonal penicillin/β-lactamase inhibitor combinations for severe nosocomial pneumonias. Monotherapy with a β-lactam (to which the organism is susceptible) is probably adequate for nosocomial pneumonias caused by *E. coli, Klebsiella,* and *Proteus* spp. Monotherapy may not be adequate, however, for pneumonia caused by *P. aeruginosa, Acinetobacter,* and *Serratia* spp. The role of specific antibiotics will be discussed in greater detail in the sections that follow.

DUAL β-LACTAM THERAPY

Dual β-lactam therapy, which combines two β-lactams (typically an antipseudomonal penicillin and third-generation cephalosporin), has been advocated by some investigators. Dual β-lactam therapy offers little over monotherapy, however, unless synergistic killing is achieved. Some β-lactam combinations are synergistic in vitro (e.g., ceftazidime and piperacillin or aztreonam plus β-lactams); however, the combination of imipenem/cilastin and another β-lactam may be antagonistic. No data are available regarding dual β-lactam therapy for pneumonia. In randomized trials in febrile, granulocytopenic patients, clinical responses with dual β-lactam combinations were similar to β-lactam/aminoglycoside regimens. Theoretically, resistance may emerge with dual β-lactam therapy because β-lactamase-producing isolates may confer resistance to both agents. Dual β-lactam therapy is expensive and we see no current role for this strategy for pneumonia.

COMBINATION OF β-LACTAM WITH AMINOGLYCOSIDE

Although aminoglycosides have potential toxicity, we believe combining a broad-spectrum β-lactam with an aminoglycoside is reasonable for serious nosocomial pneumonias (pending cultures and clarification of clinical course). Theoretic advantages of combination therapy include:

- Synergistic microbicidal activity against many bacteria can be achieved.
- Combination therapy improves survival in animal models of *P. aeruginosa* infection.
- In humans, subtherapeutic peak aminoglycoside levels correlated with reduced survival in patients with Gram-negative pneumonia.
- In a multicenter European randomized trial in granulocytopenic cancer patients with Gram-negative bacteremia, survival was superior in patients treated with ceftazidime plus long-course (10 days) amikacin compared with ceftazidime plus short-course (5 days) amikacin.
- Survival is improved in immunocompromised patients even when the infecting organisms are susceptible to both the β-lactam and the aminoglycoside.
- In a prospective study of 200 patients with *P. aeruginosa* bacteremia, mortality was higher with monotherapy using an antipseudomonal β-lactam (47% mortality) compared with the combination of a β-lactam plus aminoglycoside (27% mortality). The survival advantage was even greater among patients with pneumonia or in an ICU.
- The combination of a β-lactam/aminoglycoside may limit the emergence of antimicrobial resistance; this conceptual advantage has not yet been verified in clinical trials.

Empiric Therapy (Prior to Identification of a Specific Organism)

While optimal therapy for nosocomial pneumonia is controversial, we favor combination therapy with a broad-spectrum antipseudomonal β-lactam and aminoglycoside for patients with risk factors for acquisition of *P. aeruginosa* (e.g., mechanically ventilated patients, previous recent antibiotic therapy, prolonged hospitalization, corticosteroid use, etc.). Monotherapy with a nonpseudomonal β-lactam may be adequate for nosocomial pneumonia outside the ICU in antibiotic-naive patients at lower risk for highly virulent pathogens.

Initial Empiric Therapy for Nosocomial Pneumonia

MECHANICALLY VENTILATED PATIENTS OR PATIENTS WHO HAVE RECENTLY RECEIVED ANTIBIOTICS:

- Ceftazidime, piperacillin/tazobactam, or imipenem *plus* an aminoglycoside (if contraindications to aminoglycosides, monotherapy with ceftazidime or imipenem);
- Ciprofloxacin (alone or combined with aminoglycosides);
- Ciprofloxacin (combined with clindamycin or metronidazole) (for penicillin-allergic patients).

Note: Aminoglycosides alone are not adequate as monotherapy for pneumonia caused by EGNB but have an adjunctive role when combined with a β-lactam.

- Vancomycin should not be used routinely for empiric therapy but may be added in patients failing broad-spectrum regimens or when Gram-positive cocci are isolated by culture or observed on Gram's stain.

NONCRITICALLY ILL, NONVENTILATED PATIENTS WITH LOW RISK OF *P. AERUGINOSA:*

- Ceftriaxone or cefotaxime (monotherapy);
- Ciprofloxacin or ofloxacin (alone or combined with clindamycin or metronidazole) (for penicillin-allergic patients).

MODIFICATION OF ANTIMICROBIAL THERAPY

Initial antimicrobial therapy should be reassessed once cultural results are available (usually by 48–72 hours) and the clinical course has been clarified. The appropriate agent(s) depends on the suspected (or confirmed) organism(s) and on the microbiologic susceptibilities. For infections caused by *P. aeruginosa,* combination therapy with an extended-spectrum penicillin (e.g., piperacillin or ticarcillin), ceftazidime, or imipenem/cilastin plus an aminoglycoside is warranted. Other third-generation cephalosporins, such as cefotaxime or ceftriaxone, extended-spectrum penicillins, or imipenem/cilastin, provide excellent activity against most other EGNB. First- or second-generation cephalosporins may be substituted for more expensive agents if a specific organism has been isolated and is susceptible. For *E. coli, Klebsiella,* and *Proteus* spp., the aminoglycoside can be discontinued. For *P. aeruginosa, Serratia,* and *Acinetobacter* spp., the synergistic activity achieved with the aminoglycoside enhances outcome. Ciprofloxacin may be used for penicillin-allergic patients. When *P. aeruginosa* is isolated, addition of an aminoglycoside to confer synergy is reasonable.

DURATION

Duration of therapy for nosocomial pneumonia must be adequate to avoid recrudescent infection. Although the duration must be individualized according to clinical response and severity of the disease, treatment is usually necessary for a minimum of 10 days. A more prolonged course (extending for 14–21 days) may be appropriate for virulent pathogens, such as *P. aeruginosa,* or for complicated, severe, or protracted cases.

SPECIFIC ANTIMICROBIAL AGENTS
β-Lactams

This class of agents includes penicillins, cephalosporins, carbapenems, and monobactams. The four-membered β-lactam ring (usually fused to a second ring) is integral to the structure. Modifications or substitutions of the β-lactam ring alter antimicrobial activity or resistance to β-lactamases.

Penicillins

The penicillin group of antibiotics have excellent bactericidal activity and low toxicity. The basic structure of the penicillins consists of a β-lactam ring fused to a 5-membered thiazolidine ring; modification of side chains attached to the β-lactam ring may alter the antimicrobial spectrum, β-lactamase stability, and pharmacokinetics. The newer penicillins are modifications of ampicillin. Substituting a carboxy group for an amino group on ampicillin produced the carboxypenicillins, carbenicillin and ticarcillin. Substitution of a ureido group for the carboxy group produced the ureidopenicillins (piperacillin, mezlocillin, azlocillin).

Mechanism of Action: Penicillins interfere with bacterial cell wall (peptidoglycan) synthesis, inducing cell lysis. Killing of EGNB requires that penicillins penetrate outer portions of the bacterial cell wall and combine with key PBPs on the inner bacterial membrane. Penicillins fail to activate autolytic enzymes in enterococci and some streptococci. In such cases, an aminoglycoside or rifampin should be added to achieve bactericidal activity.

Antimicrobial Resistance: The most common mechanism of resistance to penicillins is via β-lactamases. β-Lactamases are produced by both Gram-negative and Gram-positive bacilli and hydrolyze the β-lactam ring. Additional mechanisms of resistance to penicillin can result from alterations in PBPs (resulting in decreasing affinity for penicillins) or changes in bacterial cell wall permeability. MRSA is caused by alterations in PBPs; multiresistant *P. aeruginosa* is mediated by the latter mechanism.

Toxicity: Adverse effects include maculopapular rash, eosinophilia, drug fever (particularly with ampicillin and methicillin), and seizures (particularly when high doses are given in patients with renal failure).

BENZYL PENICILLIN (PENICILLIN G)

Benzyl penicillin, or penicillin G, was introduced in 1941 and is the parent drug of the penicillin antibiotics.

Antimicrobial Spectrum: Outstanding activity against *Streptococcus pyogenes* (group A), β-hemolytic streptococci, most *Streptococcus viridans,* and group D streptococci (enterococci). In the United States, 7–12% of *S. pneumoniae* display intermediate resistance to penicillin; 1–2%, high-grade resistance. Anaerobes are exquisitely sensitive, but β-lactamase-positive *B. fragilis* are resistant. More than 80% of staphylococci are resistant. Active against *Neisseria meningitidis* and *Neisseria gonorrhoeae*. Most *M. catarrhalis* are now resistant. No significant activity against *H. influenzae* or EGNB.

Toxicity: Hypersensitivity reactions (anaphylaxis, rash) may occur with all penicillins. Gastrointestinal side effects and diarrhea are much less common than they are with extended-spectrum penicillins. No significant phlebitis.

Dosage: 4.8–10 million U of aqueous crystalline penicillin G IV daily in 4–6 divided doses. Oral penicillin VK (the potassium salt of phenoxymethyl penicillin) can be substituted once clinical response and defervescence have occurred (dose, 500 mg q.i.d.).

Indications

- Drug of choice for pneumonia caused by susceptible strains of *S. pneumoniae* or other streptococci;
- Empiric therapy for lung abscess (clindamycin may be superior);
- Infections caused by enterococci (*Streptococcus faecalis* and *Streptococcus faecium*) (must be combined with either rifampin or an aminoglycoside).

Because of its limited spectrum, penicillin G is not suitable as empiric therapy for CAP except when *S. pneumoniae* is strongly suspected and the prevalence of penicillin-resistant pneumococci in the community is low. Penicillin G has no role for nosocomial pneumonia.

ANTISTAPHYLOCOCCAL PENICILLINS

The semisynthetic penicillins were developed to treat β-lactamase-producing staphylococci resistant to penicillin G. Semisynthetic penicillins available for parenteral use are methicillin, nafcillin, and oxacillin. Cloxacillin or dicloxacillin are available for oral use.

Antimicrobial Spectrum: Active against most staphylococci, including β-lactamase-producing strains. Not active against MRSA. Less active than penicillin G against streptococci and other penicillin-susceptible organisms. No significant activity against anaerobes or EGNB.

Toxicity: Similar to penicillin but also includes interstitial nephritis and phlebitis. Nafcillin, oxacillin, and methicillin are equivalent in efficacy, but side effects (particularly interstitial nephritis) are most frequent with methicillin.

Dosage: 1–2 gm IV q4–6h. Oral cloxacillin or dicloxacillin can be substituted in some patients when clinical response has occurred (dose, 250–500 mg q.i.d.).

Indications

- In view of their narrow spectrum, antistaphylococcal penicillins should be reserved for monomicrobial pneumonia caused by susceptible strains of staphylococci.

AMINOPENICILLINS

The aminopenicillins (ampicillin, amoxicillin) were the first of the penicillins with activity against EGNB. Ampicillin was developed by adding an amino group to benzyl penicillin; amoxicillin and bacampicillin were developed later. Ampicillin and amoxicillin were widely used in the early 1970s as empiric therapy for CAP. Antimicrobial resistance to the aminopenicillins has increased dramatically over the past two decades. These gaps in the spectrum have relegated ampicillin and amoxicillin to secondary roles in the treatment of CAP. Currently, second- or third-generation cephalosporins have supplanted the aminopenicillins.

Antimicrobial Spectrum: Excellent activity against streptococci, anaerobes, and *Neisseria* spp. (comparable to penicillin G). Not active against penicillin-resistant *S. pneumoniae*. Active against β-lactamase-negative strains of *Haemophilus spp.* and *M. catarrhalis* and *Proteus mirabilis;* 30–40% of *E. coli* are resistant. No significant activity against *Klebsiella, Enterobacter, Serratia,* indole-positive *Proteus,* or *Pseudomonas* spp.

Toxicity: Similar to penicillin G except higher incidence of diarrhea and gastrointestinal symptoms (10–15%) and skin rash (3–5%).

Dosage: Ampicillin 1–2 gm IV q6h. Oral ampicillin 500 mg q.i.d. (or amoxicillin 500 mg t.i.d.) can be substituted in selected patients responding to parenteral therapy.

Indications

- Pneumonia caused by a β-lactamase negative *H. influenzae, E. coli,* or *Proteus mirabilis;*
- Infections caused by enterococci (combine with an aminoglycoside).

β-LACTAMASE INHIBITORS

Clavulanate, sulbactam, and tazobactam inhibit β-lactamases produced by certain Gram-positive and Gram-negative bacteria (e.g., staphylococci, *B. fragilis, H. influenzae, M. catarrhalis, K. pneumoniae, Proteus* spp.) but lack intrinsic antibacterial activity. The addition of β-lactamase inhibitors extends the spectrum of the parent compound (ampicillin, amoxicillin, ticarcillin, piperacillin) to include certain β-lactamase-producing strains. These β-lactamase inhibitors do not affect β-lactamases of the type 1 Richmond-Sykes classification produced by *P. aeruginosa, Enterobacter, Morganella,* or *Serratia* spp. β-Lactamase inhibitors do not improve the activity of the parent compound for β-lactamase-negative strains or bacteria that are resistant by mechanisms other than β-lactamase production. These agents have no activity against MRSA.

AMPICILLIN/SULBACTAM (UNASYN)

The addition of sulbactam to ampicillin extended the spectrum of ampicillin to include selected β-lactamase-producing organisms. Ampicillin/sulbactam is less active than third-generation cephalosporins against EGNB but has superior activity against streptococci and anaerobes. Ampicillin/sulbactam may be used as empiric therapy for CAPs caused by streptococci, anaerobes, and common respiratory bacterial pathogens.

Antimicrobial Spectrum: Excellent activity against penicillin-susceptible streptococci, anaerobes (inhibits more than 95% of strains), and methicillin-sensitive *S. aureus.* Active against *M. catarrhalis, Neisseria* spp., *H. influenzae, E. coli, Klebsiella* spp., *P. mirabilis,* and *Acinetobacter* spp. Not active against *P. aeruginosa, Serratia, Enterobacter* spp.

Dosage: Supplied as 3-gm or 1.5-gm vials for IV use in fixed 2 : 1 ratio of ampicillin to sulbactam; dose, 1.5–3 gm q6h (pharmacokinetics similar to those of ampicillin).

Indications

- Polymicrobial anaerobic infections (e.g., lung abscess, aspiration pneumonia);
- Empiric therapy for CAP (spectrum not as broad as ceftriaxone);

- Limited utility for nosocomial pneumonia (lacks activity against *P. aeruginosa* and selected EGNB).

AMOXICILLIN/CLAVULANATE (AUGMENTIN)

Amoxicillin/clavulanate, the first penicillin/β-lactamase inhibitor combination, has been available in the United States since 1984. Amoxicillin/clavulanate, available only in oral form, is as effective as oral cephalosporins or fluoroquinolones for sinusitis, bronchitis, or mild CAP.

Antimicrobial Spectrum: Expands spectrum of amoxicillin to include β-lactamase-producing strains of *H. influenzae, M. catarrhalis, B. fragilis, E. coli, Proteus, Klebsiella,* and *S. aureus.* No activity against *P. aeruginosa, Serratia, Enterobacter, Citrobacter,* or MRSA.

Toxicity: Similar to ampicillin or amoxicillin. Greater incidence of diarrhea compared with cephalosporins or penicillin VK.

Dosage: 250–500 mg t.i.d.

Indications

- Oral empiric therapy for mild CAP (in patients at low risk for EGNB or following initial parenteral therapy).

ANTIPSEUDOMONAL PENICILLINS

Carbenicillin, a carboxypenicillin produced by substituting a carboxyl group for the amino group on ampicillin, was the first penicillin with activity against *P. aeruginosa.* Substitutions on carbenicillin resulted in ticarcillin, which broadened the spectrum against EGNB. Attachment of ureido groups to the acyl side chain of ampicillin led to the ureidopenicillins; (piperacillin, mezlocillin, and azlocillin). Antipseudomonal penicillins have been extensively used to treat serious infections in granulocytopenic hosts and may be effective in severe community or nosocomial pneumonias. Currently, carbenicillin, azlocillin, and mezlocillin are rarely used. Piperacillin (alone or combined with tazobactam) or ticarcillin/clavulanate are the antipseudomonal penicillins most often used in the United States.

Antimicrobial Spectrum: Antipseudomonal penicillins are broad-spectrum agents with activity against streptococci, anaerobes, β-lactamase-negative *H. influenzae,* and most EGNB, including *P. aeruginosa.* The activity of antipseudomonal penicillins against *E. coli* is less predictable than third-generation cephalosporins (80–90% of isolates are susceptible). Twenty to forty percent of *Enterobacter* spp. are resistant. The carboxypenicillins are not reliable against *Klebsiella* spp. or *Serratia* spp. Piperacillin, has generally good activity against these pathogens. Piperacillin is the most active agent against *P. aeruginosa.* Activity of antipseudomonal penicillins against Gram-positive cocci is slightly less than that of penicillin G or ampicillin. Both ticarcillin/clavulanate and piperacillin/tazobactam have excellent activity against β-lactamase-producing strains of staphylococci or *B. fragilis,* which the parent compounds may fail to cover. MRSA are invariably resistant.

Toxicity: Similar to other penicillins. Principal side effects are skin rash, hypokalemia, and sodium load. (Carbenicillin and ticarcillin contain 4.7 mEq sodium/gm; mezlocillin and piperacillin, 1.8 mEq/gm.)

Combinations of Antipseudomonal Penicillins and β-lactamase Inhibitors

TICARCILLIN/CLAVULANATE (TIMENTIN)

Timentin is a fixed combination of 3 gm of ticarcillin and 100 mg of clavulanate potassium (a β-lactamase inhibitor). Clavulanate binds to β-lactamases secreted by selected bacteria but does not affect type 1 β-lactamases released by *P. aeruginosa, Serratia, Citrobacter,* and *Enterobacter* spp. Ticarcillin/clavulanate exhibits good activity against staphylococci (except MRSA). Activity against enterococci is modest. Ticarcillin/clavulanate has been used extensively for serious infections in both immunocompromised and immunocompetent hosts, with cure rates comparable to third-generation cephalosporins. Ticarcillin/clavulanate may be adequate for nursing home or nosocomial pneumonias. When *P. aeruginosa* is suspected, an aminoglycoside should be added.

Dosage: 3–4 gm IV q4–6h (3.1 gm q4–6h for ticarcillin/clavulanate). For *P. aeruginosa,* an aminoglycoside is added for synergy.

PIPERACILLIN/TAZOBACTAM (ZOSYN)

Piperacillin/tazobactam, a combination of piperacillin and the β-lactamase inhibitor tazobactam, was introduced in the United States in 1994. The antimicrobial spectrum of piperacillin/tazobactam is comparable to ticarcillin/clavulanate, but activity against *P. aeruginosa* and anaerobes is superior. Piperacillin/tazobactam is highly effective for serious infections (including pneumonias) in both immunocompetent and immunosuppressed hosts. Piperacillin/tazobactam was superior to ticarcillin/clavulanate for CAP in a randomized trial. Data in nosocomial pneumonia are limited, but this agent appears promising. For *P. aeruginosa* pneumonia, the dose of piperacillin/tazobactam should be increased to 4.5 gm q6h, and an aminoglycoside should be added.

Dosage: 3.375 gm q6h (for *P. aeruginosa,* the dose is 4.5 gm q6h).

Indications

- Piperacillin/tazobactam or ticarcillin/clavulanate may be used for empiric therapy of nosocomial pneumonia or serious nosocomial sepsis. An aminoglycoside should be added to provide synergy when *P. aeruginosa* is a consideration.
- Piperacillin/tazobactam or ticarcillin/clavulanate may be used for severe CAP in which polymicrobial infections (including anaerobes) are suspected.
- Antipseudomonal penicillins are not required for mild to moderate CAP (less expensive agents are usually adequate).

Cephalosporins

Since the first cephalosporin, cephalothin (Keflin), became available in the United States in 1964, the proliferation of newer agents, with differing spectra, β-lactamase stability, and pharmacokinetics, has been remarkable. All cephalosporins have the four-membered β-lactam ring bound to a six-membered dihydrothiazine ring. The cephalosporin nucleus is inherently more resistant to β-lactamases than is penicillin. Modification of position 7 of the β-lactam ring alters β-lactamase stability and antimicrobial activity. An iminomethoxy group (e.g., cefuroxime, cefotaxime, ceftizoxime, ceftriaxone) confers enhanced β-lactamase stability but slight loss of Gram-positive activity. Ceftazidime has a prophylcarboxyl group at position 7, which results in superior activity against *P. aeruginosa* but reduces antimicrobial activity against Gram-positive bacteria. The cephamycins (cefoxitin and cefotetan) contain a methoxy group at position 7, which confers resistance to Gram-negative β-lactamases (by steric hindrance) but also results in less affinity for PBPs. Substitutions at position 3 alter the pharmacokinetics without influencing antimicrobial activity; substitution at this position explains the long half-life of ceftriaxone.

Mechanism of Action: Cephalosporins bind to PBPs and interfere with bacterial cell wall (peptidoglycan) synthesis.

Antimicrobial Spectrum: Cephalosporins have broad-spectrum activity against both Gram-negative and Gram-positive bacteria. Gram-positive activity (particularly against staphylococci) is best with cefazolin and modest with succeeding generations; ceftazidime has poor activity. Cephalosporins are active against most streptococci (including *S. pneumoniae*) but generally less active than penicillins; ceftazidime is the least active agent in this class. Third-generation cephalosporins (cefotaxime, ceftriaxone) may be active against penicillin-resistant pneumococci, but cephalosporin-resistant strains have been noted with increasing frequency. Cephalosporins lack activity against enterococci or MRSA. Cefoxitin and cefotetan have excellent activity against anaerobes, but 8–30 % of isolates of *B. fragilis* are resistant. Activity of the other cephalosporins is modest and less than the penicillins. First-generation cephalosporins have marginal activity against *H. influenzae;* cefoxitin and cefotetan have modest activity. Cefuroxime and all third-generation agents are highly active. Activity against EGNB improves with each succeeding generation (particularly against Enterobacteriaceae). First-generation cephalosporins are active against most strains of *E. coli, P. mirabilis,* and *K. pneumoniae,* but do not typically cover *Enterobacter, Citrobacter, Serratia, Providencia, P. vulgaris,* or *Morganella* spp. These species are variably sensitive to cefuroxime, cefotetan, and cefoxitin; most are inhibited by third-generation agents. Only ceftazidime and cefoperazone have significant activity against *P. aeruginosa. Acinetobacter* spp. are usually resistant to cephalosporins, but some strains are susceptible to ceftazidime.

Toxicity: Hypersensitivity reactions, fever, or rash in 1–5%; gastrointestinal symptoms in 5–10%. A methylthiotetrazole group in position 3 with cefamandole, cefotetan, cefoperazone, and moxalactam is associated with hypoprothrombinemia. Only moxalactam (which is no longer used) was associated with an increased risk of bleeding.

FIRST-GENERATION CEPHALOSPORINS

First-generation cephalosporins for parenteral use include cephalothin (Keflin), cephapirin (Cefadyl), cephradine (Velosef), and cefazolin (Ancef, Kefzol). Only cefazolin is currently used. Cefazolin has limited activity against *H. influenzae;* its activity against Enterobacteriaceae is inconsistent. The spectrum of oral cephalexin (Keflex) is similarly narrow.

Dosage: Cefazolin 1 gm q8h. Oral cephalexin 500 mg q6h can be substituted in selected patients responding to parenteral therapy.

Indications

• Pneumonia caused by streptococci, *Staphylococci,* or susceptible organisms.

SECOND-GENERATION CEPHALOSPORINS

Second-generation cephalosporins for parenteral use include cefuroxime, cefamandole, cefonicid, cefoxitin, and cefotetan. Cefamandole is no longer used, and cefoxitin has largely been replaced by cefotetan. Oral agents include cefaclor, cefuroxime axetil, and ceprozil.

Antimicrobial Spectrum: Second-generation cephalosporins have superior activity against *H. influenzae* and EGNB (including most *E. coli, Klebsiella, Proteus* spp.) compared with first-generation agents. Activity against streptococci (other than enterococci) is good. Resistant strains of *S. pneumoniae* are rare, but appear to be increasing. Activity against staphylococci is modest.

CEFUROXIME (ZINACEF, KEFUROX)

Cefuroxime has excellent activity against most common respiratory pathogens and has replaced cefamandole (an earlier second-generation cephalosporin). Cefuroxime has excellent CNS penetration and exhibits greater β-lactamase stability than do earlier agents.

Antimicrobial Spectrum: Active against *S. pneumoniae, S. aureus, H. influenzae, K. pneumoniae,* and oral anaerobes.

Dosage: Cefuroxime 0.75–1.5 gm IV q8h.

Indications

• Empiric therapy of CAP in adults; (+/− macrolide to cover atypicals);
• Not recommended as empiric therapy for nosocomial pneumonia.

CEFUROXIME AXETIL (CEFTIN)

Cefuroxime axetil, formulated for oral use, is more active than cefaclor against *H. influenzae* and *M. catarrhalis* and may be used for bronchitis or mild CAP not requiring hospitalization. Cefuroxime axetil may be substituted for parenteral cefuroxime following an initial response.

Dosage: 500 mg b.i.d. for pneumonia; 250 mg b.i.d. for bronchitis.

CEFPROZIL (CEFZIL)

Cefprozil has a spectrum of activity similar to cefuroxime acetil. In randomized, double-blind trials, cefprozil has been comparable to cefaclor, cefuroxime axetil, and amoxicillin/clavulanate for bronchitis or mild CAP in adults (80–95% favorable responses).

Dosage: 500 mg b.i.d. for pneumonia; 250 mg b.i.d. for bronchitis.

CEFONICID (MONOCID)

Cefonicid, which has a prolonged half-life and can be dosed once daily, has been used sparingly for lower respiratory tract infections.

Antimicrobial Spectrum: Similar to cefuroxime but slightly less active than cefuroxime against staphylococci, *H. influenzae,* and Enterobacteriaceae.

Dosage: 1–2 gm IV/IM q24h.

Indications

• Few studies have evaluated cefonicid for pneumonia.
• Cefonicid has no advantage over cefuroxime or ceftriaxone.

CEFOTETAN (CEFOTAN)

Cefotetan, a cephamycin, has the best anaerobic activity of the cephalosporins and has largely replaced cefoxitin (an earlier cephamycin). Cefotetan has a niche for polymicrobial pneumonia caused by anaerobes and aerobic EGNB.

Antimicrobial Spectrum: Comparable to second-generation cephalosporins but superior anaerobic activity (including β-lactamase-producing *B. fragilis*); less active than cefuroxime against *H. influenzae.*

Toxicity: Has methylthiotetrazole side chain; theoretic risk for bleeding (rare).

Dosage: 1–2 gm q12h.

Indications

• Community- or nursing home-acquired pneumonias and risk factors for aspiration (alcohol abuse, esophageal disease, impaired neurologic status);
• Polymicrobial (mixed anaerobic and EGNB) pneumonias.

THIRD-GENERATION CEPHALOSPORINS

Third-generation cephalosporins available for parenteral use include cefotaxime, ceftizoxime, ceftriaxone, ceftazidime, and cefoperazone. Moxalactam is no longer used. Cefpodoxime proxetil and cefixime are available for oral use. The antimicrobial activity of cefotaxime, ceftizoxime, and ceftriaxone is similar, but cefotaxime is slightly more active against *S. aureus.* These three agents lack activity against *P. aeruginosa.* Ceftazidime and cefoperazone are the only cephalosporins with significant activity against *P. aeruginosa.* The activity of these antipseudomonal agents against anaerobes, *S. aureus,* and Gram-positive cocci is less than cefotaxime, ceftizoxime, or ceftriaxone.

Antimicrobial Spectrum: Third-generation cephalosporins extend the Gram-negative spectrum of second-generation agents to include *Serratia, Morganella morganii, Providencia* spp., and *Citrobacter* spp. Third-generation agents are extremely active against *H. influenzae* and *H. parainfluenzae,* including β-lactamase-producing isolates. Twenty to forty percent of *Enterobacter* spp. produce β-lactamases that hydrolyze cephalosporins. Liberal use of ceftazidime may foster resistance by inducible β-lactamases. Ceftazidime and cefoperazone have significant activity against *P. aeruginosa.* Most strains of *P. cepacia* and *Xanthomonas maltophilia* are resistant to cephalosporins, but some are inhibited by ceftazidime. Activity against *Acinetobacter* spp. is variable. Ceftizoxime, ceftriaxone, and cefoperazone exhibit poor activity; some strains are susceptible to cefotaxime or ceftazidime. Gram-positive activity of third-generation cephalosporins is variable. Cefotaxime is the most active; ceftazidime, the least active. Cefotaxime, ceftizoxime, and ceftriaxone are highly active against streptococci, including *S. pneumoniae.* These agents are moderately active against methicillin-sensitive *S. aureus;* activity of ceftazidime is fair to poor. MRSA and enterococci are invariably resistant to cephalosporins (irrespective of in vitro susceptibility testing). Anaerobic activity of third-generation cephalosporins is fair. Activity is modest against mouth anaerobes but is fair to poor against the *B. fragilis* group. Ceftizoxime is the most active agent in this class; ceftazidime is the least active.

CEFOTAXIME (CLAFORAN)

Cefotaxime has broad-spectrum activity, low toxicity, and is less expensive than ceftazidime. Cefotaxime may be adequate for community-acquired or nosocomial pneumonia in patients without specific risk factors for *P. aeruginosa.*

Antimicrobial Spectrum: Generally comparable to ceftriaxone and ceftizoxime; however, cefotaxime's activity against *S. aureus* may be superior to these agents.

Distinguishing Features: The desacetyl metabolite of cefotaxime (desacetylcefotaxime) has excellent antimicrobial activity similar to the parent compound, has a longer half-life, confers improved activity against staphylococci, and is synergistic with cefotaxime against susceptible strains of Enterobacteriaceae. Cefotaxime, ceftriaxone, and ceftizoxime penetrate well into the cerebrospinal fluid (CSF) and can be used to treat meningitis.

Dosage: 1–2 gm IV q8h.

Indications

- Community- or nursing home-acquired pneumonia in patients at risk for EGNB;
- Pneumonia caused by penicillin-resistant *S. pneumoniae;*
- Empiric therapy for nosocomial pneumonia arising outside the ICU;
- Pneumonia caused by *E. coli, Klebsiella, Proteus, Serratia, H. influenzae,* and other susceptible organisms;
- Not recommended for empiric treatment of pneumonia in patients with risk factors for *P. aeruginosa.*

CEFTRIAXONE (ROCEPHIN)

Because of its broad-spectrum antimicrobial activity and prolonged half-life, which permits once-daily dosing, ceftriaxone is one of the most widely used antibiotics, both in the community and in nosocomial settings. Ceftriaxone is highly efficacious for empiric therapy of community- or nursing home-acquired pneumonias (including penicillin-resistant pneumococci).

Antimicrobial Spectrum: Similar to cefotaxime and ceftizoxime.

Toxicity: Ceftriaxone is primarily eliminated by the biliary system. Compared with other cephalosporins, gastrointestinal symptoms and diarrhea are slightly more common with ceftriaxone. High concentrations in bile may lead to biliary sludge (biliary pseudolithiasis) and symptoms resembling cholelithiasis.

Dosage: 1–2 gm q24h.

Indications

- Empiric therapy of community-, nursing-home, or hospital-acquired pneumonias;
- Outpatient therapy (1 gm intramuscularly once-daily) can be initiated in the office, clinic, or emergency department. Can convert to an oral agent once improvement has occurred. This strategy may reduce the need for hospitalization;
- Pneumonia caused by *S. pneumoniae,* Enterobacteriaceae, *H. influenzae,* or susceptible pathogens;
- Pneumonia caused by penicillin-resistant *S. pneumoniae;*
- Not recommended for empiric treatment of nosocomial pneumonia in patients with risk factors for *P. aeruginosa.*

CEFTIZOXIME (CEFIZOX)

Although prospective, randomized trials have not been performed, ceftizoxime appears to be therapeutically equivalent to cefotaxime or ceftriaxone.

Dosage: 1–2 gm IV q12h.

CEFOPERAZONE (CEFOBID)

Cefoperazone is the only cephalosporin other than ceftazidime with excellent activity against *P. aeruginosa.* Cefoperazone has been successfully used as monotherapy for nursing home and nosocomial pneumonias.

Antimicrobial Spectrum: Excellent activity against *P. aeruginosa* (greater than ceftriaxone or ceftizoxime but less than ceftazidime). Less consistent activity against Enterobacteriaceae and less β-lactamase stability compared with other third-generation cephalosporins. Modest activity against anaerobes and Gram-positive bacilli (less than cefotaxime).

Toxicity: Contains methylthiotetrazole chain (potential for bleeding resulting from prothrombin deficiency).

Dosage: 1–2 gm q8h.

Indications

Cefoperazone is less active than cefotaxime against *E. coli* and *Klebsiella* spp. and is less active than ceftazidime against *P. aeruginosa.* We do not use cefoperazone; we prefer cefotaxime or ceftazidime (choice depending on susceptibilities).

- Cefoperazone has no advantage over other third-generation cephalosporins.

CEFTAZIDIME (FORTAZ, TAZIDIME, TAZICEF)

Ceftazidime is the most active cephalosporin against *P. aeruginosa* and has excellent activity against most EGNB. This agent is most appropriate when *P. aeruginosa* is a consideration. Ceftazidime has been extensively used as monotherapy for sepsis in immunocompromised hosts, with results comparable to β-lactam/aminoglycoside combinations. In several randomized trials, ceftazidime was comparable to imipenem or ciprofloxacin for nosocomial or CAP (favorable responses 78–96%). Extensive use of ceftazidime monotherapy may foster resistance, however. Plasmid-mediated extended-spectrum β-lactamase and chromosomally mediated inducible β-lactamases have emerged (particularly among Enterobacteriaceae) by selection pressure from liberal use of ceftazidime. Monotherapy has been associated with a high rate of clinical and microbiologic failures and relapses for pneumonia caused by *P. aeruginosa.*

Antimicrobial Spectrum: Excellent activity against *P. aeruginosa;* comparable to other third-generation cephalosporins against Enterobacteriaceae and aerobic EGNB. May be active against strains of *Acinetobacter, P. cepacia,* and *X. maltophilia* resistant to other cephalosporins. Ceftazidime is the least active cephalosporin against Gram-positive cocci and anaerobes.

Dosage: 1–2 gm IV q8h.

Indications

- Cornerstone of therapy for pneumonia when *P. aeruginosa* is suspected or documented (if possible, combined with an aminoglycoside for synergy);
- When *P. aeruginosa* not a consideration, use cefotaxime, ceftizoxime, or ceftriaxone;
- No role to treat CAP (except when risk factors for *P. aeruginosa,* such as cystic fibrosis or chronic bronchiectasis).

ORAL THIRD-GENERATION CEPHALOSPORINS

CEFIXIME (SUPRAX)

Cefixime, released in 1991, has a prolonged half-life that permits once-daily dosing. Cefixime is more active than second-generation agents against EGNB but has poor activity against staphylococci, anaerobes, or *Pseudomonas* spp. Apart from its favorable pharmacokinetics, cefixime has no advantage over other oral agents in treating CAP.

Dose: 400 mg once daily.

CEFPODOXIME PROXETIL (VANTIN)

Cefpodoxime proxetil, released in 1992, is highly stable against β-lactamases and has enhanced activity against EGNB compared with second-generation cephalosporins. In several randomized trials, cefpodoxime was comparable to other broad-spectrum oral agents (e.g., cefuroxime axetil, amoxicillin/clavulanate) for treatment of community-acquired bronchitis or pneumonia.

Dose: 200 mg b.i.d.

LORACARBEF (LORABID)

Loracarbef is the first of the carbacephem class of β-lactams. Its chemical structure is similar to cephalosporins, but the carbacephem ring is more stable than the cephalosporin ring. The activity of loracarbef is similar to other oral second-generation cephalosporins. In randomized trials, loracarbef 400 mg twice daily has been comparable to amoxicillin, cefaclor, and amoxicillin/clavulanate for acute bronchitis or mild CAP. Loracarbef is expensive and has no advantage over second- or third-generation oral cephalosporins.

Dose: 400 mg b.i.d.

Carbapenems

The carbapenems are a new class of β-lactams that differ from penicillins by the substitution of a carbon atom for sulphur at position 1 and an unsaturated bond between carbon atoms 2 and 3 in the five-membered ring. Carbapenems have unique side chains that confer resistance to a variety of β-lactamases and provide antipseudomonal activity.

IMIPENEM/CILASTATIN (PRIMAXIN)

Imipenem is the only carbapenem currently in clinical use. Because imipenem is hydrolyzed by renal dehydropeptidases, imipenem is combined with the dehydropeptidase inhibitor, cilastin. Imipenem/cilastin resists degradation by β-lactamases capable of hydrolyzing penicillins or cephalosporins and may be efficacious against organisms resistant to these agents. Imipenem is highly efficacious for diverse infections (including pneumonia) in both immunocompetent and immunocompromised hosts. In randomized trials, imipenem monotherapy for severe nosocomial pneumonia was associated with favorable responses in 56–84% of patients. These response rates were comparable to ceftazidime but slightly lower than ciprofloxacin. Imipenem monotherapy for *P. aeruginosa* pneumonia has been associated with a high rate of clinical failures, emergence of resistance, and relapse.

Antimicrobial Spectrum: Imipenem has the broadest spectrum of all β-lactams. Highly active against most Gram-positive cocci but not consistently active against enterococci or MRSA. Anaerobic activity (including *B. fragilis* species) is outstanding. Highly active against most EGNB, including *P. aeruginosa, Serratia* spp., and *Acinetobacter* spp. *P. cepacia* and *Xanthomonas maltophilia* are invariably resistant, however.

Toxicity: Imipenem induces seizures in less than 0.5% of patients, but the risk is higher among patients with renal failure or underlying CNS disease. Nausea is more common with imipenem compared with other β-lactams. Superinfection or colonization with *Xanthomonas maltophilia* or *Pseudomonas cepacia* complicates therapy in 1–3%.

Dosage: 0.5–1.0 IV q6h. (Higher doses for serious infections caused by *P. aeruginosa* or pathogens with a high MIC.)

Distinguishing Features: Imipenem penetrates well through the outer cell envelope of EGNB, has high affinity for PBP targets, and resists degradation by a wide variety of β-lactamases that hydrolyze penicillins, third-generation cephalosporins, and aztreonam. Imipenem is a powerful inducer of chromosomally mediated β-lactamases in *Enterobacter* and *P. aeruginosa*. Interestingly, these β-lactamases hydrolyze other β-lactams but do not affect imipenem. Overzealous use of imipenem may predispose to resistance with β-lactam-resistant organisms including *X. maltophilia, P. cepacia, P. aeruginosa, Acinetobacter* spp., and MRSA.

Indications

- Empiric therapy for severe nosocomial pneumonias in ICUs;
- Pneumonia in patients failing prior therapy with cephalosporins or extended-spectrum penicillins;
- Severe polymicrobial nosocomial pneumonia;
- Pneumonia caused by *P. aeruginosa* (combined with an aminoglycoside for synergy);
- Severe, life-threatening community- or nursing home-acquired pneumonias.

Because of its expense and potential CNS toxicity, imipenem is not indicated for uncomplicated CAP or nosocomial pneumonia susceptible to other β-lactams.

MEROPENEM (MERREM)

Meropenem is a new carbapenem recently approved by the Food and Drug Administration for treatment of adult and pediatric intraabdominal infections and pediatric meningitis. Its role as therapy for pneumonia is being evaluated in clinical trials in the United States. Meropenem is slightly less active than imipenem against Gram-positive organisms but slightly more active against EGNB; anaerobic activity is comparable. *Xanthomonas maltophilia* is usually resistant. Meropenem carries no definite risk of seizures and is a less potent inducer of β-lactamases than imipenem. Meropenem is stable to human renal dehydropeptidases and does not require concomitant administration of an enzyme inhibitor.

Monobactams

AZTREONAM (AZACTAM)

Aztreonam is the first of a generation of monobactams within the β-lactam group. Elimination of the second carbon ring leaves the β-lactam ring as a monocyclic compound. Aztreonam may be used safely in patients who are allergic to penicillins or cephalosporins because cross-reactivity does not occur. Monotherapy with aztreonam is highly effective for infections caused by EGNB but has been associated with a high rate of colonization or superinfections caused by Gram-positive cocci. Because of its narrow spectrum, aztreonam should not be used alone as therapy for pneumonia. For β-lactam allergic patients, aztreonam combined with clindamycin or vancomycin may be used as empiric treatment of nosocomial pneumonia.

Antimicrobial Spectrum: Highly active against aerobic EGNB, including most strains of *P. aeruginosa,* but no significant activity against Gram-positive cocci or anaerobes. Resists degradation by most plasmid- or chromosomally mediated β-lactamases and thus may be effective against EGNB resistant to penicillins or cephalosporins. Aztreonam may provide synergy with aminoglycosides and, in some cases, with other β-lactams.

Toxicity: Uncommon (less than 1% rash, less than 2% serious diarrhea).
Dosage: 1–2 gm q8h.

Indications

- Nosocomial pneumonia caused by aerobic EGNB;
- Pneumonia caused by susceptible pathogen in patients allergic to β-lactams;
- Empiric therapy for serious nosocomial pneumonia (should be combined with clindamycin or vancomycin to cover Gram-positive cocci);
- Alternative agents are preferred for CAP (activity against *S. pneumoniae* is minimal).

Note: A high rate of superinfections with Gram-positive organisms has been noted with aztreonam monotherapy for pneumonia.

Aminoglycosides

Aminoglycosides currently used in the United States include gentamicin, tobramycin, and amikacin. The role of aminoglycosides for pneumonia is controversial. Several factors argue against their use: high toxicity (nephrotoxicity/ototoxicity); low penetration into bronchial secretions and lung tissue; inactivation at low pH (conditions that may prevail in infected lung parenchyma); and the availability of alternative broad-spectrum agents with Gram-negative activity and less toxicity (e.g., β-lactams, quinolones). Despite these arguments, aminoglycosides are useful as adjunctive therapy (combined with a β-lactam or quinolones), primarily to achieve synergistic killing. In a nonrandomized study of *P. aeruginosa* bacteremia, mortality was significantly lower with the combination of an antipseudomonal β-lactam plus an aminoglycoside (27% mortality), compared with the β-lactam alone (47% mortality). This survival advantage was even greater among patients with pneumonia or in an ICU. Several studies have noted high rates of clinical and microbiologic failures and relapses when monotherapy is used for *P. aeruginosa* pneumonia, even when the organisms are susceptible. The synergistic killing achieved with the aminoglycosides may be important for highly virulent pathogens with high MICs but is not necessary for more susceptible pathogens. Theoretically, the use of combination therapy may reduce the emergence of resistance, although this has not yet been verified in clinical studies.

Antimicrobial Spectrum: Exceptionally broad-spectrum against aerobic EGNB; no significant activity against anaerobes. When combined with β-lactams, may confer synergistic killing against enterococci and staphylococci.

Toxicity: Nephrotoxicity and ototoxicity are most important. Risk factors for nephrotoxicity include old age, prior aminoglycoside use, preexisting renal disease, and the use of other nephrotoxic drugs concomitantly. Toxicities of tobramycin and gentamicin are comparable; both are slightly more nephrotoxic than amikacin or netilmicin. Netilmicin shows the least ototoxicity. Peak and trough serum levels are mandatory to limit toxicity. Peak levels exceeding 6 μg/mL are required for optimal microbicidal activity; trough levels greater than 2 μg/mL correlate with excessive toxicity.

Dosage: 3 mg/kg/day IV in divided doses q12h for gentamicin or tobramycin; 15 mg/kg/day for amikacin. Dose may need to be adjusted according to peak and trough serum levels. Recent studies suggest that once-daily dosing may be as effective and no more toxic (and possibly less toxic) than more frequent dosing regimens. Once-daily dosing would reduce pharmacy and nursing time and costs. Additional studies are required to evaluate the optimal aminoglycoside dosing regimen.

Nebulized Administration: Klastersky and colleagues suggested that nebulized or intratracheal aminoglycosides may improve outcome for Gram-negative lower respiratory infections. Despite extensive use of nebulized aminoglycosides for *P. aeruginosa* infections in patients with cystic fibrosis and for nosocomial Gram-negative pneumonia, no solid data affirm the efficacy of this practice. In 1990, a double-blind randomized trial in patients with Gram-negative pneumonia, intratracheal tobramycin (40 mg q8h) was no more effective than placebo in influencing clinical outcome or mortality. Parenteral β-lactam and aminoglycoside antibiotics were administered concomitantly in both groups. High-dose nebulized aminoglycosides may transiently improve symptoms and reduce bacillary load in patients with cystic fibrosis, but the impact in other patient populations is unknown. Currently, we do not use nebulized or intratracheal aminoglycosides for community- or hospital-acquired pneumonia.

Special Considerations: Gentamicin is less expensive than other aminoglycosides and is preferred unless high rates of gentamicin resistance are suspected or confirmed in the institution. Tobramycin and gentamicin are equivalent for most bacteria. For *P. aeruginosa,* MICs may be slightly lower with tobramycin than with gentamicin. Gentamicin is more active against enterococci and *S. aureus.* Amikacin is expensive and should be reserved for isolates resistant to tobramycin and gentamicin.

Indications: Aminoglycosides are inadequate as monotherapy for pneumonia but are important as adjunctive therapy in the following circumstances:

- Therapy for serious sepsis or nosocomial pneumonias caused by EGNB;
- Pneumonia caused by *Pseudomonas* spp., *Serratia,* and *Acinetobacter* spp.;
- Infections caused by enterococci (combine with penicillin or vancomycin);
- Rarely necessary for community- or nursing home-acquired pneumonias.

Macrolides

The macrolides are a class of antimicrobials characterized by substituted 14-, 15-, or 16-member rings; macrolides penetrate into tissues better than β-lactams. Erythromycin (a 14-member macrolide) was the first antibiotic of this class. Several newer 14-member macrolides with a spectrum of activity similar to erythromycin but with fewer side effects have been synthesized. Clarithromycin, azithromycin, and dirithromycin are currently available in the United States. Roxithromycin, erythromycylamine, and flurithromycin have not yet been released.

ERYTHROMYCIN

Erythromycin, first isolated in 1952, has been used extensively for community-acquired bronchitis and pneumonia for more than three decades. Erythromycin is adequate for CAP in otherwise healthy patients without risk factors for EGNB but is not adequate as monotherapy for patients with serious coexisting diseases. Erythromycin has no role in nosocomial pneumonia except when Legionellae are suspected. Its usefulness is limited by toxicity (primarily nausea and gastrointestinal symptoms).

Mechanism of Action: Interferes with microbial protein synthesis at the ribosomal level (binds to 50S ribosome subunit).

Antimicrobial Spectrum: Highly active against *S. pneumoniae, M. catarrhalis, Mycoplasma, Chlamydia,* and *Legionella* spp. Erythromycin-resistant *S. pneumoniae,* a rarity a decade ago, have been noted in 1–6% of isolates in recent studies. Erythromycin is less active than penicillins against other streptococci. Anaerobic coverage is modest (10–20% of oral anaerobes and 30–40% of *B. fragilis* are resistant). Not reliable against *S. aureus* or *S. epidermidis* (10–40% of strains are resistant). Only 40–70% of *H. influenzae* are susceptible. No significant activity against EGNB.

Toxicity: Gastrointestinal side effects (principally nausea, epigastric distress, diarrhea, and vomiting) occur in more than 20% of patients and limit its usefulness. Intravenous erythromycin is intensely irritating to veins and may cause phlebitis. Hepatotoxicity (cholestatic hepatitis) is a rare complication with the estolate form; this usually resolves with cessation of therapy.

Dosage: Intravenous dose: 500–1,000 mg q6h. Oral dose: 250–500 mg q6h. For serious infections, IV administration is recommended initially. Oral therapy may be substituted once clinical improvement has occurred.

Indications

- Bronchitis or pneumonia caused by *S. pneumoniae, Legionella, Chlamydia,* or *Mycoplasma;*
- Empiric therapy for CAP among young, previously healthy adults;
- Not adequate as monotherapy for CAP in patients at risk for EGNB;
- Nosocomial pneumonias caused by *Legionella* spp. (Add rifampin for fulminant or life-threatening cases.)

NEWER MACROLIDES

The newer macrolides currently available in the United States are clarithromycin, azithromycin, and dirithomycin. These agents require less frequent dosing and are better tolerated than erythromycin. The newer macrolides do not form the anhydrohemiketal degradation product implicated as the cause of gastrointestinal side effects seen with erythromycin. Because of their low toxicity, these agents (particularly clarithromycin and azithromycin) have supplanted erythromycin for many upper and lower respiratory tract infections caused by erythromycin-susceptible organisms.

CLARITHROMYCIN (BIAXIN)

Clarithromycin (Biaxin), introduced into the United States in 1991, may be used to treat upper or lower respiratory tract infections caused by susceptible pathogens. In randomized trials, clarithromycin was as effective as oral β-lactams or erythromycin for community-acquired bronchitis, sinusitis, or pneumonia. Clarithromycin is highly efficacious for infections caused by *Mycoplasma pneumoniae* or *C. pneumoniae*. Clarithromycin (dose 500 to 1000 mg twice daily) may be adequate for *Legionella* pneumonia, but data are limited.

Antimicrobial Spectrum: Retains the antimicrobial activity of erythromycin. The activity of clarithromycin and its 14-OH metabolite is additive against *H. influenzae*. No significant activity against EGNB.

Toxicity: Much less toxic than erythromycin; gastrointestinal adverse effects in 3–6%.

Dosage: 250–500 mg b.i.d. for 7–14 days (21 days for legionellosis).

Indications

- Bronchitis or pneumonia caused by *S. pneumoniae, H. influenzae, Legionella, Chlamydia,* or *Mycoplasma* spp.;
- Empiric therapy for CAP among young, previously healthy adults;
- Not adequate as monotherapy for CAP in patients with serious coexisting disease;
- May be added in hospitalized patients receiving parenteral β-lactams for CAP (to provide coverage against atypicals);
- No role in nosocomial pneumonia.

DIRITHROMYCIN (DYNABAC)

Dirithromycin (Dynabac) was approved by the FDA in 1995 as treatment for community-acquired bronchitis or pneumonia caused by *S. pneumoniae, Mycoplasma pneumoniae,* and *Legionella* spp. but not *H. influenzae*. Dirithomycin was comparable to erythromycin (dose 250 mg q.i.d.) in two large trials of CAP and was comparable to clarithromycin in a series of 191 patients with acute exacerbations of chronic bronchitis. Its lack of consistent activity against *H. influenzae* makes dirithromycin less attractive than clarithromycin or azithromycin for empiric therapy of CAP or bronchitis.

Antimicrobial Spectrum: Similar to erythromycin. Many strains of *H. influenzae* are resistant.

Toxicity: Similar to erythromycin, but probably fewer gastrointestinal side effects (less than 10%).

Dosage: 500 mg once daily for 7–14 days (21 days for legionellosis).

AZALIDES

The addition of a nitrogen atom to the macrolide ring (resulting in a 15-member ring) results in azalides that are far more resistant to acid hydrolysis than erythromycin or other macrolides. Azalides have greater penetration into tissues, a larger volume of distribution, and a longer half-life (more than 2 days) compared with other macrolides, β-lactams, or quinolone antibiotics. Azithromycin is the first azalide released, but several other agents are currently being studied.

AZITHROMYCIN (ZITHROMAX)

Azithromycin was released in the United States in 1992 and has been equivalent to oral β-lactams or erythromycin for treatment of bronchitis or mild to moderate CAP.

Azithromycin may be effective against *Mycoplasma* spp. and was curative in all 43 patients with *Mycoplasma pneumoniae* pneumonia in one study. Azithromycin is active against *Chlamydia* or Legionellae, but clinical data in vivo are limited.

Antimicrobial Spectrum: Bactericidal against erythromycin-sensitive streptococci and staphylococci, but slightly less active than erythromycin. Not active against erythromycin-resistant strains. MRSA and enterococci are resistant. Activity against anaerobes slightly better than erythromycin. Oral anaerobes are readily inhibited; activity against *B. fragilis* is marginal. Azithromycin is bactericidal against *H. influenzae, Neisseria* spp., and *M. catarrhalis*. Activity against *Mycoplasma pneumoniae* is similar to erythromycin. Excellent against Legionellae or *Chlamydiae* spp. but less active than clarithromycin.

Toxicity: Minor, primarily gastrointestinal (3–5%).

Dosage: 500 mg initial dose, then 250 mg once daily for 4 additional days.

Distinguishing Features: Azithromycin is more acid stable, better absorbed, and has a longer half-life than erythromycin. Azithromycin is concentrated in phagocytes and within tissues for prolonged periods. Levels of azithromycin in sputum, bronchial mucosa, and alveolar macrophages may exceed the MIC for most common respiratory pathogens for 2–4 days following a single 500-mg oral dose.

Indications

- Similar to erythromycin and clarithromycin;
- May be added in hospitalized patients receiving parenteral β-lactams for CAP (to provide coverage against atypicals);
- Not appropriate for nosocomial pneumonia.

Tetracyclines

Tetracyclines, derived from *Streptomyces* spp., were isolated in the early 1950s. Substitutions on the hydronaphthacene four-ringed nucleus differentiate the derivatives tetracycline hydrochloride, oxytetracycline, chlortetracycline, doxycycline, and minocycline. Tetracyclines are inexpensive and effective agents for bronchitis or pneumonia caused by *Mycoplasma pneumoniae* or *Chlamydia* spp. Because of the narrow spectrum, the role of tetracyclines in pneumonia is limited.

Mechanism of Action: Bind to 30S subunit of bacterial ribosomes.

Antimicrobial Spectrum: Active against most streptococci, but 10–20% of *S. pneumoniae* are resistant. Not adequate for *S. aureus* or enterococci. Anaerobic activity is modest (*B. fragilis* spp. are resistant). Marginal against *H. influenzae;* not active against aerobic EGNB. Drug of choice for *Chlamydia* and *Rickettsiae* spp.; acceptable for *Mycoplasma* and *Legionella* spp.

Toxicity: Gastrointestinal (nausea, emesis, GI distress) symptoms are common; photosensitivity (doxycycline or minocycline); discoloration of teeth or depression of bone growth in infants and children; vertigo. Outdated tetracyclines may cause renal tubular acidosis. Fatal hepatotoxicity has rarely been described.

Dosage: 250–500 mg orally q.i.d. for tetracycline, oxytetracycline, and chlortetracycline; doxycycline and minocycline 100 mg b.i.d. (oral or IV). Food binds the drug and impairs absorption; tetracyclines should be taken on an empty stomach. This effect is less problematic with doxycycline or minocycline.

Indications

- Pulmonary infections caused by *Chlamydia* or *Mycoplasma* spp.;
- Alternative to erythromycin for infections caused by Legionellae;
- Suboptimal for pneumoniae caused by *S. pneumoniae;*
- Not suitable for empiric therapy of CAP because of significant gaps in the spectrum;
- No role for nosocomial pneumonia.

Fluoroquinolones

Fluoroquinolones are derivatives of nalidixic acid and include norfloxacin, ofloxacin, ciprofloxacin, lomefloxacin, enoxacin, perfloxacin, and levofloxacin. Currently, only ciprofloxacin, norfloxacin, ofloxacin, and lomefloxacin are available in the United States. Norfloxacin is recommended only for urinary sepsis or prophylaxis. Ciprofloxacin and ofloxacin are efficacious in treating both community- and hospital-acquired pneumonias and extrapulmonary infections. Lomefloxacin may be used for bronchitis, but data on pneumonia are limited.

Antimicrobial Spectrum: Excellent potency against aerobic GNB, including most Enterobacteriaceae, *H. influenzae, Neisseria* spp., *M. catarrhalis,* and *P. aeruginosa;* less active against *P. cepacia* or *Xanthomonas maltophilia.* Good activity against *S. aureus* and *S. epidermidis,* but less active against streptococci (including *S. pneumoniae*). Minimal activity against anaerobes.

Distinguishing Features: Fluoroquinolones (with the exception of norfloxacin) achieve high concentrations in the lung, bronchial mucosa, and sputum; concentrations in the lung typically exceed serum concentrations. Concentration of quinolones in phagocytes may enhance clinical efficacy.

Mechanism of Action of Quinolones: Antagonizes bacterial DNA gyrase (interferes with DNA replication).

Antimicrobial Resistance: Resistance to quinolones can be mediated by mutations affecting DNA gyrase or drug permeability, or both. Plasmid-mediated resistance has not been observed. Chromosomal mutations that alter DNA gyrase confer resistance to quinolones alone. Changes in the bacterial outer membrane proteins confer resistance to multiple agents (including β-lactams). Resistance to *P. aeruginosa* requires multiple mutations; a single-step mutation may be sufficient to induce resistance against *S. aureus.*

CIPROFLOXACIN (CIPRO)

Ciprofloxacin was released in the United States in 1987 as the first oral antibiotic with activity against *P. aeruginosa.* By 1989, ciprofloxacin was the fourth most commonly prescribed antibiotic (more than 5 million prescriptions at a cost of $248 million). Ciprofloxacin has been extensively used to treat community-acquired, nursing home-acquired, and hospital-acquired pneumonias, and serious nosocomial infections and is as effective as broad-spectrum β-lactams. In several randomized trials of mild to moderate community- or nursing home-acquired pneumonias, ciprofloxacin was as effective as ceftazidime (more than 90% cures). In a recent multicenter randomized trial, ciprofloxacin (400 mg q8h) was superior to imipenem (1 gm q8h) for severe nosocomial pneumonia (clinical responses in 69% and 59%, respectively). Other investigators have noted cure rates exceeding 60% with ciprofloxacin monotherapy for severe nosocomial pneumonia failing prior antimicrobial therapy. Ciprofloxacin has excellent in vitro activity against *Mycoplasma pneumoniae, Legionella* spp., and *Chlamydia* spp., and anecdotal successes have been noted in open trials. Substitution of ciprofloxacin for parenteral agents is effective for both community-acquired and nosocomial pneumonias and may reduce duration of hospitalization and costs.

Antimicrobial Spectrum: Excellent activity against *H. influenzae, M. catarrhalis, Chlamydia, Legionella* spp., and aerobic EGNB (including *P. aeruginosa* and Enterobacteriaceae). Excellent against *S. aureus,* including some strains of MRSA. Marginal activity against *S. pneumoniae* and group A streptococci. Poor anaerobic activity.

Toxicity: Uncommon; GI symptoms in 3–6%; headache, dizziness, or sleep disturbance occur in 1–2%; rash, in 0.5–2%. Not recommended in children or during pregnancy.

Dosage: 200–400 mg IV q12h (doses of 400 mg q8h for organisms with a low MIC). Oral dose is 500–750 mg b.i.d.

Antimicrobial Resistance: Resistance to ciprofloxacin (particularly *S. aureus* and *P. aeruginosa*) may develop rapidly with ciprofloxacin. Risk factors for emergence of resistance include prior antimicrobial therapy, lower respiratory tract infection in the ICU, monotherapy for *P. aeruginosa,* cystic fibrosis, infections in sequestered areas (e.g., osteomyelitis), and long-term prophylaxis. Fluoroquinolone resistance has increased dramatically to *P. aeruginosa* and *S. aureus.* Although a recent survey noted resistance in fewer than 4% of Enterobacteriaceae and 1.6% of *E. coli* in the United States, resistance rates exceeding 35% have been cited in Europe following liberal use of fluoroquinolone prophylaxis. Because of the potential for emergence of antimicrobial resistance, one should be cautious about using ciprofloxacin for infections that can readily be treated with β-lactam antibiotics. Whether combining ciprofloxacin with an additional antibiotic limits or reduces the emergence of resistance is not known.

- Antimicrobial resistance may develop rapidly with monotherapy (particularly among *S. aureus* and *P. aeruginosa*).

Indications

- Nursing-home or nosocomial pneumonias provided *S. pneumoniae* has been reasonably excluded;
- Oral "step-down" therapy in hospitalized patients receiving parenteral agents (for susceptible pathogens);
- Nursing-home or nosocomial pneumonia in patients unable to tolerate β-lactams

or with organisms resistant to β-lactams. For polymicrobial pneumonias, consider adding metronidazole or clindamycin for anaerobic coverage;
- An alternative to macrolides for infections caused by Legionellae (data in vivo limited);
- Not optimal for infections caused by streptococci (including S. pneumoniae);
- Not optimal for lung abscess or aspiration pneumonia (poor activity against anaerobes).

OFLOXACIN (FLOXIN)

Ofloxacin, released in 1990, has been successfully used to treat community- or hospital-acquired pneumonia or sepsis in both immunocompetent and immunocompromised hosts. In randomized trials, ofloxacin was as effective as β-lactams, doxycycline, TMP/SMX, or erythromycin for community-acquired bronchitis or pneumonia. Ofloxacin is effective as step-down therapy in patients with community- or hospital-acquired pneumonia receiving parenteral β-lactams (provided the organisms are susceptible).

Antimicrobial Spectrum: More active than ciprofloxacin against streptococci (including S. pneumoniae) but less active against P. aeruginosa. Otherwise, antimicrobial spectrum is similar to ciprofloxacin.

Toxicity: Similar to ciprofloxacin; few serious adverse effects. Unlike ciprofloxacin, no effect on theophylline.

Dosage: Oral 400 mg q12h (98% bioavailability); IV 400 mg q12h.

Antimicrobial Resistance: As with other fluoroquinolones, resistance may be problematic with ofloxacin (particularly with P. aeruginosa and S. aureus).

Indications
- Nursing-home pneumonias (more active than ciprofloxacin against S. pneumoniae);
- Oral "step-down" therapy in hospitalized patients receiving parenteral agents;
- Nosocomial pneumonia (nonICU) in patients unable to tolerate β-lactams or with organisms resistant to β-lactams;
- For nosocomial pneumonias in the ICU, ciprofloxacin is preferred because of its superior activity against P. aeruginosa;
- An alternative to macrolides for infections caused by Legionellae (data in vivo limited);
- Not optimal for lung abscess or aspiration pneumonia (poor activity against anaerobes).

LOMEFLOXACIN (MAXAQUIN)

Lomefloxacin, a difluoroquinolone with broad-spectrum activity against both Gram-positive and Gram-negative pathogens, has a prolonged half-life, permitting once-daily dosing. Lomefloxacin is effective for acute exacerbations of chronic bronchitis caused by H. influenza or M. catarrhalis; its efficacy against S. pneumoniae has not been established. Multicenter trials in Europe in patients with acute exacerbations of chronic bronchitis noted clinical and bacteriologic cures in more than 80% of patients. When *P. aeruginosa* was isolated, eradication rates ranged from 50 to 77%. Limited data are available for pneumonia.

Antimicrobial Spectrum: Slightly less active against Gram-positive cocci than ciprofloxacin or ofloxacin. Anaerobic activity is modest. Less active against *P. aeruginosa* and EGNB than ciprofloxacin or ofloxacin.

Toxicity: Similar to the other fluoroquinolones.

Dosage: 400 mg once daily for bronchitis.

Indications

* Acute exacerbations of chronic bronchitis caused by susceptible pathogens;
* Not recommended for infections caused by *S. pneumoniae;*
* Not recommended for nosocomial pneumonia.

Other Agents

CHLORAMPHENICOL (CHLOROMYCETIN)

Chloramphenicol was an enormously popular antibiotic in the 1950s because of its broad-spectrum activity against anaerobes, Gram-positive cocci, and selected EGNB. Rare complications of aplastic anemia and the "grey baby syndrome" led to a dramatic decline in prescriptions for this agent in the 1960s. Currently, chloramphenicol is rarely used.

Mechanism of Action: Binds to 50S subunit of the 70S bacterial ribosome (blocks the attachment of aminotransfer RNA to the ribosomes).

Antimicrobial Spectrum: Broad-spectrum agent but other antimicrobials preferred for common pathogens. Excellent activity against unusual pathogens that are resistant to most antimicrobials (e.g., *Rickettsieae, Pseudomonas pseudomallei, P. cepacia,* and *Salmonella typhi*).

Toxicity: Aplastic anemia (less than 1:20,000 cases); dose-related myelosuppression; hemolytic anemia; grey baby syndrome in infants; reversible neurologic dysfunction.

Dosage: 100 mg/kg orally or IV.

Indications

* Restricted to infections resistant to alternative agents (*Rickettsieae, Pseudomonas pseudomallei, P. cepacia,* or *Salmonella typhi*).

TRIMETHOPRIM/SULFAMETHOXAZOLE (BACTRIM, SEPTRA; CO-TRIMOXAZOLE)

Trimethoprim/sulfamethoxazole (TMP/SMX), formulated as a fixed ratio of 1:5 TMP/SMX, was first introduced in the United States in 1973. TMP/SMX is used principally to treat infections caused by *Pneumocystis carinii* or *Nocardia* spp. but has a wide spectrum of activity against Gram-positive and Gram-negative organisms. TMP/SMX has been extensively used to treat bronchitis with success comparable to β-lactam and macrolide antibiotics. Few studies have assessed TMP/SMX as primary therapy for bacterial pneumonia.

Mechanism of Action: TMP and SMX interfere with bacterial cell replication by inhibiting sequential enzymes involved in the formation of tetrahydrofolic acid. The inhibition of differing enzyme steps improves antimicrobial activity and confers synergistic killing.

Antimicrobial Spectrum: Excellent activity against most Gram-positive organisms, including streptococci and staphylococci (including some MRSA). Not adequate against group A streptococci or enterococci. Recent studies have cited resistance rates of 10–20% among *S. pneumoniae.* Active against more than 99% *M. catarrhalis* and 80% of *H. influenzae.* Anaerobes are usually susceptible in vitro, but clinical data are limited. Excellent activity against Enterobacteriaceae and EGNB but *P. aeruginosa* is usually resistant. Usually active against *P. cepacia, P. pseudomallei, Xanthomonas maltophilia, Citrobacter,* and *Acinetobacter* spp. (pathogens that are often resistant to third-generation cephalosporins). Excellent activity against *Legionella* spp. in vitro and in animal models but data in humans are lacking.

Toxicity: Skin rash (3%) (usually minor); exfoliative dermatitis (Stevens-Johnson syndrome) or erythema multiforme rare (less than 1:10,000); excessive fluid when administered IV in high doses; nausea or gastrointestinal symptoms (3–10%); may contribute to marrow toxicity in patients with hematologic neoplasia or underlying marrow disorder; substantial increase in side effects in patients with acquired immunodeficiency syndrome (AIDS).

Dosage: One double-strength tablet twice daily for bronchitis; 2 ampules q8h IV for pneumonia. Single-strength tablets (80 mg TMP; 400 mg SMX) or double-strength (160/800) for oral use. For parenteral administration, 1 ampule (5 mL) contains 80 mg TMP and 400 mg SMX.

Indications

• Despite excellent in vitro susceptibility profile, limited data for pneumonia;
• Ideal for community-acquired bronchitis (because of broad spectrum and low cost);
• Acceptable for CAP or nosocomial pneumonias in patients intolerant of β-lactams.

CLINDAMYCIN (CLEOCIN)

Clindamycin, a derivative of lincomycin, has outstanding activity against anaerobes and most aerobic Gram-positive cocci (with the exception of MRSA) but lacks activity against aerobic EGNB. Because of its narrow spectrum, clindamycin has a limited role in treating pneumonia.

Mechanism of Action: Binds to 50S subunit of bacterial ribosomes and suppresses intracellular protein synthesis. Clindamycin, erythromycin, and chloramphenicol act at the same site and antagonize each other.

Antimicrobial Spectrum: Highly active against anaerobes, most streptococci (including *S. pneumoniae*), and methicillin-sensitive *S. aureus.* Enterococci and MRSA are resistant. No significant activity against aerobic EGNB, *Mycoplasma, Chlamydia,* or *Legionella* spp.

Toxicity: Skin rash (5–10%); diarrhea (2–10%); pseudomembranous colitis no more common with clindamycin than with many other antibiotics; metallic taste in mouth with IV administration (4%).

Dosage: 150–450 mg t.i.d. (orally); maximal IV dose 900 mg q8h, but 600 mg q8h is usually adequate even for serious infections. Dose must be reduced in renal failure.

Indications

- Primary therapy for community-acquired lung abscess or aspiration pneumonia;
- Nosocomial pneumonia in patients allergic to β-lactams (combine with aztreonam or a fluoroquinolone);
- Not recommended for CAP (β-lactams or macrolides are preferred).

METRONIDAZOLE (FLAGYL)

Metronidazole, a nitroimidazole introduced in 1957 to treat parasitic diseases, has been used successfully for more than three decades to treat anaerobic bacterial infections in abdominal, pelvic, and extrapulmonary sites. The role of metronidazole in pulmonary infections is controversial. A high rate of failures was noted with metronidazole as monotherapy for lung abscess or aspiration pneumonia, suggesting its lack of activity against aerobes and EGNB limit its utility in pleuropulmonary infections.

Mechanism of Action: Enters bacterial cell; reduction of the nitro group of the drug releases toxic intermediates and free radicals that damage bacterial DNA and other macromolecules.

Antimicrobial Spectrum: Limited to obligate anaerobes; lacks activity against aerobic Gram-positive organisms or EGNB.

Toxicity: Minor; gastrointestinal effects most common; CNS toxicity or peripheral neuropathy (rare); disulfiram-like effects in patients ingesting alcohol.

Dosage: Loading dose of 15 mg/kg (or 1,000 mg) IV, then 7.5 mg/kg q6h. Oral dose is 500 mg t.i.d.

Indications

- No role as monotherapy for either CAP or nosocomial pneumonia;
- Adjunctive therapy in polymicrobial aspiration pneumonia (combine with a β-lactam or fluoroquinolone);
- Community-acquired lung abscess (combine with penicillin for aerobic streptococci).

VANCOMYCIN (VANCOCIN)

Vancomycin, a glycopeptide initially isolated from *Streptomyces orientalis,* has been used since 1956 to treat staphylococcal infections. Vancomycin use declined following the introduction of methicillin but has surged dramatically over the past decade concomitant with an increased incidence of MRSA and Gram-positive bacteremias. At one university hospital, the use of parenteral vancomycin increased 161-fold from 1978 to 1992, only one-third of which was for culture-proven Gram-positive infections. Unfortunately, liberal use of vancomycin for less than rigorous indications may promote resistance.

Mechanism of Action: Multiple mechanisms include: inhibits bacterial cell wall (glycopeptide) synthesis; interferes with RNA synthesis; alters permeability of bacterial cell membrane.

Antimicrobial Spectrum: Exceptionally active against aerobic Gram-positive cocci. Bactericidal against aerobic Gram-positive organisms (*Staphylococcus epidermidis* and *S. aureus,* including MRSA), diphtheroids (e.g., *Corynebacteria*), streptococci (including all *S. pneumoniae*), and *Clostridia* spp.; bacteriostatic against enterococci. No significant activity against EGNB, anaerobes, *Mycoplasma, Chlamydia,* or *Legionella* spp.

Toxicity: Phlebitis (more than 10% in some series); maculopapular or erythematous rash (4–5%); hearing loss with high serum levels; "red man's syndrome" (erythematous flushing of the torso, neck, and face associated with pruritus, hypotension, and, rarely, cardiac arrest caused by histamine release). Nephrotoxicity is rare.

Dosage: Loading dose 15 mg/kg IV; then 500–1,000 mg q12h. Administer slowly over 60 minutes; more rapid infusion rates may be associated with red man's syndrome, pain, or hypotension. Substantial dose reductions required in renal failure. In the presence of renal failure, serum levels should be monitored (aim for peak serum concentrations of 20 to 40 μg/mL two hours postcompletion of infusion; trough levels, of 5 to 10 μg/mL). Intramuscular route not available. Oral administration does not provide adequate tissue or serum levels.

Indications

- Not adequate as empiric therapy for pneumonia (because of narrow spectrum);
- Proven or suspected infections caused by Gram-positive cocci resistant to β-lactams;
- Drug of choice for pneumonia caused by MRSA;
- Pneumonia caused by penicillin-resistant *S. pneumoniae;*
- Enterococcal infections (combine with gentamicin for bactericidal activity);
- Pneumonia failing broad-spectrum antibiotics when Gram-positive cocci are suspected.

Special Considerations: Antimicrobial resistance to vancomycin has increased dramatically in the past decade, particularly among enterococci. Risk factors for acquisition of vancomycin-resistant enterococci include residence in an ICU, serious underlying disease or debilitation, prolonged hospital stay, and prior therapy with vancomycin or multiple antimicrobials. Although enterococci rarely cause pneumonia, these resistance trends are worrisome because vancomycin-resistant genes present in Enterococci theoretically could be transferred to other Gram-positive cocci (including MRSA). Thus we reserve vancomycin for serious infections caused by Gram-positive cocci resistant or allergic to β-lactam antibiotics.

BIBLIOGRAPHY
Community-Acquired Pneumonia

Bartlett JG, Mundy LM. Community-acquired pneumonia. N Engl J Med 1996;333: 1618–1623.

Bates JH, Campbell GD, Barron AL, et al. Microbial etiology of acute pneumonia in hospitalized patients. Chest 1992;101:1005–1112.

British Thoracic Society Research Committee and the Public Health Laboratory Service. The aetiology, management, and outcome of severe community-acquired pneumonia in the intensive care unit. Respir Med 1992;86:7–13.

Campbell GD. Overview of community-acquired pneumonia: prognosis and clinical features. Med Clin North Am 1994;78:1035–1048.

Fine MF, Singer DE, Hanusa BH, Lave JR, Kapoor WN. Validation of a pneumonia prognostic index using the MedisGroups comparative hospital database. Am J Med 1993;94:153–159.

Gilbert K, Fine MJ. Assessing prognosis and predicting patient outcomes in community-acquired pneumonia. Semin Respir Infect 1994;9:140–152.

Koivula I, Sten M, Makela PH. Risk factors for pneumonia in the elderly. Am J Med 1994; 96:313–320.

Mandell LA. Community-acquired pneumonia: etiology, epidemiology, and treatment. Chest 1995;108:35S–42S.

Marrie TJ. Community-acquired pneumonia. Clin Infect Dis 1995;18:501–515.

Mcfarlane J. An overview of community-acquired pneumonia with lessons learned from the British Thoracic Society Study. Semin Respir Infect 1994;9:153–165.

Mundy LM, Auwaerter PG, Oldach D, Warner ML, et al. Community-acquired pneumonia: impact of immune status. Am J Respir Crit Care Med 1995;142:1309–1315.

Rice TL, Odeh R, Lynch JP III. Community-acquired pneumonia: examining the role of new oral antibiotics. Hosp Formul 1994;29:816–827.

Weingarten SA, Riedinger MS, Hobson P, Noah MS, et al. Evaluation of a pneumonia practice guideline in an interventional trial. Am J Respir Crit Care Med 1996;153:1110–1115.

Woodhead MA, Arrowsmith J, Chamberlain-Webber R, Wooding S, Williams I. The value of routine microbial investigation in community-acquired pneumonia. Respir Med 1991; 85:313–317.

Severe Community-Acquired Pneumonia Requiring Mechanical Ventilatory Support or ICU

Moine P, Vercken JB, Chevret S, et al. Severe community-acquired pneumonia: etiology, epidemiology, and prognostic factors. Chest 1994;105:1487–1495.

Rello J, Quintana E, Ausina V, Net A, Prats G. A three-year study of severe community-acquired pneumonia with emphasis on outcome. Chest 1993;103:232–235.

Bacterial Pneumonia Complicating HIV

Caiaffa WT, Vlahov D, Graham NM, Astemborski J, et al. Drug smoking, *Pneumocystis carinii* pneumonia, and immunosuppression increase risk of bacterial pneumonia in human immunodeficiency virus-seropositive injection drug users. Am J Respir Crit Care Med 1994;150:1493–1498.

Caiaffa WT, Graham NM, Vlahov D. Bacterial pneumonia in adult patients with human immunodeficiency virus (HIV) infection. Am J Epidemiol 1993;138:909–922.

Hirschtick RE, Glassroth J, Jordan MC, Wilcosky TC, et al. Bacterial pneumonia in persons infected with the human immunodeficiency virus. N Engl J Med 1995;333:845–851.

Keller DW, Breiman RF. Preventing bacterial respiratory tract infections among persons infected with human immunodeficiency virus. Clin Infect Dis 1995;21(suppl 1):S77–S83.

Guidelines for Initial Therapy of CAP

American Thoracic Society. Guidelines for the initial management of adults with community-acquired pneumonia: diagnosis, assessment of severity, and initial antimicrobial therapy. Am Rev Respir Dis 1993;148:1418–1428.

British Thoracic Society. Guidelines for the management of community-acquired pneumonia in adults admitted to the hospital. Br J Hosp Med 1993;49:346–350.

Fein AM, Niederman MS. Guidelines for the initial management of community-acquired pneumonia: savory recipe or cookbook for disaster? Am J Respir Crit Care Med 1995; 152:1149–1153.

Mandell LA, Niederman MS. The Canadian Community-Acquired Pneumonia Consensus Group. Antimicrobial treatment of community-acquired pneumonia in adults: a conference report. Can J Infect Dis 1993;4:25–28.

Community-Acquired Pneumonia: Radiographic Resolution

Mittle RL Jr, Schwab RJ, Duchin JS, Goin JE, Albelda SM, Miller WT. Radiographic resolution of community-acquired pneumonia. Am J Respir Crit Care Med 1994;149:630–635.

Hospital-Acquired Pneumonia

Overview and Epidemiology

Campbell GD, Niderman MS, Broughton WA, Craven DE, et al. Hospital-acquired pneumonia in adults: diagnosis, assessment of severity, initial antimicrobial therapy, and preventative strategies. A Consensus Statement. Am J Respir Crit Care Med 1996;153:1711–1725.

Chastre J, Fagon JV, Trouillet JL. Diagnosis and treatment of nosocomial pneumonia in patients in intensive care units. Clin Infect Dis 1995;21(suppl 3):S226–S237.

Fagon JY, Chastre J, Hance AJ, Montravers P, Novara A, Gibert C. Nosocomial pneumonia in ventilated patients: a cohort study evaluating attributable mortality and hospital stay. Am J Med 1993;94:281–288.

George DL. Epidemiology of nosocomial pneumonia in intensive care unit patients. Clin Chest Med 1995;16:29–44.

George DL. Epidemiology of nosocomial ventilator-associated pneumonia. Infect Control Hosp Epidemiol 1993;14:163–169.

Lynch JP III, Watts CW. Nosocomial pneumonia in the ICU: current treatment strategies. J Crit Illness 1995;10:332–353.

Maloney SA, Jarvis WR. Epidemic nosocomial pneumonia in the intensive care unit. Clin Chest Med 1995;16:209–224.

Prod-hom G, Leuenberger P, Koerfer J, Blum A, Chiolero R, Schaller MD, et al. Nosocomial pneumonia in mechanically ventilated patients receiving antacid, ranitidine, or sucralfate as prophylaxis for stress ulcer: a randomized controlled trial. Ann Intern Med 1994;120: 653–662.

Rello J, Ausina V, Ricart M, Castella J, Prats G. Impact of previous antimicrobial therapy on the etiology and outcome of ventilator-associated pneumonia. Chest 1993;104:1230–1235.

Rouby JJ, de Lassale EM, Poete P, Nicholas MH, et al. Nosocomial pneumonia in the critically ill: histologic and bacteriologic aspects. Am Rev Respir Dis 1993;103:243–247.

Differential Diagnosis

Meduri GU. Diagnosis and differential diagnosis of ventilator-associated pneumonia. Clin Chest Med 1995;16:61–93.
Rouby JJ, Laurent P, Gosnach M, Cambau E, et al. Risk factors and clinical relevance of nosocomial maxillary sinusitis in the critically ill. Am J Respir Crit Care Med 1994;150: 776–783.

Pathogenesis

Chevret S, Hemmer M, Carlet J, et al. Incidence and risk factors of pneumonia acquired in intensive care units. Intensive Care Med 1993;19:256–264.
Craven DE, Steger KA. Epidemiology of nosocomial pneumonia: new perspectives on an old disease. Chest 1995;108(suppl):1S–16S.
Craven DE, Steger KA. Nosocomial pneumonia in mechanically ventilated adult patients: epidemiology and prevention in 1996. Semin Respir Infect 1996;11:32–53.
Cunnion KM, Weber DJ, Broadhead WE, Hanson LC, et al. Risk factors for nosocomial pneumonia: comparing adult critical care populations. Am J Respir Crit Care Med 1996; 153:158–162.
Joshi N, Localio AR, Hamory BH. A predictive risk index for nosocomial pneumonia in the intensive care unit. Am J Med 1992;93:135–142.

H_2 Blockers and Antacids as Risk Factors for Nosocomial Pneumonia

Bonten MJ, Gaillard CA, Van der Geest S, Van Tiel FH, et al. The role of gastric acidity and stress ulcer prophylaxis on colonization and infection in mechanically ventilated ICU patients. Am J Respir Crit Care Med 1995;152:1825–1834.
Cook DJ, Reeve BK, Scholes LC. Histamine-2 receptor antagonists and antacids in the critically ill population: stress ulceration versus nosocomial pneumonia. Infect Control Hosp Epidemiol 1994;15:437–442.
Driks MR, Craven DE, Celli BR, Manning M, Burke RA, Garvin GM, et al. Nosocomial pneumonia in intubated patients given sucralfate as compared with antacids or histamine type 2 blockers. N Engl J Med 1987;317:1376–1382.

Gastrointestinal Versus Tracheal Colonization

Bonten MJM, Gaillard CA, van Tiel FH, Smeets HGW, van der Geest S, Stobberingh EE. The stomach is not a source of colonization of the upper respiratory tract and pneumonia in ICU patients. Chest 1994;105:878–884.
Montecalvo MA, Korsberg TZ, Farber HW, et al. Nosocomial pneumonia and nutritional

status of critical care patients randomized to gastric versus jejunal tube feedings. Crit Care Med 1992;20:1377–1387.

Palmer LB, Conelan SV, Fox G, Bellemore E, Greene WH. Gastric flora in chronically mechanically ventilated patients: relationship to upper and lower airway colonization. Am J Respir Crit Care Med 1995;151:1063–1067.

Torres A, El-ebiary M, Gonzales J, Ferrer M, et al. Gastric and pharyngeal flora in nosocomial pneumonia acquired during mechanical ventilation. Am Rev Respir Dis 1993;148:352–357.

Risk Factors for Nosocomial Pneumonia in the ICU

Centers for Disease Control and Prevention. Draft guidelines for prevention of nosocomial pneumonia. Federal Register 1994;59:4980–5021.

Dreyfuss D, Djedaini K, Gros I, Mier L, et al. Mechanical ventilation with heated humidifiers or heat and moisture exchangers: effects on patient colonization and incidence of nosocomial pneumonia. Am J Respir Crit Care Med 1995;151:986–992.

Hamill RJ, Houston ED, Georghiou PR, Wright CE, et al. An outbreak of *Burkholderia* (formerly *Pseudomonas*) *cepacia* respiratory tract colonization and infection associated with nebulized albuterol therapy. Ann Intern Med 1995;122:762–766.

Koflef MH, Shapiro SD, Fraser VJ, Silver P, et al. Mechanical ventilation with or without 7-day circuit changes. A randomized controlled trial. Ann Intern Med 1995;123:168–174.

Torres A, Gatell JM, Aznar E, El-ebiary M, et al. Re-intubation increases the risk of nosocomial pneumonia in patients needing mechanical ventilation. Am J Respir Crit Care Med 1995;152:137–141.

Valles J, Artigas A, Rello J, et al. Continuous aspiration of subglottic secretions in the prevention of ventilator-associated pneumonia. Ann Intern Med 1995;122:179–186.

Prophylaxis (SDD)

Duncan RA, Steger KA, Craven DE. Selective decontamination of the digestive tract: risks outweigh benefits for intensive care unit patients. Semin Respir Infect 1993;8:308–324.

Quinio B, Albanese J, Bues-Charbit M, Viviand X, Martin C. Selective decontamination of the digestive tract in multiple trauma patients. A prospective double-blind, randomized, placebo-controlled study. Chest 1996;109:765–772.

Selective Decontamination of the Digestive Tract Trialists' Collaborative Group. Meta-analysis of randomized controlled trials of selective decontamination of the digestive tract. Br Med J 1993;307:525–532.

Tablan OC, Anderson LJ, Arden NH, Breiman RF, et al. Guidelines for prevention of nosocomial pneumonia. The Hospital Infection Control Practices Advisory Committee, Centers for Disease Control and Prevention. Infect Control Hosp Epidemiol 1994;15:587–627.

Verhoef J, Verhage EAE, Visser MR. A decade of experience with selective decontamination of the digestive tract as prophylaxis for infections in patients in the intensive care unit: what have we learned? Clin Infect Dis 1993;17:1047–1054.

Wiener J, Itokazu G, Nathan C, Kabins SA, Weinstein RA. A randomized, double-blind, placebo-controlled trial of selective digestive decontamination in a medical-surgical intensive care unit. Clin Infect Dis 1995;20:861–867.

Diagnostic Techniques for Pneumonia

Bronchoscopy with Protected Brush

Chastre J, Fagon JV. Invasive diagnostic testing should be routinely used to manage ventilated patients with suspected pneumonia. Am J Respir Crit Care Med 1994;150:570–574.

Chastre J, Fagon JV, Bornet-Lesco M, Calvat S, et al. Evaluation of bronchoscopic techniques for the diagnosis of nosocomial pneumonia. Am J Respir Crit Care Med 1995;152:231–240.

Kollef MH, Bock KR, Richards RD, Hearns ML. The safety and diagnostic accuracy of minibronchoalveolar lavage in patients with suspected ventilator-associated pneumonia. Ann Intern Med 1995;122:743–748.

Marquette CH, Copin MC, Wallet F, Neviere R, et al. Diagnostic tests for pneumonia in ventilated patients: prospective evaluation of diagnostic accuracy using histology as a gold standard. Am J Respir Crit Care Med 1995;151:1878–1888.

Niederman MS, Torres A, Summer W. Invasive diagnostic testing is not needed routinely to manage suspected ventilator-associated pneumonia. Am J Respir Crit Care Med 1994;150: 565–570.

Papazian L, Thomas P, Garbe L, Guignon I, et al. Bronchoscopic or blind sampling techniques for the diagnosis of ventilator-associated pneumonia. Am J Respir Crit Care Med 1995; 152:1982–1991.

Torres A, Martos A, de la Bellacasa J, et al. Specificity of endotracheal aspiration, protected specimen brush, and bronchoalveolar lavage in mechanically ventilated patients. Am Rev Respir Dis 1993;147:952–957.

Quantitative Cultures of Endotracheal Aspirates

El-Ebiary M, Torres A, Gonzales J, Puig de la Bellacasa J, et al. Quantitative cultures of endotracheal aspirates for the diagnosing of ventilator-associated pneumonia. Am Rev Respir Dis 1993;148:1552–1557.

Jourdain B, Novara A, Joly-Guillou ML, Dombret MC, et al. Role of quantitative cultures of endotracheal aspirates in the diagnosis of nosocomial pneumonia. Am J Respir Crit Care Med 1995;152:241–246.

Marquette C, Georges H, Wallet P, Ramon F, et al. Diagnostic efficiency of endotracheal aspirates for the diagnosing of ventilator-associated pneumonia. Am Rev Respir Dis 1993; 148:138–144.

Pleural Space Infections

Broaddus VC. Infections in the pleural space: an update on pathogenesis and management. Semin Respir Crit Care Med 1995;16:303–314.

Bryant RE, Salmon CJ. Pleural empyema. Clin Infect Dis 1996;22:747–762.

Dorca J, Manresa F, Esteban L, Barreiro B, et al. Efficacy, safety, and therapeutic relevance of transthoracic aspiration with ultrathin needle in nonventilated patients with nosocomial pneumonia. Am J Respir Crit Care Med 1995;151:1491–1496.

Sahn SA. Management of complicated parapneumonic effusions. Am Rev Respir Dis 1993; 148:813–817.

Specific Pathogens

Acinetobacter

Anstey NM, Currie BJ, Withnall KM. Community-acquired *Acinetobacter* pneumonia in adults in Northern Territory of Australia. Clin Infect Dis 1992;14:83–91.

Lortholary O, Fagon JY, Hoi AB, Slama MA, et al. Nosocomial acquisition of multiresistant *Acinetobacter baumannii:* risk factors and prognosis. Clin Infect Dis 1995;20:790–796.

Seifert H, Strate A, Pulvererf G. Nosocomial bacteremia due to *Acinetobacter baumannii:* clinical features, epidemiology, and predictors of mortality. Medicine (Baltimore) 1995; 74:340–349.

Anaerobes

Civen R, Jousimies-Somer H, Marina M, Borenstein L, et al. A retrospective review of cases of anaerobic empyema and update of bacteriology. Clin Infect Dis 1995;20(suppl 2): S224–S229.

Dore P, Robert R, Grollier G, Rouffineau J, Lanquetot H, et al. Incidence of anaerobes in ventilator-associated pneumonia with use of a protected specimen brush. Am J Respir Crit Care Med 1996;153:1292–1298.

Finegold SM. Aspiration pneumonia. Rev Infect Dis 1991;13(suppl 9):S737–S742.

Chlamydia pneumoniae

Almirall J, Morato I, Riera F, et al. Incidence of community-acquired pneumonia and *Chlamydia* pneumonia infections: a prospective multicentre study. Eur Respir J 1993;6:14–18.

Campbell LA, O'Brien ER, Cappuccio AL, Kuo C, et al. Detection of *Chlamydia pneumoniae* in human coronary atherectomy tissues. J Infect Dis 1995;172:585–588.

Emre U, Bernius M, Roblin PM, Gaerlan PF, et al. *Chlamydia pneumoniae* infection in patients with cystic fibrosis. Clin Infect Dis 1996;22:819–823.

Grayston JT, Aldous MB, Easton A, et al. Evidence that *Chlamydia pneumoniae* causes pneumonia and bronchitis. J Infect Dis 1993;168:1231–1235.

Hammerschlag MR. Antimicrobial susceptibility and therapy of infections caused by *Chlamydia pneumoniae.* Antimicrob Agents Chemother 1994;38:1873–1878.

Kauppinen MT, Herva E, Kujala P, Leinonen M, et al. The etiology of community-acquired pneumonia among hospitalized patients during a *Chlamydia pneumoniae* epidemic in Finland. J Infect Dis 1995;172:1330–1335.

Kauppinen MT, Saikku P. Pneumonia due to *Chlamydia pneumoniae:* prevalence, clinical features, diagnosis, and treatment. Clin Infect Dis 1995;21:S244–S252.

Kern DG, Neill MA, Schachter J. A seroepidemiologic study of *Chlamydia pneumoniae* in Rhode Island: evidence of serologic cross-reactivity. Chest 1993;104:208–213.

Techniques to Diagnose Chlamydia

Gaydos CA, Fowler CL, Gill VJ, Eiden JJ, Quinn TC. Detection of *Chlamydia pneumoniae* by polymerase chain reaction-enzyme immunoassay in an immunocompromised population. Clin Infect Dis 1993;17:718–723.

Hyman CL, Roblin PM, Gaydos CA, Quinn TC, et al. Prevalence of asymptomatic nasopharyngeal carriage of *Chlamydia pneumoniae* in subjectively healthy adults: assessment by polymerase chain reaction-enzyme immunoassay and culture. Clin Infect Dis 1995;20: 1174–1178.

Enterobacter

Chow JW, Fine MJ, Shlaes, et al. *Enterobacter* bacteremia: clinical features and emergence of antibiotic resistance during therapy. Ann Intern Med 1991;115:585–590.

Haemophilus influenzae

Goetz MB, O'Brien H, Musser JM, et al. Nosocomial transmission of disease caused by nontypeable strains of *Haemophilus influenzae*. Am J Med 1994;96:342–347.

Gould IM, Forbes KJ, Gordon GS. Quinolone-resistant *Haemophilus influenzae*. J Antimicrob Chemother 1994;33:187–188.

Jorgenson JH. Update on mechanisms and prevalence of antimicrobial resistance in *H. influenzae*. Clin Infect Dis 1992;14:1119–1123.

Najm WI, Cesario TC, Spurgeon L. Bacteremia due to *Haemophilus* infections: a retrospective study with emphasis on the elderly. Clin Infect Dis 1995;21:213–216.

Rello J, Ricart M, Ausina V, Net A, Prats G. Pneumonia due to *Haemophilus influenzae* among mechanically ventilated patients. Incidence, outcome, and risk factors. Chest 1992; 102:1562–1565.

Schlamm HT, Yancovitz SR. *Haemophilus influenzae* pneumonia in young adults with AIDS, ARC, or risk of AIDS. Am J Med 1989;86:11–14

Scriver SR, Walmsley SL, Kau CL, et al. Determination of antimicrobial susceptibilities of Canadian isolates of *Haemophilus influenzae* and characterization of β-lactamases. Antimicrob Agents Chemother 1994;38:1678–1680.

Klebsiella pneumoniae

Bradford PA, Cherubin CE, Idemyor V, Rasmussen BA, Bush K. Multiple resistant *Klebsiella pneumoniae* strains from two Chicago hospitals: identification of the extended-spectrum TEM-12 and TEM-10 ceftazidime-hydrolyzing β-lactamases in a single isolate. Antimicrob Agents Chemother 1994;38:761–766.

Meyer KS, Urban C, Eagan JA, Berger BJ, Rahal JJ. Nosocomial outbreak of *Klebsiella* infection resistant to late-generation cephalosporins. Ann Intern Med 1993;119:353–358.

Legionella *(Community-Acquired)*

Blatt SP, Dolan MJ, Hendrix CW, Melcher GP. Legionnaire's disease in human immunodeficiency virus-infected patients: eight cases and review. Clin Infect Dis 1994;18:227–232.

Edelstein PH. Legionnaire's disease. Clin Infect Dis 1993;16:741–749.

Falco V, de Sevilla TF, Alegre J, Ferrer A, Vazquez JM. *Legionella pneumophila.* A cause of severe community-acquired pneumonia. Chest 1991;100:1007–1011.

Legionella

Lieberman D, Sheva B, Porath A, Schlaeffer F, et al. *Legionella* species community-acquired pneumonia: a review of 56 hospitalized adult patients. Chest 1996;109:1243–1249.

Rodero FG, de la Tabla VO, Martinez C, del Mar Masia M, et al. Legionnaire's disease in patients infected with human immunodeficiency virus. Clin Infect Dis 1995;21:712–713.

Stout JE, Yu VL, Muraca P, Joly J, Troup N, Tompkins LS. Potable water as a cause of sporadic cases of community-acquired Legionnaire's disease. N Engl J Med 1992;326: 151–155.

Legionella *(Hospital-Acquired)*

Blatt SP, Parkinson MD, Pace E, Hoffman P, et al. Nosocomial Legionnaire's disease: aspiration as a primary mode of transmission. Am J Med 1993;95:16–22.

Caratala J, Gudiol F, Pallares R, et al. Risk factors for nosocomial *Legionella pneumophila* pneumonia. Am J Respir Crit Care Med 1994;149:625–629.

Venezia RA, Agresta MD, Hanley EM, et al. Nosocomial legionellosis associated with aspiration of nasogastric feedings diluted in tap water. Infect Control Hosp Epidemiol 1994;15: 529–533.

Diagnosis of Legionella

Ingram JG, Plouffe JF. Danger of sputum purulence screens in culture of *Legionella* species. J Clin Microbiol 1994;32:209–210.

Koide M, Saito A. Diagnosis of *Legionella pneumophila* infection by polymerase chain reaction. Clin Infect Dis 1995;21:199–201.

Plouffe JF, File TM Jr, Breiman RF, Hackman BA, et al. Re-evaluation of the definition of Legionnaire's disease: use of the urinary antigen assay. Clin Infect Dis 1995;20:1286–1291.

Moraxella (Branhamella) catarrhalis

Collazos J, de Miguel J, Ayarza R. *Moraxella catarrhalis* bacteremic pneumonia in adults: two cases and review of the literature. Eur J Clin Microbiol Infect Dis 1992;11:237–240.

Fung CP, Yeo SF, Livermore DM. Susceptibility of *Moraxella catarrhalis* isolates to β-lactam antibiotics in relation to β-lactamase pattern. J Antimicrob Chemother 1994;33: 215–222.

Ioannidis JP, Worthington M, Griffiths JK, Snydman DR. Spectrum and significance of bacteremia due to *Moraxella catarrhalis*. Clin Infect Dis 1995;21:390–397.

Klingman KL, Pye A, Murphy TF, Hill SL. Dynamics of respiratory tract colonization by *Branhamella catarrhalis* in bronchiectasis. Am J Respir Crit Care Med 1995;152: 1072–1078.

Wood GM, Johnson BC, McCormack JG. *Moraxella catarrhalis:* pathogenic significance in respiratory tract infections treated by community practitioners. Clin Infect Dis 1996;22: 632–636.

Mycoplasma pneumoniae

Bebear C, Dupon M, Renaudin H, de Barbeyrac B. Potential improvements in therapeutic options for mycoplasmal respiratory infections. Clin Infect Dis 1993;17(suppl 1):S2.

Clyde WA Jr. Clinical overview of typical *Mycoplasma pneumoniae* infections. Clin Infect Dis 1993;17(suppl 1):S32–S36.

Jacobs E. Serological diagnosis of *Mycoplasma pneumoniae* infections: a critical review of current procedures. Clin Infect Dis 1993;17(suppl 1):S79–S82.

Marrie TJ. *Mycoplasma pneumoniae* pneumonia requiring hospitalization, with emphasis on infection in the elderly. Arch Intern Med 1993;153:488–494.

Pseudomonas aeruginosa

Brewer SC, Wunderink RG, Jones CB, Leeper KV Jr. Ventilator-associated pneumonia due to *Pseudomonas aeruginosa.* Chest 1996;109:1019–1029.

Dunn M, Wunderink RG. Ventilator-associated pneumonia caused by *Pseudomonas* infection. Clin Chest Med 1995;16:95–110.

Hilf M, Yu VL, Sharp JA, Zuravleff JJ, Korvick JA, Muder RR. Antibiotic therapy for *Pseudomonas aeruginosa* bacteremia: outcome correlations in a prospective study of 200 patients. Am J Med 1989;87:540–546.

Rello J, Austina V, Ricart M, Puzo C, et al. Risk factors for infection by *Pseudomonas aeruginosa* in patients with ventilator-associated pneumonia. Intensive Care Med 1994;20: 193–198.

Pseudomonas cepacia

Gladman G, Connor PJ, Williams RF, David TJ. Controlled study of *Pseudomonas cepacia* and *Pseudomonas maltophilia* in cystic fibrosis. Arch Dis Child 1992;67:192–195.

Snell GI, de Hoyos A, Krajden M, Winton T, Maurer JR. *Pseudomonas cepacia* in lung transplant recipients with cystic fibrosis. Chest 1993;103:466–471.

Steinbach S, Sun L, Jiang RZ, Flume P, et al. Transmissibility of *Pseudomonas cepacia* infection in clinic patients and lung-transplant recipients with cystic fibrosis. N Engl J Med 1994;331:981–987.

Yamagishi Y, Fujita J, Takigawa K, Negayama K, et al. Clinical features of pneumonia in an epidemic among immunocompromised patients. Chest 1993;103:1706–1709.

Staphylococcus aureus

Al-Ujayli B, Nafziger DA, Saravolatz L. Pneumonia due to *Staphylococcus aureus* infection. Clin Chest Med 1995;16:111–121.

Iwahara T, Ichiyama S, Nada T, Shimokata K, Nakashima N. Clinical and epidemiologic investigations of nosocomial pulmonary infections caused by methicillin-resistant *Staphylococcus aureus.* Chest 1994;105:826–846.

Mulligan ME, Murray-Leuisure KA, Ribner BS, Standiford HC, et al. Methicillin-resistant *Staphylococcus aureus:* a consensus review of the microbiology, pathogenesis, and epidemiology with implications for prevention and management. Am J Med 1993;94:313–328.

Rello J, Torres A, Ricart M, Valles J, Gonzalez J, Artigas A, Rodriguez-Roisin R. Ventilator-associated pneumonias by *Staphylococcus aureus:* comparison of methicillin-resistant and methicillin-sensitive episodes. Am J Respir Crit Care Med 1994;150:1545–1549.

Streptococcus pneumoniae

Afessa B, Greaves WL, Frederick WR. Pneumococcal bacteremia in adults: a 14-year experience in an inner-city university hospital. Clin Infect Dis 1995;21:345–351.

Bedos JP, Chevret S, Chastang C, Geslin P, Regnier B, et al. Epidemiological features of and risk factors for infection by *Streptococcus pneumoniae* strains with diminished susceptibility to penicillin: findings of a French survey. Clin Infect Dis 1996;22:63–72.

Davidson M, Parkinson AJ, Bulklow LR, Fitzgerald MA, Peters HV, Parks DJ. The epidemiology of invasive pneumococcal disease in Alaska, 1986–1990: ethnic differences and opportunities for prevention. J Infect Dis 1994;170:368–376.

Hoge CW, Reichler MR, Dominguez EA, et al. An epidemic of invasive pneumococcal disease in an overcrowded, inadequately ventilated jail. N Engl J Med 1994;331:643–648.

Musher DM. Infections caused by *Streptococcus pneumoniae:* clinical spectrum, pathogenesis, immunity, and treatment. Clin Infect Dis 1992;14:801–809.

Salo P, Ortqvist A, Leinonen M. Diagnosis of pneumococcal pneumonia by amplification of pneumolysin gene fragment in serum. J Infect Dis 1995;171:479–482.

Toumanen EI, Austrian R, Masure HR. Pathogenesis of pneumococcal infection. N Engl J Med 1995;332:1280–1284.

Streptococcus pneumoniae: *Antimicrobial Resistance*

Applebaum PC. Antimicrobial resistance in *Streptococcus pneumoniae:* an overview. Clin Infect Dis 1992;15:77–83.

Barnes DM, Whittier S, Gilligan PH, Soares S, et al. Transmission of multidrug-resistant serotype 23F *Streptococcus pneumoniae* in group day care: evidence suggesting capsular transformation of the resistant strain in vivo. J Infect Dis 1995;171:885–889.

Breiman RF, Butler JC, Tenover FC, Elliott JA, Facklam RR. Emergence of drug-resistant pneumococcal infections in the United States. JAMA 1994;271:1831–1835.

Coffey TJ, Dowson CG, Daniels M, Spratt B. Genetics and molecular biology of β-lactam-resistant pneumococci. Microb Drug Resist 1995;1:29–34.

Friedland IR, McCracken GH Jr. Management of infections caused by antibiotic-resistant *Streptococcus pneumoniae.* N Engl J Med 1994;331:377–382.

Hedlung J, Svenson SB, Kalin M, Henrichsen J, et al. Incidence, capsular types, and antibiotic susceptibility of invasive *Streptococcus pneumoniae* in Sweden. Clin Infect Dis 1995;21:948–953.

Hoffman J, Cetron MS, Farley MM, Baughman WS, et al. The prevalence of drug-resistant *Streptococcus pneumoniae* in Atlanta. N Engl J Med 1995;333:481–486.

Jacobs MR. Treatment and diagnosis of infections caused by drug-resistant *Streptococcus pneumoniae.* Clin Infect Dis 1992;15:119–127.

Moreno F, Crisp C, Jorgensen JH, Patterson JE. The clinical and molecular epidemiology of bacteremias at a University Hospital caused by pneumococci not susceptible to penicillin. J Infect Dis 1995;172:427–432.

Nava JM, Bella F, Garau J, et al. Predictive factors for invasive disease due to penicillin-resistant *Streptococcus pneumoniae:* a population-based study. Clin Infect Dis 1994;19:884–890.

Nissinen A, Leinonen M, Huovinen P, Herva E, et al. Antimicrobial resistance of *Streptococcus pneumoniae* in Finland, 1987–1990. Clin Infect Dis 1995;20:1275–1280.

Resistance to Cephalosporins

Klugman KP. Pneumococcal resistance to the third-generation cephalosporins: clinical, laboratory, and molecular aspects. Int J Antimicrob Agents 1994;4:63–67.

Leggiadro PJ. Penicillin- and cephalosporin-resistant *Streptococcus pneumoniae:* an emerging microbial threat. Pediatrics 1994;93:500–503.

Pallares R, Linares J, Vadillo M, Cabellos C, et al. Resistance to penicillin and cephalosporin and mortality from severe pneumococcal pneumonia in Barcelona, Spain. N Engl J Med 1995;333:474–480.

Erythromycin-resistant Pneumococci

Moreno S, Garcia-Leoni ME, Cercenado E, Diaz MD, et al. Infections caused by erythromycin-resistant *Streptococcus pneumoniae:* incidence, risk factors, and response to therapy in a prospective study. Clin Infect Dis 1995;20:1195–1200.

Pneumococcal Vaccine

Butler JC, Breiman RF, Lipman HB, Hofmann J, Facklam RR. Serotype distribution of *Streptococcus pneumoniae* infections among preschool children in the United States, 1978–1994: implications for development of a conjugate vaccine. J Infect Dis 1995;171: 885–889.

Butler JC, Breiman RF, Campbell JF, Lipman HB, et al. Pneumococcal polysaccharide vaccine efficacy: an evaluation of current recommendations. JAMA 1993;270:1826–1831.

Fedson DS. Influenza and pneumococcal vaccination in Canada and the United States, 1980–1993: what can the two countries learn from each other? Clin Infect Dis 1995;20: 1371–1376.

Fedson DS. Pneumococcal vaccine in the prevention of community-acquired pneumonia: an optimistic view of cost-effectiveness. Semin Respir Infect 1993;8:285–293.

Hirschmann JV, Lipsky BA. The pneumococcal vaccine after 15 years of use. Arch Intern Med 1994;154:373–377.

Konradsen HB. Quantity and avidity of pneumococcal antibodies before and up to five years after pneumococcal vaccination of elderly persons. Clin Infect Dis 1995;21:616–620.

Siber GR. Pneumococcal disease: prospects for a new generation of vaccines. Science 1994; 265:1385–1387.

Streptococcus Species (Not S. pneumoniae)

Jackson LA, Hilsdon R, Farley MM, Harrison LH, et al. Risk factors for group B streptococcal disease in adults. Ann Intern Med 1995;123:415–420.

Stenotrophomonas (Xanthomonas) maltophilia

Elting LS, Khardori N, Bodey GP, Fainstein V. Nosocomial infection caused by *Xanthomonas maltophilia:* a case-control study of predisposing factors. Infect Control Hosp Epidemiol 1990;11:134–138.

Khardori N, Elting L, Wong E, et al. Nosocomial *Xanthomonas maltophilia* infections in cancer patients. Rev Infect Dis 1990;12:997–1003.

Muder RR, Harris AP, Muller S, Edmond M, Chow JW, et al. Bacteremia due to *Stenotrophomononas (Xanthomonas) maltophilia:* a prospective, multicenter study of 91 episodes. Clin Infect Dis 1996;22:508–512.

Vartivarian S, Anaissie E, Bodey G, Sprigg H, Rolston K. A changing pattern of susceptibility of *Xanthomonas maltophilia* to antimicrobial agents: implications for therapy. Antimicrob Agents Chemother 1994;38:624–627.

Antimicrobial Resistance

Felmingham D. Antibiotic resistance: do we need new therapeutic approaches? Chest 1995; 108:70S–78S.

Kunin CM. Resistance to antimicrobial drugs—a worldwide calamity. Ann Intern Med 1993; 118:557–561.

Lucet JC, Chevret S, Decre D, Vanjak D, et al. Outbreak of multiply resistance Enterobacteriaceae in an intensive care unit: epidemiology and risk factors for acquisition. Clin Infect Dis 1996;22:430–436.

Pierson CL, Friedman BA. Comparison of susceptibility to β-lactam antimicrobial agents among bacteria isolated from intensive care units. Diagn Microbiol Infect Dis 1992;15: 19S–30S.

Richard P, Le Floch R, Chamoux C, Pannier M, Espaze E, Richet H. *Pseudomonas aeruginosa* outbreak in a burn unit: role of antimicrobials in the emergence of multiply resistant strains. J Infect Dis 1994;170:377–383.

Specific Antibiotics

Antibiotics (Reviews)

Mandell LA. Antibiotics for pneumonia therapy. Med Clin North Am 1994;78:997–1014.

Quenzer RU, Guay DR. Antimicrobial management strategies for patients with community-acquired respiratory tract infections. Current Ther Res 1995;56:466–477.

Ramirez JA, Srinath L, Ahkee S, Huang A, Raff MJ. Early switch from intravenous to oral cephalosporins in the treatment of hospitalized patients with community-acquired pneumonia. Arch Intern Med 1995;155:1273–1276.

Monotherapy Versus Combination Therapy

Arbo MDJ, Snydman DR. Monotherapy is appropriate for nosocomial pneumonia in the intensive care unit. Semin Respir Infect 1993;8(4):259–267.

Lynch JP III. Combination antibiotic therapy is appropriate for nosocomial pneumonia in the intensive care unit. Semin Respir Infect 1993;8:268–284.

β-Lactam Antibiotics

Penicillins

Sanders WE Jr, Sanders CC. Piperacillin/tazobactam: a critical review of the evolving clinical literature. Clin Infect Dis 1996;22:107–123.

Schlaes DM, Baughman R, Boylen CT, Chan JC, et al. Piperacillin/tazobactam compared to ticarcillin/clavulanate in community-acquired bacterial lower respiratory tract infection. J Antimicrobial Chemother 1994;34:565–577.

Wright AJ, Wilkowske CJ. The penicillins. Mayo Clin Proc 1991;66:1047–1063.

Cephalosporins

Burwen DR, Banerjee SN, Gaynes RP, et al. Ceftazidime resistance among selected nosocomial Gram-negative bacilli in the United States. J Infect Dis 1994;170:1622–1625.

Gustaferro CA, Steckelberg JM. Cephalosporin antimicrobial agents and related compounds. Mayo Clin Proc 1991;66:1064–1073.

Carbapenems (Imipenem/Cilastin)

Buckley MM, Brogden RN, Barradell LB, Goa KL. Imipenem/cilastatin: a reappraisal of its antibacterial activity, pharmacokinetic properties and therapeutic efficacy. Drugs 1992;44: 408–444.

Gaynes RP, Culver DH. Resistance to imipenem among selected Gram-negative bacilli in the United States. Infect Control Hosp Epidemiol 1992;13:10–14.

Norrby SR, Finch RG, Glauser M, et al. Monotherapy in serious hospital-acquired infections: a clinical trial of ceftazidime versus imipenem/cilastin. Antimicrob Agents Chemother 1993;31:927–937.

Monobactams (Aztreonam)

Brewer NS, Hellinger WC. The monobactams. Mayo Clin Proc 1991;66:1152–1157.

Cook JL. Gram-negative bacillary pneumonia in the nosocomial setting: role of aztreonam. Am J Med 1990;88(suppl 3C):34S–37S.

Aminoglycosides

Bates RD, Nahata MC. Once-daily administration of aminoglycosides. Ann Pharmacother 1994;28:757–766.

Edson RS, Terrell CL. The aminoglycosides. Mayo Clin Proc 1991;66:1158–1164.

Hatala R, Dinh T, Cook DJ. Once-daily aminoglycoside dosing in immunocompetent adults: a meta-analysis. Ann Intern Med 1996;124:717–725.

International Antimicrobial Therapy Cooperative Group of the European Organization for Research and Treatment of Cancer. Efficacy and toxicity of single daily doses of amikacin and ceftriaxone versus multiple daily doses of amikacin and ceftazidime for infection in patients with cancer and granulocytopenia. Ann Intern Med 1993;119:584–593.

Prins JM, Buller HR, Kuijper EDJ, et al. Once versus thrice daily gentamicin in patients with serious infections. Lancet 1993;341:335–339.

Inhaled Aminoglycosides

Brown RB, Kruse JA, Counts GW, et al. Double-blind study of endotracheal tobramycin in the treatment of Gram-negative bacterial pneumonia. Antimicrob Agents Chemother 1990; 34:269–272.
Ramsey BW, Dorkin HL, Eisenberg JD, Gibson RL, et al. Efficacy of aerosolized tobramycin in patients with cystic fibrosis. N Engl J Med 1993;328:1740–1746.

Macrolide Antibiotics

Bahal N, Nahata MC. The new macrolide antibiotics: azithromycin, clarithromycin, dirithromycin, and roxithromycin. Ann Pharmacotherapy 1992;26:46–55.

Azalides (Azithromycin)

Bohte R, van't Wout JW, Lobatto S, van Oud Alblas AB, et al. Efficacy and safety of azithromycin versus benzylpenicillin or erythromycin in community-acquired pneumonia. Eur J Clin Microbiol Infect Dis 1995;14:182–187.
Peters DH, Friedel HA, McTavish D. Azithromycin: a review of its antimicrobial activity, pharmacokinetic properties, and clinical efficacy. Drugs 1992;44:750–799.

Clarithromycin

Chien SM, Phichotta P, Siepman N, Chan CK, et al. Treatment of community-acquired pneumonia. A multicenter, double-blind, randomized study comparing clarithromycin with erythromycin. Chest 1993;103:697–701.
Hamedani P, Ali J, Hafeez S, Bachand R, Dawood G, et al. The safety and efficacy of clarithromycin in patients with *Legionella* pneumonia. Chest 1991;100:1503–1506.

Fluoroquinolones

Carratala J, Fernandez-Sevilla A, Tubau F, Callis M, Gudiol F. Emergence of quinolone-resistant *Escherichia coli* bacteremia in neutropenic patients with cancer who have received prophylactic norfloxacin. Clin Infect Dis 1995;20:557–560.
Dalhoff A. Quinolone resistance in *Pseudomonas aeruginosa* and *Staphylococcus aureus:* development during therapy and clinical significance. Infection 1994;22(suppl 2): S111–S121.
Hooper DC, Wolfson JS. Fluoroquinolone antimicrobial agents. N Engl J Med 1991;384–394.

Ciprofloxacin

Fink M, Snydman D, Niederman M, Leeper KV Jr, et al. Treatment of severe pneumonia in hospitalized patients: result of a multicenter, randomized, double-blind trial comparing intravenous ciprofloxacin with imipenem/cilastatin. Antimicrobial Agents Chemother 1994; 38(3):547–557.

Forrest A, Nix DE, Ballow CH, Goss TF, Birmingham MC, Schentag JJ. Pharmacodynamics of intravenous ciprofloxacin in seriously ill patients. Antimicrobial Agents Chemother 1993;37:1073–1081.

Paladino JA, Sperry HE, Backes JM, et al. Clinical and economic evaluation of oral ciprofloxacin after an abbreviated course of intravenous antibiotics. Am J Med 1991;91:462–470.

Ofloxacin

Gaillat J, Bru JP, Sedallian A. Penicillin G/ofloxacin versus erythromycin/amoxicillin-clavulanate in the treatment of severe community-acquired pneumonia. Eur J Clin Microbiol Infect Dis 1994;13:639–644.

Gentry LO, Rodriguez-Gomez G, Kohler RB, Khan FA, Rytel MW. Ofloxacin, parenteral followed by oral, for nosocomial pneumonia and community-acquired pneumonia requiring hospitalization. Am Rev Respir Dis 1992;145:31–35.

Jones RN, Reller B, Rosati LA, Erwin ME, et al. Ofloxacin, a new broad-spectrum fluoroquinolone. Results from a multicenter, national comparative activity surveillance study. Diagn Microbiol Infect Dis 1992;15:425–434.

Malik IA, Khan WA, Karim M, Aziz Z, Khan MA. Feasibility of outpatient management of fever in cancer patients with low-risk neutropenia: results of a prospective randomized trial. Am J Med 1995;98:224–231.

Sanders WE, Morris JF, Alessi PK, Makris AT, et al. Oral ofloxacin for the treatment of acute bacterial pneumonia: use of a nontraditional protocol to compare experimental therapy with usual care in a multicenter clinical trial. Am J Med 1991;91:261–266.

Lomefloxacin

Kemper P, Kohler D. A double-blind study of two dosage regimens of lomefloxacin in bacteriologically proven exacerbations of chronic bronchitis of Gram-negative etiology. Am J Med 1992;92(suppl 4A):98S–102S.

Mayer KH, Ellal JA. Lomefloxacin: microbiologic assessment and unique properties. Am J Med 1992;92(suppl 4A):58S–62S.

Perfloxacin

Farkas SA. Intravenous fleroxacin versus ceftazidime in the treatment of acute nonpneumococcal lower respiratory tract infections. Am J Med 1993;94(suppl 3A):142S–149S.

Other Classes of Antibiotics
Tetracyclines, Chloramphenicol, Clindamycin, and Metronidazole

Smilack JD, Wilson WR, Cockerill FR III. Tetracyclines, chloramphenicol, erythromycin, clindamycin, and metronidazole. Mayo Clin Proc 1991;66:1270–1280.

Trimethoprim/Sulfamethoxazole

Cockerill FR III, Edson RS. Trimethoprim/sulfamethoxazole. Mayo Clin Proc 1991;66: 1260–1269.

Vancomycin

CDC. Department of Health and Human Services. Centers for Disease Control and Prevention. Preventing the spread of vancomycin resistance. Federal Register 1994;59(94): 25758–25763.

Edmond MB, Ober JF, Weinbaum DL, Pfaller MA, et al. Vancomycin-resistant *Enterococcus faecium* bacteremia: risk factors for infection. Clin Infect Dis 1995;20:1126–1133.

Ena J, Dick RW, Jones RN, Wenzel RP. The epidemiology of intravenous vancomycin usage in a university hospital: a 10 year study. JAMA 1993;269:598–602.

Morris JG Jr, Shay DK, Hebden JN, McCarter RJ Jr, et al. Enterococci resistant to multiple antimicrobial agents, including vancomycin. Establishment of endemicity in a university medical center. Ann Intern Med 1995;123:250–259.

Pallares R, Dick R, Wenzel RP, Adams JR, Nettleman MD. Trends in antimicrobial utilization at a tertiary teaching hospital during a 15-year period (1978–1992). Infect Control Hosp Epidemiol 1993;14:376–382.

Shay DK, Maloney SA, Montecalvo M, Benerjee S, et al. Epidemiology and mortality risk of vancomycin-resistant enterococcal bloodstream infections. J Infect Dis 1995;172: 993–1000.

8   Fungal, Mycobacterial, and Viral Pulmonary Infections

Joseph P. Lynch, III, Galen B. Toews

Pneumocystis carinii

Epidemiology

Pneumocystis carinii, a unicellular eucaryote with features consistent with both a protozoan or fungal classification, has escalated dramatically in importance within the last decade as an opportunistic pathogen. Before 1981, fewer than 100 cases of *Pneumocystis carinii* pneumonia (PCP) were diagnosed annually in the United States. Major risk factors for PCP included iatrogenic immunosuppressive or cyto-toxic therapy, chemotherapy for hematologic malignancies, organ transplantation, primary immunodeficiency syndromes, severe malnutrition, or any disease resulting in severe and sustained deficits in cell-mediated immunity. With the advent of ac-quired immunodeficiency syndrome (AIDS), the incidence of PCP skyrocketed. PCP is the most common infection complicating human immunodeficiency virus (HIV) infection. In the absence of prophylaxis against PCP, more than 80% of HIV-infected persons develop PCP at some point in their illness. The risk of PCP in patients with HIV infection correlates with the number of CD4 cells. The risk of developing PCP within 3 years is approximately 33% among patients with CD4 counts below 200 cells/mm^3; for CD4 counts between 200 and 350, 23%; for CD4 counts exceeding 700, only 4%. Aggressive use of antimicrobial prophylaxis in patients with HIV has resulted in a steady decline in the number of cases of PCP. Nonetheless, more than 15,000 cases of PCP were reported to the Centers for Disease Control and Prevention (CDC) in 1994. A marked increase in the incidence of PCP in immunosuppressed, non–HIV-infected populations in the past 5 years has also been noted. The epide-miology and mode of transmission of *P. carinii* are poorly understood. *P. carinii* is likely acquired by inhalation and may become part of the resident microbial flora. *P. carinii* is of low virulence, and propagation and clinical infection occur only when sustained and severe impairments in host immune defenses develop. Alterna-tively, PCP may result from exposure to an exogenous source. Nosocomial outbreaks of PCP among immunosuppressed patients, the elderly, and malnourished infants suggest that person-to-person transmission may occur in at least a subset of patients.

Clinical Features

The presentation of PCP in HIV-infected patients differs from that of other immuno-suppressed patient populations. In non–HIV-infected patients, characteristic clinical features include cough, dyspnea, fever, tachypnea, crackles, and widespread alveolar or interstitial infiltrates on chest radiograph. Lobar consolidation, nodules, or cavities are virtually never seen. The course is usually rapid, progressing within 4–15 days to severe hypoxemia and respiratory failure. In contrast, in HIV-infected patients, the onset is more insidious. Low grade fever, fatigue, weight loss, mild cough, or dyspnea on exertion may be present for weeks or months. Chest radiographs are often normal or exhibit only subtle interstitial infiltrates. Serum lactate dehydrogenase is typically elevated with PCP and may be a diagnostic clue. Mortality of untreated PCP approaches 100%. With appropriate therapy, mortality rates of 5–20% have been cited. Extrapulmonary involvement was never recognized before the advent of HIV but has recently been described in patients with far-advanced AIDS. Patients receiving prophylactic aerosolized pentamidine may exhibit atypical clinical and radiographic features (e.g., extrapulmonary *P. carinii,* upper lobe predominance, pneumothoraces, lower diagnostic yield on bronchoalveolar lavage).

Diagnosis of PCP

Diagnosis of PCP requires visualizing the characteristic cysts in respiratory secretions or tissue because the organism has never been cultured. Round, helmet-shaped or crescent-shaped cysts, approximately 5–8 μm in diameter, may be identified by methenamine-silver or toluidine blue stains (within tissue) or by Papanicolaou stains (of cytologic material). The diagnostic approach to PCP has evolved considerably within the past decade. Induced sputum (using an ultrasonic nebulizer) is often the initial diagnostic test for mild cases; sensitivity in AIDS-associated PCP ranges from 47 to 94%. When sputa are nondiagnostic or when the course is acute or severe, fiberoptic bronchoscopy with bronchoalveolar lavage (BAL) should be performed (sensitivity more than 95% for HIV-associated PCP). Transbronchial biopsies add only marginally to BAL. The yield of sputum or BAL is lower in patients without AIDS because of the lower burden of organisms. Open lung biopsy is rarely warranted. Recent studies employing monoclonal antibodies or polymerase chain reaction (PCR) are promising, but their roles need to be further defined. Several studies using dihydrofolate reductase (DHFR) gene PCR have detected *P. carinii* in induced sputum, BAL, or serum, but results have been highly variable (sensitivity ranging from 10 to 86%). In a recent study, PCR amplification of internal transcribed spacers of the rRNA genes of *P. carinii* (Pc-ITS) detected the organism in 26 of 27 (96%) BAL specimens from AIDS patients with PCP. All 27 also had *P. carinii* detected in serum by Pc-ITS-PCR. In contrast, DHFR-PCR was positive in only 4 of 24 (17%) of BAL samples and in only 2 of 20 (10%) sera from patients with PCP. All specimens (BAL and sera) from 18 AIDS patients without PCP were negative by both DHFR and Pc-ITS-PCR. These data are exciting and suggest that PCR of sera may be a highly sensitive and noninvasive technique to diagnose *P. carinii,* provided the appropriate gene sequences are amplified.

Treatment of PCP

Several regimens are effective as therapy for *P. carinii.* Unfortunately, toxicity is high with all therapies and crossover to alternative agents is frequently necessary.

Trimethoprim/sulfamethoxazole (TMP/SMX) is the drug of choice for both primary therapy and prophylaxis of *P. carinii* in both HIV-infected and non–HIV-infected individuals. Pentamidine (or alternative agents) should be reserved for patients failing or experiencing side effects from TMP/SMX. Irrespective of therapeutic regimen, a 21-day course is advised to reduce the chance for relapse.

TRIMETHOPRIM/SULFAMETHOXAZOLE

Trimethoprim/sulfamethoxazole blocks folate metabolism at two sites. Sulfamethoxazole interferes with dihydrofolic synthetase, an enzyme found only in microbes. Trimethoprim inhibits both DHFR and synthetase. Bioavailability is excellent, and TMP/SMX can be administered orally or intravenously. Plasma levels of TMP/SMX do not correlate with cure rates and are not necessary to monitor efficacy. Oral TMP/SMX (10–20 mg/kg/day of the trimethoprim component) is adequate for mild to moderate PCP. Two double-strength tablets (320 mg TMP/1600 mg SMX) three times daily for adults weighing less than 80 kg is adequate; a slightly higher dose (2.5 double-strength tablets) is appropriate for adults weighing more than 80 kg. Unfortunately, side effects mandate discontinuation of therapy in 24–57% of patients with AIDS. Rash, gastrointestinal side effects, fever, neutropenia, anemia, azotemia, thrombocytopenia, or chemical hepatitis may complicate use of TMP/SMX. Adverse effects usually occur after 7 days and may preclude completing a full 21-day course of therapy. Complete blood counts, platelet counts, electrolytes, and transaminases should be monitored twice weekly during therapy. Side effects are far less common among non–HIV-infected persons. Even among patients experiencing moderate to severe adverse reactions to TMP/SMX, desensitization can be achieved in most patients by administering serial dilutions of progressively more concentrated TMP/SMX.

PENTAMIDINE ISETHIONATE

Pentamidine isethionate, an inhibitor of folate metabolism, has been extensively used for both treatment and prophylaxis of *P. carinii*. Intravenous pentamidine (4 mg/kg/day given over 60 minutes) for 21 days may be used to treat *P. carinii*. This regimen is slightly less effective than TMP/SMX. Intramuscular administration may cause abscess formation at the injection site and should be avoided. Side effects occur in up to 70% of patients receiving intravenous pentamidine. These include hypotension, dysrhythmias, nephrotoxicity, bone marrow depression, hypoglycemia, chemical hepatitis, nausea, and diabetes mellitus. Cardiac arrhythmias are rare, but management may be difficult because of the long half-life of pentamidine (up to 30 days in the lung). Aerosolized pentamidine (300 mg once monthly administered via a Respirgard II nebulizer) may be used for prophylaxis but not treatment of PCP. Aerosolized pentamidine is less effective than TMP/SMX for *P. carinii* prophylaxis and should be reserved for patients intolerant to TMP/SMX. Cough or bronchospasm occur in up to one-third of patients with long-term use of aerosolized pentamidine. Pretreatment with a β-agonist may ameliorate these symptoms. Other side effects include a bitter taste and emesis. Fewer than 5% of patients discontinue aerosolized pentamidine as a result of adverse effects. Importantly, medical personnel administering aerosolized pentamidine are at increased risk for developing asthma and infections transmitted by aerosol (including multidrug-resistant tuberculosis). In light of these concerns, aerosolized pentamidine should be used with caution and under careful supervision.

DAPSONE

Dapsone, a dihydropteroate synthetase inhibitor, when combined with sulfonamides, may be effective as therapy or prophylaxis for *P. carinii.* Dapsone has a prolonged half-life (24 hours), allowing infrequent dosing. High-dose dapsone (100 mg/day) alone is inadequate for PCP (failure rate more than 35%). The combination of oral dapsone (100 mg/day) and TMP (20 mg/kg/day), however, was as effective as oral TMP/SMX (20 and 100 mg/kg/day) for mild to moderate PCP, and was better tolerated. Drug interactions between dapsone and TMP result in increased plasma concentrations of each drug. For prophylaxis of *P. carinii,* dapsone alone or combined with pyrimethamine (a sulfonamide) may be used. Oral dapsone (100 mg/day) was as effective as TMP/SMX for *P. carinii* prophylaxis. Combining dapsone with pyrimethamine provides additional protection against toxoplasmosis. Total weekly doses of 200–300 mg dapsone and 50–75 mg pyrimethamine appear necessary for prophylaxis against *P. carinii* and *Toxoplasma gondii.* Pyrimethamine is administered once weekly; dapsone, three to seven times weekly. Dapsone is inexpensive and convenient, but adverse effects are common and are dose dependent. Methemoglobinemia and hyperkalemia occur in 50–67% of patients, but are often asymptomatic and may not require specific therapy. Hemolytic anemia may occur in patients with glucose 6-phosphate dehydrogenase (G-6-PD) deficiency. Patients should be screened for G-6-PD deficiency before initiating dapsone. Additional side effects include nausea, fever, rash, headache, hyperkalemia, or anemia; pancytopenia is a rare complication. At a dose of 100 mg weekly, fewer than 5% experience adverse effects serious enough to discontinue treatment. At doses exceeding 300 mg, one-third or more cannot tolerate therapy.

ATOVAQUONE

Atovaquone, a hydroxynaphthoquinone, is approved as therapy for mild to moderate PCP (750 mg p.o. t.i.d.) in patients unable to tolerate TMP/SMX. Atovaquone is less effective than TMP/SMX but as effective as pentamidine. Relapses have been common after initial successful therapy with atovaquone. Rash, gastrointestinal side effects, and fever are common adverse effects but require cessation of treatment in only 7% of patients. Response to atovaquone is poor in the presence of preexisting diarrhea or low plasma levels.

TRIMETREXATE

Trimetrexate, an analogue of methotrexate and a potent inhibitor of DHFR, has recently been approved as therapy for PCP. Trimetrexate (45 mg/m^2/day) plus leucovorin (20 mg/m^2 q.i.d.), however, is less effective than TMP/SMX or pentamidine as primary therapy for PCP (38% failures, up to 60% relapses). Major side effects of trimetrexate are bone marrow suppression, fever, and elevated transaminases. Concomitant administration of leucovorin minimizes toxicity.

CLINDAMYCIN/PRIMAQUINE

The combination of clindamycin/primaquine may be effective as salvage therapy for PCP failing conventional therapy. The doses are clindamycin 300–900 mg q.i.d. intravenously and primaquine 15–30 mg/day orally. Favorable responses have been noted in up to 86% of patients. An erythematous skin rash occurs in nearly 50% of patients; methemoglobinemia, in up to 25%. Fever, nausea, diarrhea, or hemolytic anemia occur in fewer than 5% of patients.

DIFLUOROMETHYLORNITHINE

Difluoromethylornithine (DFMO), administered orally once daily (400 mg/kg), has a limited role in treating PCP failing alternative therapies. DFMO is substantially less efficacious than TMP/SMX, and side effects (principally bone marrow suppression) occur in up to 60% of patients.

Preferred Therapy

- Trimethoprim/sulfamethoxazole is the treatment of choice for *P. carinii* in both HIV and non–HIV-infected patients. Treatment should be continued for 21 days.
- For severe PCP, intravenous TMP/SMX is recommended (total daily dose: 20 mg/kg, TMP; 100 mg/kg, SMX; given in four divided doses).
- For mild to moderate PCP, oral administration is preferred.
- Severe PCP or respiratory failure: add adjunctive corticosteroids.

Note: Adjunctive corticosteroids are recommended for AIDS patients with PCP and moderate or severe hypoxemia (alveolar-arterial oxygen difference greater than 35 mm Hg or a PaO_2 less than 70 mm Hg on room air). Deterioration in respiratory function, need for mechanical ventilation, and death are reduced significantly with corticosteroids. Corticosteroids should be started within 72 hours of initiating antimicrobial therapy for PCP. Although the optimal regimen has not been determined, prednisone 40 mg b.i.d. (days 1–5), 40 mg daily (days 6–10), and 20 mg daily (days 11–21) is advised.

Therapeutic Options for Patients Failing TMP/SMX or Experiencing Side Effects

- Intravenous pentamidine (4 mg/kg/day) for 21 days;
- Dapsone (100 mg/day p.o.) plus trimethoprim (20 mg/kg/day, given in four divided doses).

Salvage Regimens for Patients Failing Above Therapies

- Trimetrexate (45 mg/m^2) plus leucovorin (20 mg/m^2 q.i.d.);
- Atovaquone (dose 750 mg p.o. t.i.d.);
- Clindamycin (300–900 mg q.i.d. IV) plus primaquine (15–30 mg/day orally);
- DFMO (400 mg/kg once daily p.o.).

Prophylaxis of PCP

Primary PCP prophylaxis is recommended for patients with prior episodes of PCP, for HIV-infected patients with CD4 counts less than 200 mm^3, and for non–HIV-infected patients at risk for *P. carinii* (e.g., organ transplant recipients, intense immunosuppressive therapy, childhood leukemia). Secondary prophylaxis is advised for any patient with a prior history of PCP because the risk of relapse in this setting is high. Oral TMP/SMX is preferred unless adverse effects contraindicate it use. Single-strength (480 mg) or double-strength TMP/SMX once daily are highly efficacious (more than 99%) in preventing *P. carinii* in HIV-infected and non–HIV-infected individuals. Both regimens are also effective prophylaxis against toxoplasmosis. Thrice-weekly dosing (one double-strength tablet) appears as effective as more frequent dosing and is less toxic. Other prophylactic regimens include pentamidine (inhaled or parenteral) or dapsone (alone or combined with pyrimethamine).

Preferred Therapy for Prophylaxis of PCP

- TMP/SMX (one double-strength tablet 3–7 days per week).

Alternate Therapy

- Aerosolized pentamidine (300 mg every 4 weeks using the Respirgard II nebulizer);
- Dapsone 100 mg/day (thrice weekly may be adequate);
- Dapsone 100 mg (thrice weekly) plus pyrimethamine (50–75 mg once weekly).

FUNGAL DISEASE
Aspergillus
Epidemiology

Aspergillus spp. (*A. fumigatus, A. flavus, A. niger*) are ubiquitous in the environment, and infection with these fungi may occur via environmental exposures or endogenous reactivation of latent spores in immunocompromised hosts. With few exceptions, invasive aspergillosis develops only after severe and sustained aberrations in both cellular immunity and granulocyte number or function. Predisposing factors include organ transplantation, hematologic malignancies on chemotherapy, prior corticosteroid or immunosuppressive therapy, recent antibiotics, and severe granulocytopenia. Infection most commonly occurs by endogenous spread in immunosuppressed patients previously colonized with *Aspergillus* spp. Nosocomial outbreaks of invasive aspergillosis may result from inhalation of *Aspergillus* spores from contaminated air vents, operating rooms, and hospital wards. Duration of granulocytopenia is a critical risk factor. Among patients with hematologic malignancies, invasive aspergillosis developed in fewer than 1% of patients when granulocytopenia resolved within 2 weeks. In contrast, infection rates of 4–15% were noted when granulocytopenia persisted for more than 24–30 days. Invasive aspergillosis is a major cause of morbidity and mortality among organ transplant recipients. The incidence is highly variable among institutions and according to the transplanted organ (renal and hepatic, 1–5%; heart, heart-lung, or lung, 2–15%; bone marrow, up to 20%). Aggressive prophylaxis with antifungal agents and the use of environmental control measures to reduce exposure to *Aspergillus* spores may reduce clinical infections. Aspergillosis complicates AIDS in fewer than 1% of patients, likely reflecting the preservation of granulocyte number and function in this disorder. Only three cases of aspergillosis were described among the first 1,762 cases of AIDS reported to the CDC. The risk is greatly increased in patients with far-advanced AIDS, neutropenia, prior use of corticosteroids, or CD4 counts less than 50 mm^3.

Clinical Features

Aspergillus spp. may affect virtually any organ but have a predilection for the lungs and central nervous system. Invasive aspergillosis involves the lung (either primarily or in the context of widespread dissemination) in more than 80% of cases. Brain involvement occurs in 10–15% of cases. Prognosis with cerebral aspergillosis is grim, with a fatality rate of more than 95%. Aspergillosis involving the maxillary or ethmoidal sinuses may extend into the orbit or intracerebral vessels in neutropenic hosts. Ocular invasion may necessitate surgical enucleation in addition to medical therapy. Gastrointestinal involvement is rarely recognized antemortem but has been noted at necropsy in up to 20% of patients with disseminated aspergillosis. Virtually all such cases manifest pulmonary involvement. Primary cutaneous infection may complicate the use of Hickman catheters in granulocytopenic patients. Rare sites of involvement include the liver, spleen, upper airways, bone, wounds, epidural space, urinary tract, pericardium, and endocardium.

Bronchopulmonary Involvement

Aspergilli cause a wide spectrum of pulmonary disease, including allergic bronchopulmonary aspergillosis (ABPA), mycetoma (fungal ball), chronic necrotizing aspergillosis, invasive aspergillosis, and locally invasive endobronchial infection. ABPA is a hypersensitivity response to *Aspergillus* antigens in asthmatics. Clinical manifestations include blood and tissue eosinophilia, wheezing, pulmonary infiltrates, high serum IgE, and positive immediate skin tests to *Aspergillus*. Corticosteroids (to ablate the exaggerated antigenic response) are the mainstay of therapy. ABPA does not disseminate and antifungal therapy is not required. *Aspergillus* spp. may also infect preexisting cavities in patients with chronic granulomatous or obstructive lung disease, forming a distinct mass or fungal ball (i.e., aspergilloma or mycetoma). A crescent, with an intracavitary mass of hyphae, may be observed on chest x-rays or on computed tomographic (CT) scans. Hemoptysis may result from erosion of the fungal hyphae into pulmonary vessels. Surgical resection should be done when feasible. Specific antifungal therapy is of limited value. Chronic necrotizing aspergillosis is a rare condition, distinct from mycetoma, which may occur in immunologically normal hosts. Chronic infection with *Aspergillus* occurs within preexisting pulmo-

nary cavities and extends or invades contiguous lung parenchyma. A distinct mycetoma is not observed, and extrapulmonary spread is rare. The course of chronic
necrotizing aspergillosis is indolent and rarely fatal. Treatment with amphotericin
B or itraconazole is advised, but data affirming their efficacy are limited. In contrast
to the syndromes just reviewed, invasive aspergillosis represents tissue invasion with
Aspergillus spp. and is confined to individuals with serious deficits in immunity.
The most common initial features of invasive pulmonary aspergillosis are fever and
new or persistent infiltrate(s) on chest radiographs. Patchy bronchopneumonia, single
or multiple nodular infiltrates, or cavitary lesions may be seen. Lobar consolidation
indistinguishable from bacterial pneumonia occurs in 5–15% of patients. Diffuse
miliary or interstitial changes are unusual. Progressive parenchymal necrosis may
lead to cavitation or even mycetoma. Pleuritic chest pain and hemoptysis are common
associated symptoms. *Aspergillus* spp. have a propensity to invade pulmonary vessels; intravascular thrombosis, necrosis, or hemorrhage may result. The course of
invasive aspergillosis, in the absence of therapy, is dismal, with most patients dying
within 2–4 weeks. With aggressive medical therapy, favorable responses can be
achieved in 50–80% of patients, provided the underlying immune deficits can be
improved. Localized aspergillosis selectively invading the tracheobronchial tree may
complicate AIDS, leukemia, or organ transplantation. Bronchoscopy may demonstrate necrotizing tracheitis, destruction of cartilage, ulcerations, or pseudomembranes overlying the bronchial mucosa. Amphotericin B or itraconazole may be
effective in up to 70% of patients. Surgical debridement may be required as adjunctive therapy.

Diagnosis

Diagnosing invasive pulmonary aspergillosis is difficult, as only 10–30% of sputum
cultures are positive in this context. Furthermore, isolation of *Aspergillus* spp. from
sputum or BAL has been associated with invasive disease in only 30–80% of patients
at risk; in the remaining patients, positive cultures represent asymptomatic colonization. In patients with AIDS, isolation of *Aspergillus* spp. in BAL is highly predictive
of tissue invasion. Serologies are not helpful. Serum antibodies are neither sensitive
nor specific. Serologic studies to detect *Aspergillus* antigens by immunodiffusion or
counterimmunoelectrophoretic (CIE) techniques are of no practical value. Enzyme-
linked immunosorbent assays (ELISA) demonstrating *Aspergillus* antigen in serum
or BAL fluid are promising but are not commercially available. PCR could theoretically improve sensitivity but has the potential for false–positive reactions. A definitive diagnosis of invasive aspergillosis requires visualizing the typical septated hy-
phal forms within tissue. The fungal elements may be seen on hematoxylin-eosin
stains, but methenamine-silver stains more clearly reveal the organisms. The histopathologic response is variable; an acute suppurative response or a mixed mononuclear cell infiltrate (or both) may be observed. A frank granulomatous response is
rare. Necrosis is a hallmark; vascular invasion, with intra-arterial thrombosis, is
common. Fiberoptic bronchoscopy (to include transbronchial lung biopsies and
BAL) is the invasive procedure of choice when the disease is diffuse or when it

involves an entire segment or lobe; sensitivity ranges from 40 to 70%. Percutaneous needle aspiration is superior for small, localized, nodular densities; anticipated yields exceed 70%. Open lung biopsy is rarely required. Delay in initiation of antimycotic therapy by even a few days may markedly reduce the chance for cure. Thus, empiric treatment of suspected cases should be considered in patients at high risk for invasive disease, even though histopathologic confirmation is lacking. In granulocytopenic patients with fever or pulmonary infiltrates, isolation of *Aspergillus* from nasal or tracheobronchial secretions warrants empiric treatment with amphotericin B while awaiting the results of ancillary studies.

Treatment

Mortality from invasive pulmonary, cerebral, or disseminated aspergillosis exceeds 50–80% in most series. The most important determinants of outcome are the status of the underlying disease and the ability to restore immune function. Even with aggressive antifungal therapy, prognosis in patients with hematologic malignancies in relapse, in bone marrow transplant recipients, or in patients with AIDS is poor (more than 90% mortality). In contrast, mortality rates of less than 20% have been noted when aggressive antifungal therapy is initiated early (within 2–4 days of onset of symptoms) and remission of the underlying disease and restoration of immune function have been achieved.

Preferred Therapy

SEVERE, DISSEMINATED, OR LIFE-THREATENING INVASIVE ASPERGILLOSIS

- Amphotericin B (1–1.5 mg/kg/day for total dose of 1.5–3.0 gm), particularly in neutropenic patients or those patients at highest risk for poor outcome. Lower doses (0.5 mg/kg/day) may be adequate if the level of immunosuppression can be reduced.

ADJUNCTIVE THERAPY

- Surgical resection, drainage, or debridement of devitalized, necrotic tissue may be critical as adjunctive therapy when the disease is localized (e.g., sinusitis, skin, bone, single pulmonary cavity);
- Restore or improve immune function (or reverse underlying disease).

COMBINATION THERAPY FOR SEVERE OR FULMINANT CASES (ADD TO AMPHOTERICIN B)

- Add 5-flucytosine (5-FC). 5-FC may be synergistic with amphotericin B and penetrates well into cerebrospinal fluid, bone, and vitreous (areas in which amphotericin B achieves low concentrations). Flucytosine has potential marrow toxicity and may not be suitable for patients with limited marrow reserve.

- Add rifampin. Data from animal models and anecdotal clinical experience in humans suggest that combining rifampin and amphotericin B may be beneficial.

LOCALIZED, NONFULMINANT FORMS (OR PATIENTS FAILING AMPHOTERICIN B)

- Itraconazole (200 mg b.i.d.) is highly active against *Aspergillus* spp. and is much less toxic than amphotericin B. Oral itraconazole (200–400 mg/day) has been curative in 50–80% of cases of chronic necrotizing or invasive aspergillosis. High doses (600–800 mg/day) have been required for central nervous system involvement. Itraconazole may be used in patients failing or experiencing side effects from amphotericin B. A minimum of 6 months of therapy is recommended.
- Liposomal amphotericin B or complexes of amphotericin B with lipids may be less toxic than free amphotericin B. Data in humans are limited.

Note: Ketoconazole, miconazole, and fluconazole are not recommended for *Aspergillus* infections.

Blastomycosis

Epidemiology

Blastomycosis, produced by the soil-dwelling dimorphic fungus *Blastomyces dermatitidis,* is endemic in the central and midwestern United States and in portions of Canada. The endemic area extends eastward across the Midwest and southern United States, overlapping the endemic area for histoplasmosis. Most cases of blastomycosis occur in immunocompetent hosts. In this context, pulmonary involvement occurs in 50–80% of patients. Extrapulmonary blastomycosis involving skin, bone, or prostate occurs in more than 40% of cases. Blastomycosis is a rare opportunist, and only sporadic cases of blastomycosis complicating AIDS or organ transplantation have been described. In this context, dissemination to skin, bones, genitourinary tract, viscera, or meninges may occur.

Clinical Features

Blastomyces dermatitidis enters the host via the lung. As with other endemic fungi, most individuals infected with *B. dermatitidis* are probably asymptomatic. In immunocompetent hosts, blastomycosis typically manifests as a focal pneumonia. When symptoms are present, cough, sputum production, fever, chills, myalgias, and arthralgias are most common. Focal pneumonic infiltrates (with or without cavitation) are characteristic; miliary or interstitial patterns are observed in fewer than 20% of patients. Acute blastomycotic pneumonia may resolve spontaneously. Skin, bone, or prostate are the most common sites of extrapulmonary involvement. Liver, spleen, abdominal viscera, or central nervous system involvement is rare but may be seen in severely immunocompromised hosts.

Diagnosis

Identification of the organism by culture or histopathology is the only reliable means of diagnosing blastomycosis. *B. dermatitidis* may be identified in cytologic or histopathologic specimens as large, budding yeasts (8–20 m) with a doubly refractile cell wall. The organism may be identified by conventional KOH (10% potassium hydroxide stains) but is more clearly recognized by periodic acid-Schiff (PAS) or methenamine-silver stains. Isolation of the organism in culture requires 2–4 weeks. Histopathology usually demonstrates a suppurative response with extensive necrosis. Varying degrees of lymphocyte and mononuclear infiltration may be observed. Granulomas may be noted but are unusual.

Therapy

Amphotericin B is curative in up to 93% of patients with blastomycosis and is the treatment of choice for severe or life-threatening blastomycosis. Oral azoles may be substituted for less severe forms of blastomycosis. Randomized studies have not been performed, but itraconazole (200–400 mg daily) appears to be more effective than ketoconazole (400–800 mg daily) or fluconazole (200–400 mg daily) in open, multicenter trials. Favorable responses were noted in more than 90% of patients treated with itraconazole, compared with 80 and 65% responses with ketoconazole or fluconazole, respectively. Fluconazole penetrates well into the central nervous system, and anecdotal successes as therapy for CNS blastomycosis have been reported. Treatment with oral azoles must be prolonged (6–12 months) to minimize the chance for late relapse. Amphotericin B is warranted for patients failing oral azoles.

Preferred Therapy

IMMUNOCOMPETENT PATIENTS

- Non-life-threatening blastomycosis not involving the central nervous system: Itraconazole (400 mg/day) for at least 6 months.
- Severe, life-threatening, ventilatory failure or central nervous system involvement: Amphotericin B (0.4–0.8 mg/kg/day) to a total dose of 2 grams or until stable, then itraconazole 400 mg/day for at least 6 months.

Alternate Therapy (Less Effective than Amphotericin B or Itraconazole)

- Non-life-threatening blastomycosis not involving the central nervous system: Ketoconazole 400–800 mg/day for at least 6 months.

IMMUNOCOMPROMISED PATIENTS

- Amphotericin B (1,000–2,000 mg cumulative dose), then itraconazole (400 mg/day) for life (or until immune deficits have resolved).

Coccidioidomycosis

Epidemiology

Coccidioidomycosis is an illness caused by the dimorphic fungus *Coccidioides immitis,* which grows in the soil in endemic areas in the southwestern United States (e.g., California, Nevada, Arizona, New Mexico, and Texas). Positive skin tests for *C. immitis* (indicative of prior infection) have been noted in 1.5–25% of patients living in endemic areas. Aerosolization of the fungus by disruption of the soil by climatic conditions, construction, camping, outdoor recreational activities, excavation, or farming may lead to infection. Changes in environmental conditions markedly influence the prevalence of disease. For example, from 1986 to 1990, an average of 450 cases were reported annually in California. The incidence increased 10-fold in 1992 and 1993, following cycles of drought, rain, and disturbances in the soil. More than two-thirds of cases emanated from a single county. Clinical disease may develop following aerosolization into the lower respiratory tract. In normal hosts, immune defenses usually contain the infection, and spontaneous resolution ensues. *C. immitis* is a rare opportunist in immunocompromised hosts residing in endemic areas. Patients with defects in cellular immunity are at increased risk. Risk factors for dissemination include black or Filipino race, pregnancy, diabetes mellitus, organ transplantation, corticosteroid or immunosuppressive therapy, or AIDS. Coccidioidomycosis is a rare complication of AIDS. During a 6-year period, only 602 of 223,065 patients with AIDS (0.3%) had disseminated coccidioidomycosis. In endemic areas, 2–6% of HIV-infected patients develop coccidioidomycosis; rates as high as 25% have been noted in some endemic areas. Sporadic cases have been described in nonendemic areas, usually from laboratory hazards or exposure to contaminated material. Person-to-person transmission does not occur.

Clinical Features

Approximately 60% of infections caused by *C. immitis* are asymptomatic. Clinical features are protean, ranging from a mild influenza-like illness to severe pneumonia. Primary pulmonary involvement produces an influenza-like illness characterized by cough, fever, chest pain, headache, and sore throat. A rash is noted in approximately 50% of patients; erythema nodosum and erythema multiforme occur less frequently. Patchy infiltrates, ranging in size from segmental to lobar, are observed on chest radiographs. Pleural effusions occur in approximately 20% of patients. Primary pulmonary coccidioidomycosis usually resolves spontaneously, and most patients never seek medical attention. When the infective dose is high, however, the patient may be toxic with high fever. Persistence of pulmonary coccidioidomycosis for more than 6 weeks is referred to as chronic pulmonary coccidioidomycosis. Chest radiographs may demonstrate upper lobe infiltrates, mimicking tuberculosis (TB). Classically, thin-walled cavities may be noted. With long-standing disease, pulmonary fibrosis and calcification may develop. Symptoms include productive cough, hemoptysis, chest pain, and low grade fever. Chronic empyemas or bronchopleural fistulae are notoriously difficult to treat. Symptomatic extrapulmonary dissemination occurs in only 0.5% of infections but is more prevalent among immunosuppressed individuals. Common sites of extrapulmonary spread include meninges, bones, joints, skin, and soft tissues. Meningitis is the most dreaded complication of coccidioidal infections. Progressive and disseminated infections are nearly invariably observed in AIDS patients. In this population, pneumonia, lymphadenopathy, meningoencephalitis, hepatosplenomegaly, and multifocal spread are common.

Diagnosis

The diagnosis can be established by identifying *C. immitis* within body tissues or fluids. Histologic demonstration of a mature spherule (50–100 g) with endospores in tissue is pathognomonic. A granulomatous response may be evident. Spinal fluid examination is essential when central nervous system involvement is suspected. Complement fixation (CF) antibodies against coccidioidin are present in spinal fluid in 75% of patients. In cases of coccidioidal meningitis, large quantities of cerebrospinal fluid (CSF) may be required to confirm the diagnosis. Bone scanning is a sensitive screen for bone involvement. Serologies may aid in identifying the organism and gauging the severity and extent of disease. Serum IgM antibodies are detected in 75% of individuals with primary infections; IgG antibody is present later. The CF test is the serologic gold standard. Changes in serum CF titers may be prognostically helpful. Titers of 1:8–1:16 are common in pulmonary infection; a titer of 1:32 or greater or a rising titer suggests dissemination. If the CF test is used to guide treatment, the test must be performed in a reference laboratory and specimens must be tested together to ensure comparable results. Serologic tests in patients with AIDS may be falsely negative. Biopsy or cultures are of primary importance in these patients. Skin tests are positive in virtually all immunocompetent patients with primary infections but anergy may be seen with dissemination or preexisting immune impairment.

Therapy

Mild infections may not require therapy because spontaneous resolution frequently occurs. For severe or progressive infections, amphotericin B is the treatment of choice. Oral azoles have not yet been approved for coccidioidomycosis, but itraconazole or fluconazole are effective for mild to moderate disease not involving the central nervous system (favorable responses in more than two-thirds of patients in uncontrolled trials). Fluconazole (200–400 mg/day) is often used for empiric therapy because fluconazole is less expensive than itraconazole. For chronic pulmonary coccidioidomycosis, 1–2 years of therapy (with either agent) is advised because late relapses are common on cessation of therapy. Currently, a double-blind study comparing fluconazole with itraconazole is in progress. Traditionally, *C. immitis* meningitis has been treated with amphotericin B administered by lumbar or cisternal route. A prolonged course (more than 1 year) is warranted. Given the inconvenience and complications associated with intracisternal or lumbar routes, oral azoles are an attractive alternative for meningeal disease. Oral itraconazole or fluconazole may be adequate, but a high rate of relapse (up to 75%) has been noted when azoles are stopped.

Preferred Therapy

IMMUNOCOMPETENT PATIENTS

- Primary (focal) pulmonary infection: Observe or fluconazole (400 mg/day) for 12 months.
- Progressive or chronic pulmonary or extrapulmonary disease: Fluconazole (200–400 mg/day) or itraconazole (400 mg/day) for 1–2 years.
- Localized coccidioidomycosis in patients with risk factors for dissemination (immunosuppressive therapy, diabetes mellitus, black or Filipino race, pregnancy): Fluconazole (400 mg/day) or itraconazole (400 mg/day) for 6–12 months.
- Severe or disseminated coccidioidomycosis: Amphotericin B (2,000–3,000 mg total cumulative dose); if remission is not achieved, prolonged courses to a dose of 4,000–5,000 mg may be required.
- Coccidioidal meningitis (patient awake): Fluconazole (400–800 mg/day) or itraconazole (400 mg/day) for at least 12 months.
- Coccidioidal meningitis (patient confused): Intravenous amphotericin B (2.0–3.0 gm total cumulative dose) plus intrathecal amphotericin B (0.1–1 mg) three times weekly via an intraventricular reservoir. Continue therapy until the CSF is normal and CF titers are low or absent. After improvement, give fluconazole (400 mg/day) for 12 months.
- Adjunctive surgical resection may have a role in chronic cavitary pulmonary disease (persistent bronchopleural fistulae or localized soft tissue or bone infections refractory to medical therapy).

IMMUNOCOMPROMISED PATIENTS

- Primary (focal) pulmonary infection: Fluconazole (400 mg/day) for life (or until immune deficits have resolved).
- Diffuse pulmonary infiltrates: Amphotericin B (1500–2000 mg total cumulative dose), then fluconazole (400–800 mg/day) or itraconazole (400 mg/day) for life (or until immune deficits have resolved). Fluconazole or itraconazole alone may be efficacious for slowly progressive disease.
- Extrapulmonary focal lesions (lymphadenopathy skin lesions, osteomyelitis, meningitis). *Rapidly Progressive:* Amphotericin B (2,000–3,000 mg total dose), then fluconazole (400–800 mg/day) or itraconazole (400 mg/day) for life (or until immune deficits have resolved). *Indolent:* Fluconazole (400–800 mg/day) or itraconazole (400 mg/day) for life (or until immune deficits have resolved).

Cryptococcosis

Epidemiology

Cryptococcosis is a mycosis caused by *Cryptococcus neoformans,* an encapsulated yeast distributed worldwide in soil, avian excreta, and fruits. Two varieties of *C.*

neoformans exist. *C. neoformans* variety *neoformans* occurs worldwide; *C. neoformans* variety *gattii* occurs in subtropical or tropical climates (including southern California). Clinical infections may occur by inhalation of the yeast form into the lower respiratory tract. Direct human-to-human or animal-to-human infection is not known to occur. *C. neoformans gattii* typically infects healthy hosts and has only rarely been described in immunosuppressed patients. In contrast, *C. neoformans neoformans* usually infects immunosuppressed individuals and is the most common fungal infection complicating HIV. Dissemination and fungemia are more common with *C. neoformans* variety *neoformans*. Disease associated with the variety *gattii* is usually localized, with a longer duration of symptoms prior to presentation. Cell-mediated immunity (involving T cells and macrophages) is the paramount means of defense against *C. neoformans*. Organ transplantation, hematologic malignancies, corticosteroid or immunosuppressive therapy, and AIDS are well-recognized risk factors for cryptococcosis. No abnormality in host defenses can be found in nearly 50% of cases, however. Prior to the advent of AIDS, approximately only 400 new cases of cryptococcosis were diagnosed annually in the United States. The incidence of infections caused by *C. neoformans* ranges from 1 to 2 cases per million individuals per year among healthy hosts. In striking contrast, 6–10% of patients with AIDS develop cryptococcosis. With the advent of AIDS, the incidence of cryptococcosis has escalated dramatically.

Clinical Features

Although the lung is the portal of entry, cryptococcal meningitis occurs in more than 70% of patients and is usually the predominant feature. The avidity of *C. neoformans* for the central nervous system is not well understood. Symptoms of cryptococcal meningitis may be subtle and nonspecific (e.g., fever, headache, malaise); frank meningismus is rare. Nausea, vomiting, papilledema, obtundation, or focal neurologic findings caused by mass lesions may also occur. Cerebrospinal fluid usually demonstrates moderate lymphocytosis. Meningitis is also the most common clinical manifestation in HIV-infected patients. In patients with AIDS and meningeal cryptococcosis, extraneural cryptococcal disease (pneumonia, cryptococcemia, and skin lesions) is evident in 25–50% of cases. In non–HIV-infected patients, clinically evident pulmonary involvement occurs in only 15–40% of patients with cryptococcosis. Pulmonary manifestations are protean, ranging from cough or fever to respiratory failure. In immunocompetent hosts, focal nodules or masses are the most common findings on chest radiograph. Cavitation, lymphadenopathy, and pleural effusions are more common in HIV-infected patients than in non–HIV-infected individuals.

Diagnosis

The diagnosis of cryptococcal meningitis is based on a positive culture of CSF for *C. neoformans* and/or a positive latex agglutination test for cryptococcal antigen in CSF and serum. India ink staining is positive in 75% of patients with cryptococcal meningitis. Blood cultures are positive in more than 95% of AIDS patients with disseminated cryptococcemia. Serum antigen titers are often strikingly high (more than 1:10,000). False–positives (up to 9%) may occur in the presence of circulating rheumatoid factor. Cerebrospinal fluid cell counts may be unimpressive in cryptococcal meningitis in HIV-infected persons. In this context, cryptococcal antigen test, India ink, and cultures are invariably positive.

Diagnosis of pulmonary cryptococcosis often requires bronchoscopy because cultures and wet preparations of expectorated sputum are positive for *C. neoformans* in less than 25% of cases. Serum assays for cryptococcal antigen are often negative in non–HIV-infected persons with pulmonary cryptococcosis but are almost always positive in high titers in HIV-infected patients with cryptococcal lung disease. All patients with pulmonary cryptococcosis should have a lumbar puncture performed, even when central nervous findings are lacking. The prostate gland may be a silent reservoir of cryptococcal infection in 30% of HIV-infected patients. Prostatic massage followed by collection of a midstream urine for fungal culture may be diagnostic, especially in patients who relapse during or after therapy.

Treatment

- Pulmonary cryptococcosis usually disseminates in immunosuppressed patients and warrants antifungal therapy (even in the absence of symptoms).
- Treatment is advised even in immunologically normal hosts if pulmonary infiltrates are present on chest radiographs.
- Treatment is not necessary for immunocompetent patients with cryptococcal colonization but without radiographic lung disease.
- Normal hosts with lung nodules or masses removed surgically do not require immediate treatment but should be followed to exclude progression or relapse.

Cryptococcal meningitis in patients without HIV warrants treatment with amphotericin B (0.4 mg/kg/day) and flucytosine (150 mg/kg/day divided in four equal doses) for 6 weeks. This regimen is comparable to amphotericin B alone (0.4 mg/kg/day) for 10 weeks. Flucytosine can produce bone marrow suppression and diarrhea. Serum flucytosine levels should be monitored to maintain serum levels between 30 and 100 μg/mL two hours after a dose. Higher doses of amphotericin B (0.7 mg/kg/day) are required for immunosuppressed patients with cryptococcal meningitis. Short-course therapy (4 weeks) may be adequate in selected patients without serious underlying disease or neurologic complications. High-dose amphotericin B (1 mg/kg/day) plus flucytosine for 2 weeks, followed by itraconazole or fluconazole indefinitely, has also been successful. Fluconazole (200–400 mg/day) alone may be adequate for mild to moderate cryptococcosis but is slightly less effective than amphotericin B in severe cryptococcal meningitis. Higher doses of fluconazole (800 mg/day) may be effective as primary or salvage therapy in patients with severe cryptococcal meningitis. Fluconazole (200 mg/day indefinitely) may be used to prevent late relapses in patients with AIDS and cryptococcal meningitis following primary therapy with amphotericin B. In this context, oral fluconazole was more effective in preventing relapses and less toxic than once-weekly amphotericin B (1 mg/kg IV).

Preferred Therapy

IMMUNOCOMPETENT PATIENTS

- Pulmonary disease: Fluconazole (400 mg/day) for 6 months.
- Meningitis (patient awake, stable): Fluconazole (400 mg/day) for 6–12 months.
- Meningitis (patient confused): Amphotericin B (0.4 mg/kg/day) plus flucytosine (150 mg/kg/day) for 4 weeks.

IMMUNOCOMPROMISED PATIENTS

- Pulmonary disease: Amphotericin B (0.7 mg/kg/day) plus flucytosine (100 mg/kg/day) until stable, then fluconazole (200 mg/day) for life.
- Meningitis: Amphotericin B (0.7 mg/kg/day) plus flucytosine (100 mg/kg/day) until stable, then fluconazole (200 mg/day) for life.

Histoplasmosis

Epidemiology

Histoplasmosis, a mycosis caused by the dimorphic fungus *Histoplasma capsulatum*, is endemic in the Mississippi and Ohio River areas, where the organism resides in soil contaminated with avian excreta. Cleaning chicken houses, spelunking, excavating, or cutting or bulldozing trees contaminated by spores may lead to infection. The overall incidence of histoplasmin sensitivity in the United States is approximately 22%, but more than 90% of adults are skin-test positive in certain areas of the Mississippi and Ohio River Valleys.

Clinical Features

H. capsulatum produces a wide spectrum of clinical syndromes. Following inhalation of microconidia into the lung, the organisms multiply and spread to regional lymph nodes or via the bloodstream to the liver and spleen. Acute primary histoplasmosis occurs in individuals previously unexposed to *H. capsulatum* and is asymptomatic or produces minimal influenza-like symptoms (e.g., fever, malaise, headache, nonproductive cough). Erythema nodosum and erythema multiforme may occur during acute histoplasmosis. Primary pulmonary infections usually resolve spontaneously. Chronic progressive pulmonary histoplasmosis (lasting more than 6 weeks) may develop, particularly in patients with underlying chronic obstructive or cavitary lung disease. Upper lobe infiltrates (with or without cavitation) may mimic TB. Spontaneous resolution occurs in up to 80% of patients with noncavitary infiltrates. When cavitation is present, fewer than 20% resolve spontaneously. Symptoms of chronic pulmonary histoplasmosis include chronic sputum production, fever, weight loss, and hemoptysis. Five-year mortality rates may approach 50% in untreated patients. Progressive disseminated histoplasmosis rarely occurs in normal hosts but may occur in patients with impaired immune defenses. The incidence of disseminated histoplasmosis in HIV-infected persons is variable. In Houston and Dallas, Texas, which are on the fringe of the endemic area for histoplasmosis, the incidence is 5%. A recent study from Indianapolis, Indiana, in the heart of the endemic area, noted that 27% of HIV-infected patients developed disseminated histoplasmosis. Clinical features of disseminated histoplasmosis in HIV-infected patients included fever (75%), weight loss (58%), splenomegaly (30%), lymphadenopathy (30%), hepatomegaly (26%), anemia (30%), leukopenia (24%), and thrombocytopenia (20%). Chest radiographs demonstrated diffuse interstitial infiltrates in 70% of patients. Cough and dyspnea were noted in patients with interstitial infiltrates. Atypical presentations included skin lesions, meningitis, disseminated intravascular coagulation, and gastrointestinal ulcers.

Diagnosis

A definitive diagnosis of histoplasmosis requires identifying or culturing *H. capsulatum* in histopathologic specimens or secretions. Serologic data can provide strong confirmatory evidence in the absence of cultural data. CF is the most reliable test for detecting *H. capsulatum.* A serum CF titer to yeast-phase antigens of 1:32 or greater, or an appropriately timed fourfold increase in titer, are evidence of active or recent infection. CF titers are usually low in chronic histoplasmosis. CF titers exceeding 1:8 in CSF suggest *H. capsulatum* meningitis. Immunodiffusion assays measure precipitating antibodies to the M and H antigens. The H band is specific for active infection but is present less often than the M band. Either immunodiffusion or CF tests will be positive in 80% of patients with progressive disseminated histoplasmosis. The organisms may be visualized in peripheral blood buffy coat smears in 45% of patients with disseminated histoplasmosis. Blood cultures using the lysis centrifugation technique are positive in up to 90% of patients with disseminated disease. A radioimmunoassay for *H. capsulatum* polysaccharide antigen in urine is positive in more than 98% of patients with disseminated disease.

Treatment

IMMUNOCOMPETENT PATIENTS

- Acute primary histoplasmosis is usually self-limited and does not require treatment.
- Acute histoplasmosis with ventilatory failure: Amphotericin B (500–1000 mg total dose) or until improvement is noted.
- Cavitary disease: Itraconazole (400 mg/day) or ketoconazole (400–800 mg/day) for 6 months or amphotericin B (2,000 mg total cumulative dose).
- Progressive disseminated disease: Amphotericin B (500–1000 mg cumulative does), then itraconazole (400 mg/day) for 6 months.

IMMUNOCOMPROMISED PATIENTS

- Acute histoplasmosis: Amphotericin B (500–1000 mg cumulative dose), then itraconazole (400 mg/day) (for life or until immune deficits have resolved).

- Progressive disseminated histoplasmosis (mild): Itraconazole (400 mg/day) for life (or until immune deficits have resolved).
- Progressive disseminated histoplasmosis (severely ill): Amphotericin B (500 mg cumulative dose), then itraconazole (400 mg/day) for life (or until immune deficits have resolved).

Mucormycosis (Mucoraceae)

Mucormycosis refers to deep mycotic infection caused by nonseptated fungi belonging to the family Mucoraceae (e.g., *Rhizopus, Absidia, Cunninghamella, Mucor*). Mucoraceous infections are among the rarest of fungal infections and are confined to patients with severe impairments in both granulocyte and mononuclear phagocytic function. High-dose corticosteroid or immunosuppressive therapy, hematologic malignancies, severe granulocytopenia, diabetes mellitus, metabolic acidosis, renal failure, and chronic dialysis are important risk factors for mucormycosis. Mucormycosis rarely complicates AIDS.

Clinical Features

The major forms of mucoraceous infections include rhinocerebral, pulmonary, gastrointestinal, disseminated, and cutaneous. Rhinocerebral mucormycosis (typically involving the nasopharynx and paranasal sinuses) predominates in patients with diabetes mellitus. Extension through the ethmoids to involve the orbit, sphenoidal or cavernous sinuses, and brain may result in visual loss, cranial nerve palsies, or death. Pulmonary or disseminated mucormycosis may occur in patients with profound and global impairment in host defenses. Chest radiographs in pulmonary mucormycosis may demonstrate patchy bronchopneumonia, nodular infiltrates, consolidation, or cavities. Mucoraceae have a propensity to invade blood vessels; thrombosis, distal hemorrhagic infarction, pseudoaneurysm formation, and massive, fatal hemoptysis are well-recognized complications. Mucormycosis may involve the trachea or major bronchi, associated with pseudomembranes and extensive mucosal ulcerations. Mortality with invasive pulmonary (or endobronchial) mucormycosis exceeds 80%; only 2 of 35 patients survived among three published series.

Diagnosis

Diagnosing mucormycosis is usually difficult. In three series of pulmonary mucormycosis, the diagnosis was made at necropsy in 29 of 35 patients. Sputum cultures are positive in only 10–40% of invasive infections. Blood cultures are uniformly negative. Invasive techniques are usually required to isolate or visualize the characteristic fungal elements in tissue. Fungi of the order *Mucorales* are broad, nonseptated hyphae that branch at right angles; methenamine-silver stains more clearly demonstrate the organisms. Histologically, extensive parenchymal necrosis and hyphae invading blood vessels are typical. A neutrophilic suppurative response is characteristic; well-formed granulomata are not seen. Black necrotic pus or debris may overlie sites of necrosis or ulcerations. Isolation of Mucoraceae by culture is presumptive evidence for invasive disease; false–positives are rare. No useful serologic or skin tests exist.

Treatment

- Amphotericin B (to a minimum total dose of 2.0 gm), combined with surgical resection or debridement of involved tissue (when possible). Even with aggressive medical therapy, mortality with invasive pulmonary or disseminated mucormycosis exceeds 90% in patients with hematologic malignancies in relapse. Cures have been noted when control of the underlying disease or reduction in the level of immunosuppression has been achieved.
- Surgical debridement or resection of involved tissue may be critical to optimize outcome. This has been most evident in rhinocerebral mucormycosis in diabetic patients. Combined surgical resection and amphotericin B is advised for localized pulmonary cavitary mucormycosis.
- Other antifungal agents have no significant activity against Mucoraceae.

SPECIFIC ANTIFUNGAL DRUGS
Amphotericin B

Amphotericin B, a polyene antibiotic obtained from a strain of *Streptomyces nodosus,* has been used for more than 30 years and remains the drug of choice for severe or life-threatening invasive fungal infections. Amphotericin B is the preferred therapy for serious infections caused by aspergillosis and mucormycosis and for disseminated or life-threatening infections caused by the endemic fungi (e.g., *B. dermatitides, C. immitis, C. neoformans,* and *H. capsulatum*). Amphotericin B irreversibly binds to fungal sterols, chiefly ergosterol, to produce defects in fungal membrane function (increasing permeability). Increased membrane permeability may permit entry of other antifungal agents (e.g., flucytosine), which may further impede fungal growth.

Adverse Effects

Amphotericin B is associated with significant toxicity and requires careful monitoring. Unpleasant reactions to amphotericin B occur in approximately 70% of patients. Side effects include fever (51%), shaking chills (28%), nausea (18%), headache (9%), and thrombophlebitis (5%). Nephrotoxicity is a predictable consequence of long-term therapy with amphotericin B. Increases in serum creatinine concentrations are noted in 80% of patients. Renal dysfunction may also be manifest by hypokalemia hypomagnesemia, renal tubular acidosis, and nephrocalcinosis. Normocytic, normochromic anemia may also occur. Serum creatinine, blood urea nitrogen (BUN), electrolytes, magnesium, and a complete blood count (CBC) should be evaluated weekly during amphotericin B therapy. No adjustment in dose is required until the serum creatinine level reaches 2.5 mg/dL. Improvement in renal function usually occurs with interruption of therapy, but permanent impairment can occur with cumulative doses exceeding 3 grams. Other nephrotoxic agents should not be given concomitantly unless absolutely necessary. Potassium supplementation is required in nearly 90% of patients receiving amphotericin B.

Mode of Administration

Prolonged infusion of amphotericin B over 3–4 hours has been advised, but the frequency or severity of side effects appears to be no higher when the drug is infused over 1 hour. Because anaphylaxis may rarely complicate use of amphotericin B, a test dose (1 mg) is initiated under careful observation. Routine pretreatment with aspirin, diphenhydramine, hydrocortisone (20–50 mg), or heparin (500 units) has been advocated but may not reduce the incidence of side effects. The use of these agents should be limited to patients experiencing adverse effects or local phlebitis at the injection site. If the test dose is tolerated, the dose can rapidly be escalated to maintenance therapy. Daily therapy should be continued until a clinical response is evident (often within 1 week). Thereafter, alternate-day dosing may be adequate. Dosage should be individualized depending on clinical response and tolerance to amphotericin B. Completion of a 2-gm course of amphotericin B requires 12–18 weeks.

   Drawbacks of amphotericin B include:

* The necessity of IV administration;
* Poor penetration into CSF;
* Intolerance by many patients because of unpleasant side effects;
* Significant toxicity.

Liposomal and Colloidal Formulations of Amphotericin B

Toxicity of amphotericin B can be reduced by combining the parent compound with lipophilic molecules in a lipid-amphotericin B complex or within a liposome. Phase II and III clinical trials suggest that liposomal or lipid complex formulations allow higher doses of amphotericin B with less toxicity. The first of these compounds to be released in the United States is ABELCET, an amphotericin B-lipid complex. ABELCET was approved by the Food and Drug Administration (FDA) in November 1995 for treating aspergillosis in patients refractory to or intolerant of amphotericin B. Data from three studies involving 178 patients (of whom 111 were evaluable) noted favorable responses (partial or complete) in 39% of patients. Responses among patients previously failing amphotericin B was 28%. Responses among patients switched to ABELCET after developing nephrotoxicity from amphotericin B were higher (51%). Fever and chills were the most common adverse effects (noted in 15% of patients); nephrotoxicity was observed in 4% and was dose-dependent. The recommended daily dose of ABELCET for adults and children is 5.0 mg/kg administered as a single intravenous infusion over 2 hours. Another formulation, Amphocil, a colloidal dispersion of amphotericin B and cholesteryl sulfate in a 1:1 ratio, was effective in animal models and in a recent open-label trial (dose up to 6 mg/kg/day) in humans with documented or presumed systemic mycoses. Clinical improvement was noted in 49% of 97 evaluable patients, many of whom had failed prior therapy with intravenous amphotericin B. The drug was discontinued in 14 of 168 (8%) treated patients because of side effects (principally fever, chills, or hypotension). Clinically significant nephrotoxicity was not observed. Amphocil is not yet available in the United States. A liposomal formulation, unilamellar liposomal amphotericin B, is currently in use in several countries but is not yet available in the United States. In an open-label trial of systemic mycoses, favorable responses were achieved with unilamellar liposomal amphotericin B (AmBisome) in 49 of 64 evaluable patients (77%). These novel liposomal or colloidal preparations are promising and may be effective in patients failing to respond to or unable to tolerate conventional amphotericin B.

Oral Azole Antifungal Agents

The azole antifungals include ketoconazole, clotrimazole, miconazole, and the newer triazoles (fluconazole and itraconazole). Azoles are composed of a 5-member (azole) ring attached by a carbon or nitrogen bond to other aromatic rings. Ketoconazole is an imidazole, indicating the presence of two nitrogen atoms in the azole ring. Itraconazole and fluconazole contain three nitrogen atoms in the azole ring and are termed triazoles. All antifungal azoles impair the synthesis of ergosterol, a vital component of fungal cell membranes.

Ketoconazole

Ketoconazole is well adsorbed orally. Metabolism and excretion occurs by hepatobiliary mechanisms; urinary excretion is minimal. Ketoconazole requires gastric acidity for dissolution and absorption. Cimetidine and antacids impair absorption and should be withheld at least 2 hours after administration of ketoconazole.

Activity and Clinical Efficacy

Ketoconazole has in vitro activity against *Candida* species, *B. dermatitidis, C. immitis, H. capsulatum, Paracoccidioides brasiliensis,* and *C. neoformans.* Ketoconazole may be used to treat cavitary *H. capsulatum* and acute or chronic *B. dermatitidis* in immunocompetent hosts.

Adverse Effects

• Serious hepatotoxicity (fatal hepatotoxicity in fewer than 1:10,000 treatment courses);
• Dose-related reversible inhibition of testosterone and adrenal corticosteroid syn-

thesis (resulting in reduced libido, gynecomastia, and often impotence in males);
• Adverse interactions with other drugs.

Concurrent administration of rifampin and ketoconazole may reduce serum keto-conazole levels. Ketoconazole enhances the anticoagulant effects of coumarinlike drugs and increases blood levels of cyclosporin A. Concomitant administration of ketoconazole with phenytoin may alter the metabolism of one or both drugs. Because severe hypoglycemia has been reported in patients concomitantly receiving oral miconazole and oral hypoglycemic agents, the potential interaction of ketoconazole and oral hypoglycemic agents should be monitored.

Fluconazole

Fluconazole, a water-soluble triazole, may be administered intravenously or orally. Oral absorption is rapid (within 2 hours) and the half-life is prolonged, permitting once- or twice-daily dosing. Elimination of the drug is predominantly renal; the dose should be reduced in patients with renal insufficiency. Fluconazole penetrates well into the CSF and is an alternative to amphotericin B for treating fungal meningitis.

Activity and Clinical Efficacy

Fluconazole is highly active against *Candida* spp. and *C. neoformans* and was approved by the FDA in 1990 for treating cryptococcal meningitis and mucosal and systemic candidiasis. Fluconazole has also been used extensively for prophylaxis of infections caused by *Candida* species. Prophylactic fluconazole (400 mg/day) reduces the rate of invasive infections caused by *Candida* spp. among bone marrow transplant recipients and patients with acute leukemia. Prophylactic fluconazole has been associated with a higher rate of colonization or infection by *C. kruseii* in some studies but not in others. Fluconazole (dose 400 mg/day) has been used, with variable success, for deep mycoses caused by paracoccidioidomycosis, sporotrichosis, blasto-mycosis, coccidioidomycosis, and histoplasmosis in immunocompetent hosts. Prolonged therapy (6–12 months) is advised to reduce late relapse rate. Fluconazole should not be used for invasive infections caused by *Aspergillus* spp. Indications and optimal use of fluconazole await further controlled, prospective studies.

Adverse Effects

Fluconazole rarely causes serious toxicity. Skin rash, nausea, and elevated liver enzymes are the most common adverse effects. Hepatotoxicity has rarely been described. Alopecia may occur in 12–20% of patients with high-dose (400 mg/day) therapy for more than 2 months; this is reversible with cessation of the drug or reduction of the dose. In contrast to ketoconazole, fluconazole does not inhibit testicular or adrenal steroidogenesis and does not cause impotence. Fluconazole interferes with phenytoin, cyclosporin A, and warfarin. Drug levels of these agents should be monitored when given concomitantly with fluconazole.

Itraconazole

Itraconazole is available for oral use only. Absorption is impeded by antacids, histamines, H_2-antagonists, or omeprazole. The dose is 200 mg twice daily.

Clinical Efficacy

Itraconazole is effective against most deep fungi, including cryptococcosis, candidiasis, aspergillosis, *H. capsulatum, B. dermatitidis, C. immitis, C. neoformans, P. Brasiliensis,* and *Candida* species. Itraconazole is as effective or more effective than oral ketoconazole for non–life-threatening forms of histoplasmosis, blastomycosis, and coccidioidomycosis. Itraconazole is the treatment of choice for cavitary *H. capsulatum* or acute, chronic, pulmonary and nonmeningeal *B. dermatitidis* in immunocompetent patients. Itraconazole may be suitable to treat immunocompromised patients with the following conditions: acute and progressive disseminated *H. capsulatum;* acute, chronic, and nonmeningeal *B. dermatitidis;* coccidioidomycosis; and localized aspergillosis not involving the central nervous system.

Adverse Effects

Itraconazole is less toxic than ketoconazole. Principal side effects include nausea, vomiting, hypokalemia, gynecomastia, abnormalities in liver function tests, and hypertriglyceridemia. Serious side effects warranting discontinuation of therapy occur in fewer than 5% of patients. Effects on the endocrine system are minimal, but impotence and adrenal suppression have been described at doses exceeding 400 mg/day. Alopecia rarely complicates its use. Itraconazole markedly increases serum levels of cyclosporin A, necessitating reduction of cyclosporin A dose.

Flucytosine

5-FC, a fluorinated pyrimidine analogue, has a narrow spectrum of antimycotic activity and is never used alone because resistance develops rapidly. Flucytosine exerts its effects only in fungi that possess cytosine deaminase. This enzyme metabolizes the 5-FC to 5-fluorouracil, which is then incorporated into fungal RNA and interferes with protein synthesis. Flucytosine is water soluble, and bioavailability is excellent. Flucytosine is a small molecule and rapidly distributes to all tissues, including CSF. The kidneys secrete more than 90% of the drug unchanged. The dose is 100–150 mg/kg/day. Dose reductions are required in the presence of renal insufficiency. Serum levels should be monitored for patients at high risk for toxicity (e.g., decreased renal function, limited bone marrow reserve, concomitant therapy with amphotericin B).

Activity and Clinical Efficacy

Flucytosine is used in combination with amphotericin B. Amphotericin B, by changing fungal cell wall permeability, may enhance the uptake of flucytosine into the cell although this is controversial. Amphotericin B and flucytosine is the treatment of choice for meningitis secondary to *C. neoformans* in non–HIV-infected patients. The use of combination therapy in AIDS patients is controversial because of the high incidence of drug-induced cytopenias associated with 5-FC in these patients. If flucytosine is administered in AIDS patients, the dose should be 100 mg/day. The dose should be adjusted based on weekly serum concentration of flucytosine.

Adverse Effects

Leukopenia or thrombocytopenia occur in up to 5% of patients receiving flucytosine. Cytopenias are most common in patients with impaired renal function and correlate with high serum concentrations (usually more than 100 μg/mL).

NOCARDIA SPECIES
Epidemiology

Nocardia spp. are Gram-positive filamentous branching rods within the genus *Nocardia* and the family Actinomycetaceae. Although originally misclassified as fungi, *Nocardia* spp. are true bacteria. *Nocardia* spp. are commonly found in soil, decaying organic matter, and environmental sources, but are not part of normal human flora. Three species cause disease in humans: *N. asteroides, N. brasiliensis,* and *N. caviae.* The usual route of infection with *N. asteroides* is inhalation into the lung. Cutaneous inoculation is the predominant mechanism implicated for *N. brasiliensis. N. asteroides* accounts for 80–95% of cases of nocardiosis; *N. brasiliensis,* 3–9%; *N. caviae,* 1–3%. Nocardial infections are rare; even large referral centers encounter only 1–3 new cases per year. More than 75% of infections caused by *Nocardia* spp. occur in patients with severe defects in immunity, but infections may be noted in the absence of preexisting immunologic deficits. Risk factors for nocardiosis include high-dose corticosteroids or immunosuppressive therapy, organ transplantation, chronic granulomatous disease, and hematologic malignancies. Nocardiosis among organ transplant recipients (or other high-risk groups) has been virtually eliminated by TMP/SMX prophylaxis for *P. carinii* because TMP/SMX also inhibits *Nocardia* spp. Nocardiosis complicates AIDS in only 0.2–0.3% of cases. A recent review identified six cases of nocardiosis among 2,167 patients with AIDS at a New York Hospital between 1980 and 1989.

Clinical Features

Clinical expression of these various species differs. *N. asteroides* has a propensity to involve the lung, central nervous system, and skin. In contrast, more than half of all infections caused by *N. brasiliensis* are localized to skin or subcutaneous tissues. *N. caviae* is a rare pathogen but may cause pulmonary or disseminated disease in immunocompromised hosts. Nocardiosis involves the lung in 56–85% of cases and may appear as acute, subacute, or chronic pneumonitis. An acute, necrotizing pneumonia with chills and rigors may occur. A chronic, indolent course with symptoms progressing over several weeks, however, is more characteristic. Up to one-third of patients with pulmonary nocardiosis are asymptomatic, with incidental changes noted on chest x-ray. Solitary or multiple nodules (which may cavitate) are most characteristic, but bronchopneumonic or lobar infiltrates with consolidation may be noted. Pleural effusions are present in 20–30% of patients. Bronchopleural fistulae and empyema rarely complicate chronic pulmonary nocardiosis. Extrapulmonary involvement occurs in 20–45% of cases. The central nervous system is involved in 15% of cases. Brain abscess is the most frequent CNS manifestation, but spinal cord, epidural space, eyes, and meninges may be affected. Skin or soft tissue involvement occurs in 10–20%. Cutaneous manifestations are protean and include pustules, draining sinus tracts, subcutaneous or cutaneous nodules, mass lesions, and cellulitis. Direct inoculation of nocardial organisms into skin or soft tissue via abrasions or local trauma may result in localized infection; this is particularly characteristic of *N. brasiliensis*. Dissemination to bone, joints, heart, spleen, liver, kidney, or lymph nodes occurs in 1–4% of cases of nocardiosis (all species).

Diagnosis

The diagnosis of nocardiosis is usually difficult. Sputum smears and cultures are positive in only 20–50% of cases of pulmonary nocardiosis, even when multiple samples are obtained. Blood cultures are invariably negative. On Gram's stain, *Nocardia* spp. are Gram-positive, coccobacillary rods with a filamentous or beaded appearance. These organisms are weakly positive by Kinyoun-modified Ziehl-Neelsen acid-fast stains. *Nocardia* spp. have complex growth requirements in culture, are slow-growing, and may be overgrown by other organisms. Identification may take 1–4 weeks. Because routine cultures are often discarded after 3–4 days, the microbiologic laboratory must be specifically informed that *Nocardia* is a consideration. False–positive cultures for *Nocardia* spp. are rare. Isolation of *Nocardia* spp. from any immunocompromised host warrants treatment, even if symptoms are absent, because fatal dissemination may occur later. Invasive techniques are usually required to establish the diagnosis. Percutaneous needle aspiration is recommended for localized nodular lesions, with diagnostic yields of up to 80%. Fiberoptic bronchoscopy is preferred for diffuse disease or segmental or lobar pneumonia with consolidation. Histologically, a suppurative response, with necrosis, is characteristic. Lymphocytic and mononuclear cellular infiltrates may be observed, but well-formed granulomas are rare. *Nocardia* spp. are not visible on hematoxylin-eosin stains but may be detected on methenamine-silver stains or modified Ziehl-Neelsen stains. Sinus drainage may reveal sulfur granules from cutaneous, subcutaneous, or pleural lesions. In cases of CNS involvement, identifying *Nocardia* spp. at other sites may obviate the need to biopsy cerebral lesions. CT scans may be invaluable in detecting, staging, and following cerebral nocardiosis. An area of decreased density in the center of the lesion, surrounded by a dense ring in the periphery, is characteristic of nocardial abscess. Serologic or skin tests are not commercially available.

Treatment

- Sulfonamides, alone or in combination with trimethoprim, are the agents of choice. Controlled studies have not been performed, but sulfisoxazole, sulfadiazine, or TMP/SMX appear equally efficacious (cure rates more than 80%). The combination of TMP and SMX may be synergistic, and TMP penetrates into the CSF better than SMX. At least 12 months of therapy is advised to prevent late relapses. Most treatment failures occur in immunocompromised patients with CNS involvement or widespread disease or when treatment is delayed.

Preferred Therapy

- TMP/SMX (6–8 single-strength tablets daily in divided doses) for at least 12 months;
- Surgical resection or debridement may be critical as adjunctive therapy (particularly for cutaneous or soft tissue infections).

Alternate Therapy

- Sulfisoxazole (4–12 gm/day) or sulfadiazine (6–8 gm/day);
- Minocycline (300 mg orally b.i.d.) for cases resistant to or intolerant of sulfonamides (not reliable for CNS infections);
- Imipenem, cefuroxime, cefotaxime, ceftriaxone, amikacin, or ciprofloxacin plus TMP/SMX to confer synergy. (Reserve for patients failing TMP/SMX or minocycline or with severe infections).

MYCOBACTERIAL INFECTIONS
Mycobacterium tuberculosis

Epidemiology

Mycobacterium tuberculosis remains the most important cause of mortality resulting from infectious diseases worldwide. Globally, more than 8 million active cases occur annually, accounting for 2.9 million deaths per year. In the United States, the number of reported cases of TB annually declined steadily from 1953 (84,304 cases) to 1984 (22,255 cases). This trend reversed after 1985. Cases of TB increased by approximately 20% from 1985–1992. In 1993, 25,313 cases were reported. This resurgence in TB is largely related to the HIV epidemic and to changes in socioeconomic conditions. The number of cases of TB in patients with AIDS increased from 0.1% in 1981 to 9.5% in 1990. Additional factors contributing to this increase included homelessness, poverty, substance abuse, the influx of foreign-born immigrants from areas with high endemic rates of TB, and lack of adequate public health control measures. The proportion of cases from foreign-born immigrants increased from 22% in 1986 to 30% in 1993. Most cases among foreign-born immigrants represent reactivation rather than recent infection from the local community. Current programs to adequately identify and treat TB are inadequate. Inadequate compliance with therapeutic and prophylactic regimens has created a substantial reservoir of infected individuals with latent infection who remain at risk for reactivation. In addition, strains of *M. tuberculosis* displaying resistance to multiple antituberculous agents have increased dramatically. HIV-infected persons account for a large proportion of these drug-resistant strains; case fatality rates in this context are high. The lack of protective immunity among HIV-infected persons even after treatment for active disease puts these patients at risk for exogenous reinfection with new strains of *M. tuberculosis.*

Clinical Features

Tuberculous infection in a naive host usually produces a subclinical syndrome whose only manifestation is a positive tuberculin skin test (PPD). Primary infection may present as a lymphocyte pleural effusion, with or without a concomitant parenchymal infiltrate. Fever, sweats, chills, and a lymphocyte exudative pleural effusion suggest the diagnosis. Most cases of active TB represent reactivation of a latent (dormant) focus. In non–HIV-infected patients, reactivation TB manifests as parenchymal infiltrates in the posterior and apical segments of the upper lobes in more than 95% of patients; cavitation is frequent. Hilar or mediastinal adenopathy, localized lower or middle lobe infiltrates, or normal chest radiographs occur in fewer than 4% of cases in immunocompetent patients. Night sweats, chills, weight loss, fatigue, and cough are common associated symptoms. A productive cough (often with hemoptysis) is characteristic. Extrapulmonary involvement occurs in approximately 15% of patients with TB.

Early in the course of HIV-infection, clinical and radiographic features of TB are similar to the non–HIV-infected population. Among patients with advanced AIDS, however, cavitation is rare, and hilar adenopathy, pleural effusions, focal infiltrates, or a miliary pattern are more common. The most striking feature of TB in HIV-infected patients is the high frequency of extrapulmonary involvement. In HIV-infected patients, at least two-thirds of patients manifest extrapulmonary spread. Lymphatic involvement is most common; other sites of extrapulmonary spread include meninges, pericardium, genitourinary tract, peritonitis, bone, and skin. Vertebral TB may cause kyphosis and spinal cord symptoms. The patient typically appears after weeks to months of back pain, fever, and weight loss. Tuberculous meningitis is a dreaded complication. Fever, weight loss, and malaise usually predate CNS involvement.

Diagnosis of Active Tuberculosis

Sputum smears and cultures are the mainstay of diagnosis. Acid-fast smears of sputum are positive among 70–85% of patients with cavitary pulmonary TB; the yield is less than 40% among patients with noncavitary forms or with HIV infection. Sputum cultures are positive in 65–95% of patients with pulmonary TB. Three sputum samples (for both smear and cultures) are recommended. Conventional cultures in solid media are highly specific but require 3–6 weeks to isolate *M. tuberculosis*. More recently, radiometric techniques and nucleic acid probes (e.g., Bactec) can identify *M. tuberculosis* within 10–14 days. PCR techniques may detect *M. tuberculosis* within several hours with sensitivity comparable to conventional cultures and superior to acid-fast smears. False–positives occur in fewer than 1%. Because of its expense and complexity, however, the role of PCR in clinical practice needs to be better defined. Bronchoscopy may be considered in suspected cases of pulmonary TB when sputum smears are negative. The yield of bronchoscopic techniques varies. Sensitivity of bronchoscopic cultures in cases of active TB has ranged from 63 to 87%. Acid-fast smears, however, are positive in only 10–20%. Surprisingly, in some studies the yield of cultures of BAL was lower than that of sputum. Transbronchial lung biopsy demonstrates caseating granulomas in approximately 40% of patients with active TB and negative acid-fast smears. Although transbronchial biopsies only marginally increase the yield above sputum or BAL, the rapid diagnosis with this technique may be advantageous. Enthusiasm for bronchoscopy must be tempered by awareness of its potential for nosocomial transmission of infection, expense, and invasiveness. A recent prospective trial found that induced sputum (via an ultrasonic nebulizer) was as effective as fiberoptic bronchoscopy in patients with pulmonary TB and negative sputum smears. Sensitivity and negative predictive value of bronchoscopic cultures were 73% and 91%, respectively, compared to 87 and 96% for sputum induction. Thus, induced sputum may be a cost-effective and noninvasive means of confirming the diagnosis in smear negative but suspected cases. Other potential sites for obtaining cultures include blood (primarily in HIV-infected patients), lymph nodes, bone marrow, or clinically-infected sites. Mycobacterial blood cultures yield *M. tuberculosis* in approximately 50% of HIV-infected patients with active TB. Serologic tests are of no value.

Tuberculin Skin Tests

The tuberculin skin test (i.e., PPD) is a useful diagnostic and epidemiologic tool. Differences in the capacity to react to tuberculin skin testing has lead to differing criteria for what constitutes a positive reaction. The threshold for a positive test has recently been revised. The cutoff point is 15 mm in otherwise healthy individuals with no known contact with an active case. A cutoff of 10 mm was adopted for patients with recent skin test conversion or for patients with predisposing conditions. In contrast, 5-mm induration is considered positive in patients with HIV infection. A negative tuberculin skin test does not exclude active TB, particularly in patients with malnutrition or impairments in immunity that may lead to cutaneous anergy. The use of a second-strength tuberculin skin test in nonreactors has marginal value. Any gain in sensitivity is offset by an increased rate of false–positives.

Treatment

Antituberculous chemotherapy is based on three basic principles:

• Treatment should always include two drugs to which the organisms are susceptible;

- Prolonged treatment is required (a minimum of 6 months);
- Promoting and monitoring compliance is critical.

Tuberculous chemotherapy can be successful only if the clinical and social management of patients and their contacts is considered.

Initial (Empiric) Treatment of M. tuberculosis (While Awaiting Susceptibilities)

Treatment strategies for TB have changed in the past decade, reflecting the increased emergence of drug-resistant isolates. In 1986, the American Thoracic Society and the CDC recommended a 6-month regimen consisting of three drugs (isoniazid, rifampin, pyrazinamide). Pyrazinamide was administered for only 2 months; isoniazid and rifampin were administered for the entire 6 months. Since that time, the prevalence of strains of M. tuberculosis resistant to isoniazid, rifampin, and other antituberculous agents has increased dramatically. Currently, approximately 10% of isolates are resistant to isoniazid or rifampin. Thus, these earlier recommendations are no longer adequate. Currently, four drugs (isoniazid, rifampin, pyrazinamide, and ethambutol) are recommended as *initial* therapy for new cases of TB, while awaiting results of susceptibilities. Alternatively, isoniazid, rifampin, pyrazinamide, and streptomycin can be used. With short-course therapy (6 months), isoniazid, rifampin, pyrazinamide, and ethambutol are administered daily for 2 months, followed by twice-weekly isoniazid and rifampin for 4 months. This regimen has been effective in more than 96% of patients with TB in both immunocompetent and HIV-infected patients. Using this approach in Zaire, 96% of HIV-infected patients and 97% of HIV-negative patients with TB had responded clinically at the 6-month assessment. At 6 months, the HIV-infected patients were randomized to receive an additional 6 months of either isoniazid/rifampin or placebo. Late relapse (at 24 months) was 2% among HIV-seropositive patients receiving extended treatment, compared with 9% relapse rate among HIV-infected patients receiving placebo. Late relapse was 5.3% among HIV-negative patients who received only 6 months of therapy. Because of the potential for late relapses in HIV-infected patients, isoniazid/rifampin should be given for 12 months in this patient population.

Treatment of Susceptible Strains of M. tuberculosis

For susceptible strains of M. tuberculosis, daily administration of rifampin and isoniazid for 6–9 months is curative in 93–98% of patients (both HIV-infected or HIV-negative). For HIV-infected patients, treatment should be extended for 12 months or 6 months after organisms have been cleared from the sputum. Efficacy appears comparable with daily therapy or high-dose therapy administered two or three times per week. Fixed-dose combinations of rifampin and isoniazid or rifampin plus isoniazid and pyrazinamide are available and may encourage compliance, but they are expensive. In the United States, only 15–18% of rifampin is sold as a fixed-dose combination.

Drug-resistant Tuberculosis

The prevalence of drug-resistant organisms in the United States increased from 2% in the 1960s to 14% by 1991. Resistance is most prevalent in large urban areas, in border communities, and among ethnic or foreign-born minorities. The shift away from inpatient therapy to outpatient therapy in the 1960s set the stage for rising rates of resistance, primarily related to inadequate or erratic prior therapy. Deteriorating socioeconomic conditions and the rise in HIV-infected patients in the 1980s markedly increased the prevalence of TB in the United States. The high prevalence of TB in some institutional settings (e.g., prisons, homeless shelters, hospitals, drug treatment centers), coupled with faulty infection control practices, has further exacerbated the problem of drug resistance. Transmission of drug-resistant strains to contacts in nosocomial or institutional settings may occur. From 1988–1991, outbreaks of multidrug-resistant (MDR) TB occurred in hospitals in Miami, New York, and New Jersey, followed by similar nosocomial outbreaks elsewhere by 1992. The organisms were invariably resistant to isoniazid and rifampin but were often resistant to other first-line drugs (e.g., ethambutol, streptomycin, and pyrazinamide). More than 80% of patients in these initial outbreaks were HIV-positive, and case fatality rates were as high as 70–90%. Tuberculin skin test reactivity developed in substantial numbers of health care workers caring for infected patients. These outbreaks prompted a survey by the CDC of tuberculous cases in the United States in the first quarter of 1991. Of 3,313 isolates tested from 50 states, 14% were resistant to at least one antituberculous drug. Resistance rates to isoniazid and rifampin were 9.1% and 3.9%, respectively. Resistance to other first-line agents include ethambutol (2.4%); pyrazinamide (5.8%); streptomycin (5.7%). MDR TB, defined as resistance to both isoniazid and rifampin, was noted in 3.5% of cases. Of 114 MDR TB cases, 50% were also resistant to ethambutol and/or streptomycin. Racial or ethnic minorities accounted for 91% of MDR TB; 61% of cases were in New York City. The incidence of MDR TB was increased more than 20-fold in Hispanics, Blacks, and Asians. Development of resistance usually reflects inconsistent or erratic use of antituberculous medications. Aggregate data from the United States in 1991 noted that only 77% of patients completed a course of therapy within 12 months. Considerably high rates of noncompliance were noted in New York City and in disadvantaged populations. A recent study from Harlem noted that 89% of patients discharged on antituberculous medications were lost to follow-up, suggesting that a huge reservoir of inadequately treated patients may exist in some areas. Risk factors for resistance include HIV infection, intravenous drug abuse, previous treatment, poor compliance, interruption of therapy, and the use of less than two drugs to which the organism is susceptible. Psychiatric disease, alcoholism, drug addiction, and homelessness predict noncompliance. Race, education, socioeconomic status, or religion, however, do not reliably predict compliance.

Directly Observed Therapy

Supervised therapy (direct observation by medical personnel) reduces the frequency of primary and acquired drug resistance and relapse, and may be cost-effective.

Initial therapy is administered daily for 2–4 weeks, then twice weekly. Currently, fewer than 20% of patients infected with TB in the United States receive directly observed therapy. Given the enormous cost and morbidity associated with relapses, treatment failures, and MDR TB, greater efforts to employ this form of therapy are warranted. Directly observed antituberculous chemotherapy has been practiced in Asia and Africa for more than three decades. In 1993, the Advisory Council for the Elimination of Tuberculosis (ACET) recommended directly observed therapy as the standard of care in locales where treatment completion rates fell below 90%. Directly observed therapy by federal, state, and local health departments has been associated with significant reductions in rates of treatment failure or relapse.

Treatment of Resistant Tuberculosis

Historically, *M. tuberculosis* resistant to isoniazid alone can be adequately treated by four drug regimens incorporating rifampin. Treatment of strains resistant to both rifampin and isoniazid is more problematic, with a higher rate of treatment failures and relapses. For MDR strains, a minimum of four drugs is required, using combinations of pyrazinamide, ethambutol, fluoroquinolones, an injectable aminoglycoside, and second-line agents (e.g., capreomycin, ethionamide, cycloserine, aminosalicylic acid). These regimens are highly toxic and difficult to tolerate. Among HIV-infected patients, MDR TB has been associated with a high rate of clinical failures and mortality. Even with multiple drug regimens, median survival for MDR TB in patients with AIDS ranges from 4 to 16 weeks. For HIV-infected patients without AIDS, a median survival of 14–18 months has been cited. Even in non–HIV-infected patients, prognosis is guarded. A study of 171 HIV-negative patients with MDR TB referred to the National Jewish Center in Denver noted an overall response rate to aggressive therapy with multiple agents of 56%; overall mortality attributable to TB was 22%. These patients reflected a highly selected cohort, as virtually all had failed prior therapy, often with multiple antituberculous agents. These patients had had TB for a median of 6 years and had received a median of six drugs prior to referral. A recent study of MDR TB in New York City in non–HIV-infected patients cited favorable clinical responses in 24 of 25 patients (96%). Twenty-three patients who responded received at least three drugs with in vitro activity against the isolates, and all received prolonged treatment with a quinolone. A majority received parenteral therapy with an aminoglycoside. These favorable results were achieved in a patient population without serious preexisting immune impairments. Nineteen patients had no underlying disease prior to the diagnosis of TB. Furthermore, the disease was localized to the lung or pleura in all but four patients. This suggests medical therapy may be highly efficacious in patients without serious impairments in host defenses or widely disseminated disease. Optimal therapy has not been determined, but five or six drugs may be necessary. Resectional surgery may have an adjunctive role for patients with localized disease and adequate respiratory reserve failing medical therapy.

Retreatment

Retreatment should include a minimum of four drugs (possibly six or seven drugs). Specific regimens need to be tailored according to in vitro susceptibilities and prior drug history. At least two first-line agents (e.g., isoniazid, pyrazinamide, ethambutol, streptomycin) should be included when organisms are susceptible to these agents. Ofloxacin (400 mg b.i.d.) or ciprofloxacin (750 mg b.i.d.) are active against most strains of *M. tuberculosis,* are well-tolerated, and should be incorporated in most retreatment regimens. Combinations of second-line antituberculous agents (e.g., aminosalicylic acid, ethionamide, cycloserine, capreomycin, amikacin, kanamycin) are usually required but have considerable toxicity. Treatment with these agents should be initiated slowly; doses of individual agents should be increased with caution. Amikacin, kanamycin, and capreomycin are available for parenteral use only. Amikacin (15 mg/kg/day) is often included for the first 3–6 months for retreatment regimens. Aminosalicylic acid and ethionamide are given orally but are poorly tolerated (particularly because of gastrointestinal distress). These agents should be used only when no other options exist. Cycloserine has potential central nervous toxicity. Clofazimine, amoxicillin-clavulanate, clarithromycin, azithromycin, and rifabutin are oral agents with antituberculous activity, but clinical data on these agents is limited. Rifabutin exhibits high levels of cross-resistance with rifampin and was ineffective in a trial in Hong Kong. Because of the complexity of retreatment regimens, the design, initiation, and monitoring of therapy should be done in a center with expertise in TB. Treatment should be initiated in the hospital to assure compliance, monitor toxicities, and allow changes in regimen if required. Irrespective of specific regimen, prolonged therapy (up to 24–36 months) is desirable.

Monitoring Efficacy of Therapy

Response to antituberculous chemotherapy should be monitored by clinical features, chest radiographs, and serial sputum smears and cultures. Improvement in chest radiographs may lag behind clinical response. Diminution in fever, constitutional symptoms, and cough are indirect measures of response; bacteriologic clearing of sputum is the gold standard for documenting efficacy. Smears and cultures of sputa for acid-fast bacilli should be obtained at least monthly until negative smears and cultures are documented. More than 90% of patients revert to negative cultures within 3 months of therapy. Among patients exhibiting negative sputum cultures, follow-up cultures should be done at 6 and 12 months to exclude late relapse. Persistently positive smears at 3 months is worrisome and warrants institution of directly supervised therapy. Patients with persistently positive sputum cultures after 6 months are considered treatment failures. In this context, aggressive therapy with at least four antituberculous drugs is warranted, based on the most recent in vitro susceptibility tests for the patient's organism. Directly observed therapy is mandatory in this context.

Adverse Effects of Therapy

Hepatitis may complicate the use of isoniazid or rifampin. Elevations in transaminases occur in 18–38% of patients receiving combined therapy with isoniazid and rifampin, but severe hepatitis occurs in fewer than 6% of patients. Hepatitis is more common in the elderly (age older than 60 years) and in patients with previous liver disease or ethanol abuse. Maximal levels of transaminases are usually observed within 4 weeks of initiation of therapy. Because fatal hepatitis may complicate the use of isoniazid or rifampin, careful monitoring is required. Because of the high prevalence of asymptomatic elevation of transaminases, the American Thoracic Society, the CDC, and other societies have recently recommended against routine laboratory monitoring in patients without significant risk factors for hepatotoxicity receiving INH and rifampin. Baseline measurements of hepatic enzymes, bilirubin, serum creatinine or BUN, serum uric acid, and a CBC should be obtained, however. Patients should be monitored clinically monthly during therapy and should be specifically questioned regarding symptoms suggestive of drug toxicity. Symptoms of concern include nausea and vomiting, fatigue or weakness for more than 3 days, dark urine, icterus, rash, paresthesias, fever for more than 3 days, and right upper quadrant tenderness. Because INH-induced hepatitis is more frequent and severe in the elderly and in patients with prior liver disease or ethanol abuse, we believe transaminases should be monitored monthly in this population for the first 2 months and periodically thereafter to exclude subclinical toxicity. Elevated transaminases may in some cases decline without interruption or change in therapy. Elevations of transaminases five-fold above baseline, however, even in asymptomatic patients warrants either more careful monitoring or discontinuation of therapy. Other side effects associated with INH or rifampin include rashes (noted in 2–11% of patients) and neuropathy (with INH). More than 90% of adverse effects are noted within the first 2 months. Supplementation with vitamin B_6 (pyridoxine, 25–50 mg/day) is advised when isoniazid is given to patients with risk factors for neuropathy (e.g., substance abuse, HIV-infection, malnutrition, underlying neuropathy). Side effects from other antituberculosis agents are numerous and will not be reiterated in detail here. Major toxicities from specific first-line agents include ethambutol (ocular toxicity); streptomycin (vestibular, renal); pyrazinamide (arthralgias, hyperuricemia, hepatitis). Side effects from antituberculosis therapy are more common among HIV-infected individuals but are usually mild (e.g., rash, mild gastrointestinal distress).

Preferred Therapy

Active Tuberculosis

NONIMMUNOCOMPROMISED HOSTS (INITIAL THERAPY, PENDING CULTURES AND SUSCEPTIBILITIES)

- Four drugs, including isoniazid, rifampin, ethambutol (streptomycin can be substituted for ethambutol in patients with contraindications or experiencing adverse effects from ethambutol), and pyrazinamide for 6 months. Doses of drugs are as follows: isoniazid (300 mg/day); rifampin (600 mg/day); ethambutol (15 mg/kg/day); pyrazinamide (25 mg/kg/day, maximum 2 gm/day).

NONIMMUNOCOMPROMISED HOSTS (SUSCEPTIBLE STRAINS)

- Isoniazid, rifampin, and pyrazinamide for 2 months, then isoniazid and rifampin for the last 4 months. Isoniazid can be given daily (300 mg) or twice weekly (dose 15 mg/kg/day [maximum 900 mg/day]). Rifampin can be given daily (600 mg) or twice weekly (dose 10 mg/kg/day [maximum 600 mg/day]).
- Patients with positive sputa at 6 months are considered treatment failures.

EXTRAPULMONARY TUBERCULOSIS

- 9-month and probably 6-month regimens are effective.

MDR TB (COMPETENT OR IMMUNOCOMPROMISED HOSTS)

- Four or more antituberculous agents (active in vitro);
- Incorporating a fluoroquinolone as part of therapy is advised;
- Directly observed therapy is mandatory;
- Surgical resection may have adjunctive role for medical failures.

Preventive Therapy

Preventive therapy with isoniazid is useful in infected patients at high risk for disease progression. Priorities for preventive therapy must compare the risk of developing TB to the risk of isoniazid toxicity. Preventive therapy is advised for the following indications:

- Household members and other close associates of persons with active TB;
- Recent tuberculin convertors;
- Prior history of never-treated TB;
- Positive reaction to tuberculin skin tests and abnormal chest x-rays consistent with old but inactive TB;
- Positive tuberculin skin test and a risk factor for activation (e.g., silicosis, diabetes mellitus, prolonged therapy with corticosteroids or immunosuppressive drugs, hematologic malignancy, AIDS, end-stage renal disease, malnutrition);
- Positive tuberculin skin test, age younger than 35 years.

Prophylaxis

Isoniazid is the only medication proven to be effective for prophylaxis of TB. In tuberculin-positive patients, active disease must first be excluded before initiating prophylaxis. For immunocompetent patients, 6 months of isoniazid (300 mg/day) is adequate. In patients with HIV infection, 12 months of therapy is advised. The tuberculin skin test identifies patients at risk for reactivation. Aggressive identification and treatment of tuberculin convertors prior to developing clinical disease is critical to curtail the epidemic of TB. Approximately 10% of patients with positive tuberculin skin tests develop active TB during their lifetime. The risk is substantially greater following heavy exposure or in patients with impaired host defenses. Isoniazid prophylaxis is indicated for new PPD convertors, patients younger than 35 years of age with a positive skin test, and patients with risk factors for reactivation. Household contacts have a 2–4% risk of developing active disease in the first year. Household contacts with a 5-mm PPD should receive isoniazid prophylaxis. Initial treatment for 3 months is prudent, even if the initial PPD is negative. If the tuberculin skin test remains negative at 3 months, isoniazid can be discontinued. Exposure to heavily infected index cases in nosocomial or nursing home settings has been associated with conversion of skin tests in 16–67% of exposed tuberculin-negative individuals. Isoniazid prophylaxis (for 6 months) is indicated for PPD convertors in this context. HIV-infected persons with positive tuberculin skin tests have an 8% risk per year of developing active TB and should receive prophylaxis for 12 months.

Patients intolerant of isoniazid should receive rifampin as prophylaxis (600 mg/day for 6–12 months). Pyrazinamide or the fluoroquinolones are promising. Contacts of patients with MDR TB should receive pyrazinamide plus either ethambutol or a fluoroquinolone. Bacille Calmette-Guérin (BCG) vaccination is controversial but is of unproven efficacy. Prevention of TB among health care providers is difficult. Ultraviolet light is most effective; masks and respiratory devices are unproven.

Prophylaxis Infection Without Disease (+ PPD)

- Nonimmunocompromised: Isoniazid (300 mg/day for 6–9 months).
- AIDS: Isoniazid (300 mg/day for 12 months).
- Alternative among patients intolerant of or resistant to isoniazid: Rifampin 600 mg/day for 6–12 months.
- Contact of MDR TB (resistant to both isoniazid and rifampin): Pyrazinamide plus ethambutol or a fluoroquinolone.

Nontuberculous (Atypical) Mycobacteria

Epidemiology

Nontuberculous (atypical) mycobacteria (NTM) are ubiquitous organisms present in soil, dust, water, plants, food, and the environment. Most mycobacteria are nonpathogenic in humans, but certain species may cause clinical infections in both immunocompetent and immunocompromised hosts. Environmental sources are the reservoir for human infections. Human-to-human transmission is exceptionally rare.

Atypical Mycobacteriosis in Immunocompetent Hosts

Prior to the AIDS epidemic, NTM infection was rare in the United States, with a prevalence of 1.8 cases per 100,000 population. In immunocompetent hosts, NTM infections are usually indolent, primarily affect the lungs, and occur in older individuals. Atypical mycobacteriosis may occur in patients with preexisting lung disease (including a prior history of TB) or in previously healthy adults. Radiographic manifestations of NTM are diverse but are often similar to TB, with upper lobe pulmonary infiltrates. Widespread dissemination may occur in immunocompromised hosts but is rare in patients with intact immune defenses. A review of clinical infections caused by NTM in the United States from 1979–1980 (prior to the AIDS epidemic) disclosed the following distribution: *Mycobacterium avium* complex, 61%; rapidly growing mycobacteria (*M. fortuitum* and *M. abscessus*), 19%; *M. kansasii,* 10%; other mycobacteria (e.g., *M. chelonae, M. marinum, M. smegmatis, M. scrofulaceum, M. xenopi*) accounted for the remaining cases. Marked geographic variability exists in the prevalence of atypical mycobacteria. *M. avium* complex and the rapidly growing mycobacteria (e.g., *M. abscessus, M. fortuitum*) predominate in the southeastern USA and Texas; *M. kansasii* is more common in the central United States.

Atypical Mycobacteriosis in Immunocompromised Hosts

The advent of AIDS dramatically increased the incidence and nature of NTM disease. Disseminated NTM disease develops in 30–50% of patients with far-advanced AIDS (typically when CD4 counts fall below 50 mm^3). *M. avium-intracellulare* complex (MAC) accounts for more than 95% of NTM infections in AIDS patients. Typical presenting features include fever, weight loss, constitutional and gastrointestinal symptoms. Pulmonary involvement occurs in only 5–22% of AIDS patients with disseminated MAC and is rarely severe.

Clinical Features of NTM in Immunocompetent Hosts

In immunocompetent hosts, chronic pulmonary disease is the most common manifestation of NTM. Atypical mycobacteriosis may complicate cystic fibrosis, end-stage emphysema or other chronic disorders, or patients with immune deficits. Recent studies, however, have cited atypical mycobacteriosis in older individuals (typically women) without prior lung disease or immune impairments. *M. kansasii* and MAC are the most common NTMs affecting the lungs. Rapidly growing mycobacteria (e.g., *M. fortuitum, M. abscessus*) have recently been recognized as rare, but important, pulmonary pathogens. Symptoms of pulmonary NTM infections include cough, sputum production, dyspnea, hemoptysis, malaise, and fatigue. Fever and weight loss are less common and less severe than with *M. tuberculosis.* Cultures are sporadically positive, yet progressive destruction may occur with persistent bronchopulmonary infection. Early reports of radiographic features of NTM emphasized thin-walled cavities, often involving the anterior and apical segments of the upper lobes, in up to 40% of cases. Noncavitary infiltrates occur in approximately 60% of cases. More recent reports of NTM in previously healthy nonsmoking elderly adults cited localized infiltrates in the right middle lobe or lingula in up to 80% of cases. Scattered parenchymal nodules may also be evident. Chest radiographs may be normal in

2–4% of cases. Pleural effusions are rare. Thin-section, high-resolution CT scans may show bronchiectasis and small pulmonary nodules. Bronchiectasis may result from prolonged infection with mycobacteria. The lung nodules represent granulomas.

The natural history of pulmonary disease caused by NTM in non–HIV-infected individuals is variable. *M. kansasii* tends to affect older adults and is more common in the central United States. The disease usually progresses gradually over months or years. Treatment is usually efficacious. MAC and rapidly growing mycobacteria usually run an indolent course but may progressively destroy lung parenchyma over months or even years. Pulmonary disease caused by rapid growers is usually seen in adults older than 50 years of age (particularly females) with no antecedent pulmonary disease. Other risk factors include esophageal disease and cystic fibrosis. *M. abscessus* and *M. fortuitum* account for more than 95% of pulmonary infections caused by the rapid growers. Pulmonary involvement is infrequent with other species of mycobacteria. *M. chelonae* and *M. marinum* typically cause localized skin, soft tissue, or wound infections. *M. scrofulaceum* may cause cervical lymphadenitis in children, although MAC predominates in this setting.

Clinical Features of NTM in Immunocompromised Hosts

Disseminated mycobacteriosis is a rare opportunist in non–HIV-infected patients with serious impairments in host defenses (e.g., hairy cell leukemia, organ transplant recipients). In 1980, prior to the AIDS epidemic, only 24 published cases of disseminated NTM caused by MAC had been described. By 1990, more than 12,000 cases of disseminated NTM (principally MAC) complicating AIDS had been reported to the CDC, for a cumulative incidence of 7.6%. Subsequent studies cited an incidence of disseminated mycobacteriosis of 15–40% among patients with far-advanced AIDS and CD4 counts below 50 mm^3. Infection is rare in patients with CD4 counts above 100. MAC accounts for more than 95% of NTM infections in patients with AIDS. NTM infections in patients with AIDS are usually disseminated, with predominantly extrapulmonary manifestations. Fever, weight loss, night sweats, diarrhea, abdominal pain, anemia, or elevated alkaline phosphatase are characteristic features. The gastrointestinal tract appears to be the most common portal of entry. The most commonly affected organs are blood, bone marrow, liver, spleen, and lymph nodes. Clinical pulmonary involvement occurs in 5–22% of patients with AIDS-associated NTM. Untreated MAC has been associated with a poor prognosis; mortality exceeds 50% within 6 months. Aggressive treatment for MAC, employing two or more agents, may improve symptoms and prolong survival.

Diagnosis

Conventional acid-fast smears (by Ziehl-Neelson or fluorochrome methods) and media used to culture *M. tuberculosis* are satisfactory to identify atypical mycobacteria in clinical specimens. Positive cultures may reflect true infection, asymptomatic colonization, or environmental contamination. Persistently positive smears or cultures, in the appropriate clinical context, strongly suggest clinical disease. The American Thoracic Society suggested the diagnosis of pulmonary infection with NTM could be presumed when the following criteria are satisfied: (a) at least two sputa (or bronchial washings) are acid-fast smear positive and cultures demonstrate moderate to heavy growth of NTM; (b) the clinical context is appropriate; and (c) alternative etiologies have been reasonably excluded. Identification of NTM on transbronchial or open lung biopsy may substantiate the diagnosis when sputa are negative. Growth of NTM in conventional solid culture media requires 2–4 weeks, with the exception of rapid growers, which may be evident within 7 days. For *M. avium* and *M. intracellulare,* growth can be detected by 7 days with radiometric culture systems (e.g., Bactec system). Biochemical tests (e.g., niacin test) or Bactec using selective growth inhibitors may distinguish *M. tuberculosis* from NTM. Species-specific DNA probes may identify *M. avium* and *M. intracellulare* within 4 hours when sufficient colony growth is evident in agar or broth but are not available for other NTM. Cultures of bone marrow, blood, or involved extrapulmonary sites may be diagnostic in patients with AIDS and disseminated NTM. Skin tests or serologies are not helpful to diagnose NTM.

Treatment of NTM

In Vitro Susceptibility Testing for NTM

Routine susceptibility testing of NTM against conventional antituberculous drugs is not always necessary because drug patterns are predictable for certain species. *M. kansasii* is routinely susceptible to rifampin and ethambutol; susceptibility to isoniazid is variable. More than 90% of isolates of MAC are resistant to isoniazid, rifampin, pyrazinamide, and streptomycin. The rapidly growing mycobacteria (e.g., *M. fortuitum, M. abscessus,* and *M. chelonae*) are invariably resistant to first-line antituberculous agents. For these species, susceptibility testing should be performed to antibiotics such as amikacin, doxycycline, fluoroquinolones, macrolides, and sulfonamides. For *M. kansasii* and MAC, susceptibility testing to conventional antituberculous agents or other antibiotics (e.g., fluoroquinolones, macrolides, sulfonamides, doxycycline) should be done under the following circumstances: failing regimens, a history of prior treatment, when *M. tuberculosis* is suspected, for isolates resistant to rifampin.

Therapy of M. kansasii

M. kansasii is usually susceptible to rifampin, isoniazid, ethambutol, and streptomycin and may be susceptible to macrolides, sulfonamides, amikacin, and rifabutin. *M. kansasii* is predictably resistant to pyrazinamide. Although randomized controlled trials have not been performed, preferred therapy is isoniazid, rifampin, and ethambutol daily for 18–24 months. This regimen can usually be initiated without in vitro susceptibility testing. With this regimen, more than 95% of patients respond favorably, and the rate of relapse is low. Streptomycin may be substituted in patients intolerant of isoniazid. Short-course or intermittent therapy have not been adequately studied. Other regimens that have been used include ethambutol and rifampin for 9 months, and daily high-dose isoniazid (900 mg), pyridoxine (50 mg), high-dose ethambutol (25 mg/kg), and sulfamethoxazole (3.0 gm) for 18–24 months.

Preferred Therapy for M. kansasii

- Isoniazid (300 mg), rifampin (600 mg), and ethambutol (15 mg/kg) daily for 18–24 months;
- Streptomycin may be substituted for patients intolerant of isoniazid.

Alternative Therapies (Less Data)

- Ethambutol and rifampin for 9 months;
- Isoniazid (900 mg), ethambutol (25 mg/kg), and sulfamethoxazole (3 gm) daily.

Treatment of Mycobacterium Avium-intracellulare Complex in Immunocompetent Hosts

Susceptibility patterns of MAC are extremely diverse, and the role of in vitro susceptibility in determining therapy is controversial. Treatment of MAC has not been evaluated in randomized trials. Unfortunately, first-line antituberculosis agents are not active against MAC. Second-line agents (e.g., ethionamide and cycloserine) have greater in vitro activity but have considerable toxicity. Treatment for MAC requires prolonged therapy (18–24 months) with multiple agents and is toxic. Some patients remain stable clinically and radiographically for years; cautious observation may be appropriate in these patients. Treatment in immunocompetent patients should be reserved for patients with symptomatic or progressive disease. Every regimen should include a macrolide (either clarithromycin or azithromycin). Most investigators add ethambutol as a second drug. Some investigators initiate therapy with a macrolide antibiotic for the first 4 months and then add streptomycin (for 3 months), rifabutin, and ethambutol. The decision to use additional drugs can be individualized. For severe or progressive disease, at least two of the following drugs should be added: rifampin or rifabutin; clofazimine; ciprofloxacin; streptomycin or amikacin (for the first 2–6 months). Ototoxicity may complicate the use of streptomycin or amikacin; these agents may be reserved for patients failing to respond to oral agents. Clarithromycin is slightly more active than azithromycin against MAC in vitro and has been used more extensively. Rifabutin (formerly ansamycin) may be used in place of rifampin in non–HIV-infected patients with chronic MAC pulmonary disease. Rifabutin is well tolerated in doses up to 450 mg/day, but adverse effects are noted in most patients receiving doses of 600 mg/day or concomitant macrolide antibiotics. The combination of rifabutin and clarithromycin has been associated with a high incidence of adverse effects (up to 77%) in both HIV- and non–HIV-infected patients. Leukopenia was the most common adverse effect; other side effects include nausea, vomiting, or diarrhea (42%); diffuse polyarthralgia syndrome (19%); hyperpigmentation (15%); and anterior uveitis (8%). Uveitis has only been noted in patients with AIDS. These adverse effects reflect complex interactions between rifabutin and macrolides. Rifabutin reduces clarithromycin levels while clarithromycin increases tissue rifabutin levels and enhances rifabutin toxicity. Azithromycin may have less effects on rifabutin metabolism than clarithromycin. When rifabutin is administered with clarithromycin, the initial dose of rifabutin should be 300 mg/day with increments only in patients failing to respond. CBCs should be obtained monthly for patients receiving rifabutin and macrolide-containing regimens. Ciprofloxacin has excellent in vitro activity against MAC and is usually well tolerated. Clofazimine is another antimycobacterial agent with excellent activity against most MAC. Clofazimine may be combined with clarithromycin and ethambutol plus (for the first 2–6 months only) an injectable aminoglycoside (i.e., streptomycin or amikacin). Irrespective of specific therapeutic regimen, treatment of MAC disease should be given for a minimum of 18–24 months. Therapy may be discontinued in patients failing to respond within 12 months. Additional treatment options for patients failing four drug regimens include combinations of five or six drugs (e.g., cycloserine, ethionamide, streptomycin, amikacin, clofazamine, macrolides, or ciprofloxacin). For patients failing medical therapy, surgical resection may be required, provided the disease is localized to one lobe of the lung. In this context, antimycobacterial therapy should be given prior to and following surgery.

Treatment of Disseminated MAC in AIDS

Optimal therapy for disseminated MAC in AIDS is controversial. In nonrandomized trials, four drug regimens employing combinations of ethambutol, rifampin (or rifabutin), ciprofloxacin, and either amikacin or clofazamine were effective, but toxicity mandated discontinuation of therapy in 37–46% of patients. Less aggressive regimens with fewer side effects may improve compliance. Most current regimens use either clarithromycin (1000 mg/day) or azithromycin (500 mg/day) plus ethambutol as part of initial therapy. Monotherapy is not adequate because it fails to eradicate MAC and may facilitate resistance. Additional agents (e.g., clofazamine, rifabutin, rifampin, ciprofloxacin, or amikacin) may be added as deemed appropriate. Isoniazid or pyrazinamide has no role in treating MAC. Rifabutin, combined with clofazimine and ethambutol, was superior to placebo in treating MAC bacteremia in patients with AIDS. A retrospective analysis of disseminated MAC complicating AIDS noted longer mean survival (255 days) among patients receiving three or more antimycobacterial agents active in vitro against MAC compared with untreated patients (145 day survival). Patients receiving clarithromycin or azithromycin as part of the regimen had a longer survival compared with patients not receiving macrolide antibiotics. Irrespective of specific regimen, HIV-infected patients with MAC responding to therapy should be treated for life unless adverse effects preclude continuation.

Preferred Therapy for M. Avium-intracellulare

Treatment for Disseminated MAC in AIDS

- Clarithromycin or azithromycin plus ethambutol (10 mg/kg) as initial therapy for non–life-threatening cases;
- Rifabutin or rifampin (600 mg); clofazimine (100–200 mg); ciprofloxacin (1,500 mg), ethambutol (10 mg/kg); azithromycin (500 mg) or clarithromycin (1,000 mg) daily.

Prophylaxis of MAC in AIDS

Oral rifabutin (300 mg/day) is effective for prophylaxis of MAC in patients with advanced AIDS. In 1993, the U.S. Public Health Service and the CDC recommended prophylaxis for all AIDS patients when CD4 counts fall below 100/uL. Other experts suggest initiating rifabutin only when CD4 counts fall below 50. Prophylaxis is not necessary for AIDS patients with CD4 counts above 100 because MAC infection is rare above this threshold. Rifabutin prophylaxis should be continued indefinitely unless side effects develop. Rifabutin may promote the emergence of rifampin resistance among patients with *M. tuberculosis*. Before rifabutin is initiated, disseminated MAC and active TB should be excluded. Rifabutin is usually well tolerated but neutropenia, thrombocytopenia, rash, and gastrointestinal symptoms each occur in 2–4% of patients. Uveitis occurs in 0.3% of AIDS patients receiving rifabutin, but the incidence is higher among patients receiving concomitant macrolide antibiotics. A recent double-blind, placebo-controlled multicenter trial found that prophylactic clarithromycin (500 mg b.i.d.) reduced MAC bacteremia and mortality in AIDS patients with CD4 counts below 100. Studies evaluating azithromycin or ethambutol, alone or in combination with rifabutin, are in progress.

Prophylaxis of MAC in AIDS

- Rifabutin (300 mg daily indefinitely) when CD4 counts fall below 100 mm^3.

Rapidly Growing Mycobacteria

Optimal therapy of pulmonary disease caused by rapidly growing mycobacteria (e.g., *M. fortuitum, M. abscessus,* and *M. chelonae*) is not clear. A paucity of clinical data are available but randomized therapeutic trials have not been performed. Conventional antituberculous agents have no role because these organisms are invariably resistant. Rapidly growing mycobacteria may be susceptible to traditional antibiotics (e.g., amikacin, cefoxitin, doxycycline, fluoroquinolones, imipenem, macrolides, and sulfonamides). Therapy should be based on in vitro susceptibilities. Isolates of *M. fortuitum* are predictably susceptible to the newer oral macrolide antibiotics, fluoroquinolones, and selected parenteral agents (i.e., amikacin, imipenem, and cefoxitin). Ninety percent of isolates of *M. abscessus* and *M. chelonae* are susceptible to amikacin and cefoxitin; the majority are also susceptible to the oral macrolides. *M. abscessus* and *M. chelonae* are usually resistant to other oral antibiotics (including the fluoroquinolones). For severe infections caused by rapidly growing mycobacteria, initial therapy with intravenous amikacin and cefoxitin for 2–6 weeks is reasonable. Once clinical improvement has been achieved, therapy may be changed to a combination of at least two oral agents to which the organisms are susceptible. Unfortunately, clinical failures and relapses are common, particularly with *M. abscessus*. *M. fortuitum* lung disease is less virulent than *M. abscessus* and can usually be cured with prolonged antibiotic therapy (6–18 months). In contrast, *M. abscessus* is rarely cured with medical therapy alone. Surgical resection, together with antibiotic therapy, may be required for localized pulmonary disease caused by *M. abscessus*. Data regarding therapy for *M. chelonae* are sparse. Even aminoglycoside-containing regimens have had poor success. Anecdotal successes have been described with combinations of an oral agent (e.g., macrolide or ciprofloxacin) and cefoxitin.

Miscellaneous Mycobacteria

Mycobacterium simiae, a mycobacterium in Runyon's classification group I (along with *M. kansasii* and *M. marinum*), may rarely cause disease in humans. Sporadic cases of clinical disease caused by *M. simiae* have been described in Cuba, Israel, and the southern United States (mainly Texas). *M. simiae* is a rare cause of chronic pulmonary disease in patients with previous TB or malignancy. More recently, *M. simiae* has been implicated as a cause of pulmonary and extrapulmonary disease in HIV-infected patients in Texas and endemic areas. Distinguishing colonization from infection is difficult; only 10–25% of isolates are associated with clinical disease. Optimal therapy has not been determined because *M. simiae* are invariably resistant to conventional antituberculous agents in vitro (although 31% were susceptible to streptomycin in a recent study). Combination therapy with an oral macrolide (azithromycin or clarithromycin), a quinolone, and clofazimine is advised, but data are limited.

VIRAL INFECTIONS
RNA Viruses

Infections caused by RNA viruses (e.g., influenza A and B, parainfluenza, respiratory syncytial virus) may cause lower respiratory tract infections in immunocompetent adults. RNA viruses are not opportunists but may also infect patients with impaired host defenses.

Influenza Virus
Epidemiology

Influenza remains an important cause of morbidity and mortality, particularly in the elderly or in patients with underlying cardiopulmonary disease or impairments in host defenses. More than 10,000 excess deaths annually were attributed to each of the 19 epidemics of influenza in the United States from 1957 to 1986. Most deaths were a result of pneumonia or exacerbations of cardiopulmonary disease; more than 80% of fatalities occurred in adults older than 65 years of age. Recent data from the CDC noted an increase in the number of deaths attributed to influenza and pneumonia in the United States from 1979 to 1994. The crude death rate for pneumonia and influenza increased from 20.0 to 31.8 deaths per 100,000 from 1979 to 1994; age-adjusted mortality increased 22%. Since the proportion of individuals older than 65 years of age continues to increase, these trends underscore the need for aggressive prophylaxis (with both influenza and pneumococcal vaccines) in high-risk groups. Minor changes in surface antigens (i.e., hemagglutinin or neuraminidase) cause new epidemics annually; major shifts appear in 9- to 39-year intervals and may result in pandemics. Epidemics of influenza in the Northern Hemisphere peak from December through March.

Clinical Features

Influenza virus infection produces an acute viral syndrome characterized by prominent myalgias, headache, coryza, fever, and cough. Pneumonia is a frequent complication in the elderly or in patients with preexisting pulmonary disease. Influenza may cause a primary viral pneumonia or may predispose to secondary bacterial bronchitis or pneumonia. Primary influenza pneumonia is more common in children and typically presents with peribronchiolar or interstitial infiltrates. In adults, secondary bacterial pneumonias caused by *Streptococcus pneumoniae, H. influenzae,* or *S. aureus* may complicate influenza. Cough, dyspnea, purulent sputum, or fever may develop 7–14 days after the initial viral syndrome has abated or resolved. The link between influenza and subsequent exacerbations of chronic pulmonary disease is well recognized. Hospitalizations for acute exacerbations of chronic pulmonary diseases, bronchitis, pneumonia, and congestive heart failure are markedly increased during influenza epidemics.

Prophylaxis

Influenza vaccination is the mainstay of prophylaxis and may avert the need for treatment. Influenza vaccine is a heat-killed virus containing two subtypes of influenza A and one subtype of influenza B. The influenza vaccination is noninfectious and can be administered to pregnant women. Local side effects (e.g., soreness or redness at the vaccination site for 1–2 days) occur in up to one-third of recipients. Vaccines are 70–80% effective in normal hosts; lower efficacy can be expected in immunocompromised or elderly individuals. Vaccination in patients older than 65 years of age reduces the rate of hospitalization for pneumonia, influenza, acute chronic and respiratory conditions, and congestive heart failure; importantly, a significant reduction of mortality from respiratory or cardiac causes during influenza seasons has also been noted. Annual vaccination of high-risk patients not only reduces morbidity and mortality but also may markedly reduce health care costs.

Recently, Medicare approved influenza vaccination as a reimbursable service for elderly adults. A recent randomized trial in healthy, working adults (age range 18–64 years) without comorbidities found that vaccinated individuals had fewer upper respiratory illnesses, sick days, and physician's visits for upper respiratory illnesses compared with placebo-treated controls. The authors suggested that vaccination may be cost effective, even in healthy young adults. Despite these important protective effects, influenza vaccination is greatly underused. In the United States, approximately 30% of persons older than 65 years of age and only 9–13% of high-risk adults younger than 65 years of age are vaccinated. Vaccination rates in excess of 60% for targeted populations have been achieved with organized programs and in some health maintenance organizations. Vaccinating high-risk groups during hospitalizations or health care visits during influenza seasons should be encouraged. Influenza virus vaccine can be given simultaneously with pneumococcal vaccine, but different sites should be used. Side effects with influenza vaccination are rare apart from local discomfort at the injection site. Vaccination is recommended in the following populations:

PATIENTS AT INCREASED RISK FOR COMPLICATIONS OF INFLUENZA

- Preexisting cardiac or pulmonary disease;
- Residents of nursing homes or chronic care facilities;
- Age older than 65 years;
- Chronic metabolic disorder (e.g., diabetes mellitus, renal failure, hemoglobinopathy, immunosuppression);
- Children and teenagers receiving chronic aspirin therapy.
- Health care workers in hospitals or nursing homes;
- Home care providers to high-risk persons;
- Members of households with high-risk patients.

For high-risk or exposed patients refusing vaccination, amantadine or rimantadine may be used as prophylaxis against influenza A.

Treatment of Established Influenza A Infections

Amantadine and rimantadine, antiviral agents that inhibit early stages of viral replication, are effective as prophylaxis or treatment of influenza A but have no activity against influenza B. Both are well absorbed orally. Extensive experience has been gained with amantadine; rimantadine has only recently been approved for use in the United States. The dose of amantadine is 200 mg once daily in healthy young adults and 100 mg for adults older than 65 years of age. While influenza vaccination is the preferred method for prophylaxis of influenza A infections, amantadine or rimantadine may be in used in the following circumstances: high-risk patients refusing vaccination; patients with impaired immune response to vaccine; high-risk patients awaiting humoral antibody response to the vaccine. Amantadine or rimantadine are 70–90% effective in preventing laboratory-induced influenza A. Both agents, when administered as prophylaxis during the influenza season, markedly reduce outbreaks of influenza in nursing home, nosocomial, and closed population settings. Prophylactic treatment in household contacts following exposure to the virus has been less consistently effective. Amantadine may enhance the protective effect of influenza vaccine in patients with AIDS, chronic renal failure, or impaired immunity. In addition, a 2-week course of amantadine following influenza vaccination may be considered in high-risk patients after influenza A has been encountered in the community, to confer protection while awaiting the antibody response. For treatment of established influenza A infection, amantadine is most effective when given within 48 hours of the onset of symptoms. Its efficacy in preventing or treating pneumonia caused by influenza A is not clear. Since rigorous diagnostic confirmation is difficult and expensive, therapy may be given empirically in patients with a clinical syndrome consistent with influenza A in communities where influenza is endemic. In adults younger than age 65, the dose of amantadine is 100 mg twice daily for 5–7 days. In adults older than 65 years of age, the dose is 100 mg/day. Amantadine is usually well tolerated, but insomnia, lightheadedness, or difficulty concentrating occur at doses exceeding 200 mg/day (or even more than 100 mg in the elderly). The dose must be reduced in patients with renal failure. Minor gastrointestinal side effects (e.g., nausea, anorexia) may occur; serious renal, hepatic, or bone marrow toxicity have not been reported. An acute overdose of amantadine results in anticholinergic syndrome (e.g., dry mouth, pupillary dilatation, toxic psychosis, urinary retention). Rimantadine, a structural analogue of amantadine, has been associated with fewer central nervous side effects than amantadine; gastrointestinal toxicity is similar. The dose of rimantadine is similar to amantadine. Although experience with rimantadine is less extensive than with amantadine, rimantadine may be preferred in patients with severe renal failure or central nervous system disease or in elderly adults because of its lower toxicity. The prevalence of resistance to amantadine or rimantadine is unknown, but resistance may develop in nursing home or household settings following use of either agent.

Respiratory Syncytial Virus

Epidemiology

Respiratory syncytial virus (RSV) is highly contagious and is the most common cause of community-acquired croup, bronchiolitis, and pneumonia in infants and children. Infections caused by RSV are seasonal, occurring from November through March. In children less than 5 years of age, hospitalization rates for respiratory conditions correlate with epidemics of RSV, parainfluenza, and influenza viruses. The incidence and severity of RSV infections are increased in infants with bronchopulmonary dysplasia, congenital heart disease, recent surgery, or immunosuppression. RSV infections have infrequently been reported in adults, which in part may reflect lack of surveillance. RSV has been implicated in fewer than 2–5% of community-acquired pneumonias in adults, but some studies have found RSV in up to 10% of community-acquired pneumonias when both viral cultures and serologies were performed. Similar to influenza A, the rate of hospitalization and deaths in adults caused by respiratory failure is increased during peaks of RSV infections. Most RSV infections are self-limited, but respiratory failure and fatalities may occur. The severity of RSV infections may be enhanced in the elderly or in patients with preexisting cardiopulmonary disease. Epidemics of respiratory infections caused by RSV may occur in nursing home and nosocomial settings (particularly in immuno-compromised hosts) and may be severe.

Clinical Features

Clinical manifestations of RSV infections are nonspecific and may be indistinguishable from influenza A. Coryza, cough, and low grade fever may be prominent. In children, wheezing, dyspnea, and interstitial infiltrates on chest radiographs reflect bronchiolar involvement. In adults, wheezing or cough may occur in up to one-third of infected patients. The diagnosis of RSV infections in adults is difficult. Nasal swabs and cultures are the best means to diagnose RSV. Commercial rapid antigen tests, the mainstay of diagnosis in children, may be less sensitive in adults. In one study of 140 RSV infections in the elderly, rapid antigen tests were positive in only 28. For severe pneumonia, bronchoscopy with BAL and appropriate cultures and rapid antigen tests may be diagnostic. Serologies (a fourfold rise in IgG or high titer IgM) may substantiate the diagnosis in epidemiologic studies but have no practical role in individual patients.

Therapy

Aerosolized ribavirin may be effective for children with RSV pneumonitis, and anecdotal successes have been noted in adults. Administration, however, is logistically difficult, expensive, and inconvenient. Delivery requires a small-particle aerosol generation via a face mask, ventilator, or infant oxygen hood, with measures to prevent escape of the drug. Aerosolization is usually given for 12–18 hours daily for 3–7 days. In uncontrolled trials, shorter duration (2 hours t.i.d.) was as effective as 12–18 hours treatment.

Prophylaxis of RSV

Initial efforts to produce a killed vaccine were disastrous, with worsening bronchiolitis and pneumonia in response to subsequent exposure to wild type RSV among vaccinated (as compared with nonimmunized) children. In 1993, Groothuis and colleagues reported that immune globulin with higher titers of neutralizing antibodies to RSV reduced and attenuated RSV infections among high-risk children. Immune globulin is promising but is also expensive, requires intravenous administration, and its niche needs to be further delineated.

Parainfluenza Virus

Epidemiology

Parainfluenza virus, an RNA virus of the paramyxovirus family, is a common cause of lower respiratory tract infections in children less than 6 years of age. Clinical features include sinusitis, croup, bronchiolitis, and pneumonia. With increasing age, the incidence and severity of infections caused by parainfluenza diminishes. Outbreaks of severe parainfluenza pneumonia have been described in bone marrow transplant recipients and immunocompromised hosts but have only been implicated as causes of pneumonia in immunocompetent adults in the community.

Clinical Features

Symptoms are similar to RSV. Upper respiratory tract involvement is common, with coryza and sinusitis. Mild cough, wheezing, and dyspnea may be noted when the process extends to the lower airways. In contrast to influenza, myalgias or arthralgias are usually absent. In most patients the disease is mild and self limited; however, in immunocompromised patients, fulminant, fatal respiratory failure has been described. Conventional cultures are positive in only 28–40% of cases and may require several days to isolate the organism. Techniques using monoclonal antibodies or nucleic acid probes have been developed, but their role needs to be clarified. Nasopharyngeal swabs are preferred site to culture. BAL may be required to substantiate the diagnosis in patients with lower respiratory tract involvement. Histologic features of involved lung are variable and include diffuse alveolar damage, giant cell interstitial pneumonitis, and viral inclusions.

Treatment

Data evaluating therapy are sparse, but anecdotal responses have been noted with aerosolized ribavirin.

Rhinovirus

Rhinoviruses account for approximately one-third of "common colds" and may infect the upper or lower respiratory tracts. Coryza, cough, and mild upper respiratory tract illness are typical features of rhinovirus infections. Hoarseness occurs in nearly half of infected patients. Fever is usually absent or low grade. The rate of infection is highest in young children, but all ages may be affected. Rhinovirus infections may precipitate exacerbations of asthma or bronchitis in both children and adults. Pneumonia is rare but may occur in debilitated patients, in nursing home residents with chronic pulmonary disease, in the elderly, or in infants. More than 100 rhinovirus serotypes exist, so immunity is only partially protective. No specific therapy is available, but symptoms usually spontaneously abate within a few days.

Hantavirus

Epidemiology

Hantaviruses, single-stranded RNA viruses of the family Bunyaviridae that are transmitted to humans by inhalation excreta or by secretions of rodents, have only recently been implicated as causes of pneumonia in the United States. In May 1993, an outbreak of illness characterized by a prodrome of fever and myalgias followed by the abrupt onset of adult respiratory distress syndrome (usually within 24 hours) occurred in the southwestern United States. The outbreak was linked to Hantaviruses and was termed the Hantavirus Pulmonary Syndrome (HPS). Sporadic cases of HPS have since been noted in other areas of the United States (including the northeast). As of April 10, 1995, 106 confirmed cases of HPS had been identified in the United States. Planting, hand plowing, and domestic activities that expose patients to contaminated rodent excreta are risk factors for acquisition. Person-to-person transmission does not occur. The incubation period ranges from 4 to 42 days (average 2 weeks). The outbreak of Hantavirus in the spring and summer of 1993 may reflect an unusual increase in Hantavirus-infected deer mice. Subclinical Hantavirus infection appears to be rare; only approximately 1% of residents in the southwestern United States have detectable IgG or IgM antibodies.

Clinical Features

Common clinical features include myalgias (88%), nausea or vomiting (75%), headache (63%), dizziness (38%), arthralgias (25%), and abdominal pain (21%). In contrast to influenza, sore throat or nasal symptoms occur in fewer than 20% of cases. Cough, a common early symptom of influenza, was rarely a presenting feature of HPS. By the time cough develops, the disease is usually far advanced. Within 12–24 hours, shock and pulmonary edema typically develop. Laboratory aberrations reported in HPS include elevated serum lactate dehydrogenase (100%), low serum bicarbonate (less than 21 mEq/L in 77%), thrombocytopenia (67%), and hematocrit more than 48% (55%). Chest radiographs in HPS demonstrate bilateral alveolar or interstitial infiltrates; lobar pneumonia is rare. The pathophysiology of HPS represents a progressive interstitial capillary-leak syndrome rather than a focal pneumonia. In fact, a lobar process suggests an alternative etiology (such as pneumococcal pneumonia). Serologic assays using ELISA, Western blot, or PCR can confirm the diagnosis within 24 hours.

Therapy

No treatment is available. Intravenous ribavirin has been tried but has been ineffective. Disease prevention requires eliminating rodents from human environments.

DNA Viruses

Serious infections with DNA viruses (e.g., cytomegalovirus, herpes simplex, varicella zoster, adenovirus) occur primarily in immunocompromised hosts and may cause serious pneumonias.

Cytomegalovirus

Serious cytomegalovirus (CMV) infections are almost exclusively confined to individuals with severe impairments in host defenses (e.g., AIDS, organ transplant recipients, intensive chemotherapy or immunosuppressive therapy). CMV rarely causes clinical infections in normal hosts; however, serum antibodies are present in 45–80% of normal adults, indicating that asymptomatic infection occurs commonly. CMV infections complicate 5–70% of allogeneic bone marrow transplant recipients; among solid organ transplant recipients, the incidence ranges from 40 to 80%. Ten to thirty percent of CMV-infected patients develop clinical pneumonitis. Rates of CMV pneumonia are even higher among lung or heart–lung allograft recipients. Predisposing factors for CMV infections among organ transplant recipients include receipt of CMV-infected organs or blood products or prior seropositivity. Primary infections (i.e., arising from donor organ or blood products in seronegative recipients) typically are far more severe than secondary infections (reactivation) in previously seropositive recipients. Among organ transplant recipients, virtually all CMV infections occur from 30 to 120 days post transplantation (mean of 40–55 days). CMV infections before day 21 or after 6 months are rare. Late relapse may occur in patients receiving cytolytic agents (e.g., ALG, OKT3), intensified immunosuppression, or following discontinuation of prior ganciclovir prophylaxis.

Clinical Features

The manifestations of CMV infections are diverse. Asymptomatic viral shedding (i.e., viruria, viremia) is frequent among organ transplant recipients. The most common manifestation of CMV infection in immunocompromised patients is an atypical mononucleosis syndrome with fever, atypical lymphocytes in peripheral blood, anemia, leukopenia, and abnormal liver function tests. Disseminated or fulminant CMV disease may be fatal. Pneumonia occurs in 10–30% of CMV-infected patients. Diffuse interstitial or alveolar infiltrates on chest radiographs are characteristic, but focal infiltrates mimicking bacterial pneumonia may be observed. A miliary pattern reflects hematogenous spread. Large nodular infiltrates or cavities are virtually never seen with CMV pneumonitis. Viremia is noted in more than 80% of patients with CMV pneumonitis, and usually antedates the pulmonary infection by 7–14 days. Mortality of untreated CMV pneumonitis may exceed 50%; with treatment, mortality rates of less than 15% are typical. Infection with CMV interferes with cell-mediated immunity and has been associated with a high rate of opportunistic superinfections. CMV upregulates class II HLA antigen expression and may potentiate allograft dysfunction and rejection.

Diagnosis

The diagnosis of CMV pneumonitis can be established by demonstrating large CMV-infected cells in tissue or cytologic specimens. Basophilic intranuclear inclusions (an "owl's eye" appearance) can be demonstrated readily by hematoxylin-eosin,

Wright's, Giemsa, or Papanicolaou's stains; multiple smaller cytoplasmic inclusion bodies are also present. Conventional viral cultures are positive in 70–90% of confirmed cases but take 2–6 weeks to grow. Immunofluorescent studies using monoclonal antibodies against CMV antigens (shell vial cultures) are preferred. These techniques are superior to conventional cytologic and cultural techniques and enable a rapid diagnosis (within 24 hours). In situ hybridization with cDNA probes against CMV-viral DNA appear comparable to immunofluorescent techniques but are cumbersome and require 2–3 days to complete. Surveillance cultures of buffy coat blood cells, urine, or BAL may demonstrate CMV even prior to developing clinical symptoms; however, blood cultures may be negative in up to 80% of patients with CMV pneumonitis.

Therapy

Ganciclovir [9-(1–3-dihydroxy-2-propoxymethyl)guanine] is the treatment of choice for CMV infections. Favorable responses have been noted in 60–90% of organ transplant recipients treated with intravenous ganciclovir. The initial dose is 5 mg/kg twice daily for 2–3 weeks, followed by less intense therapy (e.g., 5 mg/kg/day five to seven times per week) for variable periods as maintenance or prophylactic therapy. The propensity for relapse on cessation of therapy has led some investigators to advocate prolonged low dose maintenance therapy (up to 3–6 months) among patients at high risk. CMV infections in patients with AIDS are suppressed, but not cured, by ganciclovir. Daily intravenous ganciclovir is associated with significant cost, inconvenience, and risk of catheter-related complications. Oral ganciclovir, approved for use by the FDA in December 1994, has been used as chronic suppressive therapy for CMV retinitis in patients with AIDS, following initial therapy with intravenous ganciclovir. Oral ganciclovir (dose 3000 mg/day) has fewer side effects than the intravenous form but bioavailability is only 9%, and the need for dosing six times daily is logistically difficult. Additional studies are required to determine its role. Intravenous foscarnet (trisodium phosphonoformate) may be used in patients with CMV infections failing or experiencing side effects from ganciclovir. Foscarnet has considerable toxicity (e.g., nausea, hypomagnesemia, hypocalcemia, nephrotoxicity, seizures) and is reserved for ganciclovir failures. Acyclovir is not adequate for established CMV infections.

Preferred Therapy

- Ganciclovir IV (initial dose of 10 mg/kg/day for 14–21 days): consider long-term prophylaxis for 2–6 months (5 mg/kg/day for 5 days weekly) in high-risk patients;
- Ganciclovir IV (10 mg/kg/day for 14–21 days), followed by high-dose acyclovir (3,200 mg/day) for 2–6 months.

Alternate Therapy

- Foscarnet sodium (60 mg/kg q8h for 21 days, followed by maintenance);
- Oral ganciclovir (3000 mg/day in six divided doses).

Prophylaxis

Prophylaxis against CMV has been used primarily among organ transplant recipients at high risk. Patients at highest risk are seronegative recipients receiving organs from CMV-positive donors. Prophylactic strategies continue to evolve. Passive immunization with high-titer anti-CMV immunoglobulin ("hyperimmune") globulin, high-dose acyclovir, ganciclovir, or combinations of antiviral agents have all been tried. Hyperimmune globulin was ineffective in seropositive bone marrow or lung allograft recipients but was protective in renal transplant recipients. Efficacy among seropositive liver or heart transplant recipients is controversial. In one multicenter, placebo-controlled, randomized trial reported by Snydman and colleagues, multiple doses of hyperimmune globulin (administered up to 16 weeks posttransplantation) reduced the rate of severe CMV disease among liver transplant recipients but did not affect the overall rate of infections. This strategy, however, was ineffective in the patient group at highest risk (donor (+), recipient (–)). Furthermore, the cost of this prophylactic strategy was approximately $13,000 per patient. In some studies, the combination of hyperimmune globulin combined with acyclovir reduced serious CMV infections among high-risk hepatic and cardiac transplant recipients; other studies have failed to demonstrate benefit. High-dose oral acyclovir (1600–3200 mg/day for 12 weeks) reduced the incidence and severity of CMV infections in seropositive renal transplant recipients but was ineffective among lung allograft recipients. Disparate results have been reported using this approach for seropositive bone marrow transplant recipients. In a randomized, double-blind trial involving 18 European centers, intravenous acyclovir (500 mg/m^2 every 8 hours for 1 month) followed by oral acyclovir for an additional 6 months reduced the incidence of CMV pneumonia and reduced mortality in seropositive allogenic bone marrow recipients. In contrast, a recent retrospective analysis from Seattle found no difference in the incidence of CMV pneumonia or mortality among autologous marrow recipients given IV acyclovir (500 mg/m^2 every 8 hours) from day 5 pretransplantation to day 30 posttransplantation. Alternative prophylactic strategies with IV ganciclovir have been tried in high-risk organ transplant recipients. "Preemptive" therapy with ganciclovir in asymptomatic patients at high risk for CMV may reduce morbidity and mortality in bone marrow, heart, and lung allograft recipients. These strategies involve administering ganciclovir for prolonged periods (ranging from 30 to 120 days). Unfortunately, all of these prophylactic strategies are expensive, logistically difficult, and have potential toxicity. At present, optimal prophylaxis for CMV is controversial. Ganciclovir is most effective, but optimal duration of therapy needs to be further defined. Some centers initiate ganciclovir prophylaxis in patients at highest risk for CMV (i.e., donor (+)/recipient (–)) within 7 days of transplantation. Ganciclovir is initiated at full dose for 14–21 days, followed by low-dose maintenance therapy (5 mg/kg/day) for an additional 30–120 days. Oral ganciclovir has not been studied in this context. Substituting oral ganciclovir (3000 mg/day) or high-dose acyclovir (1,600–3,200 mg daily) may be considered following initial therapy (14–21 days) with IV ganciclovir, but limited data are available regarding the efficacy of these strategies. Additional studies are required to affirm optimal prophylactic regimens in various organ transplant recipients.

Herpes Simplex Virus (HSV)

Herpes simplex virus type 1 (HSV-1) is a common cause of mucocutaneous infections worldwide in all patient populations. More than 80% of adults in the United States are seropositive for HSV-1. Pneumonitis caused by HSV-1 is rare but may occur in up to 5% of immunocompromised patients with severe cutaneous or disseminated HSV infections. Risk factors for dissemination or pneumonitis include organ transplantation, hematologic malignancies, high-dose corticosteroid or immunosuppressive therapy, AIDS, etc. Lower respiratory tract infection (including pneumonia) may occur in patients with adult respiratory distress syndrome (ARDS) and in nonimmunocompromised patients following surgery or prolonged mechanical ventilatory support. Instrumentation and mechanical trauma of the airways are risk factors for herpetic pulmonary infections.

Clinical Features

Asymptomatic infection is characteristic, with prolonged periods of latency. Reactivation in immunocompetent hosts is characterized by mucosal ulcers (fever blisters) involving the lips or oropharynx. Visceral involvement, pneumonitis, or widespread dissemination may occur in patients with severe impairments in host defenses. Clinical manifestations of HSV lower respiratory infections range from mild pharyngitis or bronchitis to severe hemorrhagic pneumonitis. Characteristic findings of HSV pneumonitis include fever, leukocytosis, bronchospasm, cough, and dyspnea. Oropharyngeal herpetic lesions are present concomitantly in more than 80% of patients. Chest radiographs reveal focal or diffuse interstitial infiltrates; cavitation does not occur. Punctate ulcerations of tracheal or bronchial mucosa, edema, and pseudomembranes may be noted on bronchoscopic examination. Fulminant HSV pneumonitis may cause pulmonary edema and hemorrhage. In some series of HSV pneumonitis, mortality rates as high as 40–70% have been cited. Bacterial or fungal superinfection complicates HSV pneumonitis in up to 50% of patients and may contribute to mortality.

Diagnosis

Herpes simplex viruses may be demonstrated by cytologies, biopsies, or cultures. Eosinophilic intranuclear inclusions and multinucleated (syncytial) giant cells are the cardinal histologic features. HSV-1 may colonize the lower respiratory tract as a saprophyte; distinguishing colonization from infection is difficult.

Therapy

Acyclovir (Zovirax) is the cornerstone of therapy. Intravenous acyclovir is recommended for pneumonitis, visceral, or disseminated HSV (dose 250 mg/m^2 q8h). Oral acyclovir may be used for mucocutaneous infections (dose 400 mg t.i.d.). Outcome depends on the immune status of the host and the presence or absence of complicating superinfections. Acyclovir is effective prophylaxis against HSV in high-risk patient populations (e.g., organ transplant recipients) (dose 200 mg t.i.d or 400 mg b.i.d.). Foscarnet may be used for acyclovir-resistant isolates. Famciclovir is active in vitro against HSV-1, but clinical data are limited.

Preferred Therapy
For Severe Infections

- Intravenous acyclovir 250 mg/m^2 q8h for 7–10 days;
- Reduce level of immunosuppression when possible;
- Oral acyclovir 400 mg t.i.d. may be used for mild to moderate infections.

Alternative Therapy

- Foscarnet (for patients failing acyclovir).

Prophylaxis

- Oral acyclovir 200 mg t.i.d. or 400 mg b.i.d. as prophylaxis in high-risk patients.

Varicella Zoster

Varicella or chicken pox is a common childhood exanthem characterized by fever and a generalized, pruritic vesicular rash. Primary varicella is almost exclusively a childhood disease. The disease is usually benign and self-limited; however, pneumonia or encephalitis are rare but potentially fatal complications in adults or immunocompromised hosts. Herpes zoster or shingles, a cutaneous exanthem caused by reactivation of the varicella zoster virus (VZV), occurs in approximately 15% of adults during their lifetime. Latent VZV within the dorsal root ganglia of cutaneous nerves may be reactivated during periods of impaired cellular immunity. The incidence of VZV is increased in the elderly and occurs in 10–25% of patients receiving aggressive immunosuppressive or cytotoxic therapy.

Clinical Features

Clinically, VZV infections present as a painful rash with grouped vesicles on an erythematous base, often confined to a dermatome in immunocompetent hosts. Postherpetic neuralgia lasting for more than two months occurs in nearly 50% of patients with cutaneous VZV infections. Pneumonia, resulting from hematogenous dissemination, is a rare complication in immunocompromised hosts. The cutaneous exanthem usually precedes pulmonary manifestations by 1–7 days. Chest radiographs in VZV pneumonia typically demonstrate interstitial infiltrates with a peribronchiolar distribution. Lobar pneumonia is rare. Histologic and cytologic features of VZV pneumonia are identical to those of HSV pneumonitis. Mortality of untreated VZV pneumonia in immunocompromised patients ranges from 15 to 25%. With acyclovir, mortality is less than 10%.

Therapy

Routine treatment of varicella is not necessary; however, acyclovir is advised for varicella infections in immunocompromised hosts or for severe infections in immunocompetent patients. Oral acyclovir (800 mg five times daily) is effective for primary varicella (for those patients requiring treatment) or reactivation cutaneous infections (shingles). A 7–10 day course is usually adequate. In a recent prospective randomized trial, 21 days of acyclovir or the combination of oral prednisolone and acyclovir was no more effective than 7 days of acyclovir alone in reducing the frequency of postherpetic neuralgia and was of marginal benefit in reducing pain during the early phases. Corticosteroid-treated patients experienced more adverse effects. Corticosteroids should not be used to treat VZV infections because toxicity and the risk of dissemination are increased. Famciclovir, the oral form of penciclovir, is active against VZV, herpes simplex types 1 and 2, and Epstein-Barr virus. Famciclovir has excellent bioavailability and low toxicity and was approved by the FDA in June 1994 for treatment of acute herpes zoster. In a placebo-controlled trial of acute herpes zoster in immunocompetent adults, oral famciclovir (500 or 750 mg t.i.d. for 7 days) accelerated lesion healing and viral clearance and reduced the duration of postherpetic neuralgia. Penciclovir triphosphate (the active metabolite of famciclovir) persists in virus-infected cells 10 times longer than does acyclovir triphosphate. These favorable properties suggest that famciclovir may have some advantages over acyclovir for VZV infections. Data evaluating therapy for VZV pneumonia are limited. Because of the potential lethality of VZV pneumonia, we advise initial treatment with high-dose intravenous acyclovir (800 mg q5h). Renal failure may complicate the use of intravenous acyclovir, presumably by precipitation of the drug in the renal tubules. This does not occur with oral acyclovir. Oral acyclovir may be substituted once clinical improvement is evident. Because of the high cost of acyclovir, the course should be limited to 7 days in patients with mild to moderate VZV infections. Therapy may be extended for an additional 7–14 days in patients with severe, disseminated, or slowly resolving disease. Reducing the level of immunosuppressive or corticosteroid therapy may accelerate healing and prevent dissemination. For seropositive patients at high risk for reactivation (e.g., organ transplant recipients), prophylactic acyclovir 200 mg t.i.d. is highly effective.

Preferred Therapy for Pneumonia, Severe, or Disseminated VZV

- Intravenous acyclovir (5–10 mg/kg q8h for 7 days) (up to 14–21 days for severe or protracted disease);
- Reduce level of immunosuppression (when possible).

Therapy for Milder Cases or Following Initial Response to Intravenous Acyclovir

- Oral acyclovir (800 mg five times daily for 7 days);
- Famciclovir (500 or 750 mg t.i.d. for 7 days) (for acute cutaneous herpes zoster).

Prophylaxis

- Oral acyclovir 200 mg t.i.d (in selected high-risk patients).

Adenovirus

Adenovirus may cause lower or upper respiratory tract infections in both normal and compromised hosts. Fatal, hemorrhagic pneumonia may occur. Adenovirus is a rare opportunist. Adenovirus was isolated from 5% of 1,050 bone marrow transplant recipients in one series and was implicated in 15 clinical infections (including 12 pneumonias) during an 11-year period at UCLA. Pneumonia caused by adenovirus is characterized histologically by interstitial infiltrates and necrosis, sloughing of bronchial mucosa, pulmonary edema, and alveolar hemorrhage. Chest x-rays typically demonstrate diffuse interstitial or alveolar infiltrates. CNS involvement with diffuse meningoencephalitis and progressive hepatic necrosis are rare complications. Unfortunately, no specific therapy is available.

BIBLIOGRAPHY

Overview of Pulmonary Opportunistic Infections

Jolis R, Castella J, Puzo C, Coll P, Abeledo C. Diagnostic yield of protected BAL in diagnosing pulmonary infections in immunocompromised patients. Chest 1996;109:601–607.
Shelhamer JH, Gill VJ, Quinn TC, Crawford SW, et al. The laboratory evaluation of opportunistic pulmonary infections. Ann Intern Med 1996;124:585–599.

Pneumocystis carinii
Risk Factors, Epidemiology, and Clinical Features

Hoover DR, Saah AJ, Bacellar H, et al. Clinical manifestations of AIDS in the era of Pneumocystis prophylaxis. N Engl J Med 1993;329:1922–1926.
Lundgren JD, Barton SE, Lazzarin A, Danner S, et al. Factors associated with the development of *Pneumocystis carinii* pneumonia in 5,025 European patients with AIDS. Clin Infect Dis 1995;21:106–113.
Yale SH, Limper AH. *Pneumocystis carinii* pneumonia in patients without acquired immunodeficiency syndrome: associated illnesses and prior corticosteroid therapy. Mayo Clin Proc 1996;71:25–31.

Pneumocystis carinii *Pneumonia in Non-HIV-infected Patients*

Godeau B, Coutant-Perronne V, Huong DLT, et al. *Pneumocystis carinii* pneumonia in the course of connective tissue disease: report of 34 cases. J Rheumatol 1994;21:246–251.

Ognibene FP, Shelhamer JH, Hoffman GS, Kerr GS, et al. *Pneumocystis carinii* pneumonia: a major complication of immunosuppressive therapy in patients with Wegener's granulomatosis. Am J Respir Crit Care Med 1995;151:795–799.

Sepkowitz KA, Brown AE, Armstrong D. *Pneumocystis carinii* pneumonia without acquired immunodeficiency syndrome. Arch Intern Med 1995;155:1125–1129.

Varthalitis I, Aoun M, Daneau D, Meunier F. *Pneumocystis carinii* pneumonia in patients with cancer: an increasing incidence. Cancer 1993;71:481–485.

Diagnosis of PCP

Horner RD, Bennett CL, Rodriguez D, Weinstein RA, et al. Relationship between procedures and health insurance for critically ill patients with *Pneumocystis carinii* pneumonia. Am J Respir Crit Care Med 1995;152:1435–1442.

Huang L, Hecht FM, Stansell JD, Montanti R, Hadley WK, Hopewell PC. Suspected *Pneumocystis carinii* pneumonia with a negative induced sputum examination: is early bronchoscopy useful? Am J Respir Crit Care Med 1995;151:1866–1871.

Tu JV, Biem J, Detsky AS. Bronchoscopy versus empirical therapy in HIV-infected patients with presumptive *Pneumocystis carinii* pneumonia: a decision analysis. Am Rev Respir Dis 1993;148:370–377.

Diagnostic Techniques: PCR to Detect PCP

Atzori C, Lu JJ, Jiang B, Bartlett MS, et al. Diagnosis of *Pneumocystis carinii* pneumonia in AIDS patients by using polymerase chain reactions on serum specimens. J Infect Dis 1995;172:1623–1626.

Olsson M, Elvin K, Lofdahl S, Linder E. Detection of *Pneumocystis carinii* DNA in sputum and bronchoalveolar lavage samples by polymerase chain reaction. J Clin Microbiology 1993;31:221–226.

Predicting Outcome (Clinical Course)

Bennett CL, Weinstein RA, Shapiro MF, Kessler HA, et al. A rapid preadmission method for predicting inpatient course of disease for patients with HIV-related *Pneumocystis carinii* pneumonia. Am J Respir Crit Care Med 1994;150:1503–1507.

Treatment of PCP Pneumonia

Bozzette SA, Finkelstein DM, Spector SA, et al. A randomized trial of three antipneumocystic agents in patients with advanced human immunodeficiency virus infection. N Engl J Med 1995;332:693–699.

Iannnidis JP, Cappelleri JC, Skolnik PR, Lau J, Sacks HS. A meta-analysis of the relative efficacy and toxicity of *Pneumocystis carinii* prophylactic regimens. Arch Intern Med 1996; 156:177–188.

Moe AA, Hardy WD. *Pneumocystis carinii* infection in the HIV-seropositive patient. Infect Dis Clin North Am 1994;8:331–364.

Safrin S, Finkelstein DM, Feinberg J, Frame P, et al. Comparison of three regimens for treatment of mild to moderate *Pneumocystis carinii* pneumonia in patients with AIDS. A double-blind, randomized trial of oral trimethoprim/sulfamethoxazole, dapsone/trimethoprim, and clindamycin/primaquine. Ann Intern Med 1996;124:792–802.

TMP/SMZ Adverse Effects

Hughes W, LaFon SW, Scott JD, Masur H. Adverse effects associated with trimethoprim/ sulfamethoxazole and atovaquone during the treatment of AIDS-related *Pneumocystis carinii* pneumonia. J Infect Dis 1995;l171:1295–1301.

Atovaquone

Dohn MN, Weinberg WG, Torres RA, et al. Oral atovaquone compared with intravenous pentamidine for *Pneumocystis carinii* pneumonia in patients with AIDS. Ann Intern Med 1994;121:174–180.

Hughes W, Leoung G, Kramer F, Bozzette SA, et al. Comparison of atovaquone (566C80) with trimethoprim/sulfamethoxazole to treat *Pneumocystis carinii* pneumonia in patients with AIDS. N Engl J Med 1993;328:1521–1527.

Trimetrexate with Leucovorin Versus TMP/SMZ

Sattler FR, Frame P, Davis R, et al. Trimetrexate with leucovorin versus trimethoprim/sulfamethoxazole for moderate-to-severe episodes of *Pneumocystis carinii* pneumonia in patients with AIDS: a prospective, controlled, multicenter investigation of the AIDS Clinical Trials Group Protocol. J Infect Dis 1994;170:165–172.

Clindamycin/Primaquine

Noshkin GA, Murphy RL, Balck JR, Phair JP. Salvage therapy with clindamycin/primaquine for *Pneumocystis carinii* pneumonia. Clin Infect Dis 1992;14:183–188.

Corticosteroids for PCP

Caumes E, Roudier C, Rogeaux O, et al. Effect of corticosteroids on the incidence of adverse cutaneous reactions to trimethoprim/sulfamethoxazole during treatment of AIDS-associated *Pneumocystis carinii* pneumonia. Clin Infect Dis 1994;18:319–323.

Sleasman JW, Hemenway C, Kelin AS, Barrett DJ. Corticosteroids improve survival of children with AIDS and *Pneumocystis carinii* pneumonia. AJDC 1993;147:1451–1457.

Prophylaxis of PCP

Simonds RJ, Lindegren ML, Thomas P, Hanson D, et al. Prophylaxis against *Pneumocystis carinii* pneumonia for children with perinatally acquired human immunodeficiency virus infection in the United States. N Engl J Med 1995;332:786–790.

Simonds RJ, Hughes WT, Feinberg J, Navin TR. Preventing *Pneumocystis carinii* pneumonia in persons infected with the human immunodeficiency virus. Clin Infect Dis 1995;21(suppl 1):S44–S48.

TMP/SMX

Schneider MM, Nielsen TL, Nelsing S, Hoepelman AI, et al. Efficacy and toxicity of two doses of trimethoprim/sulfamethoxazole as primary prophylaxis against *Pneumocystis carinii* pneumonia in patients with human immunodeficiency virus. J Infect Dis 1995;171: 1632–1635.

TMP/SMX in Patients Previously Intolerant

Gluckstein D, Ruskin J. Rapid oral desensitization to trimethoprim/sulfamethoxazole (TMP/SMZ): use in prophylaxis for *Pneumocystis* pneumonia in patients with AIDS who were previously intolerant to TMP/SMX. Clin Infect Dis 1995;20:849–853.

Aerosolized Pentamidine

Hardy WD, Feinberg J, Finkelstein D, et al. A controlled trial of trimethoprim/sulfamethoxazole or aerosolized pentamidine for secondary prophylaxis of *Pneumocystis carinii* pneumonia in patients with human immunodeficiency syndrome. N Engl J Med 1992;327: 1842–1848.

May T, Beuscart C, Reynes J, Marchou B, et al. Trimethoprim/sulfamethoxazole versus aerosolized pentamidine for primary prophylaxis of *Pneumocystis carinii* pneumonia: a prospective, randomized, controlled clinical trial. LFPMI Study Group. J Acquir Immune Defic Syndr 1994;7:457–462.

Schnieder MM, Hoepelman AI, Eeftinck Schattenkerg JK, et al. A controlled trial of aerosolized pentamidine or trimethoprim/sulfamethoxazole as primary prophylaxis of *Pneumocystis carinii* pneumonia in patients with human immunodeficiency virus syndrome. N Engl J Med 1992;327:1836–1841.

Dapsone Versus TMP/SMX

Jorde UP, Horowitz HW, Wormser GP. Utility of dapsone for prophylaxis of *Pneumocystis carinii* pneumonia in trimethoprim/sulfamethoxazole-intolerant, HIV-infected individuals. AIDS 1993;7:355–359.

Dapsone Versus Aerosolized Pentamidine

Girard PM, Landman R, Gaudebout C, Olivares R, Saimot AG, Jelazko P, et al. Dapsone/pyrimethamine compared with aerosolized pentamidine as primary prophylaxis against

Pneumocystis carinii pneumonia and toxoplasmosis in HIV infection. The PRIO Study Group. N Engl J Med 1993;328:1514–1520.

Opravil M, Hirschel B, Lazzarin A, Heald A, et al. Once weekly administration of dapsone/ pyrimethamine versus aerosolized pentamidine as combined prophylaxis for *Pneumocystis carinii* pneumonia and toxoplasmic encephalitis in human immunodeficiency virus-infected patients. Clin Infect Dis 1995;20:531–541.

Salmon-Ceron D, Fontbonne A, Saba J, et al. Lower survival in AIDS patients receiving dapsone compared with aerosolized pentamidine for secondary prophylaxis of *Pneumocystis carinii* pneumonia. J Infect Dis 1995;172:656–664.

Torres RA, Barr M, Thorn M, Gregory G, Kiely S, Chanin E, et al. Randomized trial of dapsone and aerosolized pentamidine for the prophylaxis of *Pneumocystis carinii* pneumonia and toxoplasmic encephalitis. Am J Med 1993;95:573–583.

Dapsone Versus TMP/SMX

Podzamczer D, Salazar A, Jimenez J, Consiglio E, et al. Intermittent trimethoprim/sulfamethoxazole compared with dapsone/pyrimethamine for the simultaneous primary prophylaxis of *Pneumocystis* pneumonia and toxoplasmosis in patients infected with HIV. Ann Intern Med 1995;122:755–761.

Fungal Disease

Jarvis WR. Epidemiology of nosocomial fungal infections, with emphasis on *Candida* species. Clin Infect Dis 1995;20:1526–1530.

Rossetti F, Brawner DL, Bowden R, Meyer WG, et al. Fungal liver infection in marrow transplant recipients: prevalence at autopsy, predisposing factors, and clinical features. Clin Infect Dis 1995;20:801–811.

Sarosi GA, Ampel N, Cohn DL, Dismukes WE, et al. Fungal infections in HIV-infected persons. Am J Respir Crit Care Med 1995;152:816–822.

Walsh TJ, Gonzalez C, Roilides E, Mueller BU, et al. Fungemia in children infected with the human immunodeficiency virus: new epidemiologic patterns, emerging pathogens, and improved outcome with antifungal therapy. Clin Infect Dis 1995;20:900–906.

Aspergillus
Clinical Epidemiology and Reviews

Denning DW, Stevens DA. Antifungal and surgical treatment of invasive aspergillosis: review of 2,121 published cases. Rev Infect Dis 1990;12:1147–1201.

Lortholary O, Meyohas MC, Dupont B, Cadranel J, et al. Invasive aspergillosis in patients with acquired immunodeficiency syndrome: report of 33 cases. Am J Med 1993;95:177–187.

Miller WT Jr, Sais GJ, Frank I, Gefter J, et al. Pulmonary aspergillosis in patients with AIDS. Clinical and radiographic correlations. Chest 1994;105:37–44.

Aspergillus: Techniques for Diagnosis

Horvath JA, Dummer S. The use of respiratory tract cultures in the diagnosis of invasive pulmonary aspergillosis. Am J Med 1996;100:171–178.

Patterson TF, Miniter P, Patterson JE, Rappeport JM, Andriole VT. *Aspergillus* antigen detection in the diagnosis of invasive aspergillosis. J Infect Dis 1995;171:1553–1558.

Spreadbury C, Holden D, Aufauvre-Brown A, Bainbridge B, Cohen J. Detection of *Aspergillus fumigatus* antigen by polymerase chain reaction. J Clin Microbiol 1993;31:615–621.

Aspergillus: *Itraconazole Therapy*

Caras WE, Pluss JL. Chronic necrotizing pulmonary aspergillosis: pathologic outcome after itraconazole therapy. Mayo Clin Proc 1996;71:25–30.

Denning DW, Lee JY, Hostetler JS, Pappas P, Kauffman CA, et al. NIAID Mycoses Study Group multicenter trial of oral itraconazole therapy for invasive aspergillosis. Am J Med 1994;97:135–144.

Sanchez C, Mauri E, Dalmau D, Quintana S, et al. Treatment of cerebral aspergillosis with itraconazole: do high doses improve the prognosis? Clin Infect Dis 1995;21:1485–1487.

Blastomycosis

Bradsher RW. Histoplasmosis and blastomycosis. Clin Infect Dis 1996;22(suppl 2):S102–111.

Pappas P, Pottage JC, Powderly WG, et al. Blastomycosis in patients with the acquired immunodeficiency syndrome. Ann Intern Med 1992;116:847–853.

Pappas PG, Threlkeld MG, Bedsole GD, Cleveland KO, et al. Blastomycosis in immunocompromised patients. Medicine (Baltimore) 1993;72:311–325.

Fluconazole for Blastomycosis

Pappas P, Bradsher RW, Chapman SW, Kauffman CA, et al. Treatment of Blastomycosis with fluconazole: a pilot study. Clin Infect Dis 1995;20:267–271.

Itraconazole for Blastomycosis and Histoplasmosis

Dismukes WE, Bradsher RW Jr, Cloud GC, Kauffman CA, et al. Itraconazole therapy for blastomycosis and histoplasmosis: NIAID Mycoses Study Group. Am J Med 1992;93:489–497.

Candida

Haron E, Vartivarian S, Anaissie E, Dekmezian R, Bodey GP. Primary *Candida* pneumonia: experience at a large cancer center and review of the literature. Medicine (Baltimore) 1993;72:137–142.

Pfaller MA. Nosocomial candidiasis: emerging species, reservoirs, and modes of transmission. Clin Infect Dis 1996;22:S89–S94.

Shelly MA, Poe RH, Kapner LB. Pulmonary mycetoma due to *Candida albicans:* case report and review. Clin Infect Dis 1996;22:133–135.

Fluconazole for Candidiasis

Rex JH, Bennett JE, Sugar AM, Pappas PG, et al. A randomized trial comparing fluconazole with amphotericin B for the treatment of candidemia in patients without neutropenia. N Engl J Med 1994;331:1325–1330.

Coccidioidomycosis

Ampel NM, Dols CL, Galgiani JN. Coccidioidomycosis during human immunodeficiency virus infection: results of a prospective study in a coccidioidal endemic area. Am J Med 1993;94:235–240.

DiTomasso JP, Ampel NM, Sobonya RE, Bloom JW. Bronchoscopic diagnosis of pulmonary coccidioidomycosis: comparison of cytology, culture, and transbronchial biopsy. Diagn Microbiol Infect Dis 1994;18:83–87.

Jones JL, Fleming PL, Ciesielski CA, Hu DJ, et al. Coccidioidomycosis among persons with AIDS in the United States. J Infect Dis 1995;171:961–966.

McNeil MM, Ampel NM. Opportunistic coccidioidomycosis in patients infected with human immunodeficiency virus. Clin Infect Dis 1995;21(suppl 1):S111–S113.

Standaert SM, Schaffner W, Galgiani JN, Pinner RW, et al. Coccidioidomycosis among visitors to a *Coccidiodes immitis*-endemic area: an outbreak in a military reserve unit. J Infect Dis 1995;171:1672–1675.

Stevens DA. Coccidioidomycosis. N Engl J Med 1995;332:1077–1082.

Fluconazole for Coccidioidomycosis

Catanzaro A, Galgiani JN, Levine BE, Sharkey-Mathis PK, et al. Fluconazole in the treatment of chronic pulmonary and nonmeningeal disseminated coccidioidomycosis. Am J Med 1995;98:249–256.

Galgiani JN, Catanzaro A, Cloud GA, et al. Fluconazole therapy for coccidioidal meningitis. The NIAID Mycoses Study Group. Ann Intern Med 1993;119:28–35.

Perez JA, Johnson RH, Caldwell JW, Arsura EL, Nemecheck P. Fluconazole therapy in coccidioidal meningitis maintained with intrathecal amphotericin B. Arch Intern Med 1995; 155:1665–1669.

Cryptococcosis

Epidemiology of Cryptococcosis

Meyohas MC, Roux P, Bollens D, Chouaid C, et al. Pulmonary cryptococcosis: localized and disseminated infections in 27 patients with AIDS. Clin Infect Dis 1995;21:628–633.

Rozenbaum R, Goncalves ARR. Clinical epidemiological study of 171 cases of cryptococcosis. Clin Infect Dis 1994;18:369–380.

Speed B, Dunt D. Clinical and host differences between infections with the two varieties of *Cryptococcus neoformans*. Clin Infect Dis 1995;21:28–34.

Cryptococcal Antigen

Baughman RP, Rhodes JC, Dohn MN. Detection of cryptococcal antigen in bronchoalveolar lavage fluid: a prospective study of diagnostic utility. Am Rev Respir Dis 1992;145: 1226–1229.

Treatment of Cryptococcosis

de Lalla F, Pellizzer G, Vaglia A, Manfrin V, et al. Amphotericin B as primary therapy for cryptococcosis in patients with AIDS: reliability of relatively high doses administered over a relatively short period. Clin Infect Dis 1995;20:263–266.

Dismukes WE. Management of cryptococcosis. Clin Infect Dis 1993;17(suppl 2):S507–S512.

Pinner RW, Hajjeh RA, Powderly WG. Prospects for preventing cryptococcosis in persons infected with the human immunodeficiency virus. Clin Infect Dis 1995;21(suppl 1): S103–S107.

Fluconazole for Cryptococcal Meningitis

Dromer F, Mathoulin S, Dupont B, Brugiere O, et al. Comparison of the efficacy of amphotericin B and fluconazole in the treatment of cryptococcosis in human immunodeficiency virus negative patients: retrospective analysis of 83 patients. Clin Infect Dis 1996;22:S154–S160.

Haubrich RH, Haghighat D, Bozzette SA, Tilles J, et al. High-dose fluconazole for treatment of cryptococcal disease in patients with human immunodeficiency virus infection. J Infect Dis 1994;170:238–242.

Menichetti F, Fiorio M, Tosti A, Gatti G, et al. High-dose fluconazole therapy for cryptococcal meningitis in AIDS. Clin Infect Dis 1996;22:838–840.

Nightingale SD. Initial therapy for acquired immunodeficiency syndrome-associated cryptococcosis with fluconazole. Arch Intern Med 1995;155:538–540.

Powderly WG, Saag MS, Cloud GA, et al. A controlled trial of fluconazole or amphotericin B to prevent relapse of cryptococcal meningitis in patients with the acquired immunodeficiency syndrome. N Engl J Med 1992;326:793–798.

Saag MS, Powderly WG, Cloud GA, Robinson P, et al. Comparison of amphotericin B with fluconazole in the treatment of AIDS-associated cryptococcal meningitis. N Engl J Med 1992;326:83–89.

Itraconazole for Cryptococcal Meningitis

de Gans J, Portegies P, Tiessens G, et al. Itraconazole compared with amphotericin B plus flucytosine in AIDS patients with cryptococcal meningitis. AIDS 1992;6:185–190.

Histoplasmosis

Hajjeh RA. Disseminated histoplasmosis in persons infected with human immunodeficiency virus. Clin Infect Dis 1995;21(suppl 1):S108–S111.

Wheat LJ. Histoplasmosis in Indianapolis. Clin Infect Dis 1992;14(suppl 1):S91–S97.

Fluconazole for Histoplasmosis

Norris S, Wheat J, McKinsey D, Lancaster D. Prevention of relapse of histoplasmosis with fluconazole in patients with acquired immunodeficiency syndrome. Am J Med 1994;96: 504–508.

Itraconazole for Histoplasmosis

Wheat J, Hafner R, Wulfsohn M, Spencer P, et al. Prevention of relapse of histoplasmosis with itraconazole in patients with the acquired immunodeficiency syndrome. Ann Intern Med 1993;118:610–616.

Wheat LJ, Hafner RE, Korzun A, et al. Itraconazole therapy of histoplasmosis in patients with the acquired immunodeficiency syndrome. Am J Med 1995;98:336–342.

Mucormycosis

Coffey MJ, Fantone J III, Stirling MC, Lynch JP III. Pseudoaneurysm of pulmonary artery in mucormycosis. Am Rev Respir Dis 1992;145:1487–1490.

Hopkins RJ, Rothman M, Fiore A, Boldblum SE. Cerebral mucormycosis associated with intravenous drug usc: three case reports and review. Clin Infect Dis 1994;19:1133–1137.

Morrison VA, McGlave PB. Mucormycosis in the BMT population. Bone Marrow Transplant 1993;11:383–388.

Singh N, Gayowksi T, Singh J, Yu VL. Invasive gastrointestinal zygomycosis in a liver transplant recipient: case report and review of zygomycosis in solid-organ transplant recipients. Clin Infect Dis 1995;20:617–620.

Tedder M, Spratt JA, Anstadt MP, Hegde SS, Tedder SD, Lower JE. Pulmonary mucormycosis: results of medical and surgical therapy. Ann Thorac Surg 1994;57:1044–1050.

Antifungal Drugs

Overview

Sarosi GA, Davies SF. Therapy for fungal infections. Mayo Clin Proc 1994;69:1111–1117.

Amphotericin B

Gallis HA. Amphotericin B: a commentary on its role as an antifungal agent and as a comparative agent in clinical trials. Clin Infect Dis 1996;22:S144–S147.

Goodwin SD, Cleary JD, Walawander CA, Taylor JW, Grasela TH Jr. Pretreatment regimens for adverse events related to infusion of amphotericin B. Clin Infect Dis 1995;20:755–761.

Meyer RD. Current role of therapy with amphotericin B. Clin Infect Dis 1992;14(suppl 1): 154–160.

Liposomal Amphotericin B

Bowden RA, Cays M, Gooley T, Mamelok RD, van Burik JA. Phase I study of amphotericin B colloidal dispersion for the treatment of invasive fungal infections after marrow transplant. J Infect Dis 1996;173:1208–1215.

Graybill JR. Lipid formulations for amphotericin B: does the emperor need new clothes? Ann Intern Med 1996;124:921–923.

Hiemenz JW, Walsh TJ. Lipid formulations of amphotericin B: recent progress and future directions. Clin Infect Dis 1996;22:S133–S145.

Kline S, Larsen TA, Fieber L, Fishbach R, et al. Limited toxicity of prolonged therapy with high doses of amphotericin B lipid complex. Clin Infect Dis 1995;21:1153–1158.

Oppenheim BA, Herbrecht R, Kusne S. The safety and efficacy of amphotericin B colloidal dispersion in the treatment of invasive mycoses. Clin Infect Dis 1995;21:1145–1153.

Sharkey PK, Graybill JR, Johnson ES, Hausrath SG, et al. Amphotericin B lipid complex compared with amphotericin B in the treatment of cryptococcal meningitis in patients with AIDS. Clin Infect Dis 1996;22:315–321.

Oral Azole Drugs

Como JA, Dismukes WE. Oral azole drugs as systemic antifungal therapy. N Engl J Med 1994;330:263–272.

Kauffman CA. Role of azoles in antifungal therapy. Clin Infect Dis 1996;22:S148–S153.

Fluconazole

Diaz M, Negroni R, Montero-Gei F, et al. A Pan-American 5-year study of fluconazole therapy for deep mycoses in the immunocompetent host. Clin Infect Dis 1992;14(suppl 1);S68–S76.

Pappas PG, Kauffman CA, Perfect J, Johnson PC, et al. Alopecia associated with fluconazole therapy. Ann Intern Med 1995;123:354–357.

Fluconazole for Prophylaxis of Fungal Infections

Schaffner A, Schaffner M. Effect of prophylactic fluconazole on the frequency of fungal infections, amphotericin B use, and health care costs in patients undergoing chemotherapy for hematologic neoplasias. J Infect Dis 1995;172:1035–1042.

Slavin MA, Osborne B, Adams R, Levenstein MJ, et al. Efficacy and safety of fluconazole prophylaxis for fungal infections after marrow transplantation—a prospective, randomized, double-blind study. J Infect Dis 1995;171:1545–1552.

Nocardia

Coker RJ, Bignardi G, Horner P, et al. *Nocardia* infection in AIDS: a clinical and microbiologic challenge. J Clin Pathol 1992;45:821–822.

Javaly K, Horowitz HW, Wormser GP. Nocardiosis in patients with human immunodeficiency virus infection. Medicine (Baltimore) 1992;71:128–138.

Rolfe MW, Strieter RM, Lynch JP III. Nocardiosis. Semin Respir Med 1992;13:216–233.

Tuberculosis

Castro KG. Tuberculosis as an opportunistic disease in patients infected with human immunodeficiency virus. Clin Infect Dis 1995;21(suppl 1):S66–S71.

Perlman DC, Salomon N, Perkins MP, Yancovitz S, Paone D, Des Jarlais DC. Tuberculosis in drug users. Clin Infect Dis 1995;21:1253–1264.

Epidemiology and Transmission of TB

Burwen DR, Block AB, Griffin LD, Ciesielski CA, et al. National trends in the concurrence of tuberculosis and acquired immunodeficiency syndrome. Arch Intern Med 1995;155:1281–1286.

Friedman LN, Williams MT, Singh TP, Frieden TR. Tuberculosis, AIDS, and death among substance abusers on welfare in New York City. N Engl J Med 1996;334:828–833.

McKenna MT, McCray E, Onorato I. The epidemiology of tuberculosis among foreign-born persons in the United States, 1986 to 1993. N Engl J Med 1995;332:1071–1076.

Raviglione MC, Snider DE Jr, Kochi A. Global epidemiology of tuberculosis: morbidity and mortality of a worldwide epidemic. JAMA 1995;273:220–226.

Shafer RW, Edlin BR. Tuberculosis in patients infected with human immunodeficiency virus: perspective on the past decade. Clin Infect Dis 1996;22:682–704.

Small PM, Hopewell PC, Singh SP, Paz A, et al. The epidemiology of tuberculosis in San Francisco. A population-based study using conventional and molecular methods. N Engl J Med 1994;330:1703–1709.

Nosocomial Tuberculosis

McGowan JE JR. Nosocomial tuberculosis: new progress in control and prevention. Clin Infect Dis 1995;21:489–505.

Menzies D, Fanning A, Yuan L, Fitzgerald M. Tuberculosis among health care workers. N Engl J Med 1995;332:92–98.

Sepkowitz KA. Tuberculosis and the health care worker: a historical perspective. Ann Intern Med 1994;120:71–79.

Sepkowitz KA. AIDS, tuberculosis, and the health care worker. Clin Infect Dis 1995;20:232–242.

Shafer RW, Small PM, Larkin C, Singh SP, et al. Temporal trends and transmission patterns during the emergence of multidrug-resistant tuberculosis in New York City: a molecular epidemiologic assessment. J Infect Dis 1995;171:170–176.

Stead WW. Management of health care workers after inadvertent exposure to tuberculosis: a guide for the use of preventive therapy. Ann Intern Med 1995;122:906–912.

TB: Health Care Costs

Brown RE, Miller B, Taylor WR, Palmer C, et al. Health care expenditures for tuberculosis in the United States. Arch Intern Med 1995;155:1595–1600.

Diagnosis of TB

Anderson C, Inhaber N, Menzies R. Comparison of sputum induction and fiberoptic bronchoscopy in the diagnosis of tuberculosis. Am J Respir Crit Care Med 1995;152:1570–1574.

Chin DP, Yajko DM, Hadley K, Sanders CA, et al. Clinical utility of a commercial test based on the polymerase chain reaction for detecting *Mycobacterium tuberculosis* in respiratory specimens. Am J Respir Crit Care Med 1995;151:1872–1877.

Schluger NW, Rom WN. Current approaches to the diagnosis of active pulmonary tuberculosis. Am J Respir Crit Care Med 1994;149:264–267.

Shinnick TM, Good RC. Diagnostic mycobacteriology laboratory practices. Clin Infect Dis 1995;21:291–299.

Therapy

Overview of Therapy of TB

Bass JB Jr, Farer LS, Hopewell PC, O'Brien R, et al. Treatment of tuberculosis and tuberculosis infection in adults and children. American Thoracic Society and the Centers for Disease Control and Prevention. Am J Respir Crit Care Med 1994;149:1359–1374.

Iseman MD. Treatment of multidrug-resistant tuberculosis. N Engl J Med 1993;329:784–791.

Directly Observed Therapy of TB

Bayer R, Wilkinson D. Directly observed therapy for tuberculosis: history of an idea. Lancet 1995;345:1545–1548.

Weis SE, Slocum PC, Blais FX, King B, et al. The effect of directly observed therapy on the rates of drug resistance and relapse in tuberculosis. N Engl J Med 1994;330:1179–1184.

Short Course Therapy of TB

Perriens JH, St. Louis ME, Mukadi YB, Brown C, Prignot J, Puthier F, et al. Pulmonary tuberculosis in HIV-infected patients in Zaire. A controlled trial of treatment for either 6 or 12 months. N Engl J Med 1995;332:779–784.

Fixed Drug Combination Therapy of TB

Moulding T, Dutt AK, Reichman LB. Fixed-dose combinations of antituberculous medications to prevent drug resistance. Ann Intern Med 1995;122:951–954.

Drug-resistant Tuberculosis

Bloch AB, Cauthen GM, Onorato IM, et al. Nationwide survey of drug-resistant tuberculosis in the United States. JAMA 1994;271:665–671.

Edlin BR, Tokars JI, Grieco MH, et al. An outbreak of multi-drug resistant tuberculosis among hospitalized patients with the acquired immunodeficiency syndrome. N Engl J Med 1992;326:1514–1521.

Goble M, Iseman MD, Madsen LA, Waite D, Ackerson L, Horsburgh CR Jr. Treatment of 171 patients with pulmonary tuberculosis resistant to isoniazid and rifampin. N Engl J Med 1993;328:527–532.

Mahmoudi A, Iseman MD. Pitfalls in the care of patients with tuberculosis: common errors and their association with acquisition of drug resistance. JAMA 1993;270:65–68.

Park MM, Davis AL, Schluger NW, Cohen H, Rom WN. Outcome of MDR TB patients, 1983–1993: prolonged survival with appropriate therapy. Am J Respir Crit Care Med 1996; 153:317–324.

Salomon N, Perlman DC, Friedmann P, Buchstein S, Kresiwirth BN, Mildvan D. Predictors and outcome of multidrug-resistant tuberculosis. Clin Infect Dis 1995;21:1245–1252.

Telzak EE, Sepkowitz K, Alpert P, Mannheimer S, et al. Multidrug-resistant tuberculosis in patients without HIV infection. N Engl J Med 1995;333:907–911.

Turett GS, Telzak EE, Torian LV, Blum S, et al. Improved outcomes in patients with multi-drug-resistant tuberculosis. Clin Infect Dis 1995;21:1238–1244.

Ofloxacin and Ciprofloxacin for Mycobacterial Infections

Berning SE, Madsen L, Iseman MD, Peloquin CA. Long-term safety of ofloxacin and ciprofloxacin in the treatment of mycobacterial infections. Am J Respir Crit Care Med 1995; 151:2006–2009.

Kennedy N, Berger L, Curram J, Fox R, et al. Randomized controlled trial of a drug regimen that includes ciprofloxacin for the treatment of pulmonary tuberculosis. Clin Infect Dis 1996;22:827–833.

Surgical Management of Drug-resistant TB

Pomerantz M, Madsen L, Goble M, Iseman M. Surgical management of resistant mycobacterial tuberculosis and other mycobacterial pulmonary infections. Ann Thorac Surg 1991; 52:1108–1112.

Tuberculosis and HIV

Jones BE, Otaya M, Antoniskis D, Sian S, et al. A prospective evaluation of antituberculosis therapy in patients with human immunodeficiency virus infection. Am J Respir Crit Care Med 1994;150:1499–1502.

Public Health Policy

Earnest MA, Sbarbaro JA. Defining the issues: returning patients with tuberculosis to institutional settings. Clin Infect Dis 1995;20:497–500.

Prevention of TB

ACCP Consensus Statement. Institutional control measures for tuberculosis in the era of multiple drug resistance. ACCP/ATS Consensus conference. Chest 1995;108:1690–1710.

Centers for Disease Control and Prevention. Guidelines for preventing the transmission of *Mycobacterium tuberculosis* in health care facilities, 1994. MMWR Morb Mortal Wkly Rep 1994;43(RR–13):1–132.

Huebner RE, Schein MR, Bass JB Jr. The tuberculin skin test. Clin Infect Dis 1993;17: 968–975.

Pesanti EL. The negative tuberculin skin test: tuberculin, HIV, and anergy panels. Am J Respir Crit Care Med 1994;149:1699–1709.

Schluger N, Ciotoli C, Cohen D, Johnson H, Rom WN. Comprehensive tuberculosis control for patients at high risk for noncompliance. Am J Respir Crit Care Med 1995;151: 1486–1490.

Isoniazid Preventive Therapy

Passannante MR, Gallagher CT, Reichman LB. Preventive therapy for contacts of multidrug-resistant tuberculosis. Chest 1994;106:431–434.

Sterling TR, Brehm WT, Frieden TR. Isoniazid preventive therapy in areas of high isoniazid resistance. Arch Intern Med 1995;155:1622–1628.

van den Brande P, Steenberger WV, Verwoort G, Demedts M. Aging and hepatotoxicity of isoniazid and rifampin in pulmonary tuberculosis. Am J Respir Crit Care Med 1995;152: 1705–1708.

Question Role of BCG for Prevention of TB

Colditz GA, Brewer TF, Berkey CS, et al. Efficacy of BCG vaccine in the prevention of tuberculosis: meta-analysis of the published literature. JAMA 1994;271:698–702.

Brewer TF, Colditz GA. Bacille Calmette-Guérin Vaccination for the prevention of tuberculosis in health care workers. Clin Infect Dis 1995;20:136–142.

Overview of Atypical Mycobacteriosis

Choudhri S, Manfreda J, Wolfe J, Parker S, Long R. Clinical significance of nontuberculous mycobacteria isolates in a Canadian tertiary care center. Clin Infect Dis 1995;21:128–133.

Kennedy TP, Weber DJ. Nontuberculous mycobacteria: an underappreciated cause of geriatric lung disease. Am J Respir Crit Care Med 1994;149:1654–1658.

Sison JP, Yao Y, Kempei CA, Hamilton JR, et al. Treatment of *Mycobacterium avium* complex infection: do the results of in vitro susceptibility tests predict therapeutic outcome in humans? J Infect Dis 1996;173:677–683.

Wolinsky E. Mycobacterial diseases other than tuberculosis. Clin Infect Dis 1992;15:1–12.

Mycobacterium avium *Complex*

Benson CA, Ellner JJ. *Mycobacterium avium* complex infections and AIDS: advances in theory and practice. Clin Infect Dis 1993;17:7–20.

Chin DP, Hopewell PC, Yajko DM, et al. *Mycobacterium avium* complex in the respiratory or gastrointestinal tract and the risk of *M. avium* complex bacteremia in patients with human immunodeficiency virus infection. J Infect Dis 1994;169:289–295.

Kalayjian RC, Toossi Z, Tomashefski JF Jr, Carey JT, et al. Pulmonary disease due to infection by *Mycobacterium avium* complex in patients with AIDS. Clin Infect Dis 1995;20: 1186–1194.

Swensen SJ, Hartman TE, Williams DE. Computed tomographic diagnosis of *Mycobacterium avium-intracellulare* complex in patients with bronchiectasis. Chest 1994;105:49–52.

Specific Therapy for Mycobacterium avium

Dautzenberg B, Piperno D, Benite P, Diot P, Truffot-Pernot C, Chauvin JP. Clarithromycin in the treatment of *Mycobacterium avium* lung infection in non-AIDS patients. Chest 1995; 107:1035–1040.

Griffith DE, Brown BA, Girard WM, Wallace RJ Jr. Adverse events associated with high-dose rifabutin in macrolide-containing regimens for the treatment of *Mycobacterium avium* complex lung disease. Clin Infect Dis 1995;21:594–598.

Hopewell P, Cynamon M, Starke J, Iseman M, O'Brien R. Evaluation of new anti-infective drugs for the treatment and prevention of infections caused by the *Mycobacterium avium* complex. Clin Infect Dis 1992;15(suppl 1):S296–S306.

Masur H. Recommendation on prophylaxis and therapy for disseminated *Mycobacterium avium* complex disease in patients infected with the human immunodeficiency virus. Public Health Task Force of Prophylaxis and Therapy for *Mycobacterium avium* complex. N Engl J Med 1993;329:898–904.

Nightingale SD, Cameron DW, Gordin FM, Sullam PM, et al. Two controlled trials of rifabutin prophylaxis against *Mycobacterium avium* complex in AIDS. N Engl J Med 1993;329: 828–833.

Ostroff SM, Spiegel RA, Feinberg J, Benson CA, Horsburgh CR Jr. Preventing disseminated *Mycobacterium avium* complex disease in patients infected with human immunodeficiency virus. Clin Infect Dis 1995;21(suppl 1):S72–S76.

Shafran SD, Deschenes J, Miller M, Phillips P, Toma E. Uveitis and pseudojaundice during a regimen of clarithromycin, rifabutin, and ethambutol. N Engl J Med 1994;330:438–439.

Sullam PM, Gordin FM, Wynne BA. The Rifabutin Treatment Group. Efficacy of rifabutin in the treatment of disseminated infection due to *Mycobacterium avium* complex. Clin Infect Dis 1994;19:84–86.

Wallace RJ Jr, Brown BA, Griffith DE, et al. Initial clarithromycin monotherapy for *Mycobacterium avium-intracellulare* complex lung disease. Am J Respir Crit Care Med 1994;149: 1335–1341.

Wallace RJ Jr, Brown BA, Griffith DE, Girard W, Tanaka K. Reduced serum levels of clarithromycin in patients treated with multi-drug regimens including rifampin or rifabutin for *Mycobacterium avium-intracellulare* infection. J Infect Dis 1995;171:747–750.

Mycobacterium kansasii

Bamberger DM, Driks MR, Gupta MR, et al. *Mycobacterium kansasii* among patients infected with human immunodeficiency virus in Kansas City. Clin Infect Dis 1994;18:395–400.

Parenti DM, Symington JS, Keiser J, Simon GL. *Mycobacterium kansasii* bacteremia in patients infected with human immunodeficiency virus. Clin Infect Dis 1995;21:1001–1003.

Wallace RJ Jr, Dunbar D, Brown BA, et al. Rifampin-resistant *Mycobacterium kansasii*. Clin Inf Dis 1994;18:736–743.

Witzig RS, Fazal BA, Mera RM, Mushatt DM, et al. Clinical manifestations and implications of coinfection with *Mycobacterium kansasii* and human immunodeficiency virus type 1. Clin Infect Dis 1995;21:77–85.

Rapid Growing Mycobacteria

Griffith DE, Girard WM, Wallace RJ Jr. Clinical features of pulmonary disease caused by rapidly growing mycobacteria. Am Rev Respir Dis 1993;147:1271–1278.

Griffith DE. Lung disease caused by rapidly growing mycobacteria. Clin Pulmonary Med 1995;2(5):258–266.

Mycobacteria

Valero G, Peters J, Jorgensen JH, Graybill JR. Clinical isolates of *Mycobacterium simiae* in San Antonio, Texas. An 11-year review. Am J Respir Crit Care Med 1995;152:1555–1557.

Viruses

RNA viruses

Overview

Denny FW Jr. The clinical impact of human respiratory virus infection. Am J Respir Crit Care Med 1995;152:S4–S12.

Mahmood W, Sacks SL. Anti-infective therapy for viral pneumonia. Semin Respir Infect 1995;10:270–281.

McIntosh K, Halonen P, Ruuskanen O. Report of a workshop on respiratory viral infection: epidemiology, diagnosis, treatment, and prevention. Clin Infect Dis 1993;16:151–164.

Yang E, Rubin BK. "Childhood viruses" as a cause of pneumonia in adults. Semin Respir Infect 1995;10:232–243.

Influenza

LaForce FM, Nichol KL, Cox NJ. Influenza: virology, epidemiology, disease, and prevention. Am J Prev Med 1994;10(suppl):31–44.

Scheiblauer H, Reinacher M, Tashiro M, Rott R. Interactions between bacteria and influenza A virus in the development of influenza pneumonia. J Infect Dis 1992;166:783–791.

Sullivan KM, Monto AS, Longini IM Jr. Estimates of the US health impact of influenza. Am J Public Health 1993;83:1712–1716.

Influenza Vaccination

Fedson DS. Influenza and pneumococcal vaccination in Canada and the United States, 1980–1993: what can the two countries learn from each other? Clin Infect Dis 1995;20: 1371–1376.

Gross PA, Hermogenes AW, Sacks HS, Lau J, Levandowski RA. The efficacy of influenza vaccine in elderly persons. A meta-analysis and review of the literature. Ann Intern Med 1995;123:518–527.

Nichol KL, Margolis KL, Wuorenma J, Von Sternberg T. The efficacy and cost-effectiveness of vaccination against influenza among elderly persons living in the community. N Engl J Med 1994;331:778–784.

Nichol KL, Lind A, Margolis KL, Murdoch M, et al. The effectiveness of influenza vaccination against influenza in health, working adults. N Engl J Med 1995;333:889–893.

Prevention and control of influenza: recommendations of the Immunization Practices Advisory Committee (ACIP). MMWR Morb Mortal Wkly Rep 1995;44(RR13):535–537.

Influenza Treatment with Amantadine

Houck P, Hemphill M, LaCroix S, Hirsh D, Cox N. Amantadine-resistant influenzae A in nursing homes. Arch Intern Med 1995;155:533–537.

Influenza Treatment with Rimantadine

Piedra PA. Influenza virus pneumonia: pathogenesis, treatment, and prevention. Semin Respir Infect 1995;10:216–223.

Parainfluenza Virus

Heilman CA. Respiratory syncytial and parainfluenza viruses. J Infect Dis 1990;161:402–406.
Wendt CH, Hertz MI. Respiratory syncytial virus and parainfluenza virus infections in the immunocompromised host. Semin Respir Infect 1995;10:224–232.

Respiratory Syncytial Virus (RSV)

Falsey AR, Cunningham CK, Barker WH, Kouides RW, et al. Respiratory syncytial virus and influenza A infections in the hospitalized elderly. J Infect Dis 1995;172:389–394.
Whimbey E, Cough RB, Englund JA, Andreff M, et al. Respiratory syncytial virus pneumonia in hospitalized patients with leukemia. Clin Infect Dis 1995;21:376–379.

Rhinoviruses

Wald TG, Schult P, Krause P, Miller BA, et al. A rhinovirus outbreak among residents of a long-term care facility. Ann Intern Med 1995;123:588–594.

DNA Viruses

Cytomegalovirus (CMV)

CMV Complicating Transplantation

Duncan SR, Paradis IL, Yousem SA, Similo SL, et al. Sequelae of cytomegalovirus pulmonary infections in lung allograft recipients. Am Rev Respir Dis 1992;146:1419–1425.
Ettinger NA, Bailey TC, Trulock EP, Storch GA, Anderson D, Raab S, et al. Cytomegalovirus infection and pneumonitis. Impact after isolated lung transplantation. Am Rev Respir Dis 1993;147:1017–1023.
Kanj SS, Sharara AI, Clavien PA, Hamilton JD. Cytomegalovirus infection following liver transplantation: review of the literature. Clin Infect Dis 1996;22:537–549.
Kirklin JK, Naftel DC, Levin TB, Bourge RC, et al. Cytomegalovirus after heart transplantation. Risk factors for infection and death: a multi-institutional study. J Heart Lung Transplant 1994;13(3):394–404.
Ljungman P, Biron P, Bosi A, et al. Cytomegalovirus interstitial pneumonia in autologous bone marrow transplant recipients. Bone Marrow Transplant 1994;13:209–212.

CMV Complicating AIDS

Drew WL. Cytomegalovirus infection in patients with AIDS. Clin Infect Dis 1992;14: 608–615.

OKT3 as Risk Factor for CMV Infection

Portela D, Patel R, Larson-Keller JJ, Ilstrup DM, et al. OKT3 treatment for allograft rejection is a risk factor for cytomegalovirus disease in liver transplantation. J Infect Dis 1995;171: 1014–1018.

PCR to Diagnosis CMV

Patel R, Smith TF, Espy M, Portela D, et al. A prospective comparison of molecular diagnostic techniques for the early detection of cytomegalovirus in liver transplant recipients. J Infect Dis 1995;171:1010–1014.

Ganciclovir Therapy

Faulds D, Heel RC. Ganciclovir: a review of its antiviral activity, pharmacokinetic properties, and therapeutic efficacy in cytomegalovirus infections. Drugs 1990;39:597.

Ganciclovir Prophylaxis

Duncan SR, Paradis IL, Dauber JH, Yousem SA, Hardesty RL, Griffith BP. Ganciclovir prophylaxis for cytomegalovirus infections in pulmonary allograft recipients. Am Rev Respir Dis 1992;146:1213–1215.

Hibberd PL, Tolkoff-Rubin NE, Conti D, Stuart F, et al. Preemptive ganciclovir therapy to prevent cytomegalovirus disease in cytomegalovirus antibody-positive renal transplant recipients. A randomized controlled trial. Ann Intern Med 1995;123:18–26.

Merigan TC, Renlund DG, Keay S, Bristow MR, et al. A controlled trial of ganciclovir to prevent cytomegalovirus disease after heart transplantation. N Engl J Med 1992;326: 1182–1186.

Valenza M, Czer LS, Pan SH, Aleksic I, et al. Combined antiviral and immunoglobulin therapy as prophylaxis against cytomegalovirus infection after heart transplantation. J Heart Lung Transplant 1995;14:659–665.

Winston DJ, Ho WG, Bartoni K, Du Mond C, et al. Ganciclovir prophylaxis of cytomegalovirus infection and disease in allogenic bone marrow transplant recipients. Results of a placebo-controlled, double-blind trial. Ann Intern Med 1993;118:179–184.

Oral Ganciclovir

Anderson RD, Griffy KG, Jung D, Dorr A, et al. Ganciclovir absolute bioavailability and steady-state pharmacokinetics after oral administration of two 3000 mg/d dosing regimens in human immunodeficiency virus- and cytomegalovirus-seropositive patients. Clin Ther 1995;17:425–432.

Drew WL, Ives D, Lalezari JP, Crumpacker C, et al. Oral ganciclovir as maintenance treatment for cytomegalovirus retinitis in patients with AIDS. N Engl J Med 1995;333:615–620.

The Oral Ganciclovir European and Australian Cooperative Study Group. Intravenous versus oral ganciclovir: European/Australian comparative study of efficacy and safety in the prevention of cytomegalovirus retinitis recurrence in patients with AIDS. AIDS 1995;9: 471–477.

Prophylactic Acyclovir

Bailey TC, Ettinger NA, Storch GA, Trulock EP, Hanto DW, Dunagan WC, et al. Failure of high-dose oral acyclovir with or without immune globulin to prevent primary cytomegalovirus disease in recipients of solid organ transplants. Am J Med 1993;95:273–277.

Boeckh M, Gooley TA, Reusser P, Bucker CD, Bowden RA. Failure of high-dose acyclovir to prevent cytomegalovirus disease after autologous marrow transplantation. J Infect Dis 1995;172:939–943.

Prentice HG, Gluckman E, Powles RL, Ljungman P, et al. Impact of long-term acyclovir on cytomegalovirus infection and survival after allogeneic bone marrow transplantation. Lancet 1994;343:749–753.

Singh N, Yu VL, Mieles L, Wagener MM, et al. High-dose acyclovir compared with short-course preemptive ganciclovir therapy to prevent cytomegalovirus disease in liver transplant recipients. A randomized trial. Ann Intern Med 1994;120:375–381.

Prophylactic-immune Globulin

Snydman DR, Werner BG, Dougherty NN, Griffith J, et al. Cytomegalovirus immune globulin prophylaxis in liver transplantation. A randomized, double-blind, placebo-controlled trial. Ann Intern Med 1993;119:984–991.

Herpes Simplex Virus

Schuller D, Spessert C, Fraser VJ, Goodenberger DM. Herpes simplex virus from respiratory tract secretions: epidemiology, clinical characteristics, and outcome in immunocompromised and nonimmunocompromised hosts. Am J Med 1993;94:29–33.

Stewart JA, Reef SE, Pellett PE, Corey L, Whitley RJ. Herpesvirus infections in persons infected with human immunodeficiency virus. Clin Infect Dis 1995;21(suppl 1): S114–S120.

Herpes Varicella/Zoster Virus

Donahue JG, Choo PW, Manson JE, Platt R. The incidence of herpes zoster. Arch Intern Med 1995;155:1605–1612.

Glesby MJ, Moore RD, Chaisson RE. Clinical spectrum of herpes zoster in adults infected with human immunodeficiency virus. Clin Infect Dis 1995;21:370–375.

Wallace MR, Bowler WA, Murray NB, Brodine SK, Oldfield EC III. Treatment of adult varicella with oral acyclovir. A randomized, placebo-controlled trial. Ann Intern Med 1992; 117:358–363.

Wood MJ, Johnson RW, McKendrick MW, Taylor J, Mndal BK, Crooks J. A randomized trial of acyclovir for 7 days or 21 days with and without prednisolone for treatment of acute herpes zoster. N Engl J Med 1994;330:896–900.

Wood MJ, Kay R, Dworkin RH, Soong SJ, Whitley RJ. Oral acyclovir therapy accelerates pain resolution in patients with herpes zoster: a meta-analysis of placebo-controlled trials. Clin Infect Dis 1996;22:341–347.

Herpes Zoster: Famciclovir

Tyring S, Barbarash RA, Nahlik JE, Cunningham A, et al. Famciclovir for the treatment of acute herpes zoster: effects on acute disease and postherpetic neuralgia. A randomized, double-blind, placebo-controlled trial. Ann Intern Med 1995;123:89–97.

Adenovirus

Hogg JC, Hegele RG. Adenovirus and Ebstein-Barr virus in lung disease. Semin Respir Infect 1995;10:244–253.

Hantavirus

Auwaerter PG, Oldach D, Mundy LM, Burton A, et al. Hantavirus serologies in patients hospitalized with community-acquired pneumonia. J Infect Dis 1996;173:237–239.

Butler JC, Peters CJ. Hantaviruses and Hantavirus pulmonary syndrome. Clin Infect Dis 1994; 19:387–395.

Duchin JS, Koster FT, Peters CJ, Simpson GL, et al. Hantavirus pulmonary syndrome: a clinical description of 17 patients with a newly recognized disease. N Engl J Med 1995; 330:949–955.

Levy H, Simpson SQ. Hantavirus pulmonary syndrome. Am J Respir Crit Care Med 1994; 149:1710–1713.

Moolenaar RL, Dalton C, Lipman HB, Umland ET, et al. Clinical features that differentiate Hantavirus pulmonary syndrome from three other acute respiratory illnesses. Clin Infect Dis 1995;21:643–649.

White DJ, Means RG, Birkhead GS, Bosler EM, et al. Human and rodent Hantavirus infection in New York State. Public Health significance of an emerging infectious disease. Arch Intern Med 1996;156:722–726.

Zeitz PS, Butler JC, Cheek JE, Samuel MC, et al. A case-control study of Hantavirus Pulmonary Syndrome during an outbreak in the Southwestern United States. J Infect Dis 1995; 171:864–870.

Antiviral Agents

Acyclovir

Whitley RJ, Gnann JW Jr. Acyclovir: a decade later. N Engl J Med 1992;327:782–789.

Forscarnet

Chrisp P, Clissold SP. Foscarnet: a review of its antiviral activity, pharmacokinetic properties, and therapeutic use in immunocompromised patients with cytomegalovirus retinitis. Drugs 1991;41:104–109.

9 Pleural Diseases, Pleural Effusions

Richard W. Light

Approximately 1 million patients in the United States develop a pleural effusion each year. Any time a patient with an abnormal chest x-ray is evaluated, the possibility of a pleural effusion should be considered. Increased densities on the chest x-ray are frequently attributed to parenchymal infiltrates, although they actually represent pleural fluid. The earliest radiologic sign of a pleural effusion is blunting of the posterior costophrenic sulcus on lateral x-ray. If this angle is blunted, bilateral decubitus chest x-rays should be obtained to ascertain whether free pleural fluid is present. The presence of pleural fluid can be documented by one of the following:

- Bilateral decubitus x-rays of the chest (see Chapter 1);
- Computerized tomographic (CT) scan of the chest;
- Ultrasonic examination of the chest.

PHYSIOLOGY OF PLEURAL FLUID FORMATION

Fluid can enter the pleural space from:

- Interstitial spaces of the lung;
- Capillaries in the parietal pleura;
- Capillaries in the visceral pleura;
- The peritoneal cavity.

Pleural fluid accumulates when the rate of fluid formation exceeds the rate of fluid absorption. This situation can be caused by either an increased rate of formation or a decreased rate of absorption. Rate of formation is normally 0.01 mL/kg/hr, whereas capacity for absorption is 0.20 mL/kg/hr.

- Absorption is almost exclusively via the lymphatics in the parietal pleura;
- Lymphatics in the visceral pleura do not communicate with the pleural space;
- Little fluid exits the pleural space via capillaries.

Fluid entry into the pleural space from the capillaries follows Starling's equation. The following factors increase the rate of pleural fluid formation from the capillaries:

- Increased hydrostatic pressure in the capillaries in either the visceral or the parietal pleura;
- Decreased pressure in the pleural space;
- Decreased oncotic pressure in the blood;
- Increased oncotic pressure in the pleural fluid.

451

The rate of fluid entry into the pleural space from the interstitial spaces of the lungs increases when:

- Interstitial fluid is increased;
- The lymphatics that normally drain the lung become disrupted, such as occurs with lung transplantation.

CLINICAL FEATURES
Symptoms of Pleural Effusion

- Dyspnea on exertion;
- Chest tightness;
- Pleuritic chest pain.

Signs of Pleural Effusion

- Dullness to percussion over fluid;
- Absent tactile fremitus over effusion;
- Decreased breath sounds over effusion.

APPROACH TO PATIENTS WITH PLEURAL EFFUSION

Pleural effusions can occur as complications of many different diseases (Table 9.1). The vigor with which various diagnoses are pursued depends on the likelihood that the individual has that particular disease. Rough estimates on the incidence of the most common causes of pleural effusions are provided in Table 9.2.

When a patient has a pleural effusion that measures more than 10 mm on the decubitus x-ray, a diagnostic thoracentesis usually should be performed. If the patient has obvious congestive heart failure, consideration can be given to postponing the thoracentesis until the heart failure is treated. The characteristics of pleural fluid change little with diuresis over several days. If, however, such a patient is febrile or has pleuritic chest pain, or if the effusions are not of comparable size on both sides, a thoracentesis should be performed without delay.

Performing a Diagnostic Thoracentesis

This procedure is usually performed while the patient sits upright. A table should be available for the patient to rest his arms on. The patient's back should remain relatively vertical; if the patient leans forward too far, the lowest part of the hemithorax may move anteriorly and no fluid will remain posteriorly.

The site for insertion of the needle should be determined with care.

Table 9.1. Differential Diagnoses of Pleural Effusions

Transudative Pleural Effusions
- Congestive heart failure
- Cirrhosis
- Peritoneal dialysis
- Nephrotic syndrome
- Superior vena cava obstruction
- Fontan procedure
- Urinothorax
- Myxedema
- Pulmonary emboli

Exudative Pleural Effusions
- Neoplastic diseases
  - Metastatic disease
  - Mesothelioma
- Infectious diseases
  - Bacterial infections
  - Tuberculosis
  - Fungal infections
  - Viral infections
  - Parasitic infections
- Pulmonary embolization
- Gastrointestinal disease
  - Acute pancreatitis
  - Chronic pancreatic pleural effusion
  - Esophageal perforation
  - Intra-abdominal abscesses
  - Diaphragmatic hernia
  - Postabdominal surgery
  - Endoscopic variceal sclerotherapy
  - After liver transplant
- Collagen vascular diseases
  - Rheumatoid pleuritis
  - Lupus erythematosus
  - Churg-Strauss syndrome
  - Familial Mediterranean fever
  - Immunoblastic lymphadenopathy
- Drug-induced pleural disease
  - Nitrofurantoin
  - Dantrolene
  - Methysergide
  - Bromocriptine
  - Procarbazine
  - Amiodarone
  - Methotrexate
- Asbestos exposure
- Postcardiac injury syndrome
- Pericardial disease
- Postcoronary artery bypass surgery
- Uremia
- Yellow nail syndomre
- Sarcoidosis
- Trapped lung
- Meigs' syndrome
- After lung transplant
- Ovarian hyperstimulation syndrome
- Hemothorax
- Chylothorax

- Insert the needle posteriorly where the ribs are easily palpable and where the fluid gravitates.
- Make the first attempt one interspace below the level where the tactile fremitus is lost.
- Most unsuccessful thoracentesis procedures result from attempting to perform the thoracentesis at a level that is too low.
- Insertion of the needle at a low level is dangerous because the spleen or liver may be lacerated.
- Evaluate with ultrasound if fluid is not obtained after two or three attempts.

Table 9.2. Approximate Annual Incidence of Various Types of Pleural Effusions in the United States

Causes	Incidence (Reported Cases)
Congestive heart failure	500,000
Pneumonia (bacterial)	300,000
Malignant disease	200,000
lung	60,000
breast	50,000
lymphoma	40,000
other	50,000
Pulmonary embolization	150,000
Viral disease	100,000
Cirrhosis with ascites	50,000
Gastrointestinal disease	25,000
Collagen vascular disease	6,000
Asbestos exposure	2,000
Mesothelioma	1,500
Tuberculosis	1,000

The actual performance of the procedure is as follows:

- Thoroughly cleanse the skin over the site.
- Anesthetize the skin with lidocaine using a short 25-gauge needle.
- Anesthetize the periosteum of the underlying rib and the parietal pleura by performing the following steps with a 22-gauge needle 1.5 inches long. Move the needle up and over the rib with frequent injections of small amounts (approximately 0.1 mL) of lidocaine. Once superior to the rib, slowly advance the needle toward the pleural space, with aspiration followed by the injection of 0.1–0.2 mL lidocaine every 1–2 mm. Once pleural fluid is obtained through the anesthetizing needle, withdraw the needle.
- Withdraw the fluid by using a second 22-gauge needle attached to a 50–60-mL syringe that contains 0.5–1.0 mL heparin. Slowly insert the needle along the same tract with constant aspiration until pleural fluid is obtained. Continue aspiration until the syringe is filled.
- Withdraw the needle.

If more than 60 mL of pleural fluid is to be removed, a plastic catheter rather than a sharp needle should be used.

Complications of thoracentesis include:

- Pneumothorax, which occurs in 10% of patients; 20% of these patients require a chest tube;
- Infection of the pleural space;

- Hemothorax from laceration of an intercostal artery or vein, the spleen, or the liver;
- Seeding of the needle tract with tumor cells;
- Vasovagal reaction with bradycardia and hypotension.

Separating Transudative from Exudative Pleural Effusions

The first question to be answered with a diagnostic thoracentesis is whether the patient has a transudative or an exudative pleural effusion. An exudative effusion results from increased permeability of the pulmonary or pleural capillaries, whereas a transudative effusion results from imbalances of the hydrostatic and osmotic forces in the pleural or pulmonary capillaries.

This differentiation can be made by simultaneous analysis of the protein and lactic acid dehydrogenase (LDH) levels in the pleural fluid and in the serum. Exudative pleural effusions meet at least one of the following criteria, whereas transudative pleural effusions meet none:

- Ratio of pleural fluid to serum protein more than 0.5;
- Ratio of pleural fluid to serum LDH more than 0.6;
- Absolute level of pleural fluid LDH more than two-thirds upper normal limit for serum.

If none of the above criteria is met, the patient has a transudative pleural effusion, and the pleura itself can be ignored while the congestive heart failure, cirrhosis, or nephrosis is treated. Remember, however, that transudative pleural effusion can result from pulmonary embolization.

If a transudative pleural effusion is probable, the most cost-effective use of the laboratory is initially to measure only the pleural fluid protein and LDH levels. Other diagnostic tests, such as cytology, cell count, and differential, amylase, glucose, and cultures, are obtained only if the patient is proved to have an exudative pleural effusion.

TRANSUDATIVE PLEURAL EFFUSIONS
Congestive Heart Failure

Congestive heart failure is the disease most responsible for pleural effusions.

Pathophysiology

The accumulation of pleural fluid in patients with congestive heart failure appears to be related more to left ventricular than to right ventricular failure.

- Left ventricular failure leads to increased interstitial fluid, which then traverses the visceral pleura to enter the pleural space. In animal experiments, approximately 25% of pulmonary edema fluid moves directly from the lung into the pleural space.

Clinical Features

Patients with pleural effusions secondary to congestive heart failure usually have other signs and symptoms.

- Increasing dyspnea on exertion;
- Increasing peripheral edema and orthopnea or paroxysmal nocturnal dyspnea;
- Auscultation may reveal an S_3 gallop and crepitations (crackles), as well as signs of the pleural effusions (see Chapter 5);
- The chest x-ray usually reveals cardiomegaly (see Chapter 5);
- Pleural effusions are usually bilateral and roughly equivalent in size;
- The pleural fluid is a transudate.

Diagnosis and Treatment

The diagnosis is usually suggested by the clinical picture of congestive heart failure.

- Perform thoracentesis to demonstrate that fluid is a transudate when the patient does not respond to therapy, when effusions are not roughly the same size, when the patient is febrile, or when the patient has pleuritic chest pain.
- If the effusion meets the criteria for exudates as outlined above but the serum albumin minus the pleural fluid albumin is more than 1.2 gm/dL, the patient in all probability has a transudative effusion.
- Treatment consists of digitalis, diuretics, and afterload reduction.
- A rare patient has dyspnea from a large persistent pleural effusion despite optimal medical therapy. If dyspnea is relieved by a therapeutic thoracentesis, consideration can be given to attempting a pleurodesis with a sclerosing agent.

Hepatic Hydrothorax

Pleural effusions sometimes develop in patients with cirrhosis, particularly if ascites is present. The incidence of pleural effusion is approximately 6% in patients with cirrhosis and ascites but is less than 1% in patients with cirrhosis with hypoalbuminemia but without ascites.

Pathophysiology

The predominant mechanism is the movement of the ascitic fluid directly from the peritoneal cavity through the diaphragm into the pleural space.

- Small pores in the diaphragm have been demonstrated.

Clinical Features

The pleural effusion with hepatic hydrothorax tends to be large because of the large reservoir of fluid in the peritoneal cavity that can flow directly into the pleural space with its lower pressure.

- Usually, tense ascites is present, but occasionally the ascites is subclinical.
- A large effusion may produce severe dyspnea.
- The pleural effusions are usually right-sided (67%) but may be left-sided (16%) or bilateral (17%).

Diagnosis and Treatment

In a patient with cirrhosis, tense ascites, and a pleural effusion, the diagnosis is easy.

- Both a paracentesis and a thoracentesis should be performed to ascertain that both fluids are transudates. The pleural fluid protein level, although usually slightly higher than the ascitic fluid protein level, is still less than 3.0 gm/dL.
- Patients with hepatic hydrothoraces are prone to develop bacterial infections of the pleural space.
- Primary treatment is geared toward treatment of the ascites because the hydrothorax is an extension of the peritoneal fluid. A low-salt diet is recommended and diuretics should be administered judiciously. Serial therapeutic thoracenteses are not indicated because the pleural fluid rapidly reaccumulates and the thoracenteses deplete the patient of body protein.

If the pleural effusion persists despite optimal therapy directed toward the ascites, three therapeutic options, none of which is ideal, are available.

- Tube thoracostomy followed by the injection of a sclerosing agent; however, electrolyte depletion can lead to death.
- Implantation of a peritoneal-to-venous shunt; however, these shunts frequently do not control the effusion.
- Thoracotomy with surgical repair of the diaphragmatic leak; however, thoracotomy is a major surgical procedure.

Other Transudative Pleural Effusions

Although congestive heart failure and hepatic hydrothorax account for most transudative pleural effusions, the following conditions also cause transudative pleural effusions.

Peritoneal Dialysis

Large pleural effusions occasionally complicate peritoneal dialysis.

- Dialysate appears to move directly through the diaphragm.
- Incidence is 10% in those patients on continuous ambulatory peritoneal dialysis.

- The effusion is almost always on the right side.
- The pleural fluid has biochemical characteristics between those of the dialysate and those of the serum.
- Treat with chemical pleurodesis combined with a short period of small-volume, intermittent peritoneal dialysis.

Nephrotic Syndrome

Pleural effusion occurs in approximately 20% of patients with the nephrotic syndrome.

- Effusions are usually bilateral transudates because of the low oncotic pressure in the serum.
- Pulmonary embolus must be ruled out in this situation because emboli are common in patients with the nephrotic syndrome.
- Primary treatment is aimed at treating the nephrotic syndrome, but chemical pleurodesis occasionally may be performed.

Superior Vena Cava Syndrome

Pleural effusions are not present in most patients with superior vena cava obstruction.

- Pleural effusions do occur in neonates with superior vena cava thrombosis, however.

Fontan Procedure

This procedure is used to treat infants and children with hypoplastic right ventricles.

- The right ventricle is bypassed with an anastomosis between the superior vena cava, the right atrium, or the inferior vena cava and the pulmonary artery.
- Almost all patients develop bilateral pleural effusions postoperatively, which are frequently large and clinically significant.
- With refractory effusions, consider chemical pleurodesis or a pleuroperitoneal shunt.

Urinothorax

Pleural fluid can accumulate in the presence of retroperitoneal urinary leakage secondary to urinary obstruction, trauma, or retroperitoneal inflammatory or malignant processes.

- Effusion develops within hours of the precipitating event.
- Pleural fluid looks and smells like urine.
- Diagnosis is confirmed by demonstrating a higher creatinine level in the pleural fluid than in the serum.
- Effusion resolves once urinary tract obstruction is relieved.

Myxedema

Pleural effusions occasionally occur as a complication of myxedema.

- Incidence is probably less than 5%.
- Pleural fluid may have biochemical characteristics of either a transudate or an exudate.

Miscellaneous Causes of Transudative Pleural Effusions

- Approximately 20% of the pleural effusions secondary to pulmonary embolism are transudative.
- Although pleural effusions secondary to Meigs' syndrome and sarcoidosis have been described as transudative, this is probably not the case.

EXUDATIVE PLEURAL EFFUSIONS

Once a patient is known to have an exudative pleural effusion, one should attempt to determine which of the diseases listed in Table 9.1 is responsible. Pneumonia, malignant disorders, and pulmonary embolization account for most exudative pleural effusions. The following tests should be performed on the pleural fluid from a patient with an exudative pleural effusion of unknown origin: glucose level, amylase level, LDH level, differential cell count, microbiologic studies, and cytology. In selected patients, other tests on the pleural fluid, such as pH level, antinuclear antibody (ANA) level, adenosine deaminase (ADA) level, rheumatoid factor level, and lipid analysis, may be of value.

Tests on Pleural Fluid

Appearance

The gross appearance of the pleural fluid should always be described and its odor noted.

- Bloody fluid: Obtain hematocrit. If hematocrit is more than 50% that of peripheral blood, hemothorax is present and tube thoracostomy should be considered.
- Cloudy fluid: Centrifuge fluid. If supernatant is clear, the initial cloudiness was caused by cells or debris. If supernatant is cloudy, the initial cloudiness was caused by high lipid levels and the patient has chylothorax or pseudochylothorax.
- Putrid odor indicates bacterial infection (probably anaerobic) of the pleural space.
- Urinelike odor strongly suggests urinothorax.

Glucose

Measurements of the pleural fluid glucose level are indicated because a reduced level (less than 60 mg/dL) narrows the diagnostic possibilities to the following seven conditions:

- Parapneumonic effusion;
- Malignant effusion;
- Tuberculous effusion;
- Rheumatoid effusion;
- Hemothorax;
- Churg-Strauss syndrome;
- Paragonimiasis.

Amylase

Measurement of the pleural fluid amylase level is indicated because an elevated level (above the upper normal limit of serum) indicates that the patient has one of the following three diseases:

- Esophageal perforation: Important to establish diagnosis early because mortality is high if not properly treated.
- Pancreatic disease: Patients with chronic pancreatic pleural effusions often appear to have cancer.
- Pleural malignancy: Salivary type amylase in this situation.

LDH

The pleural fluid LDH level is not used in the differential diagnosis of exudative pleural effusion. Nevertheless, a pleural fluid LDH level should be measured every time a diagnostic thoracentesis is performed because it is a good indicator of the degree of inflammation in the pleural space. Increasing levels with serial thoracenteses indicate that the degree of inflammation is worsening and one should pursue the diagnosis more aggressively.

White Blood Cell Count and Differential Cell Count

The absolute pleural fluid white blood cell count has limited utility.

- Counts more than $10,000/mm^3$ are most common with parapneumonic effusions but are also seen with pancreatitis, pulmonary embolism, collagen vascular disease, malignant disorders, and tuberculosis.
- The differential cell count on the pleural fluid is of more utility than the absolute cell count.
- Presence of predominantly polymorphonuclear leukocytes indicates an acute disease process, such as pneumonia, pulmonary embolization, pancreatitis, intra-abdominal abscess, or early tuberculosis.
- Presence of predominantly mononuclear cells indicates a chronic disease process, such as malignant disease, tuberculosis, or a resolving acute process.
- Presence of predominantly small lymphocytes indicates that the patient probably has tuberculosis or a malignant disease.
- Presence of more than 10% eosinophils usually indicates that the patient has had

either blood or air in the pleural space. If neither air nor blood has been present in the pleural space, several unusual diagnoses should be considered: benign asbestos pleural effusions, pleural effusions caused by drug reactions, paragonimiasis, or Churg-Strauss syndrome. Diagnosis is never determined for approximately 20% of exudative pleural effusions, and, interestingly, pleural fluid eosinophilia is found in approximately 40% of these effusions.

- The presence of more than 5% mesothelial cells in the pleural fluid basically rules out a diagnosis of pleural tuberculosis.

Cytology

Pleural fluid cytology is useful in establishing the diagnosis of malignant pleural effusion.

- Cytologic results are positive in 40–90% of malignant pleural effusions and depend on the type of tumor (difficult with lymphomas), the amount of fluid submitted (more fluid, higher yield), and the skill of the cytologist.
- Immunohistochemical tests using monoclonal antibodies are complementary to cytology.
- Flow cytometry can demonstrate abnormal numbers of chromosomes in approximately two-thirds of patients with malignant pleural effusions. The number of chromosomes is normal in benign cells.
- Diagnosis of malignancy can be facilitated via electron microscopy.

Culture and Bacteriologic Stains

The following pleural fluid cultures should be obtained on patients with undiagnosed exudative pleural effusions:

- Aerobic and anaerobic bacterial cultures plus a Gram's stain;
- Mycobacterial cultures;
- Fungal cultures and fungi.

pH

The pleural fluid pH is most useful in determining whether chest tubes should be inserted in patients with parapneumonic effusions.

- If the pleural fluid pH is less than 7.00, tube thoracostomy should be instituted.
- If the pleural fluid pH is more than 7.20, the patient probably does not require tube thoracostomy.

The reduction of pleural fluid pH to less than 7.20 can occur with nine other conditions:

- Systemic acidosis (pleural fluid pH approximates blood pH normally);
- Esophageal rupture in which case the low pH is caused by concurrent infection;

- Rheumatoid pleuritis;
- Tuberculous pleuritis;
- Malignant pleural disease (if pleural tumor burden is large);
- Hemothorax;
- Paragonimiasis;
- Churg-Strauss syndrome (the patient also has asthma);
- Urinothorax (protein and LDH levels may be low).

When the pleural fluid pH is used as a diagnostic test, the pleural fluid must be measured with the same care as arterial pH.

- The fluid should be collected anaerobically in a heparinized syringe.
- The fluid should be placed in ice between collection and analysis.
- The analysis should be performed with a blood gas machine.

Immunologic Studies

Patients with systemic lupus erythematosus (SLE) or rheumatoid arthritis may have a pleural effusion during the course of their disease.

- The best screening test for lupus pleuritis is the pleural fluid ANA titer. With lupus pleuritis, the pleural fluid ANA titer is more than or equal to 1:160 or more than or equal to the serum titer. The test is both sensitive and specific.
- Only patients with rheumatoid pleuritis have a pleural fluid rheumatoid factor titer more than or equal to 1:320 or more than or equal to the serum titer.

Other Diagnostic Tests

Several other tests are useful at times in the differential diagnosis of pleural effusions.

- Pleural fluid ADA levels. Levels more than 70 U/L are virtually diagnostic of tuberculous pleuritis, whereas levels less than 40 U/L virtually rule out this diagnosis.
- Pleural fluid lipid analysis. A pleural fluid triglyceride level more than 110 mg/dL is diagnostic of chylothorax. With pseudochylothorax, the pleural fluid cholesterol level is elevated.
- Perform lipoprotein analysis of the pleural fluid if there is confusion about whether the patient has a chylothorax or a pseudochylothorax. The demonstration of chylomicrons in the pleural fluid establishes the diagnosis of chylothorax.
- Measurements that have not been unequivocally demonstrated to be of value in the differential diagnosis of pleural effusions are carcinoembryonic antigen, hyaluronic acid, lysozyme, alkaline phosphatase, and acid phosphatase.

Invasive Tests for Undiagnosed Exudative Pleural Effusions

In most patients, the cause of the pleural effusion is apparent after the initial clinical assessment and a diagnostic thoracentesis. If the diagnosis is not apparent, the following invasive tests might be considered: needle biopsy of the pleura, thoracoscopy, bronchoscopy, and open biopsy of the pleura. Because pulmonary embolism is one of the leading causes of pleural effusion, this diagnosis should be considered in all patients with an undiagnosed pleural effusion.

- Perfusion lung scan is the best screening test.
- Pulmonary angiography is often necessary (see Chapter 13).

A diagnosis is never established for approximately 20% of the exudative pleural effusions that resolve spontaneously, leaving no residua. Three factors should influence the vigor with which one pursues the diagnosis in patients with undiagnosed exudative effusions:

- The symptoms and clinical course of the patient: If the symptoms are minimal or improving, a less aggressive approach is indicated.
- The trend of the pleural fluid LDH level: If the pleural fluid LDH tends to increase with serial thoracenteses, a more aggressive approach is indicated because the process is getting worse.
- The attitude of the patient: If the patient is desperate to know why a pleural effusion has developed, an aggressive approach should be taken.

Needle Biopsy

With special needles, small specimens of the parietal pleura can be obtained relatively noninvasively.

- Useful mainly to establish the diagnosis of malignant or tuberculous pleural effusion.
- The initial biopsy is positive for granulomas in 50–80% of patients with pleural tuberculosis. The demonstration of granulomas on the pleural biopsy is virtually diagnostic of tuberculous pleuritis. Culture of a portion of the pleural biopsy specimen for mycobacteria increases the diagnostic yield.
- The initial biopsy is positive in approximately 40% of patients with malignant pleural disease.
- Overall, the yield from pleural fluid cytology is higher than that obtained by needle biopsy in patients with malignant disease.
- When malignant disease is strongly suspected, pleural biopsy should be performed only if initial cytology is nondiagnostic.

Thoracoscopy

Although thoracoscopy has been a part of thoracic surgical practice for many years, the advent of video-assisted techniques has greatly expanded the indications and uses of this procedure. With this procedure, a scope is introduced through the chest wall into the pleural space after a pneumothorax has been induced on the side of the pleural effusion.

- The view of the thoracic cavity with video-assisted thoracoscopy is as good as it is with a limited thoracotomy.
- The diagnosis is established in patients with malignant effusions more than 90% of the time.
- Diagnoses of benign disease are rarely made.

The following is the indication for thoracoscopy in patients with an undiagnosed pleural effusion:

- An unresolving undiagnosed pleural effusion in a patient who has had at least two nondiagnostic pleural fluid cytologies and one nondiagnostic needle biopsy of the pleura.
- A procedure such as talc insufflation of pleural scarification should be carried out at the time of the thoracoscopy to prevent recurrence of the effusion.

Bronchoscopy

Bronchoscopy is at times useful in the evaluation of patients with an undiagnosed exudative pleural effusion. The procedure is recommended for undiagnosed pleural effusions in the following situations:

- Parenchymal infiltrate is apparent on chest x-ray or CT scan;
- Presence of hemoptysis;
- Large pleural effusion;
- Diagnostic yield should exceed 70% in these three situations.

Open Biopsy

Thoracotomy with direct biopsy of the pleura is the most invasive procedure used to diagnose pleural effusion.

- This invasive procedure does not provide a definitive diagnosis in a substantial percentage of patients.
- In facilities without the capacity to do videothoracoscopy, open biopsy should be done for the same indications as is thoracoscopy.

MALIGNANT PLEURAL EFFUSIONS

The annual incidence of malignant pleural effusions is approximately 200,000 in this country. The three tumors that cause approximately 75% of all malignant pleural effusions are lung carcinoma (30%), breast carcinoma (25%), and tumors of the lymphoma group (20%).

Pathophysiology

The initial step in the development of pleural metastases is the embolization of the tumor to the lung and/or visceral pleura.

- Parietal pleura is involved via secondary seeding from the visceral pleura or the pleural fluid.

Direct mechanisms responsible for accumulation of pleural fluid:

- Pleural metastases can increase the permeability of the pleural surfaces so that more fluid is formed.
- Lymphatic involvement can lead to decreased pleural fluid clearance.
- The thoracic duct can be interrupted, thereby leading to a chylothorax.
- Bronchial obstruction can lead to markedly decreased pleural pressure and a pleural effusion.
- Pericardial involvement with a malignant tumor is frequently associated with the accumulation of pleural fluid.

Indirect mechanisms:

- Hypoproteinemia can decrease the serum oncotic pressure and lead to pleural effusion.
- Patients with a malignant disorder have a higher incidence of pulmonary embolism, which may cause a pleural effusion.
- The postobstructive pneumonia secondary to bronchogenic carcinoma may cause a parapneumonic effusion.
- The therapy for the tumor (radiation or chemotherapy) may itself cause the effusion.

Clinical Features

The most common symptom reported by patients with malignant pleural effusions is dyspnea, which occurs in approximately 50% of patients.

- Only approximately 25% of patients with malignant pleural effusions have chest pain. The pain is usually dull and aching rather than pleuritic in nature.
- Symptoms attributable to the tumor itself are frequent (e.g., weight loss in 32%, malaise in 21%, and anorexia in 14%).
- The pleural fluid is an exudate.
- The ratio of pleural fluid to serum protein level is less than 0.5 in approximately 20% of patients with pleural malignancy, but the LDH ratio is more than 0.60, or the absolute pleural fluid LDH meets exudative criteria in this 20%.
- The fluid may be serous or bloody.
- The predominant cells can be lymphocytes, other mononuclear cells, or polymorphonuclear leukocytes.
- Pleural fluid eosinophilia is uncommon.
- The pleural fluid glucose level is reduced to less than 60 mg/dL in 15–20% of malignant pleural effusions, and this is a marker that the patient has a large tumor burden. Mean survival is less than 2 months. (The pleural fluid pH is also reduced in most patients with a low glucose malignant pleural effusion.)

Diagnosis

The diagnosis of a malignant pleural effusion is established by demonstrating malignant cells in the pleural fluid or in the pleura itself.

- Diagnosis is most commonly established with pleural fluid cytology, which is positive in approximately 60% of patients.
- Needle biopsy of pleura is positive in 40% of patients.
- Immunohistochemical tests using monoclonal antibodies directed against various antigens are useful in differentiating malignant from benign pleural effusions, and adenocarcinomas from mesotheliomas.
- Chromosomal abnormalities demonstrated by flow cytometry are highly suggestive of malignant disease.
- Thoracoscopy effectively establishes the diagnosis, as does open biopsy.

Treatment

The initial step is to identify the location of the primary tumor.

- The clinician must determine whether the tumor is of a type that is responsive to chemotherapy. Small-cell lung carcinoma, lymphomas, leukemias, and, rarely, germ-cell tumors, may have an associated pleural effusion and may respond to chemotherapy.

Indication for pleurodesis or the removal of fluid via a pleuroperitoneal shunt:

- The patient's lifestyle is compromised by dyspnea;
- The dyspnea improves after a therapeutic thoracentesis.

Contraindications for pleurodesis:

- Shift of mediastinum toward the side of the effusion;
- Life expectancy less than 30 days.

Selection of agent for pleurodesis:

- Tetracycline is no longer available;
- The tetracycline derivatives doxycycline (500 mg) or minocycline (300 mg) appear to be as effective as tetracycline;
- Talc (5 gm) administered either as a slurry or insufflated is the most effective, but there are concerns about its association with the development of acute respiratory distress syndrome;
- Bleomycin (60 IU) intrapleurally is less effective and more expensive than either the tetracycline derivatives or talc.

The goal of a chemical pleurodesis is to obliterate the pleural space so that there is no place for the pleural fluid to reaccumulate. The following procedure is recommended to produce the intense inflammatory response that results in fusion of the visceral and the parietal pleurae and obliteration of the intervening space.

- A chest tube should be inserted.
- Systemic sedation and local anesthesia (4 mg/kg lidocaine) should be given because the procedure at times is painful.
- The sclerosing agent (doxycycline 500 mg or talc 5 gm in a total volume of 50 mL) should be injected only if the underlying lung has expanded.
- After injection, the chest tube is clamped for 1–2 hours.
- Suction is then maintained for at least 48 hours and until the pleural drainage is less than 150 mL/day.

Pleurodesis effectively controls the pleural effusions in 70–90% of properly selected patients. Most failures occur because of poor patient selection; either the mediastinum is shifted toward the side of the pleural effusion or the lung does not expand after the chest tube is inserted.

An alternative to pleurodesis is a pleuroperitoneal shunt.

- This device consists of two catheters connected with a valved pump chamber. The two one-way valves in the pump chamber are positioned so that fluid can flow only from the pleural space to the pump chamber to the peritoneal cavity. The pumping chamber must be used to move fluid from the pleural cavity to the peritoneal cavity because the pleural pressure is lower than the peritoneal pressure.
- Advantages of the shunt are that total hospitalization time is less than that required for chemical pleurodesis; the amount of pain is less than that caused by tetracycline pleurodesis; the procedure can be done on an outpatient basis; and the procedure can be effective even if the underlying lung does not completely reexpand.
- The disadvantages of the shunt are that the shunt becomes obstructed in some patients; insertion of the pump frequently requires general anesthesia; and the patient must use the pump daily.

Malignant Mesothelioma

These highly malignant tumors are thought to arise from the mesothelial cells that line the pleural cavities.

- Malignant mesothelioma is much more common in individuals with a history of asbestos exposure; 75% of patients with mesothelioma have a history of exposure to asbestos. The current incidence is 1,500 cases per year.
- The usual presentation is the insidious onset of chest pain or shortness of breath. Pain is usually nonpleuritic and is frequently referred to the upper abdomen or shoulder.
- The chest x-ray almost always reveals a pleural effusion and frequently the effusion is large, occupying 50% or more of the hemithorax. The CT scan is suggestive of the diagnosis.
- The fluid is exudative and has lower mean glucose and pH levels than does the fluid from metastatic carcinoma.
- The diagnosis of malignant mesothelioma is difficult and usually requires either thoracoscopy or an open pleural biopsy.

- Malignant mesothelioma has no effective treatment. Patients are best managed symptomatically; oxygen is administered for dyspnea and opiates are given to help to relieve chest pain.

PARAPNEUMONIC EFFUSIONS AND BACTERIAL INFECTIONS OF THE PLEURAL SPACE

A parapneumonic effusion is any pleural effusion associated with bacterial pneumonia, lung abscess, or bronchiectasis. Parapneumonic effusions are probably the most common exudative pleural effusions in the United States. Approximately 40% of the 1.2 million individuals who develop a bacterial pneumonia in the United States each year have a pleural effusion.

The subcategories of parapneumonic effusions are:

- Complicated parapneumonic effusions, which require tube thoracostomy for their resolution;
- An empyema, which is an exudative effusion on which the Gram's stain of the pleural fluid is positive.

Pathophysiology

The evolution of a parapneumonic effusion can be divided into three stages that represent a continuous spectrum:

- The exudative stage is the first stage and is characterized by the collection of sterile fluid in the pleural space. The pleural fluid in this stage is an exudate with primarily polymorphonuclear leukocytes, a normal glucose level, and a normal pH level. Appropriate antibiotic therapy effects resolution of both the pneumonic process and the pleural disease.
- The fibropurulent stage is the next stage and is characterized by infection with the offending bacteria of the previously sterile pleural fluid. The pH and glucose levels of the pleural fluid become progressively lower while the LDH level of the pleural fluid becomes progressively higher. As this stage progresses, the pleural space becomes loculated as the result of the formation of fibrin membranes.
- The organization stage is the final stage and is characterized by fibroblasts growing into the exudate from both the visceral and the parietal pleural surfaces to produce an inelastic membrane called the pleural peel. This peel encases the lung and renders it nearly functionless.

Bacteriology

Prior to the antibiotic era, *Streptococcus pneumoniae* or hemolytic streptococci were responsible for most empyemas.

- At present, anaerobic organisms, aerobic organisms, and mixed infections with aerobes and anaerobes each account for approximately one-third of culture-positive parapneumonic effusions.

Clinical Features

The clinical picture depends on whether organisms are aerobic or anaerobic.

- If aerobic, an acute febrile illness with chest pain, sputum production, and leukocytosis ensues.
- If anaerobic, a subacute illness with weight loss, anemia, and leukocytosis ensues. Most patients also have a history of an episode of unconsciousness or some other factor that predisposes them to aspiration and anaerobic pneumonia.

Diagnosis

The possibility of a parapneumonic effusion should be considered whenever a patient with a bacterial pneumonia is initially evaluated.

- Obtain bilateral decubitus chest x-rays if either of the posterior costophrenic angles is blunted on the lateral chest x-ray or if either diaphragm is not visible throughout its length.
- Semiquantitate the amount of pleural fluid by measuring the distance between the inside of the chest wall and the outside of the lung. If the thickness of the fluid is less than 10 mm, the effusion is not clinically significant and a thoracentesis is not indicated. If the thickness of the fluid is more than 10 mm, a diagnostic thoracentesis should be performed immediately.

Treatment

One can identify a complicated parapneumonic effusion only by examining the pleural fluid. A diagnostic thoracentesis should be performed as soon as the presence of a significant amount of pleural fluid is demonstrated.

- Aliquots of the pleural fluid should be sent for measurement of the pleural fluid glucose, LDH, amylase and protein levels, pH, a differential and total white blood cell count, Gram's stain, and aerobic and anaerobic bacterial cultures.
- Usually the fluid also is submitted for mycobacterial and fungal smears and cultures, as well as for cytologic studies.

At the time of the initial evaluation, the pleural effusion of some patients with parapneumonic effusions is already loculated.

- Ultrasonic examinations of the pleural space are effective in distinguishing loculated fluid from pneumonic infiltrates.
- Perform thoracentesis with ultrasonic guidance.
- Loculated fluid by itself is not an indication for tube thoracostomy.

When a patient with pneumonia and pleural effusion is initially evaluated, the decision whether to initiate tube drainage of the pleural space must be made and an appropriate antibiotic must be selected.

- Individuals who require tube thoracostomy must be identified immediately. A delay of even 24 hours increases morbidity and mortality.
- Indications for chest tube insertion are the presence of gross pus in the pleural space, organisms on the pleural fluid Gram's stain, pleural fluid glucose less than 60 mg/dL, and pleural fluid pH less than 7.00.

Even when none of these criteria is met, tube thoracostomy should still be considered if the pleural fluid pH is less than 7.20 or if the pleural fluid LDH is more than 1,000 IU/L.

- In borderline cases, serial thoracenteses at 12- to 24-hour intervals are useful in deciding whether to place chest tubes. If the pleural fluid LDH tends to decrease and the pleural fluid pH and glucose levels tend to increase with serial thoracenteses, the patient is improving and tube thoracostomy is not indicated. Alternatively, if the LDH is increasing and the pH and glucose levels are decreasing, tube thoracostomy should be performed without delay.

If the fluid is thick and viscid, a relatively large chest tube should be used; if the fluid is thin, a small tube will work satisfactorily.

- Position tube in the most dependent part of the effusion. This is probably best done by the interventional radiologist.
- Leave the tube in place until the volume of the pleural drainage is less than 50 mL/24 hr and until the draining fluid becomes clear yellow.

If clinical and radiologic improvement does not occur within 24 hours, either the pleural drainage is unsatisfactory or the patient is receiving the wrong antibiotic.

- Review culture results.
- Check position of chest tube.
- If drainage is inadequate because of loculation of the pleural fluid, administer a thrombolytic agent (streptokinase or urokinase) intrapleurally.
- If drainage is still inadequate, consider thoracoscopy with the breakdown of adhesions or thoracotomy with decortication.

Certain factors can help to predict whether closed tube drainage will be sufficient therapy for a complicated parapneumonic effusion. In general, when a patient has a purulent empyema that is loculated, chest tubes alone usually are not sufficient therapy. The following scheme is a useful classification of complicated parapneumonic effusions:

- Class I, low pH pleural effusion: Pleural fluid pH is less than 7.20, but pleural fluid cultures are negative. Tube thoracostomy by itself is usually successful.
- Class II, classic empyema: Pleural fluid cultures are positive, but no loculations. Patient may need thrombolytic therapy in addition to chest tubes.

- Class III, complicated empyema: Multiple loculations on chest x-ray, initially or subsequently, or trapped lung. Almost all patients require thrombolytic therapy and many require decortication or open drainage procedure.

TUBERCULOUS PLEURAL EFFUSIONS

In many parts of the world, the most common cause of an exudative pleural effusion is tuberculosis. Such pleural effusions, however, are relatively rare in the United States, with an annual incidence of 1,000 cases.

Tuberculous pleural effusions are thought to result when a subpleural caseous focus in the lung ruptures into the pleural space.

- Delayed hypersensitivity is responsible for pleural effusion.
- Tuberculous pleuritis can appear as an acute or chronic illness. The acute presentation is characterized by cough and chest pain; the chronic presentation is characterized by low grade fever, weakness, and weight loss.
- The effusion is almost always unilateral and is usually small to moderate in size, although at times it may be massive. One-third of patients have concurrent parenchymal infiltrates.
- When untreated, the effusion resolves, but most patients subsequently develop tuberculosis.
- Pleural fluid is an exudate with predominantly small lymphocytes.
- The diagnosis is established by needle biopsy of the pleura demonstrating granuloma or positive mycobacterial cultures of the pleural fluid or pleural biopsy specimen. Elevated levels of ADA or gamma interferon in the pleural fluid are suggestive of the diagnosis.
- Patients with tuberculous pleuritis should be treated the same as patients with pulmonary tuberculosis (see Chapter 8). All patients with an undiagnosed exudative pleural effusion and a positive purified protein derivative (PPD) should be treated for pleural tuberculosis unless their pleural fluid ADA is below 40 U/L.

PLEURAL EFFUSIONS IN PATIENTS WITH AIDS

- Pleural effusions are uncommon in patients with AIDS.
- The most common cause is Kaposi's sarcoma (KS). Diagnosis is difficult, and open biopsy usually is required.
- Parapneumonic effusions are the second most common cause, followed by tuberculosis, cryptococcosis, and lymphoma.
- Effusions are unusual with *Pneumocystis carinii* infection.
- Patients with AIDS and pleural effusion should undergo diagnostic thoracentesis. If no diagnosis, a needle biopsy of pleura is performed if fluid is exudative. If still no diagnosis, one should consider treatment for tuberculosis. If the patient is

symptomatic, a pleuroperitoneal shunt should be implanted or chemical pleurodesis should be attempted.

PLEURAL EFFUSIONS CAUSED BY PULMONARY EMBOLIZATION

Although pulmonary embolism is one of the most common causes of pleural effusion (Table 9.2), it is frequently not considered in the differential diagnosis of pleural effusion.

- Effusion may be either a transudate or an exudate with any cell type. Pleural fluid may or may not be bloody.
- Patients have usual symptoms of pulmonary embolization.
- Parenchymal infiltrate is also apparent in 50% of patients.
- The initial diagnostic study is usually a perfusion lung scan. If the perfusion scan is abnormal, a ventilation lung scan should be obtained. If doubt still exists after these tests, a pulmonary arteriogram should be performed (see Chapter 30).
- The treatment is the same as that for any patient with a pulmonary embolus. If effusion enlarges during treatment, thoracentesis should be repeated to rule out infection or hemothorax.

PLEURAL EFFUSIONS CAUSED BY DISEASES OF THE GASTROINTESTINAL TRACT

Several different gastrointestinal diseases may have an associated pleural effusion.

Acute Pancreatitis

Approximately 20% of patients with acute pancreatitis have an exudative pleural effusion.

- The effusion probably results from diaphragmatic inflammation.
- Occasionally chest symptoms dominate the clinical picture.
- The pleural fluid is an exudate with predominantly polymorphonuclear leukocytes and an elevated amylase.
- The effusion does not alter the treatment plan for a patient with acute pancreatitis.

Chronic Pancreatic Pleural Effusion

The possibility of a chronic pancreatic pleural effusion should be considered in all patients who seem to have a malignant pleural effusion but in whom the pleural fluid cytologic results are negative.

- Results from a sinus tract leading from the pancreas through the aortic or esophageal hiatus into the mediastinum.
- Clinical picture is dominated by chest symptoms, such as dyspnea, cough, and chest pain.
- Effusion is usually large and recurs rapidly after a therapeutic thoracentesis.
- A markedly elevated pleural fluid amylase level is key to the diagnosis.
- Usually therapy requires abdominal exploration with ligation or excision of the sinus tract and drainage or partial resection of the pancreas.

Esophageal Perforation

This diagnosis should be considered in all acutely ill patients with exudative pleural effusions because if this condition is not treated rapidly and appropriately, mortality approaches 100%.

- Usually follows instrumentation of esophagus but may occur spontaneously.
- Severe symptoms result from intense infection of the mediastinum.
- Pleural fluid amylase level is a good screening test. The amylase level is markedly elevated because saliva, with its high amylase content, enters the mediastinum through a hole in the esophagus. The diagnosis is confirmed with contrast studies of the esophagus.
- The treatment of choice for esophageal perforation is exploration of the mediastinum with primary repair of the esophageal tear and drainage of the pleural space and mediastinum.

Intra-abdominal Abscess

Approximately 80% of subphrenic abscesses, 40% of pancreatic abscesses, 30% of splenic abscesses, and 20% of intrahepatic abscesses have an accompanying pleural effusion.

- Effusion results from diaphragmatic irritation.
- The possibility of an abscess should be strongly considered in any patient with an undiagnosed exudative pleural effusion containing predominantly polymorphonuclear leukocytes when pulmonary parenchymal infiltrates are absent.
- The diagnosis of intra-abdominal abscess is best established with abdominal CT scanning.
- Treatment consists of drainage of the abscess.

PLEURAL DISEASE CAUSED BY COLLAGEN VASCULAR DISEASES
Rheumatoid Pleuritis

Approximately 5% of patients with rheumatoid arthritis develop a pleural effusion in the course of their disease.

- The pleural effusion usually develops only after the arthritis has been present for several years.
- Most patients are male, older than 35 years of age, and have subcutaneous nodules.
- The pleural fluid is characterized by a glucose level less than 30 mg/dL, a LDH level more than 700 IU/L, a pH less than 7.20, and a rheumatoid factor titer more than 1:320.
- No treatment has proved effective for rheumatoid pleuritis.

Lupus Pleuritis

The incidence of pleural effusion with either systemic or drug-induced lupus erythematosus is approximately 40%.

- Arthritis or arthralgias are usually present before effusion develops.
- Almost all patients with lupus pleuritis have pleuritic chest pain, and most are also febrile.
- Many different drugs have been incriminated for producing drug-induced lupus erythematosus. Hydralazine, procainamide, isoniazid, phenytoin, and chlorpromazine are most commonly indicated. The presenting signs, symptoms, and radiographic abnormalities are similar to those of spontaneous lupus.
- The pleural fluid is an exudate that may have predominantly polymorphonuclear leukocytes or lymphocytes. The pleural fluid glucose level is usually more than 60 mg/dL, the LDH level is less than 500 IU/L, and the pH is more than 7.20.
- Measurement of the level of ANA in the pleural fluid is the best test for lupus pleuritis. With lupus, the ANA titer is equal to or greater than 1:160 or the pleural fluid to serum ANA ratio is equal to or greater than 1.
- Oral corticosteroids are effective therapy for lupus pleuritis.

PLEURAL EFFUSIONS CAUSED BY DRUG REACTIONS

Administration of the following drugs has been associated with the development of a pleural effusion:

- Nitrofurantoin, the urinary antiseptic;
- Dantrolene, the muscle relaxant;
- Methysergide, the antimigraine drug;
- Bromocriptine, the antiParkinson's drug;
- Procarbazine, the antineoplastic drug;
- Amiodarone, the antiarrhythmic drug.

Individuals with drug-induced pleural effusions may appear with acute, subacute, or chronic illnesses.

- Concomitant pulmonary infiltrates are sometimes present.
- Characteristics of fluid are poorly described, but it is frequently eosinophilic.

BIBLIOGRAPHY

Broaddus VC, Wiener-Kronish JP, Staub NC. Clearance of lung edema into the pleural space of volume-loaded anesthetized sheep. J Appl Physiol 1990;68:2623–2630.

Broaddus VC, Wiener-Kronish JP, Berthiauma Y, Staub NC. Removal of pleural liquid and protein by lymphatics in awake sheep. J Appl Physiol 1988;64:384.

Harris RJ, Kavuru MS, Rice TW, Kirby TJ. The diagnostic and therapeutic utility of thoracoscopy: a review. Chest 1995;108:828–841.

Landreneau RJ, Keenan RJ, Hazelrigg SR, Mack MJ, Naunheim KS. Thoracoscopy for empyema and hemothorax. Chest 1996;109:18–24.

Lee KA, Harvey JC, Reich H, Beattie EJ. Management of malignant pleural effusions with pleuroperitoneal shunting. J Am Coll Surg 1994;178:586–588.

Light RW. A new classification of parapneumonic effusions and empyema. Chest 1995;108: 299–301.

Light RW. Pleural diseases. Philadelphia, Pa: Williams & Wilkins, 1995.

Shinto RA, Light RW. The effects of diuresis upon the characteristics of pleural fluid in patients with congestive heart failure. Am J Med 1990;88:230.

Van Way C III, Narrod J, Hopeman A. The role of early limited thoracotomy in the treatment of empyema. J Thorac Cardiovasc Surg 1988;96:433.

Walker-Renard PB, Vaughan LM, Sahn SA. Chemical pleurodesis for malignant pleural effusions. Ann Intern Med 1994;120:56–64.

10 Acid-Base Disorders

David Nierman, Paul L. Marino

Although the interpretation and management of acid-base disorders is an essential skill in patient care, physician performance in acid-base disturbances has been far from skilled. In one study of physician attitudes about computerized acid-base interpretations, 70% of the physicians surveyed claimed they were competent in acid-base interpretations and did not need computer assistance. This same group of physicians, however, correctly identified only 39% of the acid-base disorders from a sample of arterial blood gas measurements. Another report from a university-affiliated hospital shows a diagnostic accuracy of only 17% for physician interpretation of combined acid-base disorders. Finally, an audit of physician performance in life-threatening situations at a university-affiliated hospital revealed that 33% of the therapeutic decisions made by physicians in response to life-threatening blood gas abnormalities were inappropriate or untimely. These reports show a disturbing lack of knowledge in acid-base balance, and they are mentioned here to emphasize the need for clinicians to maintain a working knowledge of the information presented in this chapter.

RULE-BASED ACID-BASE INTERPRETATIONS

Acid-base regulation is a well-defined process that allows for a highly organized approach to identifying acid-base disorders. A "rule-based" method is used in the acid-base interpretations in this chapter. This method creates predictions based on the observed behavior of acid-base regulation, and these predictions are used as statements or instructions (rules) that will identify acid-base abnormalities. Rules create rigid guidelines that reduce uncertainty and simplify the problem-solving process; these attributes can improve the accuracy of acid-base interpretations.

Acid-Base Relationships

The principal features of acid-base regulation are defined by the chemical relationship among pH, carbon dioxide, and bicarbonate ions in the extracellular fluid. This relationship is expressed below, using the partial pressure of carbon dioxide (PCO_2) and the concentration of bicarbonate ions [HCO_3] and hydrogen ions [H^+] in circulating blood.

$$[H^+] \text{ (mEq/L)} = 24 \times (PCO_2/[HCO_3])$$

This relationship defines the PCO_2/HCO_3 ratio as the principal factor in determin-

477

Table 10.1. Expected Compensatory Responses

Primary Disorder	Expected Response
Metabolic acidosis	Expected PCO_2 = 1.5 × HCO_3^- + 0.8 (+2)
Metabolic alkalosis	Expected PCO_2 = 0.7 × HCO_3^- + 20 (+1.5)
Respiratory acidosis	$\Delta pH/\Delta PCO_2$ = $\begin{matrix} 0.008 \text{ (acute)} \\ 0.003 \text{ (chronic)} \end{matrix}$
Respiratory alkalosis	$\Delta pH/\Delta PCO_2$ = $\begin{matrix} 0.008 \text{ (acute)} \\ 0.017 \text{ (chronic)} \end{matrix}$

ing the acid-base properties of extracellular fluid. As such, the PCO_2/HCO_3 ratio can be used to describe the different types of acid-base disorders (Table 10.1). The "primary" acid-base disorders are defined by the component of the PCO_2/HCO_3 ratio that is initially altered or is altered by the greatest magnitude; that is, the "respiratory" acid-base disorders indicate a primary change in PCO_2, and the "metabolic" acid-base disorders identify HCO_3 as the primary abnormality. "Secondary" or compensatory adjustments are identified as a decrease in the magnitude of change in PCO_2/HCO_3 produced by the primary acid-base disorder.

Compensatory Changes

The goal of acid-base regulation is to reduce or eliminate the change in pH (i.e., change in PCO_2/HCO_3 ratio) produced by an acid-base disturbance. This is accomplished by compensatory adjustments to primary acid-base changes, and these adjustments are aimed at reducing the change in the PCO_2/HCO_3 ratio produced by the primary disturbance. For example, an increase in PCO_2 (primary respiratory acidosis) must be accompanied by an increase in HCO_3 (compensatory metabolic alkalosis) to limit the change in the PCO_2/HCO_3 ratio caused by the change in PCO_2. In other words, compensatory responses to primary respiratory acid-base disorders will involve changes in serum bicarbonate levels in the same direction as the PCO_2 changes. These adjustments in serum bicarbonate are produced in the kidneys and represent changes in urinary bicarbonate excretion. These renal adjustments require 3 to 5 days for completion, thus creating a period of "partial compensation." Table 10.1 shows the changes in pH associated with partial and full compensation. Note that the compensatory changes are not enough to maintain constant pH (i.e., compensation differs from correction).

Compensation for primary metabolic acid-base disorders involves a change in ventilation that changes the arterial PCO_2 in the same direction as the original change in serum bicarbonate level. These responses are mediated by chemoreceptors that respond to changes in pH and modulate the activity of the respiratory centers in the lower brainstem. Metabolic acidosis produces an increase in ventilation and a decrease in PCO_2; metabolic alkalosis depresses ventilation and raises the PCO_2. Table 10.1 shows the expected changes in PCO_2 in each type of metabolic acid-base disorder. Note that there is no period of partial compensation (i.e., the respiratory response is fully developed at onset).

Rules for Acid-Base Disorders

The equations in Table 10.1 define the changes expected in the different types of acid-base disorders. These relationships have been used to generate the following rules.

Rule 1. A primary metabolic disorder is present if:

A. The pH and PCO_2 change in the same direction, or

B. The pH is abnormal but the PCO_2 is normal.

Rule 2. In primary metabolic disorders, a secondary disturbance is identified by a difference between the PCO_2 expected from respiratory compensation and the PCO_2 measured in arterial blood.

A. For primary metabolic acidosis, expected $PCO_2 = 1.5(HCO_3) + 8(\pm 2)$

B. For primary metabolic alkalosis, expected $PCO_2 = 0.7(HCO_3) + 20(\pm 1.5)$*

Measured $PCO_2 >$ expected PCO_2 = associated respiratory acidosis

Measured $PCO_2 <$ expected PCO_2 = associated respiratory alkalosis

Rule 3. A primary respiratory disorder is present if the pH and PCO_2 change in opposite directions.

Rule 4. In primary respiratory disorders, the relative changes in pH and PCO_2 will determine the extent of compensation and identify secondary metabolic disturbances, using the following guidelines:

A. For respiratory acidosis:

pH/PCO_2	Disorder
> 0.008	Associated metabolic acidosis
0.008	Acute uncompensated acidosis
0.003–0.008	Partially compensated acidosis
< 0.003	Associated metabolic acidosis

B. For respiratory alkalosis:

pH/PCO_2	Disorder
> 0.008	Associated metabolic alkalosis
0.008	Acute uncompensated alkalosis
0.002–0.008	Partially compensated acidosis
< 0.002	Associated metabolic acidosis

* The respiratory response to metabolic alkalosis can be variable and unpredictable, creating some concern about the validity of the expected PCO_2 in metabolic alkalosis. Several equations are available for predicting the PCO_2 in metabolic alkalosis; this one was selected because it is currently the most popular. The accuracy of this relationship when the HCO_3 exceeds 40 mEq/L is not known.

Rule 5. A mixed metabolic-respiratory disorder is present if the pH is normal and the PCO_2 is abnormal.

Acid-Base Interpretations

The rules in the previous section are now applied to acid-base interpretations; the flow diagrams for this approach are shown in Figures 10.1 and 10.2. These interpretations are based on the relationships between pH and PCO_2 and are organized according to the change in pH. The normal ranges for acid-base parameters in arterial blood are as follows: pH = 7.36 to 7.44; PCO_2 = 36 to 44 mm Hg; HCO_3 = 22 to 26 mEq/L.

If pH is LOW:
A. A low or normal PCO_2 indicates a primary metabolic acidosis (see rules 1A and 1B).
   1. The equation in rule 2A [PCO_2 = 1.5(HCO_3) + 8(±2)] is then used to identify an associated respiratory disorder.
B. A high PCO_2 indicates a primary respiratory acidosis (see rule 3).

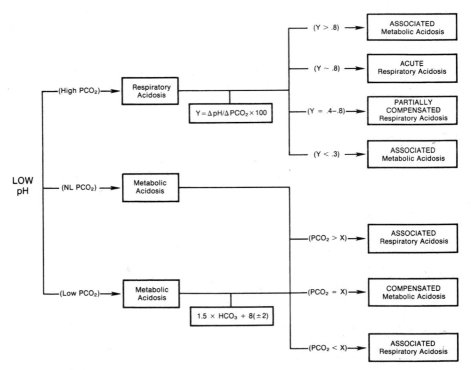

Figure 10.1. Flow diagram for acid-base interpretation when arterial pH is below normal. (See text for explanation.) (From Marino PL. The ICU book. Philadelphia, PA: Lea & Febiger, 1997, In Press. Reprinted with permission.)

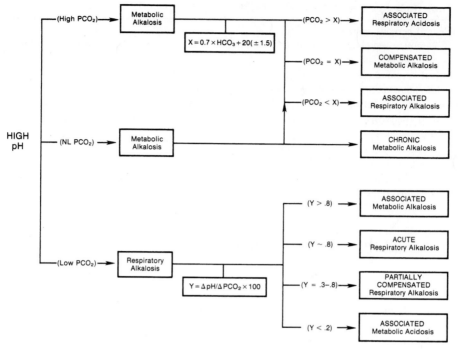

Figure 10.2. Flow diagram for acid-base interpretation when arterial pH is above normal. (See text for explanation.) (From Marino PL. The ICU book. Philadelphia, PA: Lea & Febiger, 1997, In Press. Reprinted with permission.)

1. The change in the pH/PCO$_2$ ratio is then used to determine the degree of compensation and to identify an associated metabolic disorder (see rule 4).

If pH is HIGH:

A. A high or normal PCO$_2$ indicates a primary metabolic acidosis (see rules 1A and 1B).
   1. The equation [PCO$_2$ = 0.7(HCO$_3$) + 20($\pm$1.5)] in rule 2B is then used to identify an associated respiratory disorder.
B. A low PCO$_2$ indicates a primary respiratory alkalosis (see rule 3).
   1. The pH/PCO$_2$ ratio is then used to determine the degree of compensation and to identify an associated metabolic disorder (see rule 4B).

If pH is NORMAL:

A. A high PCO$_2$ indicates a mixed respiratory acidosis–metabolic alkalosis (see rule 5).
B. A low PCO$_2$ indicates a mixed respiratory alkalosis–metabolic acidosis (see rule 5).
C. A normal PCO$_2$ may indicate normal acid-base status but does not rule out combined metabolic acidosis–metabolic alkalosis. In this situation, the anion gap can prove to be valuable.

Table 10.2. Respiratory Acidosis

Central nervous system depression:
  Narcotics, sedatives, head trauma, CNS infections, CVAs, cerebral ischemia, obesity-hypo-
    ventilation syndrome
Spinal cord and peripheral nerve disease:
  Guillain-Barre syndrome, myasthenia gravis, botulism
Musculoskeletal disorders:
  Kyphoscoliosis, flail chest, bilateral phrenic nerve damage, polymyositis
Pleural disease:
  Massive pleural effusion, pneumothorax
Intrinsic lung disease:
  COPD, advanced ARDS, large pulmonary emboli, severe pneumonia, severe pulmonary
    edema, stage IV asthma

RESPIRATORY ACIDOSIS

Respiratory acidosis, defined as an increased PCO_2, results from alveolar hypoventilation. Physiologically, there will be either decreased total minute ventilation V_E (e.g., narcotic overdose or neuromuscular weakness) or increased physiologic dead space (e.g., increased V_D/V_T ratio as in COPD) (Table 10.2). Distinguishing the underlying physiology becomes important when deciding on diagnosis and treatment. To differentiate these two physiologic causes, the alveolar-arterial (A-a) gradient can be calculated on room air ($FIO_2 = 0.21$) using the shortened alveolar gas equation:

$$PAO_2 = 150 - PCO_2/0.8$$
$$\text{A-a gradient} = PAO_2 - PaO_2$$

If the increased PCO_2 is from a decreased minute ventilation, the A-a gradient will be normal. If it is from ventilation-perfusion abnormalities, however, the A-a gradient should be increased.

RESPIRATORY ALKALOSIS

Respiratory alkalosis, defined as a decreased PCO_2, occurs as a result of increased alveolar ventilation from hyperventilation (Table 10.3).

Table 10.3. Respiratory Alkalosis

Central nervous system disease or stimulants:
  Anxiety (voluntary hyperventilation), fever, pain, third trimester pregnancy, salicylates,
    progesterone, sepsis, liver cirrhosis, brain trauma, infection, CVAs, tumors
Thoracic disease:
  Small to moderate pleural effusion, pneumothorax
Intrinsic lung disease:
  Interstitial fibrosis, pneumonia, mild pulmonary edema, stages I + II asthma

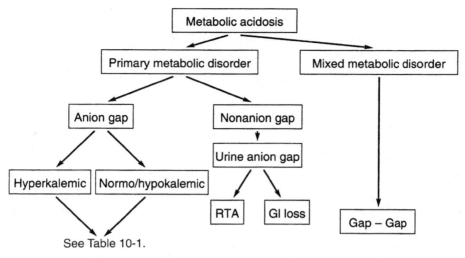

Figure 10.3. Diagnostic evaluation of metabolic acidosis.

METABOLIC ACIDOSIS

Metabolic acidosis is defined as a primary decrease in plasma bicarbonate and is caused by either the accumulation of fixed exogenous inorganic or endogenous organic acids or the loss of HCO_3^- buffer, as in diarrhea. Acidemia refers to a plasma pH that is decreased. Interpretation of a metabolic acidosis follows a straightforward algorithm (Fig. 10.3).

Anion Gap

First, decide whether there is a normal or increased anion gap (Fig. 10.4). The anion gap, calculated by $[Na^+ - (Cl^- + HCO_3^-)]$, is normally 12 ± 4 mEq mmol/L and is composed of negatively charged proteins (largely albumin), phosphate, sulfate, and other organic anions. When a fixed acid donates a proton (H^+) to the serum, the bicarbonate should decrease 1 mEq/L for every 1 mEq/L of H^+ added. Therefore, the anion gap should increase by the same amount, and an increase in the anion gap almost always indicates acid accumulation. In contrast, if bicarbonate is lost in the urine or stool, the kidneys will hold on to chloride to compensate, thereby maintaining the total negative equivalency and keeping the calculated anion gap normal.

The sensitivity of the anion gap in stratifying metabolic acidoses has been questioned. The main problem is which value to choose as the upper limit of normal. Most laboratories currently use ion-selective electrodes to measure Na^+, K^+, and Cl^-. This technology frequently gives higher Cl^- levels and lower Na^+ levels than do older photometric or colorimetric assays, yielding a consistently smaller normal anion gap. Using this new technology, the upper limit of normal for the anion gap is often ≤ 6 mmol/L and practically always ≤ 11 mmol/L. Yet, even when using

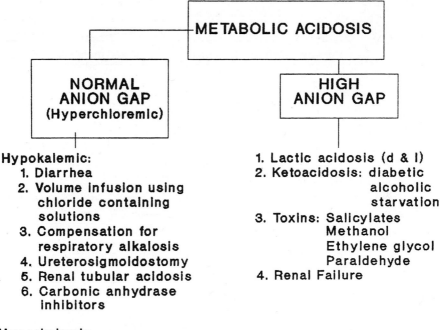

Figure 10.4. Classification of metabolic acidosis.

11 as the upper limit of normal, 29% of surgical ICU patients with elevated lactate levels were not identified. The anion gap was least sensitive for patients with mildly elevated lactate levels between 2.5 and 4.9 mmol/L.

Hypoalbuminemia

The serum albumin contributes approximately half (11 mEq/L out of a total of 23 mEq/L) of the total unmeasured anion pool. Assuming normal serum electrolytes, a 50% reduction in serum albumin will reduce the calculated anion gap by 5–6 mEq/L; this should be added to the calculated number when deciding in which category to place the acidosis. Because hypoalbuminemia is common in ICU patients, this correction should be kept in mind whenever the calculation is made because it may help recategorize a previously unsuspected elevated anion gap acidosis.

Hyponatremia

For unclear reasons, hyponatremia may also decrease the calculated anion gap. Because most causes of hyponatremia occur from net increases in free water, one would expect that the serum chloride would drop as much as the sodium, yielding a normal calculated anion gap. The chloride often does not drop equally, however. It may be that other unmeasurable anion concentrations, such as albumin, also decrease.

Urinary Anion Gap

The next step in interpretation is to further subcategorize these two broad groups. Normal anion gap acidoses are subdivided into hypokalemic and hyperkalemic groups (Fig. 10.4). In patients with a normal anion gap and hypokalemic hyperchloremic acidosis, the urinary anion gap can help differentiate a renal tubular acidosis from gastrointestinal bicarbonate loss (Fig. 10.4). The major unmeasured cation in the urine is ammonium, which is the excretable form of titratable acid. When urine acidification is deranged and the kidneys are unable to excrete acid, the urine anion gap becomes more positive. Measuring the urinary anion gap requires a spot urine for Na^+, K^+, Cl^-, and pH.

Urinary Anion Gap: Total Anions − Total Cations

$UA + Cl^- = Na^+ + K^+ + UC$

Anion gap: $UA - UC = (Na^+ + K^+) - Cl^-$

Urine anion gap	Urine pH	Diagnosis
Negative	< 5.5	Normal
Positive	> 5.5	RTA
Negative	> 5.5	Diarrhea

Ratio of Anion Gap Excess to Decrease in Serum Bicarbonate

The final step in analysis is to look at the ratio of anion gap excess to the decrease in serum bicarbonate, referred to as the "gap–gap" ratio (Fig. 10.5).

Gap–gap ratio: AG excess/HCO_3 deficit = $[AG - 12/24 - HCO_3]$

This ratio has the following three uses:

- To determine whether there is a mixed metabolic acidosis, which is a common occurrence in the ICU. When an organic acid such as lactic acid is added to blood, there will be an equal drop in HCO_3 for every mEq acid added to the anion gap, and the gap–gap ratio will remain 1. When there is a hyperchloremic acidosis from loss of HCO_3, the numerator remains low as the denominator increases, and the ratio will approach zero. When there is a mixed metabolic acidosis, the ratio will fall between 0 and 1.
- To follow responses to treatment in diabetic ketoacidosis. Prior to treatment, when serum ketones are elevated and serum bicarbonate is low, the gap–gap ratio will be high. Once treatment has begun with fluids and insulin, the ketone level drops,

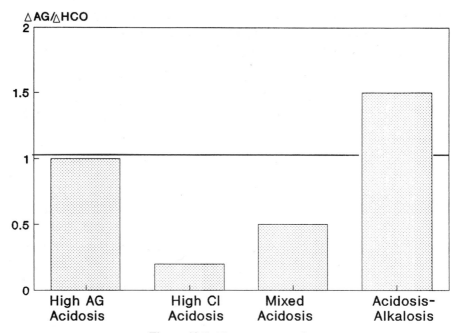

Figure 10.5. The gap − gap ratio.

but the serum HCO_3 may remain low because of the dilutional effect of intravenous fluids. Although this low HCO_3 may be incorrectly interpreted as an inadequate response to treatment, the drop in gap–gap ratio actually indicates that the ketones are being cleared and that the acidosis is changing from a high gap acidosis to a low one.

- To evaluate the presence of a mixed metabolic acidosis and alkalosis. In the presence of a high anion gap acidosis, adding alkali will make the gap–gap ratio greater than 1.

LACTIC ACIDOSIS

Lactic acidosis is a common cause of acute metabolic acidosis in critically ill patients and usually results from inadequate cellular oxygenation.

Lactate is produced within all cells in the body by the conversion of pyruvate to lactate, a reaction catalyzed by the enzyme lactate dehydrogenase (LDH). Cellular levels of lactate are mainly determined by mitochondrial function; therefore, states of impaired mitochondrial function (such as cellular hypoxia) will cause cellular levels of lactate to increase, which will then be added to the circulation. Hyperlactatemia is not synonymous with lactic acidosis. In situations such as beriberi or Reye's syndrome, lactate accumulation without an acidosis can occur (formerly referred to as type B1 lactic acidosis). Although all cells except red blood cells are capable of extracting lactate from the circulation, most is removed by the liver and kidneys and converted back to pyruvate via LDH for either gluconeogenesis or energy production. A normal liver is capable of increasing lactate clearance to 10 times the baseline.

Normal serum lactate levels are 2 mEq/L or less (normal arterial blood is less than 1.5 mmol/L, and normal venous blood is less than 2.0 mM/L). Increased production by the tissues and/or decreased clearance of lactate by the liver will result in increased serum levels. Although alterations in liver function may delay lactate clearance, in the absence of shock, however, near total destruction of the liver is necessary before lactate levels markedly increase.

Cardiogenic shock and septic shock are common states in which the oxygen supply may be inadequate to meet the oxygen needs of the tissues. Lactate levels are generally higher in hemorrhagic shock than in septic shock. Although there may not be frank hypotension (a common criterion used to indicate systemic shock), elevated lactate levels with acidosis in these settings still imply shock at a cellular level. In any case of clinical shock, an elevated lactate level carries a poor prognosis.

When discussing an imbalance between oxygen supply and oxygen demand, it is worthwhile to review the determinants of oxygen delivery:

$$\dot{D}O_2 = (\text{cardiac output}) \times [(Hb)(\text{saturation})(1.34) + (pO_2)(0.003)]$$

Lack of adequate cardiac output resulting in a peripheral low flow state is the most important contributor to the development of lactic acidosis. Although hypoxemia (a low PO_2) is commonly listed as a cause of lactic acidosis, patients with respiratory insufficiency have been shown to tolerate an arterial PO_2 as low as 22 mm Hg without developing an acidosis. Although anemia is also listed as a cause of lactic acidosis, there are many patients (e.g., Jehovah's Witnesses) who are able to tolerate hemoglobins as low as 3.0 g/dL without this happening, as long as the cardiac output can increase to compensate. If the cardiac output in an anemic patient cannot appropriately increase to compensate for the drop in delivery, a lactic acidosis may appear.

Thiamine Deficiency

Another cause of lactic acidosis that is being increasingly recognized in ICU patients is thiamine deficiency. Thiamine causes increased lactates by reducing the mitochondrial oxidation of pyruvate. Pyruvate, instead of being converted to acetyl CoA, is diverted into the production of lactate. In patients with elevated lactate levels out of proportion with the degree of clinical hemodynamic instability, serum thiamine levels should be checked while empiric thiamine is given.

D-Lactic Acidosis

A diagnostic entity that physicians should be aware of is D-lactic acidosis. Lactate is a stereoisomer and exists in L and D forms. Anaerobic human cells produce the L-isomer, a molecule that is readily metabolized by L-lactate dehydrogenase. Anaerobic bacteria, such as *Bacteroides fragilis, Eubacterium, Lactobacillus, Bifidobacterium,* and some enteric aerobes, such as *E. coli,* produce both L and D isomers. Some patients who have undergone extensive bowel surgery, when exposed to high carbohydrate enteral diets, can develop a syndrome of ''D-lactate-associated encephalopathy.'' In this setting, large amounts of D-lactate are produced by these enteric bacteria, which are then absorbed into the bloodstream and distributed across the extracellular fluid compartment, including the cerebrospinal fluid. Because mammalian cells lack D-lactate dehydrogenase, and D-lactate is slowly metabolized through unclear enzymatic pathways, D-lactate accumulates.

Patients with this syndrome present with slurred speech, confusion, lethargy, ataxia, and changed mental status and are frequently thought to be drunk or intoxicated. Laboratory tests show an increased anion gap acidosis with normal L-lactate levels. When suspected, special D-lactate levels may be measured by the laboratory, either by enzymatic means using an in vitro kit with D-lactate dehydrogenase or by nuclear magnetic resonance spectrophotometry. Treatment is effective and consists of oral nonabsorbable antibiotics and a carbohydrate-restricted diet.

Because human cells are unable to produce D-lactate, an intriguing area of investigation is the possible use of D-lactate levels in the blood or urine of patients as a marker for bacterial infection. Rats have been shown to develop detectable blood levels of D-lactate following experimentally produced *Klebsiella* peritonitis. This remains a future area of research.

LACTIC ALKALOSIS

Severe alkalosis (pH > 7.6) can cause increased lactate production by red blood cells, probably by enhancing certain pH-dependent enzymes in the glycolytic pathway. In normal flow states, the liver is usually able to handle the increased lactate production. In low flow states in which hepatic clearance is reduced, however, serum lactate levels may climb, particularly with exogenous alkali therapy.

Diagnosis

Intensivists should have a low threshold for obtaining serum lactate levels. Although the patient with a high anion gap acidosis in circulatory shock will clearly have an elevated lactate level, so might the patient with a relatively normal anion gap and only mildly lowered bicarbonate. There are no distinctive clinically significant features that suggest L-lactic acidosis, and patients with levels elevated only slightly to 2.5 mmol/L already have a marked increase in mortality. In any patient suspected of having inadequate tissue oxygen supply, lactate levels are essential for diagnosis and management.

Arterial blood will reflect both systemic production and clearance of lactate, whereas blood drawn from a peripheral vein will only reflect regional production. Excellent correlation has been shown between arterial blood and either superior vena cava or pulmonary artery blood (mixed venous), and these sites can be used. The blood sample should be either placed immediately on ice or drawn into a vacuum tube containing a glycolytic inhibitor, such as sodium fluoride, to limit further lactate production by the red blood cells.

KETOACIDOSIS

Ketoacidosis is characterized by the metabolism of free fatty acids by the liver with the generation of acetoacetate, β-hydroxybutyric acid, and acetone. There are two requirements that must be met for ketoacidosis to occur. First, there must be increased delivery of free fatty acids from the peripheral adipose tissue to the liver, a process primarily induced by relative or absolute insulin deficiency. Second, the liver must channel these fatty acids into ketone bodies rather than through the normal pathway of triglyceride synthesis, a process apparently induced by a rise in the ratio of glucagon to insulin in portal blood.

There are three ketoacidoses:

- *Diabetic ketoacidosis:* The result of either an absolute or relative insulinopenia. Concentrations of free fatty acids may reach two to four times that of a normal fasting state, which drives ketone production and results in a metabolic acidosis. Treatment of diabetic ketoacidosis consists of two simultaneous goals: the correction of the ketoacidosis by adequate exogenous insulin and the correction of fluid and electrolyte deficits. Even with a severe acidemia, the infusion of exogenous bicarbonate is not recommended. Bicarbonate infusion can lead to increased levels of acetoacetate and β-hydroxybutyric acid, possibly secondary to hepatic ketogenesis, and may delay improvement in ketosis.
- *Alcoholic ketoacidosis:* Usually arises in alcoholics who abstain from alcohol 1 or more days prior to presentation and requires three simultaneous factors to occur. First, low caloric intake leads to reduced liver glycogen stores and decreased insulin. Second, dehydration decreases renal clearance of ketone bodies. Finally, oxidation of ethanol impairs hepatic gluconeogenesis and increases the NADH: NAD ratio, which results in the conversion of acetoacetate to β-hydroxybutyrate. Alcoholic ketoacidosis usually resolves within 24 hours with an infusion of saline and glucose and does not require additional insulin.
- *Starvation ketoacidosis:* Occurs from the mobilization of fatty acids from peripheral tissues and is usually mild. In prolonged fasting, serum insulin levels, although low, are present and are enough to prevent free fatty acid levels in plasma from continuing to increase.

Diagnosis

Diagnosis of a ketoacidosis is made by a positive nitroprusside test. This colorimetric reaction, in which either a nitroprusside tablet or stick turns purple, only measures serum acetoacetate at levels over 3 mEq/L; it does not measure β-hydroxybutyric acid. Acetoacetate and β-hydroxybutyric acid exist in equilibrium with each other, with their interconversion catalyzed by the enzyme β-hydroxybutyrate dehydrogenase.

$$\text{Acetoacetate} + \text{NADH} + \text{H}^+ \xrightarrow{\text{BHBDH}} \beta\text{-hydroxybutyrate} + \text{NAD}^+$$

Tissue hypoxia can lead to decreased availability of intracellular NADH. This will increase the ratio of NADH/NAD$^+$, which drives the above reaction to the right. Because the nitroprusside reaction does not occur with β-hydroxybutyrate, it is possible to have severe ketoacidosis and hypoxia yet a negative or trace positive nitroprusside test.

TREATMENT
Should a Metabolic Acidosis Be Treated?

Metabolic acidosis has established detrimental effects, especially on cardiovascular function. In vivo, myocardial dysfunction, a reduced threshold for ventricular fibrillation, direct arterial vasodilation, indirect sympathetic-mediated vasoconstriction, and direct venous vasoconstriction can occur. In addition, metabolic acidosis can cause marked increases in pulmonary vascular resistance, resulting in increased right heart afterload. Finally, although mild acidosis causes tachycardia secondary to catecholamine release, as the acidosis worsens, bradycardia occurs. Despite all this, it is not clear if these experimental observations are clinically applicable. Acidemia causes catecholamine release and the vasodilation may counteract the drop in cardiac output. Acidemia may also improve O_2 availability by causing a right shift of the oxyhemoglobin dissociation and may protect cellular metabolism in hypoxic conditions. Clinically, patients with diabetic ketoacidosis can tolerate pH levels as low as 7.0 without cardiovascular compromise.

Some data suggests that elevated blood lactate can have harmful negative inotropic effects independent of pH. Increased intracellular lactate suppresses the activity of glyceraldehyde 3-phosphate dehydrogenase, thereby inhibiting glycolysis and limiting myofibril ATP production.

Although avoiding the detrimental effects of a severe acidosis may be desirable, no clear consensus exists concerning when or how to treat. Any treatment decision must be made in the context of what is causing the acidosis, whether the accumulation is of inorganic or organic acids and whether it is a primary process (as with poisonings) or a reflection of other pathology (as in lactic acidosis or ketoacidosis). Appearance of a lactic acidosis in a critically ill patient usually indicates inadequate oxygen delivery to meet the metabolic oxygen demand of the tissues. Therefore, the focus of treatment should not be on exogenous bicarbonate replacement but on aggressively correcting $\dot{V}O_2/\dot{D}O_2$ imbalances.

Is Bicarbonate Beneficial?

A debate has raged for years over the use of sodium bicarbonate to correct lactic acidosis. Bicarbonate therapy can produce a number of harmful effects, including hyperosmolarity, hypercapnia aggravation of intracellular acidosis, hypotension, and ionized hypocalcemia. In hypoxic dogs, bicarbonate therapy has been shown to worsen lactic acidosis. Most important, the use of bicarbonate has never been shown to either improve hemodynamics in critically ill patients with lactic acidosis or improve the outcome.

When lactic acid is buffered by sodium bicarbonate, CO_2 is generated by the following process:

$$\text{Lactate} - H^+ + NaHCO_3 \rightarrow Na^+\text{lactate}^- + H_2O + CO_2.$$

In shock situations in which microvasculature circulation is decreased or in other settings in which ventilation is fixed (e.g., the patient has been deliberately paralyzed), CO_2 will accumulate in the tissues, rapidly pass into cells, and cause an intracellular acidosis, with harmful effects. A clear example of this has been shown in cardiac arrest. Closed cardiac massage can, at most, generate 20–25% of the normal cardiac output. Arterial blood drawn at this time will reveal a normal to low $PaCO_2$ (depending on the effectiveness of ventilation). Mixed venous blood drawn simultaneously will show a markedly elevated PCO_2, reflecting tissue respiratory acidosis. Administered exogenous bicarbonate is converted to CO_2 in the tissues; this adds to venous acidosis and worsens the situation.

Other alkalinizing agents have been developed that do not cause this undesirable CO_2 production.

- *Carbicarb:* Carbicarb, (Table 10.4), which consists of one-third M Na_2CO_3 and one-third M $NaHCO_3$ and has the same alkalinity as bicarbonate, has been found to raise blood pH without raising PCO_2. Clinical experience with carbicarb is limited at present, but the preliminary results are encouraging.
- *Dichloroacetate:* Sodium dichloroacetate stimulates pyruvate dehydrogenase and diverts pyruvate away from lactate production and toward mitochondrial oxygenation. Although DCA has been shown to decrease serum lactate levels, this has not translated into improved clinical outcome. In a recent prospective, multicenter, controlled study of the use of dichloroacetate in patients with lactate acidosis,

Table 10.4. Alkali Solutions

	Carbicarb	*NaHCO₃*
Na^+	1,000	1,000 (mmol/L)
HCO_3	333	1,000
CO_3^{2-}	333	0
PCO_2	3	over 200 (mm Hg)
pH 25 C°	9.6	8.0
Osmolality	1,667	2,000 (mOsm/kg)

From Sun JH, Filley GF, Hord K. Carbicarb: an effective substitute for NaHCO₃ for the treatment of acidosis. Surgery 1987;102:835. Reprinted with permission.

although patients who received dichloroacetate had an increase in pH and decrease in lactate levels, there was no improvement in either hemodynamics or survival.

If bicarbonate is to be used, the standard recommendation is to keep the serum pH above 7.2. To calculate the approximate amount to give, the space of distribution is approximately 0.5% of body weight, but this may be twice as large with severe acidosis. With a normal PCO_2, a goal of a serum bicarbonate of 15 mEq/L should be sufficient.

$$HCO_3 \text{ deficit} = 0.5 \times \text{wt (kg)} \times (\text{desired } HCO_3 - \text{serum } HCO_3)$$

One-half of the calculated deficit is given IV bolus and the rest is added to hyponatremic solution and run over 4 to 6 hours. Periodic determinations of acid-base balance are necessary to titrate therapy.

The treatment for lactic acidosis resulting from cellular hypoxia is correction of the cellular hypoxia. There should be aggressive attempts to increase flow to the tissues, preferably guided by invasive hemodynamic monitoring. The $\dot{V}O_2$, the $\dot{D}O_2$, and the extraction ratio are closely followed. A lower than normal extraction ratio in the setting of lactic acidosis implies that the peripheral tissues are unable to remove the required oxygen from the circulation, probably because of an endothelial defect. This is a poor sign. If oxygen delivery is low and the extraction ratio is normal or high, the next step is to try to increase the delivery. First, volume load with colloid or crystalloid and follow the above parameters. A hematocrit of 30 is adequate in this setting. If the $\dot{D}O_2$ remains low despite volume loading, add inotropic agents.

The use of exogenous alkalinizing agents for a lactic acidosis is a temporizing measure and is doomed to failure unless the cause of the acidosis is resolved.

METABOLIC ALKALOSIS

Metabolic alkalosis is the most common acid-base disorder in hospitalized patients. The hallmark of a metabolic alkalosis is a serum bicarbonate that is greater than expected for the patient's PCO_2. While a drop of pH to between 7.0 and 7.2 may be tolerated by many patients without adverse effects, a pH above 7.55 has an associated mortality of 40% in the critically ill. Overall, the most common causes of metabolic alkalosis in the ICU are loss of gastric juice protons and chloride through either NG suction or vomiting and renal retention of bicarbonate secondary to hypovolemia and chloride depletion.

Metabolic alkalosis can be categorized into three broad groups for both diagnosis and treatment strategies. Differentiating these groups requires a spot urinary chloride (Fig. 10.6).

- Chloride-responsive: Urinary chloride < 15 mEq/L. Chloride is the only nonbicarbonate anion that contributes to ECF volume. Therefore, in conditions where chloride is depleted, the kidney holds on to bicarbonate as compensation to maintain the total anion equivalency.

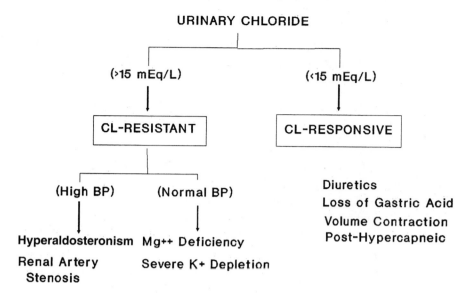

Figure 10.6. Classification of metabolic alkalosis.

(a) Gastric acid loss: Will cause depletion of both H^+ and Cl^- ions.

(b) Diuretics: Cause loss of K^+, Mg^{++}, and, most important, Cl^-. By contributing to an increase in renal acid excretion, diuretics lead to a disproportionate loss of fluid rich in Cl^- and a transcellular shift of hydrogen ions. Some of potassium loss can be prevented by either using or adding potassium-sparing diuretics, such as triamterene or spironolactone.

(c) Extracellular volume contraction.

(d) Post hypercapnic.

- Chloride-resistant: Urinary chloride > 15 mEq/L. The chloride-resistant alkaloses are usually mild and hypervolemic, and treatment is directed toward the underlying disorder. These alkaloses are generated and maintained by the kidneys and result from either a chloride-reabsorptive defect (i.e., Bartter's syndrome) or a hypermineralocorticoid state (i.e., hyperaldosteronism, Cushing's syndrome).

- Alkali administration: Exogenous bicarbonate administration rarely causes a metabolic alkalosis, secondary to the kidneys' tremendous ability to excrete excess bicarbonate.

Complications

- Hypoventilation: The ventilatory response to a metabolic alkalosis is variable and may be absent. The following equation shows that there must be a relatively severe metabolic alkalosis to cause significant CO_2 retention (e.g., a HCO_3 of 40 only results in a PCO_2 of 49).

$$\text{Expected } PCO_2 = 0.7 \times HCO_3 + 20(\pm 1.5)$$

A more important respiratory consequence of a metabolic alkalosis is shift of the oxyhemoglobin dissociation curve to the left, therefore making less oxygen available to the peripheral tissues.

- Neuromuscular: When the pH is greater than 7.55, neuromuscular irritability may occur, ranging from a positive Chvostek or Trousseau sign, to muscle cramping and spasms, to frank tetany (at a pH $>$ 7.55–7.6), and finally to lethargy, stupor, and coma. The central nervous system manifestations are more common in those patients with low ionized Ca^{2+} levels, prior seizures, or cerebrovascular disease.
- Myocardial irritability: Includes increased digitalis toxicity.
- Decreased ionized Ca^{2+}: Although the total calcium may remain normal, alkalosis causes increased binding of the ionized fraction to plasma proteins. It is not clear whether this is clinically significant.

Once a metabolic alkalosis is established, a vicious cycle may ensue. The combination of extracellular fluid contraction, hypokalemia, and chloride depletion results in a secondary hyperaldosteronism, which leads to more alkalosis. This self-perpetuating cycle may be the most important aspect of this acid-base disorder, with treatment required to break the cycle.

Treatment

Fluid Therapy

Most of the metabolic alkalosis encountered in the intensive care unit and practically all of the serious alkaloses ($HCO_3 > 40$) belong in the hypovolemic chloride-responsive group. Therefore, initial treatment strategies first involve chloride replacement using either NaCl, KCl, HCl, or combinations of these three.

- NaCl: Patients who are volume depleted generally respond well to treatment with 0.9% NaCl. The chloride deficit is calculated by the following equation:

$$\text{Cl deficit (mEq)} = 0.27 \times \text{wt (kg)} \times (100 - \text{present Cl})$$

Because a liter of 0.9% saline contains 154 mEq of Cl^-, the volume of NaCl needed is:

$$\text{0.9\% saline replacement (L)} = \text{Cl deficit}/154$$

- KCl: Because of the prohibitive amount of K^+ that would be needed, KCl alone is not adequate to provide adequate chloride replacement. If hypokalemia is present, however, it must be corrected because hypokalemia will sustain the metabolic alkalosis even after the calculated Cl^- deficit has been replaced. Correction of hypokalemia has a crucial important role in the treatment of metabolic alkalosis.
- HCl: In severe alkalosis, dilute hydrochloric acid may be necessary. Hydrochloric acid must be administered through a central line to avoid its sclerosing actions, glass bottles must be used, and the IV tubing must be changed frequently. The

solution that is used is 0.1 N HCl, which contains 100 mEq H^+/L. To calculate the amount needed, the following equations are used:

$$H^+ \text{ deficit (mEq)} = 0.5 \times \text{wt (kg)} \times (\text{present } HCO_3 - \text{ desired } HCO_3)$$

$$\text{Volume (L) of 0.1N HCl} = H^+ \text{ deficit}/100$$

$$\text{Infusion rate} = 0.2 \text{ mEq/kg/hr}$$

Arginine HCl, lysine HCl, and NH_4Cl are solutions that were previously used but are no longer commercially available.

Drug Therapy

Drug therapy has a role when there is a chloride-responsive metabolic alkalosis in normovolemic or hypervolemic patients. Neither Diamox nor H_2 blockers will correct a preexisting alkalosis.

- Acetazolamide: Diamox (250 1,000 mg/day divided doses), a carbonic anhydrase inhibitor, blocks bicarbonate resorption in the proximal tubule and may be useful when extracellular volume is high. Unfortunately, Diamox may also cause additional K^+ and volume depletion, which, as mentioned above, can perpetuate an alkalosis.
- H_2 blockers: Can be used to prevent H^+ loss with loss of gastric juice and may have a particular role in normovolemic chronic renal failure patients. It is important to first check the gastric secretions to identify the presence of acid. The treatment goal is to keep the pH greater than 5. Because of concerns about gastric superinfection, aspiration, and translocation of bacteria through the gut, the use of H_2 blockers in the ICU should be avoided.

Dialysis

A final option for a severe metabolic alkalosis in patients with renal failure is hemodialysis with a high chloride, low acetate bath. If the patient has a normal or high volume status, another alternative is to use CVVH with simultaneous IV chloride replacement using 0.9% NaCl.

BIBLIOGRAPHY

Broughton JO, Kennedy TC. Interpretation of arterial blood gases by computer. Chest 1984; 85:148–149.

Cooper DJ, Walley KR, Wiggs BR, Russell JA. Bicarbonate does not improve hemodynamics in critically ill patients who have lactic acidosis. Ann Intern Med 1990;112:492–498.

Hindman BJ. Sodium bicarbonate in the treatment of subtypes of acute lactic acidosis: physiologic considerations. Anesthesiology 1990;72:1064–1076.

Hingston DM. A computerized interpretation of arterial pH and the blood gas data: do physicians need it? Respir Care 1982;27:809–815.

Iberti TJ, Leibowitz AB, Papadakos PJ, Fischer EP. Low sensitivity of the anion gap as a screen to detect hyperlactatemia in critically ill patients. Crit Care Med 1990;18:275–277.

Kokko JP, Tannen RL, eds. Fluids and electrolytes. Philadelphia, PA: WB Saunders Company, 1990:27–53.

Kruse JA, Carlson RW. Lactate metabolism. Crit Care Clin 1987;5(4):725–726.

Kucera RR, Shapiro JI, Whalen MA, et al. Brain pH effects of $NaHCO_3$ and Carbicarb in lactic acidosis. Crit Care Med 1989;17:1320–1323.

Marino PL. The ICU Book. Philadelphia, PA: Lea & Febiger, 1991.

McLaughlin ML, Kassirer JP. Rational treatment of acid-base disorders. Drugs 1990;39: 841–855.

Okuda Y, Adrogue HJ, Field JB, Nohara H, Yamashita K. Counterproductive effects of sodium bicarbonate in diabetic ketoacidosis. J Clin Endocrinol Metab 1996;81:314–320.

Quintanilla A, Singer I. Metabolic alkalosis in the patient with uremia. Am J Kidney Dis 1991;XVII(5):591–595.

Riley LJ, Ilson BE, Narins RG. Acute metabolic acid-base disorders. Crit Care Clin 1987;5: 699–746.

Schreck DM, Zacharias D, Grunau CFV. Diagnosis of complex acid-base disorders: physician performance vs. the microcomputer. Ann Emerg Med 1986;15:164–170.

Smith SM, Eng RHK, Buccini F. Use of D-lactic acid measurements in the diagnosis of bacterial infections. J Infect Dis 1986;154(4):658–664.

Stacpoole PW, Lorenz AC, Thomas RG, Harman EM. Dichloroacetate in the treatment of lactic acidosis. Ann Intern Med 1988;108:58–63.

Stacpoole PW, Wright EC, Baumgartner TG, et al. A controlled clinical trial of dichloroacetate for treatment of lactic acidosis in adults. N Engl J Med 1992;327:1564–1569.

Vincent J-L. Lactate levels in critically ill patients. Acta Anaesthesiol Scand Suppl 1995; 107:261–266.

Winter SD, Pearson JR, Gabow PA, et al. The fall of the serum anion gap. Arch Intern Med 1990;150:311.

11 Acute Lung Injury and Acute Respiratory Distress Syndrome

Borna Mehrad, John G. Weg

The acute respiratory distress syndrome (ARDS) was first recognized as "traumatic wet lung" in soldiers during World War II. Its recent prominence can be traced to an article published in the *Lancet* in 1967, which described a group of 12 patients with the syndrome. Later publications on the subject have referred to this entity as the adult (rather than acute) respiratory distress syndrome to distinguish it from the respiratory distress syndrome of the newborn. The syndrome has repeatedly been observed in children, however, and the current recommendation is a return to the original term, acute respiratory distress syndrome.

DEFINITION

ARDS has been difficult to define because of its many predisposing factors and various clinical manifestations. It is further complicated by the fact that ARDS is often one manifestation of a systemic process, affecting a number of other organ systems. Indeed, ARDS may be a window to many cases of multiple organ dysfunction syndrome (MODS). Prospective studies of patients at risk for developing ARDS have shown a continuum of clinically evident lung injury, making any cutoff point for its definition arbitrary. Many of the affected patients have been found to have less severe versions of the syndrome, and only some progress to full-blown ARDS.

Past attempts at defining ARDS have included the criteria of intrapulmonary shunting, diffuse radiographic infiltrates, reduced pulmonary compliance, and "normal" pulmonary artery wedge pressure in various combinations and scoring systems.

In 1994, an American–European consensus conference developed a standard definition for ARDS:

- The term "acute lung injury" (ALI) was used to describe the continuum of the pathologic process;
- The term "acute respiratory distress syndrome" was reserved for the most severe end of this spectrum.

ALI was defined as "a syndrome of inflammation and increased permeability that is associated with a constellation of clinical, radiologic, and physiologic abnormalities that cannot be explained by, but may coexist with, left atrial hypertension." This is manifest by a combination of impaired gas exchange and accumulation of

497

Table 11.1. Definition of Acute Lung Injury and ARDS

	Oxygenation	Chest Radiograph	PAWP
ALI	$PaO_2/FiO_2 < 300$ regardless of PEEP	Bilateral infiltrates on frontal radiograph	< 18 cm or no clinical evidence of left atrial hypertension
ARDS	$PaO_2/FiO_2 < 200$ regardless of PEEP	Bilateral infiltrates on frontal radiograph	< 18 cm or no clinical evidence of left atrial hypertension

From Bernard BR, et al and the Consensus Committee. Am J Respir Crit Care Med 1994;149:818–824. Reprinted with permission.

solute in airspaces. As shown in Table 11.1, the degree of impairment of gas exchange was quantified as a ratio of the partial pressure of arterial oxygen to the fraction of inspired oxygen (PaO_2/FiO_2), regardless the amount of positive end-expiratory pressure (PEEP) used. Both ALI and ARDS were defined as acute in onset and persistent, lasting days to weeks.

EPIDEMIOLOGY
Incidence
The 1972 report of the National Heart and Lung Institute Task Force On Respiratory Diseases estimated the incidence of ARDS at 150,000 cases per year (or 70 per 100,000) in the United States. This value has been questioned in several subsequent studies, including a recent report that estimated the incidence at 4.8–8.3 cases per 100, 000 in Utah. Other studies performed in many different populations have yielded similar results. This discrepancy may in part relate to the different definitions of ARDS used in the various studies, to incorrect estimation in some reports, or may reflect an actual change in the true incidence of the syndrome over time. In addition, subsets of certain populations may be at unusually high risk for developing ARDS, thus skewing the incidence rate for that population. For example, a study done in San Francisco in the 1980s reported *Pneumocystis carinii* pneumonia as the cause of ARDS in 20% of their patients.

Mortality
The mortality rate from ARDS has been variously reported as 30 to 60%, with a rate of 40% quoted in most recent studies. Although some of this variation relates to dissimilarities in studied populations and to the lack of a uniform definition of ARDS, this downward trend likely reflects improvement in various aspects of supportive care. A recent study from the University of Washington reported a reduction in ARDS mortality from 60 to 36% over the 10-year period of 1983 to 1993. This reduction in mortality was attributable to improved survival in patients with sepsis syndrome who were less than 60 years of age. The multicenter evaluation of synthetic surfactant in ARDS found a mortality rate of 40% in 725 patients studied

in 1992–1993. Development of ARDS has been shown to be a predictor of mortality in ICU patients with Gram-negative sepsis, multiple transfusions, and trauma.

Among patients who have developed ARDS, retrospective analyses have identified several parameters that predict higher mortality; these include:

- Age greater than 60;
- Relative paucity of immature neutrophils on the peripheral smear;
- Acidemia despite mechanical ventilation;
- Low serum bicarbonate level;
- Need for multiple blood transfusions.

Many parameters are notable for their inability to predict mortality in patients with ARDS: lung injury scoring systems; physiologic parameters such as PaO_2, FiO_2, and PEEP; smoking; gender; and chronic diseases.

ARDS patients who do not have dysfunction of other organ systems have a relatively low mortality rate. Patients who develop ARDS as a result of aspiration of gastric contents, opiate overdose, and fat embolism have a better prognosis; ARDS caused by sepsis, bone marrow transplantation, and opportunistic pneumonia yields the poorest outcome. Similarly, trauma patients with ARDS have a lower mortality rate compared with "medical" patients, who are more prone to multiple organ dysfunction. In addition, patients with ARDS who develop complications of secondary sepsis syndrome or multiorgan failure (particularly liver failure) have a higher mortality rate.

In one study of causes of death in ARDS, the majority of deaths within the first three days of diagnosis were caused by the underlying disease or injury; after the first three days, most deaths were attributable to sepsis, cardiac dysfunction, or irreversible respiratory failure. Patients who died of central nervous system damage sustained during the precipitating event, however, often died after the third day. Sepsis syndrome has been reported as the leading cause of death after the first three days. Death from respiratory failure alone is relatively uncommon, accounting for 16% of deaths in large series.

PREDISPOSITION

ARDS has been associated with numerous heterogeneous conditions (Table 11.2). In studies that addressed the incidence of ARDS after specific insults, sepsis syndrome and aspiration of gastric contents were found to lead to ARDS in approximately one-third of instances. Multiple transfusions and chest trauma with pulmonary contusion resulted in ARDS in 20–25% of patients. Moreover, the presence of more than one risk factor has an additive effect on the risk of ALI. In one study, the incidence of ARDS was 25% in patients with one predisposing factor, 42% with two predisposing factors, and 85% if three coexisted.

Both systemic and pulmonary infections can precipitate ALI. The incidence of pneumococcal pneumonia is highest in the elderly, but younger patients are more likely to develop ARDS as a consequence of it. *Pneumocystis carinii,* primary influ-

Table 11.2. Conditions Leading to ARDS

Predisposing Factors	Incidence of ARDS (%)
Direct lung insults	
Aspiration of gastric contents	30–36
Pneumonia	12
Inhalation lung injury (smoke, crack cocaine)	
Near drowning	
High-altitude pulmonary edema	
Pulmonary contusion	
Reexpansion lung injury	
Radiation	
Systemic insults	
Sepsis syndrome	25–43 (ALI in 60%)
Shock	
Nonthoracic trauma	17–40
Burns	
Pancreatitis	2
Uremia	
Diabetic ketoacidosis	
Acute neurologic insult (e.g. SAH, head trauma)	
Disseminated intravascular coagulation	22
Multiple transfusions	5–40
Cardiopulmonary bypass	
Systemic drug toxicity (see Table 11.3)	
Oxygen toxicity	
Thromboembolism	
Fat embolism	
Air embolism	
Complications of pregnancy	
Carcinomatosis	

Table 11.3. Partial List of Drugs That Can Cause ARDS

Opiate analgesics	Cytosine arabinoside
Naloxone	Vinca alkaloids
Methadone	Mitomycin
Heroin	Salicylates
Thiazide diuretics	Tricyclic antidepressants
Hydrochlorothiazide	Miscellaneous
Immunomodulators	Protamine
Interleukin-2	Ethchlorvynol
Cyclosporin	Propoxyphene
Antineoplastic agents	Paraldehyde
Bleomycin	Colchicine
Methotrexate	

enza pneumonia, and, more recently, pulmonary Hantavirus are well-documented examples of nonbacterial causes of pneumonia that may progress to ARDS.

Although chronic conditions have not been shown to predispose patients to ARDS after a systemic insult, a recent study found that patients with a history of heavy alcohol consumption were more likely to develop ARDS and had a higher in-hospital mortality.

Relationship of ARDS with Sepsis and MODS

Sepsis syndrome is both the most common predisposing event and an important cause of death in ARDS. Gram-negative bacteria are the most common cause of sepsis syndrome. In a study of patients with bacterial sepsis and ALI, mortality was higher if the source of the sepsis was a pneumonia or if the source could not be found.

In patients with ARDS, the incidence of renal failure is 40–55%, liver failure 12–95%, and cardiac failure 10–23%. These observations have led to the increasing recognition that ARDS may be the pulmonary manifestation of MODS. The commonest cause of MODS is systemic inflammatory response syndrome (SIRS), defined as two or more of the following: fever or hypothermia, tachypnea, tachycardia, leukocytosis or leukopenia, or greater than 10% bandemia. Although SIRS can have a noninfectious cause, sepsis is defined as SIRS with a proven or suspected microbial etiology.

It has been suggested that local or systemic insults evoke regulatory antiinflammatory as well as proinflammatory responses. Both pathways have beneficial effects initially but have deleterious consequences if the response is excessive or the balance between them lost. SIRS is the consequence of an unregulated proinflammatory response. An unbalanced antiinflammatory response leads to immunosuppression—a state referred to as compensatory antiinflammatory response syndrome (CARS). A final stage, termed "immunologic dissonance," is believed to represent continued excess of either proinflammatory or antiinflammatory mediators, or both. Although unproven, this model provides an explanation for the failure of recent studies aiming to inhibit various proinflammatory mediators. It also serves to focus on the possibility that inhibition of certain mediators, whether proinflammatory or antiinflammatory, may negatively impact survival.

HISTOPATHOLOGIC FEATURES

The morphologic changes of ARDS have been labeled diffuse alveolar damage (DAD). During the entire course of ARDS, proteinaceous fluid is found within the alveoli and there is an increased number of macrophages and neutrophils.

Histopathologic changes in ARDS have been divided into three phases:

- The acute phase (the first week);
- The subacute phase (days 4 to 10);
- The chronic phase (beyond the 8th day).

The acute, or exudative, phase is characterized by increased permeability of the alveolar-capillary membrane. The earliest changes are capillary congestion and interstitial and alveolar edema. The alveoli contain leukocytes, red cells, and cellular debris. There is extensive necrosis of the alveolar epithelium with denudation of the basement membrane. The hallmark of this phase, the eosinophilic hyaline membrane, is associated with damage to type I pneumocytes and is most prominent in the alveolar ducts. It is composed of fibrin and cellular debris.

In the subacute, or proliferative, phase, there is less edema and vascular congestion. Type II pneumocytes proliferate along the previously denuded epithelium. Hyaline membranes are seldom found after the 10th day of ARDS. Fibroblasts proliferate and migrate into the alveolar exudate, and there is evidence of early fibrosis. Connective tissue forms in the airspaces, interstitium, respiratory bronchioles, and walls of intra-acinar microvessels.

Fibrosing Alveolitis

The late phase of ARDS, if resolution does not occur, is the result of ongoing fibroproliferation, leading to extensive remodeling of lung parenchyma. It is characterized by prominent fibrosis, which may cause obliteration of alveolar spaces. Areas of microcystic airspaces alternate with areas of scarring. Intra-alveolar fibrosis predominates over interstitial fibrosis, and there is marked widening of the alveolar septa by dense, hypocellular, and eosinophilic collagenous connective tissue.

In autopsy studies of ARDS patients, type III collagen, which is newly formed and more susceptible to enzyme digestion, predominates in the early proliferative phase. The wider and less digestible fibers of type I collagen predominate in the fibrotic phase.

Vascular Pathology

In the acute phase there is evidence of capillary engorgement and microvascular thromboemboli. These changes persist into the intermediate stage, when fibrocellular proliferation of small arteries and veins develops. In the late stage, vascular remodeling results in distortion of blood vessels and reduced numbers and dilatation of capillaries. All of these changes are thought to contribute to the pulmonary hypertension of ARDS.

PATHOPHYSIOLOGY

The basic pathophysiologic processes of ARDS are:

- An increase in alveolar-capillary barrier permeability;
- A decrease in lung compliance;
- Intrapulmonary shunt and ventilation/perfusion mismatch;
- Increased pulmonary vascular resistance.

These findings are often superimposed on the effects of other concomitant processes, such as sepsis or underlying cardiac disease. It is, nonetheless, useful to consider the physiologic aberrations of patients with "pure" ARDS.

Microvascular Permeability

The normal alveolar-capillary membrane is relatively impermeable to intravascular macromolecules, and the hydrostatic force promoting efflux of liquid into lung parenchyma is balanced by the osmotic force exerted by the high concentration of intravascular macromolecules. This balance is disrupted when the inflammatory process damages the endothelial membrane and renders it permeable to macromolecules. As a result, movement of fluid into the lung parenchyma becomes a function of microvascular pressure. The resultant pulmonary edema causes reduced lung compliance—thus increasing the work of breathing in unventilated patients—and leads to a decrease in ventilation/perfusion ratio and intrapulmonary shunting.

Oxygen Delivery

One of the cardinal clinical features of ARDS is hypoxemia refractory to high concentrations of inspired oxygen. The mechanism of the hypoxemia is absent or inadequate ventilation of alveolar units that continue to receive perfusion. The reason for the compromised ventilation is partial or complete alveolar filling with edema fluid, inflammatory exudate, or scar tissue. Studies using the multiple inert gas elimination technique (MIGET) have demonstrated that 18 to 68% of cardiac output in ARDS perfuses unventilated lung and is, therefore, effectively shunted from the right to left heart. Approximately half of the studied patients had low ventilation to perfusion ratios, accounting for the small improvement in oxygenation often seen with increasing FiO_2. Close agreement between the measured and calculated arterial pO_2 in these studies argues against a significant diffusion barrier between the alveoli and capillaries as a cause of hypoxemia in ARDS. Approximately half of the cardiac output in ARDS perfused areas with a normal or high ventilation to perfusion ratio. These areas of "dead space" ventilation necessitate a higher minute ventilation to maintain a given pCO_2. In unventilated patients, this adds to increased oxygen consumption by the respiratory muscles without contributing to arterial oxygenation.

In normal individuals, an increase in oxygen consumption ($\dot{V}O_2$) results in an increase in cardiac output (CO), an increase in oxygen extraction as measured by the difference between arterial and mixed-venous oxygen content ($C_{a-\bar{v}}O_2$), and an increase in ventilation. According to the Fick equation:

$$CO = \dot{V}O_2/C_{a-\bar{v}}O_2 \quad \text{or}$$

$$\dot{V}O_2 = (CO)\,(C_{a-\bar{v}}O_2)$$

Normal individuals display physiologic dependence of oxygen consumption ($\dot{V}O_2$) on oxygen delivery ($\dot{D}O_2$) only in states of very low oxygen delivery. Oxygen delivery is calculated as follows:

$$\dot{D}O_2 = CO \cdot (CaO_2 + 0.003 \ PaO_2)$$

$$= CO \cdot [1.34 \ (SaO_2 \cdot Hb\%) + 0.003 \ PaO_2]$$

where CaO_2 is arterial oxygen content, $0.003 \ PaO_2$ is fraction of oxygen dissolved in plasma, SaO_2 is arterial oxygen saturation, and Hb% is concentration of hemoglobin in g/dL.

Pathologic dependence of oxygen consumption on oxygen delivery is defined as a state where oxygen consumption varies directly with oxygen delivery, with resulting compromise in tissue oxygenation. A pathologic dependence of $\dot{V}O_2$ on $\dot{D}O_2$ has been described, although not uniformly, in ARDS, sepsis, and other critical illnesses. When this occurs, mixed venous oxygen saturation becomes an unreliable index of tissue oxygen requirement.

Pulmonary Hypertension and Cardiac Function

Pulmonary artery pressures are generally mildly elevated in the first days after the onset of ARDS but often increase to high levels in the ensuing days. This pulmonary hypertension is caused by a combination of hypoxic pulmonary vasoconstriction, collapse of pulmonary microvasculature as a result of PEEP, and in situ thrombosis of pulmonary microvasculature. The presence of these thrombi on pulmonary angiography has been shown to correlate with pulmonary hypertension.

These changes contribute to an increase in right ventricular afterload, causing a compensatory increase in right ventricular end-diastolic volume to maintain right ventricular output (Frank-Starling's law). As right ventricular afterload increases, a point is reached at which the right ventricular output falls, thus failing to provide adequate left ventricular filling. Failure of the right ventricle may be related to myocardial ischemia caused by increasing wall stress.

Reduced right-sided cardiac output causes a reduction in left ventricular cardiac output. In addition, right ventricular enlargement may result in the shifting of the interventricular septum to the left, resulting in reduced left ventricular compliance and therefore reduced left ventricular diastolic filling, further compromising left ventricular cardiac output. In compensation, heart rate and peripheral vascular resistance increase to maintain systemic blood pressure. In the absence of coexisting disease or PEEP, however, left ventricular contractility is normal in most patients with ALI.

CELLULAR PATHOPHYSIOLOGY

Figure 11.1 denotes a simplified flow diagram of the pathophysiology of ARDS at a cellular level.

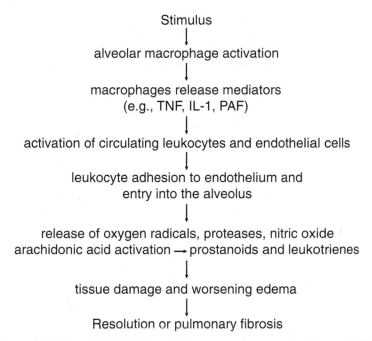

Stimulus

alveolar macrophage activation

macrophages release mediators
(e.g., TNF, IL-1, PAF)

activation of circulating leukocytes and endothelial cells

leukocyte adhesion to endothelium and
entry into the alveolus

release of oxygen radicals, proteases, nitric oxide
arachidonic acid activation → prostanoids and leukotrienes

tissue damage and worsening edema

Resolution or pulmonary fibrosis

Figure 11.1. Simplified depiction of the pathogenic process leading to ARDS.

Cytokines

Interleukin-1 (IL-1) and tumor necrosis factor-alpha (TNF-α) are two of the primary products secreted by macrophages in response to stimuli such as endotoxin. Although structurally different, these so-called ''early response'' cytokines have very similar activity at a cellular level. Their activity is concentration-dependent in that, at low concentrations, they produce only local inflammation; at higher concentrations they produce systemic effects typical of SIRS and MODS.

In ARDS, IL-1 and TNF-α activate the capillary endothelial cells to express specific adherence molecules (intercellular adhesion molecule-1 or ICAM-1, and members of the selectin family) on their surface, thus recruiting circulating neutrophils and monocytes to the site of injury. IL-1 and TNF-α may also play a role in priming the recruited neutrophils, preparing them for a burst of metabolic activity.

Another group of cytokines, the CXC superfamily, plays a central role in inducing adhering neutrophils to migrate into the alveolus. Members of this group of cytokines, such as IL-8, are relatively resistant to enzymatic degradation and to changes in pH, thus exerting a sustained effect at the site of inflammation. Neutrophils express the adhesion molecule β-2 integrin under the influence of IL-8, which, through interaction with ICAM-1, initiates neutrophil migration into the alveolus.

Although not a cytokine, platelet-activating factor (PAF) is also an early inflammatory mediator in ARDS. It is a phospholipid metabolite released by many cells, including neutrophils, platelets, and endothelial cells. It augments superoxide production by neutrophils, enhances platelet aggregation, and induces synthesis of eicosanoids. It also increases endothelial permeability, thus contributing to tissue edema.

Eicosanoids

Arachidonic acid, the precursor of the eicosanoids, is readily available in the cell membrane. In the setting of inflammation, it is metabolized by the enzyme cyclooxygenase into many products, including thromboxane A_2 (TX-A_2), which is released by macrophages and platelets. These cyclooxygenase products are increased in both animal models and human studies of ARDS. TX-A_2 is a potent vasoconstrictor and also contributes to aggregation of platelets and neutrophils. Prostacyclin, another cyclooxygenase product elaborated by endothelial cells, acts as a vasodilator and platelet deaggregator, attenuating the effects of TX-A_2. The opposing vascular effects of these products are thought to play a role in hypoxic pulmonary vasoconstriction and systemic vasodilatation seen in ARDS.

Arachidonic acid is also metabolized by another enzyme, 5-lipoxygenase, producing the leukotriene family of eicosanoids. Some members of this family, including leukotrienes D_4 and E_4, have been implicated in reactive airways disease. Although these products have been detected in large amounts in animal models of ALI, their precise role in this setting has not been elucidated.

Nitric Oxide

Nitric oxide is synthesized by many types of cells, including endothelial cells, macrophages, platelets, and smooth muscle cells. Its homeostatic role occurs at relatively low concentrations and involves dynamic regulation of blood flow and modulation of airway tone, acting as a bronchodilator in the lungs and as a vasodilator in both the pulmonary and systemic vascular beds. In higher concentrations, such as in the setting of inflammation, it has cytopathic properties, including inactivation of enzymes involved with cellular respiration and reacting with molecular oxygen to produce reactive oxygen species.

Synthesis of nitric oxide in the presence of inflammation is induced by the "early response" cytokines such as TNF and IL-1. The cytopathic properties of nitric oxide may contribute to host defense in infections. These properties augment the damaging effects of inflammation on host cells, however.

Reactive Oxygen Species

Once activated, inflammatory cells such as neutrophils and macrophages release oxygen radicals, such as superoxide and hydrogen peroxide. These are chemically unstable molecules with unpaired electrons, which have strong oxidative properties. They cause oxidative damage to cell membrane phospholipids and induce protein oxidation and DNA hydroxylation. Products of lipid oxidation have been found in bronchoalveolar lavage (BAL) in patients with ARDS. The deleterious effects of these molecules are prevented by endogenous antioxidants, such as glutathione, superoxide dismutase, catalase, and vitamin E. These molecules preferentially react with oxygen radicals, preventing oxidative damage to neighboring molecules. ARDS is an example of a setting in which these antioxidant defenses are overwhelmed by an excess of oxygen radicals.

In addition to the mediators already mentioned, inflammatory cells release a number of proteolytic enzymes, resulting in the activation of kinins, the complement cascade, and coagulation and fibrinolytic pathways, causing further amplification of the inflammatory process and tissue damage.

CLINICAL FEATURES
Presentation

Although symptoms may develop immediately after certain insults, such as aspiration of gastric contents, there is frequently a delay of hours:

- Patients develop worsening respiratory distress, initially manifested as increasing tachypnea;
- There is usually little or no sputum production, and there is a paucity of specific physical findings.

Natural History

A pattern of clinical evolution has been described in ARDS. The initial presentation is characterized by dyspnea, tachypnea, widening of alveolar-arterial oxygen gradient, and respiratory alkalosis. As the syndrome progresses, hypoxia becomes less responsive to supplemental oxygen, and decreased lung compliance becomes evident as extravascular fluid accumulates. Subsequently, a hyperdynamic state develops, with increased cardiac output, reduced systemic vascular resistance, and arterial hypoxemia.

Patients who survive this period usually have a gradual improvement in oxygenation and return of lung compliance to near-normal levels over several weeks, eventually returning to near-normal lung function over several months. A considerably smaller group develops increasing pulmonary fibrosis with progressive respiratory failure reminiscent of idiopathic pulmonary fibrosis. This group cannot be weaned from mechanical ventilation and eventually succumb.

Conventional Diagnostic Studies
Chest Radiography

The chest radiograph may show only minimal changes for several hours following the acute insult, despite clinical evidence of increasing respiratory distress and hypoxemia:

- Lung volumes may be decreased, indicating diffuse microatelectasis.
- Early evidence of increased pulmonary interstitial fluid may include peribronchial haziness.
- In instances in which ARDS is incited by direct lung insult, there may be radiologic evidence of the primary insult (e. g., evidence of airspace disease after aspiration).
- Infiltrates progress over the ensuing 24 hours as diffuse lung injury leads to increased-permeability pulmonary edema. These infiltrates have been characterized as a dense, patchy alveolar consolidation. The involvement is bilateral and usually symmetrical.
- Pleural effusions have been demonstrated in both clinical and animal models of ARDS.
- Subsequently, interstitial and ground glass patterns may develop.
- Extra-alveolar collections of air, known as interstitial emphysema, may be visible as parenchymal stippling in areas of prior consolidation.
- Discrete cysts resembling pneumatoceles may develop and sometimes enlarge markedly.
- The addition of PEEP to mechanical ventilation may produce an improved radiologic appearance.

Differentiation of ALI and cardiogenic pulmonary edema on the basis of radiographic features is a common clinical problem and has been addressed in many studies. Some studies have found that dense perihilar and gravitationally dependent infiltrates, redistribution of blood flow to the upper lobes, and wider vascular pedicles indicate cardiogenic pulmonary edema. Several studies, however, have failed to make this determination based on readings of single radiographs. Given the variations in radiographic technique, position of the patient, and various methods of ventilatory support, the chest radiograph has little utility in making the distinction between cardiogenic pulmonary edema and ARDS.

Hemodynamic Monitoring

Peripheral artery catheterization is commonly performed in patients with ARDS to simplify repeated arterial blood gas analysis, as well as for continuous monitoring of systemic blood pressure. The pulmonary artery balloon catheter has become an integral part of the care of patients with ARDS. Monitoring of the pulmonary artery occlusion (or "wedge") pressure (PAWP) is indicated in the majority of patients with ALI.

The PAWP provides information about left ventricular preload by measuring the left atrial end-diastolic filling pressure—if the compliance of the chambers remains stable, the LVEDP is proportional to the left ventricular end-diastolic volume, or preload. The PAWP also reflects the pulmonary capillary hydrostatic pressure, which is the principal force driving fluid into the extravascular space. Pulmonary artery systolic and diastolic pressures and the calculated pulmonary vascular resistance provide information about right ventricular afterload. Oximetric PA catheters can be used to determine mixed venous oxygen saturation, which can be used as an index of oxygen delivery in some patients. A decrease in mixed venous saturation reflects greater tissue oxygen extraction, suggesting reduced cardiac output. The utility of this in patients with sepsis or ALI is extremely limited, however, because changes in cardiac output may result in a reduction of oxygen consumption.

In patients with acute diffuse pulmonary infiltrates, PAWP helps to differentiate ARDS from cardiogenic pulmonary edema, thus dictating the course of therapy—PAWP of 18 cm or less is part of the consensus definition of ALI and ARDS. In addition, in patients with ALI, intravascular volume expansion leads to elevated pulmonary microvascular pressures, exacerbating leakage of fluid into the extravascular space.

Several pitfalls complicate the use of pulmonary artery catheters in the setting of ARDS. A common error is to interpret the PAWP without consideration of surrounding alveolar pressure. The PAWP approximates the left ventricular end-diastolic pressure when the alveolar pressure is at or near atmospheric. The most consistent values can be obtained when it is measured at the end expiration. With PEEP, the end-expiratory alveolar pressure may be greater than atmospheric pressure. The degree to which PEEP increases end-expiratory alveolar pressure is variable and depends on lung compliance. This effect of PEEP is small in the stiff lungs of ARDS. Interrupting mechanical ventilation or PEEP for measurement of PAWP is not recommended.

Another potential difficulty in the interpretation of the PAWP is related to catheter position: accurate PAWP can only be measured in zone 3 conditions (pulmonary arterial > pulmonary venous > alveolar pressure), in which the pulmonary venous pressure is greater than alveolar pressure and the pulmonary venules remain patent throughout the respiratory cycle. Balloon-tipped catheters will usually lodge in a zone 3 area initially because these areas have the highest blood flow, but changes in alveolar or venous pulmonary pressure may change a given area from zone 3 to zone 1 (alveolar pressure > pulmonary arterial > pulmonary venous pressures) or zone 2 (pulmonary arterial > alveolar > pulmonary venous pressures). This can be suspected if the PAWP varies greatly with respiration or is greater than pulmonary artery diastolic pressure.

Lastly, left ventricular end-diastolic pressure is proportional to end-diastolic volume (preload) only if chamber compliance remains constant. As such, unexplained change in PAWP should prompt consideration of causes of change in left ventricular compliance, such as myocardial ischemia.

Such considerations have led critics to voice concern over whether the use of pulmonary artery catheters improves survival in critically ill patients enough to offset morbidity of potential complications of its insertion. A recent large, multicenter prospective cohort study of ICU patients, many of whom met the definition of ALI, correlated the outcomes of patients to the use of pulmonary artery catheters on the first ICU day. Using case-matching and multivariate regression models, including a "propensity score" of the likelihood of PA catheter insertion, this study found a small but significant increase in mortality, as well as increased cost, associated with the use of the catheter. Randomized studies are needed, however, before these results are applied to patient care.

Experimental Diagnostic Studies

Bronchoalveolar Lavage

The findings of BAL fluid in ARDS are characteristic of acute inflammation and are nonspecific. Neutrophils increase up to 80% of all cells, in contrast to the normal 2 to 3%. Various studies have shown elevated levels of peroxides, elastase, proteolytic enzymes, complement fragments, and inflammatory mediators (such as TNF-α, IL-1, and eicosanoids) in BAL fluid in patients with ARDS.

These findings have helped elucidate the pathophysiologic processes at the alveolar level but do not have diagnostic or prognostic value. A recent study, however, found low concentrations of antiinflammatory cytokines interleukin-10 and interleukin-1 receptor antagonist to be associated with poor prognosis. Another study found that an elevated concentration of type III procollagen predicted mortality in patients with established ARDS. Type III procollagen is an index of pulmonary fibrosis, and it is surmised that elevated levels identify patients at risk for progression to fibrosing alveolitis and persistent respiratory failure.

Membrane Barrier Function and Extravascular Lung Water

Although not routinely performed, the integrity of the pulmonary alveolar-capillary membrane can be indirectly measured by evaluating the composition of pulmonary edema fluid. A pulmonary edema to plasma protein ratio of 0.75 or greater has been shown to reliably distinguish ARDS from cardiogenic pulmonary edema if the fluid is collected within the first half hour of its development and is therefore unaffected by alveolar fluid clearance. More direct measures of the integrity of the alveolar-capillary membrane have included measurement of accumulation of radiolabeled macromolecules in the lung.

Given that presence of pulmonary edema is integral to all definitions of ARDS, several methods of measuring extravascular lung water (EVLW) have been developed. These include indicator dilution, CT and MRI, impedance plethysmography, and radioisotope techniques. Although used in experimental settings, the quantity of EVLW has not been found to have clinical implications beyond lung compliance measurements derived from ventilator parameters.

Computed Tomography

CT, especially thin-section studies, has been used to characterize the parenchymal abnormalities of ARDS. Early CT studies reported a nonuniform pattern of interstitial and alveolar disease, with predominant involvement of dependent areas. More recent studies, however, have shown that increasing levels of PEEP produce a more homogenous distribution. At a PEEP of 20 cm H_2O, the distribution of ventilation is almost uniform in ventral and dorsal areas of lung. CT scans of the late, fibroproliferative

ARDS show a ground glass appearance with occasional reticular or reticulonodular infiltrates, without evidence of gravitational distribution.

THERAPY
Conventional Mechanical Ventilation

Mechanical ventilation is the cornerstone of management of patients with ARDS. Its goal is to provide adequate ventilation (CO_2 removal) and oxygenation. Conventional mechanical ventilation employs tidal volumes of 10–15 mL/kg and a respiratory rate sufficient to maintain normocapnia. Although there has been a recent interest in using lower tidal volumes (7–10 mL/kg), surveys have shown that the majority of patients with ARDS are treated with higher volumes.

PEEP is employed to improve oxygenation and to reduce the theoretical risk of oxygen toxicity. PEEP improves oxygenation by recruiting closed alveoli and forcing alveolar liquid into the pulmonary interstitium. Keeping the alveoli open results in an increase in the functional residual capacity, contributes to improvement in lung compliance, reduces the potential for sheer stress, and allows more homogenous ventilation from the dorsal to ventral portions of the lung.

The major disadvantage of using PEEP is reduction in cardiac output, which may occur because of increased intra-alveolar pressure, leading to collapse of intrapulmonary microvasculature and increased pulmonary vascular resistance. If severe enough, the resultant pulmonary hypertension can force the interventricular septum to bulge to the left, thereby reducing left ventricular end-diastolic dimensions, reducing the left ventricular output. In addition, PEEP may decrease venous return by compression of the inferior vena cava.

These considerations have lead investigators to advocate a level of PEEP that maximizes various physiologic parameters. For example, "best PEEP" is defined as the PEEP at which lung compliance is maximized; "optimal PEEP" as the PEEP at which the shunt fraction is minimized; "preferred PEEP" allows maximal tissue oxygen delivery; and "least PEEP" is the minimum necessary PEEP to reduce FiO_2 to 50% while maintaining a PaO_2 greater than 59 mm Hg. In our intensive care unit, hemodynamic parameters (PAWP, cardiac output, arterial blood gas, and static lung compliance) are measured at baseline and with increasing increments of 2 to 3 cm of PEEP. The goal is to achieve the best oxygen delivery at the lowest PAWP and FiO_2 ("preferred PEEP"). There is currently insufficient data to recommend supranormal oxygen delivery.

Experimental Strategies in Mechanical Ventilation
Permissive Hypercapnia

Permissive hypercapnia aims to prevent alveolar overdistension by reducing pulmonary inflation pressures to less than 35 cm H_2O. This is achieved by using a tidal volume of 5 to 9 mL/kg, resulting in a lower minute ventilation. This frequently causes a respiratory acidosis, with a $PaCO_2$ as high as 100 mm Hg and pH as low as 7.20. Many animal studies as well as some uncontrolled clinical trials have shown a survival advantage with permissive hypercapnia when compared with conventional mechanical ventilation, but its definitive role awaits evaluation in randomized controlled trials. Potential complications of acute respiratory acidosis, such as decrease in myocardial contractility, increased sympathetic tone, cerebral edema, pulmonary vasoconstriction, and hyperkalemia, may limit the use of permissive hypercapnia, especially in specific patient populations (e.g., in patients with intracranial hypertension).

Patient Positioning

Small studies have shown improved oxygenation in ARDS with lateral decubitus or prone positioning. The mechanism of this is thought to be a combination of improved perfusion of ventilated areas, postural drainage of secretions, and possibly improved diaphragmatic function.

Inverse Ratio Ventilation

In conventional mechanical ventilation, as in spontaneous breathing, inspiration occurs in the first one-third of the breathing cycle and expiration in the last two-thirds (I:E ratio of 1:2). "Inverse ratio" ventilation (IVR) refers to ventilation with a relatively prolonged inspiratory phase (I:E ratio greater than 1:1). A longer inspiratory phase produces a higher mean airway pressure while allowing lower peak pressures. In addition, sustained inspiratory pressure has been postulated to ventilate otherwise atelectatic alveoli, thus improving gas exchange. Although it can be used in pressure- or volume-cycled ventilatory modes, most studies have used IVR in conjunction with pressure-controlled ventilation. IVR produces a variable and generally unknown amount of PEEP. Sedation and neuromuscular blockade are usually required to ventilate patients effectively in this mode; they carry the risk of prolonged ventilator dependence. There are no randomized controlled studies comparing IVR with conventional ventilation.

High Frequency Ventilation

High frequency ventilation provides alveolar ventilation without large volume changes and with lower intratracheal pressures. This is achieved in one of three ways: high frequency positive pressure ventilation uses tidal volumes of 3 to 4 mL/kg and respiratory rates of 60 to 100 breaths/min with passive exhalation; high frequency oscillation uses tidal volumes of 1 to 3 mL/kg and respiratory rates of 60 to 3600 breaths/min, but both inhalation and exhalation are active. High frequency jet ventilation uses a pulsating jet of gas (1–5 mL/kg) emitted from a small-bore cannula placed in the trachea at rates of 180 to 600 breaths/min. High frequency jet ventilation has not been shown to confer any advantage over conventional mechanical ventilation in four clinical trials and was associated with a higher incidence of pneumothoraces in some trials.

"Open Lung" Ventilation

The open lung approach to mechanical ventilation uses sufficient PEEP to maintain the lung above the lower inflection point while using very low tidal volumes (approximately 6 mL/kg) to minimize "cyclic parenchymal stretch." In a small randomized study, this method showed a trend toward lowering mortality; it is currently the subject of a prospective randomized trial by the National Heart, Lung, and Blood Institute (NHLBI) ARDS network.

Extracorporeal Gas Exchange

Extracorporeal membrane oxygenation (ECMO) uses veno-venous or veno-arterial bypass to pump blood through an external membrane oxygenator. A prospective, controlled randomized trial in 1979 and a smaller retrospective analysis in 1988 did not show any advantage to ECMO in comparison with standard mechanical ventilation. In addition, both studies showed a significant incidence of bleeding complications in patients receiving ECMO, all of whom required full anticoagulation.

Extracorporeal CO_2 removal ($ECCO_2R$) uses a lower flow rate through veno-venous bypass and relies on low frequency mechanical ventilation and intratracheal gas insufflation for oxygenation. A randomized controlled trial in 1994 showed equivalent outcomes when $ECCO_2R$ was compared with pressure-controlled IVR.

Intravenous oxygenation (IVOX) involves the percutaneous placement of an intravascular oxygenation device, made up of multiple hollow filaments with gas-permeable walls, into the inferior vena cava. The utility of this device is yet to be determined.

Partial Liquid Ventilation

Ventilation with perfluorocarbons has several potential advantages. Perfluorocarbons are inert liquids with 25 times more oxygen solubility, three times more CO_2 solubility, and one-fourth of the surface tension of water. After instillation of a volume of perfluorocarbon approximating the functional residual capacity, a standard mechanical ventilator is used for ventilation. Nonrandomized studies in a small number of patients with ARDS and in premature infants have shown encouraging results. A randomized trial is currently under way.

Other Supportive Therapy
Fluid Management

The goal of fluid management in ARDS is to maintain an adequate cardiac output and tissue oxygen delivery at the lowest possible PAWP. In the presence of a damaged alveolar-capillary membrane, elevation of the pulmonary microvascular pressure exacerbates the leakage of intravascular fluid into the extravascular space. Several studies have shown a correlation between such increases in EVLW and mortality. In addition, intravascular volume expansion may contribute to right ventricular end-diastolic volume overload, which in turn leads to increased wall stress and oxygen requirement of the right ventricle.

Using colloids is not recommended in ARDS. Albumin or synthetic colloid solutions rapidly enter the pulmonary extravascular space because the pulmonary alveolar-capillary barrier is rendered permeable to these macromolecules in ARDS. It is advisable to use blood transfusion to maintain a hematocrit of 40 to 45% to maximize oxygen-carrying capacity in patients who remain hypoxic or when there is difficulty maintaining oxygen delivery (Fig 11.2). Supranormal hematocrits increase blood viscosity and reduce central nervous system perfusion and may reduce cardiac output.

There is disagreement in the literature whether it is preferable to maintain very low levels of PAWP (5–8 mm Hg) while maintaining cardiac output with pressors or to maintain near-normal PAWP (10–14 mm Hg) with less reliance on pressors. The higher PAWP results in higher EVLW; the use of pressors may affect cardiac function and splanchnic blood flow. To date, randomized studies have not compared these strategies.

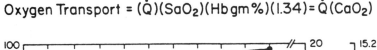

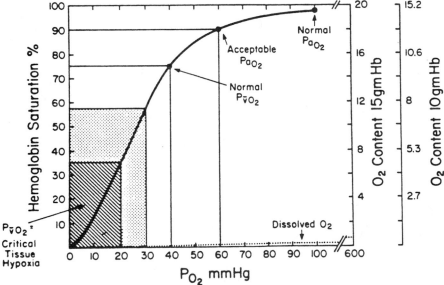

Figure 11.2. Diagram of oxyhemoglobin dissociation curve and relationships of PO_2 hemoglobin saturation and content, PVO_2, and oxygen content measurements. The PO_2 of 600 torr (79.8 kPa) is the PaO_2 expected in a normal individual breathing an FiO_2 of 1.0. The values of PVO_2 in the striped area represent tissue hypoxia; the values of PVO_2 in the stippled area represent potentially critical values in some tissues or organs, e.g., heart and brain. (From Weg JG. Crit Care Med 1991;19(5):655. Reprinted with permission.)

Experimental Pharmacotherapy

Given that only a minority of patients with ARDS die of respiratory failure, it can be argued that improvement in ventilatory support is not likely to have a large impact on outcome. Potential therapeutic interventions are being developed as the cellular mechanism of ARDS is elucidated.

Surfactant

Prematurely born infants with respiratory distress have long been recognized to have a deficiency of surfactant. Studies have shown surfactant to be functionally abnormal in ARDS and there are conflicting reports regarding whether its amount is reduced. Although preliminary observations had shown encouraging results, a large, blinded, randomized controlled trial showed that continuous aerosolized synthetic surfactant did not improve outcome compared with placebo in patients with sepsis-induced ARDS.

Corticosteroids

Despite their theoretical benefits in the prevention and treatment of ARDS, randomized controlled trials have shown increased mortality with use of corticosteroids in sepsis, no effect on the rate of development of ARDS in susceptible patients, and no improvement in recovery or survival in early ARDS. Recent uncontrolled reports of improved outcome have rekindled interest in the use of corticosteroids in the late fibrotic phase of ARDS (5–10 days after onset). Patients with established ARDS and peripheral or BAL eosinophilia have been shown to have a better prognosis and more rapid rate of recovery. A randomized trial to evaluate the use of corticosteroids in late ARDS is currently being conducted by the NHLBI ARDS network.

Nitric Oxide

Previously known as "endothelium-derived relaxing factor," nitric oxide has emerged as a potent mediator in many systems, including the lung, where it acts as a microvascular vasodilator. Nonrandomized studies in ARDS have shown that nitric oxide inhaled in minute concentrations (5 to 80 parts per million) causes vasodilatation and increases perfusion to ventilated alveolar units. When administered continuously, it improves ventilation/perfusion matching and oxygenation and reduces pulmonary vascular resistance without affecting other hemodynamic variables. The molecule is metabolized locally and, at low concentrations, has no discernible systemic effect. Optimism regarding the utility of nitric oxide in ARDS is tempered by concern regarding its prominent role as a mediator of inflammation and sepsis. Controlled randomized studies are required to establish the role of nitric oxide in the management of ARDS.

Eicosanoids

Ketoconazole is an oral imidazole, which was originally developed as an antifungal agent. It is also a potent inhibitor of thromboxane synthetase and 5-lipoxygenase, and therefore inhibits the production of thromboxane A_2, thromboxane B_2, leukotriene B_4, and procoagulant activity (PCA). Two small studies have shown a reduction in the incidence of ARDS in at-risk patients treated prophylactically with ketoconazole. The efficacy of this therapy in established ARDS is currently under evaluation in a randomized double-blinded multicenter study (NHLBI ARDS network).

Nonsteroidal antiinflammatory drugs such as indomethacin and ibuprofen inhibit cyclooxygenase, inhibiting the production of prostacyclin and thromboxane A_2. Studies in animal models of sepsis have shown some encouraging results when these drugs were given before the insult. Human data has been limited to small studies in sepsis and in ARDS and has yielded conflicting results.

Prostaglandin E_1 (alprostadil) is a vasodilator and an antiinflammatory mediator, inhibiting neutrophil chemotaxis and degranulation and preventing platelet aggregation. It was shown to improve hemodynamic parameters and reduce oxygen requirement in small studies, but in a randomized blinded trial it caused systemic hypotension and diarrhea without conferring a survival advantage. More recently, a small randomized trial of liposomal prostaglandin E_1 showed the beneficial effects on hemodynamics and oxygenation with little side effects, but was too small to detect a survival difference.

Antioxidants

One of the mechanisms of lung injury in ARDS is through release of reactive oxygen species, which damage membranes and result in cell death. Studies of a number of antioxidant molecules, including animal studies with superoxide dismutase and catalase, and human studies with N-acetylcysteine have not shown any benefit to this mode of therapy.

Anticytokines and Antiendotoxin Antibodies

The interaction between endotoxin and cytokines is central in the pathogenesis of SIRS and sepsis, the most frequent cause of ARDS. Animal studies have shown that administration of antagonists before, with, or very shortly after the inflammatory stimulus may protect against SIRS or sepsis. Despite promising results of early studies, however, larger trials failed to demonstrate beneficial effects with monoclonal antiendotoxin antibodies in human sepsis. Similarly, a randomized trial of anti–TNF-α antibody did not show any survival advantage, and a trial of soluble TNF receptor showed increased mortality associated with the use of the drug. Two phase III trials of IL-1 receptor antagonist showed no difference between the treatment and placebo groups.

Some animal studies suggest that antagonism of cytokines may be useful in preventing the development of SIRS and ARDS. Human studies to evaluate the prophylactic use of antagonists have not been published. Because bacterial infection frequently complicates ARDS and some cytokines have a protective role in the setting of sepsis, there is concern that inhibition of these may lead to deleterious results.

Other Agents

Pentoxiphylline is a phosphodiesterase inhibitor that reduces neutrophil chemotaxis, degranulation, and adherence to endothelium in animal models. A pilot study has shown it to be safe in ARDS, but clinical trials of its efficacy have not yet been published.

Adhesion molecules mediate neutrophil adhesion to the endothelium, an important step in their recruitment in ARDS. Monoclonal antiadhesion molecule antibodies are currently under investigation in prevention of ARDS in trauma patients.

COMPLICATIONS AND OUTCOME OF ACUTE LUNG INJURY

Air Leaks (Barotrauma)

Barotrauma, more appropriately termed "air leaks," is defined as extrusion of air outside the tracheobronchial tree:

- Air leaks occur in approximately 10% of patients with ARDS.
- The site of disruption is at the border between the alveolar base and the vascular sheath, with subsequent dissection of air along the vascular sheaths.
- Air trapped in the pulmonary interstitium can produce the radiologic appearance of parenchymal stippling, termed pulmonary interstitial emphysema.
- Intraparenchymal pseudocysts are localized air collections resembling pneumatoceles, but pathologically do not have an epithelial lining.
- Proximal tearing of the attachment of sheaths to mediastinal pleura leads to pneumomediastinum, often the first indication of air leaks.
- Further dissection of air along facial planes causes subcutaneous emphysema and, less commonly, retroperitoneal or intraperitoneal air.

We analyzed the 725 patients in the database of the artificial surfactant in sepsis-induced ARDS trial for evidence of air leaks. We were unable to show any correlation between peak airway pressure, mean airway pressure, tidal volume, or minute ventilation and pneumothorax or other air leaks. There were no differences in the distribution of pressures or volumes in patients with and without air leaks. No difference in mortality was detected between the groups with and without pneumothoraces and those with or without air leaks.

In addition to air leaks, animal models have been shown to develop pathologic changes indistinguishable from ARDS on exposure to very high ventilatory volumes (equivalent of 3-liter tidal volume in a 70 kg man). Whether high inflation pressures and PEEP contribute to clinical worsening of established ARDS in humans is controversial and is the subject of a multicenter randomized trial.

Nosocomial Pneumonia

Nosocomial ventilator-associated pneumonia has been reported at autopsy in as many as 73% of patients with ARDS. Although it is associated with increased mortality, establishing a causal relationship has been difficult because of confounding variables. Nosocomial pneumonia is a common cause of sepsis complicating ARDS, although it rarely produces bacteremia. Autopsy studies of patients with ARDS have shown that one-third of patients with clinically suspected pneumonia did not have histologic evidence of disease and that pneumonia was undiagnosed in one-third of patients with proven histologic disease. Clinical signs of pneumonia, such as fever, leukocytosis, and purulent sputum, are nonspecific and insensitive in the setting of mechanical ventilation and ARDS. The bilateral pulmonary infiltrates of ARDS make the detection of a new process very difficult.

The airways of all intubated patients are colonized by Gram-negative bacteria within 24 hours of entering the ICU, making Gram's stain and culture of secretions not helpful in diagnosis. Bronchoscopic sampling of the lower respiratory tract with a protected brush or BAL and quantitative culture techniques have been advocated for the diagnosis of ventilator-associated pneumonia. The utility of this approach is limited by the difficulty in preventing upper airway contamination of samples, and is not useful in patients on antibiotics.

Bedside clinical findings of purulent sputum, fever, and new infiltrates remain the mainstay of the diagnosis of ventilator-associated pneumonia in ARDS, despite their limitations. Antibiotic therapy, based on local sensitivity patterns, should be initiated as soon as pneumonia is clinically suspected. We recommend empiric therapy with a β-lactam and an aminoglycoside as a starting regimen. Sputum culture sensitivities can be used to guide antibiotic therapy. There is no role for prophylactic administration of antibiotics.

Long-term Sequelae in Survivors

Pulmonary function testing performed shortly after recovery shows a restrictive ventilatory defect that persists in at least one-third of patients for three months. Improvement in the restrictive defect continues such that the majority of patients have near-normal lung volumes by six months. Although the number of patients with residual defects at 1 year is small, little improvement usually occurs beyond that time.

Another common early feature of pulmonary function tests after ARDS is impaired gas transfer, as evidenced by a reduced DL_{CO}. This abnormality usually persists beyond 6 months but is generally mild and asymptomatic. A minority of patients have oxygen desaturation on exercise testing, and an even smaller number have resting hypoxemia.

Survivors of ARDS do not, as a rule, have a reduction in FEV_1 or FEV_1/FVC ratios. Decreased mid-expiratory flow rates have, however, been reported in up to one-half of the survivors. These changes may not be observed until the third month after discharge, but often persist or worsen in severity. Affected patients have evidence of airway hyperreactivity, with partial improvement with inhaled bronchodilators.

SUMMARY: AN APPROACH TO ARDS

ALI and ARDS represent an inflammatory response of the lung to systemic or direct insults. Because the utility of many of the treatment modalities used in this syndrome has not been fully evaluated in a scientific manner, this section summarizes the available literature:

- Patients with ALI require close monitoring in an ICU.
- Pulmonary arterial and central venous catheters, arterial catheters, and urinary catheters are indicated for monitoring oxygen delivery, cardiac output, PAWP, venous access, ease of frequent blood draws, and blood pressure and urine output monitoring.
- A diligent search for the precipitating event, particularly occult infections, should be undertaken at the outset and appropriate treatment initiated.
- All patients meeting the definition of ARDS will require mechanical ventilation.
- Assist-control volume ventilation with tidal volume of 10–15 mL/kg and a respiratory rate set to maintain near-normal pH and pCO_2 are recommended.
- Begin with no PEEP and an FiO_2 of 100% and attempt to reduce the FiO_2 while maintaining the PaO_2 at approximately 60 mm Hg.
- Add PEEP in 2–3-cm increments while monitoring cardiac output to assure good $\ddot{O}_2$.
- In patients who cannot be adequately oxygenated by this method, attempt lateral decubitus or prone positioning.
- In patients with adequate oxygenation, reduce the FiO_2 in increments to less than 60%. PEEP is then reduced in increments of 2–3 cm H_2O every 30 to 60 minutes. Although there are proponents of various other ventilatory modes, none of these other modes have been shown to be superior to assist-control ventilation with PEEP to date.
- Most patients require regular sedation.
- Fluid management should aim to maintain the lowest possible PAWP without compromising the cardiac output.
- Intravascular volume overload should be avoided.
- Routine care should include nutrition and prophylaxis against thromboembolic disease.
- Daily portable radiographs should be examined for evidence of pneumothoraces and worsening infiltrates.
- Febrile patients should be evaluated for source of infection, with particular attention to pneumonia and intravascular catheter infection.

BIBLIOGRAPHY

Introduction and Definition

Ashbaugh DG, Bigelow DG, Petty TL, Levine BE. Acute respiratory distress in adults. Lancet August 1967;12:319–323.

Bernard GR, Artigas A, Brigham KL, Carlet J, Falke K, Hudson L, Lamy M, Legall JR, Morris A, Spragg R, and the Consensus Committee. The American–European Consensus Conference on ARDS: definitions, mechanisms, relevant outcomes, and clinical trial coordination. Am J Respir Crit Care Med 1994;149:818–824.

Fowler AA. Adult respiratory distress syndrome: does it really exist? Semin Respir Crit Care Med 1994;15(4):250–253.

Knaus WA, Sun X, Hakim RB, Wagner DP. Evaluation of definitions for adult respiratory distress syndrome. Am J Respir Crit Care Med 1994;150:311–317.

Moss M, Goodman PL, Heinig M, Barkin S, Ackerson L, Parsons PE. Establishing the relative accuracy of three new definitions of the adult respiratory distress syndrome. Crit Care Med 1995;23(10):1629–1637.

Murray JF, Matthay MA, Luce JM, Flick MR. An expanded definition of the adult respiratory distress syndrome. Am Rev Respir Dis 1988;138:720–723.

Schuster DP. What is acute lung injury? What is ARDS? Chest 1995;107:1721–1726.

Epidemiology

Baughman RP, Gunther KL, Rashkin MC, Keeton D, Pattishall EN. Changes in the inflammatory response of the lung during acute respiratory distress syndrome: prognostic indicators. Am J Respir Crit Care Med 1996;154:76–81.

Burkhardt MJ, et al. Update: Hantavirus infection: United States, 1993. MMWR 1993;42:517–519 (JAMA 1993;270(4):429, 432).

Dorinsky PM, Gadek JE. Multiple organ failure. Clin Chest Med 1990;11(4):581–591.

Doyle RL, Szaflarski N, Modin GW, Wiener-Kronish JP, Matthay MA. Identification of patients with acute lung injury: predictors of mortality. Am J Respir Crit Care Med 1995;152:1818–1824.

Eriksen NL, Parisi VM. Adult respiratory distress syndrome and pregnancy. Semin Perinatol 1990;14(1):68–77.

Fowler AA, Hamman RF, Zerbe GO, Benson KN, Hyers TM. Adult respiratory distress syndrome: prognosis after onset. Am Rev Respir Dis 1985;132:472–478.

Fruchtman SM, Gombert ME, Lyons HA. Adult respiratory distress syndrome as a cause of death in pneumococcal pneumonia. Chest 1983;83:598–601.

Hankins GDV, Nolan TE. Adult respiratory distress syndrome in obstetrics. Obstet Gynecol Clin North Am 1991;18(2):273–287.

Heffner JE, Brown LK, Barbieri CA, Harpel KS, DeLeo J. Prospective validation of an acute respiratory distress syndrome predictive score. Am J Respir Crit Care Med 1995;152:1518–1526.

Hudson LD. Epidemiology of adult respiratory distress syndrome. Semin Respir Crit Care Med 1994;15(4):254–260.

Hudson LD. Multiple systems organ failure (MSOF): lessons learned from the adult respiratory distress syndrome (ARDS). Crit Care Clin 1989;5(3):697–705.

Hudson LD, Milber JA, Anardi D, Maunder RJ. Clinical risks for development of the acute respiratory distress syndrome. Am J Respir Crit Care Med 1995;151:293–301.

Hyers TM, Fowler AA. Adult respiratory distress syndrome: causes, morbidity, and mortality. Fed Proc 1986;45:25–29.

Kreuzfelder E, Joka T, Keinecke HO, Obertacke U, Schmit-Neuerburg KP, Nakhosteen JA, Paar D, Scheiermann N. Adult respiratory distress syndrome as a specific manifestation of a general permeability defect in trauma patients. Am Rev Respir Dis 1988;137:95–99.

Malouf M, Glanville AR. Blood transfusion-related adult respiratory distress syndrome. Anaesth Intensive Care 1993;21(1):44–49.

Milberg JA, Davis DR, Steinberg KP, Hudson LD. Improved survival of patients with acute respiratory distress syndrome (ARDS): 1983–1993. JAMA 1995;273:306–309.

Mojica B, et al. Hantavirus pulmonary syndrome: Northeastern United States, 1994. MMWR 1994;43:548–549, 555–556 (JAMA 1994;272(13):997–998).

Montgomery AB, Stager MA, Carrico CJ, Hudson LD. Causes of mortality in patients with the adult respiratory distress syndrome. Am Rev Respir Dis 1985;132:485–489.

Moolenaar RL, Dalton C, Lipman HB, et al. Clinical features that differentiate Hantavirus pulmonary syndrome from three other acute respiratory illnesses. Clin Infect Dis 1995;21:643–649.

Moss M, Bucher B, Moore FA, Moore EE, Parsons PE. The role of chronic alcohol abuse in the development of acute respiratory distress syndrome in adults. JAMA 1996;275:50–54.

Pepe PE, Potkin RT, Reus DH, Carrico CJ. Clinical predictors of the adult respiratory distress syndrome. Am J Surg 1982;144:124–130.

Perl TM, Dvorak L, Hwang T, Wenzel RP. Long-term survival and function after suspected Gram-negative sepsis. JAMA 1995;274:338–345.

St. John RC, Dorinsky PM. Multiple organ dysfunction: pathogenesis and approach to therapy. Semin Respir Crit Care Med 1994;15(4):325–334.

Suchyta MR, Clemmer TP, Orme JF Jr, Morris AH, Elliott G. Increased survival of ARDS patients with severe hypoxemia (ECMO criteria). Chest 1991;99:951–955.

Thomsen GE, Morris AH. Incidence of the adult respiratory distress syndrome in the state of Utah. Am J Respir Crit Care Med 1995;152:965–971.

Weiss SM, Hudson LD. Outcome from respiratory failure. Crit Care Clin 1994;10(1):197–215.

Histopathologic Features

Gattinoni L, Bombino M, Pelosi P, Lissoni A, Pesenti A, Rumagalli R, Tagliabue M. Lung structure and function in different stages of severe adult respiratory distress syndrome. JAMA 1994;271:1772–1779.

Lamy M, Fallat RJ, Koeniger E, Dietrich HP, Ratliff JL, Eberhart RC, Tucker HJ, Hill JD. Pathologic features and mechanisms of hypoxemia in adult respiratory distress syndrome. Am Rev Respir Dis 1976;114:267–284.

Martin C, Papazian L, Payan MJ, Saux P, Gouin F. Pulmonary fibrosis correlates with outcome in adult respiratory distress syndrome. Chest 1995;107:196–200.

Meduri GU, Eltorky M, Winer-Muram HT. The fibroproliferative phase of late adult respiratory distress syndrome. Semin Respir Infect 1995;10(3):154–175.

Myrick B. Pathology of the adult respiratory distress syndrome. Crit Care Clin 1986;2(3):405–428.

Tomashefski JF Jr. Pulmonary pathology of the adult respiratory distress syndrome. Clin Chest Med 1990;11(4):593–619.

Tomashefski JF Jr, Davies P, Boggis C, Green R, Zapol W, Reid LM. The pulmonary vascular lesions of the adult respiratory distress syndrome. Am J Pathol 1983;112:112–126.

Pathophysiology

Bone RC. Immunologic dissonance: a continuing evolution in our understanding of the systemic inflammatory response syndrome (SIRS) and the multiple organ dysfunction syndrome (MODS). Ann Intern Med 1996;125(8):680–687.

Danek SJ, Lynch JP, Weg JG, Dantzker DR. The dependence of oxygen uptake on oxygen delivery in the adult respiratory distress syndrome. Am Rev Respir Dis 1980;122:387–395.

Marini JJ. Lung mechanics in adult respiratory distress syndrome. Clin Chest Med 1990; 11(4):673–690.

Meduri GU, Kohler G, Headley S, Tolley E, Stentz F, Postlethwaite A. Inflammatory cytokines in the BAL of patients with ARDS: persistent elevation over time predicts poor outcome. Chest 1995;108:1303–1314.

Melot C. Ventilation-perfusion relationships in acute respiratory failure. Thorax 1994;49: 1251–1258.

Pelosi P, D'Andrea L, Vitale G, Pesenti A, Gattinoni L. Vertical gradient of regional lung inflation in adult respiratory distress syndrome. Am J Respir Crit Care Med 1994;149: 8–13.

Reid PT, Donnelly SC, Haslett C. Inflammatory predictors for the development of the adult respiratory distress syndrome. Thorax 1995;50:1023–1026.

Ronco JJ, Phang PT, Walley KR, Wiggs B, Fenwick JC, Russell JA. Oxygen consumption is independent of changes in oxygen delivery in severe adult respiratory distress syndrome. Am Rev Respir Dis 1991;143:1267–1273.

Rossaint R, Hahn SM, Pappert D, Falke KJ, Radermacher P. Influence of mixed venous PO_2 and inspired O_2 fraction on intrapulmonary shunt in patients with severe ARDS. Am J Physiol 1995:1531–1536.

Strieter RM, Kunkel SL. Acute lung injury: the role of cytokines in the elicitation of neutrophils. J Investig Med 1994;42(4):640–651.

Weg JG. Oxygen transport in adult respiratory distress syndrome and other acute circulatory problems: relationship of oxygen delivery and oxygen consumption. Crit Care Med 1991; 19(5):650–657.

Presentation, Natural History, and Studies

Aberle DR, Brown K. Radiologic considerations in the adult respiratory distress syndrome. Clin Chest Med 1990;11(4):737–754.

Bone RC. The ARDS lung: new insights from computed tomography. JAMA 1993;269(16): 2134–2135.

Clark JG, Milberg JA, Steinberg KP, Hudson LD. Type III procollagen peptide in the adult respiratory distress syndrome: association of increased peptide levels in bronchoalveolar lavage fluid with increased risk for death. Ann Intern Med 1995;122:17–23.

Connors AF, Speroff T, Dawson NV, et al. The effectiveness of right heart catheterization in the initial care of critically ill patients. JAMA 1995;276:889–897.

Demling RH. The modern version of adult respiratory distress syndrome. Annu Rev Med 1995;46:193–202.

Gattinoni L, Pelosi P, Crotti S, Valenza F. Effects of positive end-expiratory pressure on distribution of tidal volume and recruitment in adult respiratory distress syndrome. Am J Respir Crit Care Med 1995;151:1807–1814.

Goldenheim PD, Kazemi H. Cardiopulmonary monitoring of critically ill patients (Pt. 1). N Engl J Med 1984;311(11):717–720.

Goldenheim PD, Kazemi H. Cardiopulmonary monitoring of critically ill patients (Pt. 2). N Engl J Med 1984;311(12):776–780.

Matthay MA. Fibrosing alveolitis in the adult respiratory distress syndrome. Ann Intern Med 1995;122:65–66.

Maunder RJ, Shuman WP, McHugh JW, Marglin SI, Butler J. Preservation of normal lung regions in the adult respiratory distress syndrome: analysis by computed tomography. JAMA 1986;255:2463–2465.

Wiedemann HP, Matthay MA, Matthay RA. Cardiovascular-pulmonary monitoring in the intensive care unit (Pt. 1). Chest 1984;85(4):537–549.

Wiedemann HP, Matthay MA, Matthay RA. Cardiovascular-pulmonary monitoring in the intensive care unit (Pt. 2). Chest 1984;85(5):657–668.

Mechanical Ventilation and Supportive Therapy

Amato MBP, Barbas CSV, Medeiros DM, et al. Beneficial effects of the "open lung approach" with low distending pressures in acute respiratory distress syndrome: a prospective randomized study on mechanical ventilation. Am J Respir Crit Care Med 1995;152:1835–1846.

Bidani A, Tzouanakis AE, Cardenas VJ, Zwischenberger JB. Permissive hypercapnia in acute respiratory failure. JAMA 1994;272:957–962.

Bishop MH, Shoemaker WC, Appel, PL, et al. Prospective, randomized trial of survivor values of cardiac index, oxygen delivery, and oxygen consumption as resuscitation endpoints in severe trauma. J Trauma 1995;38:780–787.

Boyd O, Grounds RM, Bennett ED. A randomized clinical trial of the effect of deliberate perioperative increase of oxygen delivery on mortality in high-risk surgical patients. JAMA 1993;270:2699–2707.

Clevenger FW, Acosta JA, Osler TM. Barotrauma associated with high-frequency jet ventilation for hypoxic salvage. Arch Surg 1990;125:1542–1545.

Cujec B, Polasek P, Mayers I, Johnson D. Positive end-expiratory pressure increases the right-to-left shunt in mechanically ventilated patients with patent foramen ovale. Ann Intern Med 1993;119:887–894.

DiRusso SM, Nelson LD, Safesak K, Miller RS. Survival in patients with severe adult respiratory distress syndrome treated with high-level positive end-expiratory pressure. Crit Care Med 1995;23(9):1485–1496.

Gattinoni L, Brazzi L, Pelosi P, et al. A trial of goal-oriented hemodynamic therapy in critically ill patients. N Engl J Med 1995;333:1025–1032.

Gattinoni L, Pesenti A, Mascheroni D. Low-frequency positive pressure ventilation with extracorporeal CO_2 removal in severe acute respiratory failure. JAMA 1986;256:881–886.

Gattinoni L, Pesenti A, Avalli L, Rossi F, Bombino M. Pressure-volume curve of total respiratory system in acute respiratory failure: computed tomographic scan study. Am Rev Respir Dis 1987;136:730–736.

Gattinoni L, D'Andrea L, Pelosi P, Vitale G, Pesenti A, Fumagalli R. Regional effects and mechanism of positive end-expiratory pressure in early adult respiratory distress syndrome. JAMA 1993;269(16):2122–2127.

Gattinoni L, Pelosi P, Crotti S, Valenza F. Effects of positive end-expiratory pressure on regional distribution of tidal volume and recruitment in adult respiratory distress syndrome. Am J Respir Crit Care Med 1995;151:1807–1814.

Gauger PG, Pranikoff T, Schreiner RJ, Moler FW, Hirschl RB. Initial experience with partial liquid ventilation in pediatric patients with the acute respiratory distress syndrome. Crit Care Med 1996;24(1):16–22.

Hayes MA, Timmins AC, Yau EHS, Palazzo M, Hinds CJ, Watson D. Elevation of systemic oxygen delivery in the treatment of critically ill patients. N Engl J Med 1994;330: 1717–1722.

Hayes MA, Yau EHS, Timmins AC, Hinds CJ, Watson D. Response of critically ill patients to treatment aimed at achieving supranormal oxygen delivery and consumption: relationship to outcome. Chest 1993;103:886–895.

Hickling KG. Extracorporeal CO_2 removal in severe adult respiratory distress syndrome. Anaesth Intensive Care 1986;14(1):45–63.

Hickling KG, Walsh J, Henderson S, Jackson R. Low mortality rate in adult respiratory distress syndrome using low-volume, pressure-limited ventilation with permissive hypercapnia: a prospective study. Crit Care Med 1994;22:1566–1578.

Hirschl RB, Pranikoff T, Wise C, et al. Initial experience with partial liquid ventilation in adult patients with the acute respiratory distress syndrome. JAMA 1996;275:383–389.

Hirschl RB, Merz SI, Montoya JP, Parent A, Wolfson MR, Shaffer TH, Bartlett RH. Development and application of a simplified liquid ventilator. Crit Care Med 1995;23(1):157–163.

Hudson LD. New therapies for ARDS. Chest 1995;108(suppl 2):79S–91S.

Kacmarek RM, Kirmse M, Nishimura M, Mang H, Kimball WR. The effects of applied vs auto-PEEP on local lung unit pressure and volume in a four-unit lung model. Chest 1995; 108(4):1073–1079.

Kuo PH, Wu HD, Yu CJ, Yang SC, Lai YL, Yang PC. Efficacy of tracheal gas insufflation in acute respiratory distress syndrome with permissive hypercapnia. Am J Respir Crit Care Med 1996;154:612–616.

Leach CL, Greenspan JS, Rubenstein SD, Shaffer TH, Wolfson MR, Jackson JC, DeLemos R, Fuhrman BP. Partial liquid ventilation with perflubron in premature infants with severe respiratory distress syndrome. N Engl J Med 1996;335(11):761–767.

Lewandowski K. Permissive hypercapnia in ARDS: just do it? Intensive Care Med 1996;22: 179–181.

Ludwigs U, Klingstedt C, Baehrendtz S, Wegenius G, Hedenstierna G. Volume-controlled inverse ratio ventilation in oleic acid-induced lung injury: effects on gas exchange, hemodynamics, and computed tomographic lung density. Chest 1995;108:804–809.

Mang H, Kacmarek RM, Ritz R, Wilson RS, Kimball WP. Cardiorespiratory effects of volume- and pressure-controlled ventilation at various I/E ratios in an acute lung injury model. Am J Respir Crit Care Med 1995;151:731–736.

Marcy TW, Marini JJ. Inverse ratio ventilation in ARDS: rationale and implementation. Chest 1991;100:494–504.

Marini JJ. Inverse ratio ventilation—simply an alternative, or something more? Crit Care Med 1995;23(2):224–228.

Merritt TA, Heldt GP. Partial liquid ventilation—the future is now. N Engl J Med 1996; 335(11):812–815.

Morris AH, Wallace CJ, Menlove RL, et al. Randomized clinical trial of pressure-controlled inverse ratio ventilation and extracorporeal CO_2 removal for adult respiratory distress syndrome. Am J Respir Crit Care Med 1994;149:295–305.

Nelson LD. High-inflation pressure and positive end-expiratory pressure: injurious to the lung? No. Crit Care Clin 1996;12:603–625.

Papadakos PJ, Apostolakos MJ. High-inflation pressure and positive end-expiratory pressure: injurious to the lung? Yes. Crit Care Clin 1996;12:627–634.

Pappert D, Rossaint R, Slama K, Grüning T, Falke KJ. Influence of positioning on ventilation-perfusion relationships in severe adult respiratory distress syndrome. Chest 1994;106: 1511–1516.

Petty TL, Bone RC, Gee MH, Hudson LD, Hyers TM. Contemporary clinical trials in acute respiratory distress syndrome. Chest 1992;101:550–552.

Ranieri VM, Mascia L, Fiore T, et al. Cardiorespiratory effects of positive end-expiratory pressure during progressive tidal volume reduction (permissive hypercapnia) in patients with acute respiratory distress syndrome. Anesthesiology 1995;83(4):710–720.

Romand JA, Shi W, Pinsky MR. Cardiopulmonary effects of positive pressure ventilation during acute lung injury. Chest 1995;108:1041–1048.

Roupie E, Dambrosio M, Servillo G, et al. Titration of tidal volume and induced hypercapnia in acute respiratory distress syndrome. Am J Respir Crit Care Med 1995;152:121–128.

Shoemaker WC, Appel PL, Kram HB, Waxman K, Lee TS. Prospective trial of supranormal values of survivors as therapeutic goals in high-risk surgical patients. Chest 1988;94: 1176–1186.

Slutsky AS. Mechanical ventilation. Chest 1993;104(6):1833–1859.

Tharratt RS, Allen RA, Albertson TE. Pressure-controlled inverse ratio ventilation in severe adult respiratory failure. Chest 1988;94:755–762.

Thorens JG, Jolliet P, Ritz M, Chevrolet JC. Effects of rapid permissive hypercapnia on hemodynamics, gas exchange, and oxygen transport and consumption during mechanical ventilation for the acute respiratory distress syndrome. Intensive Care Med 1996;22: 182–191.

Tuchschmidt J, Fried J, Astiz M, Rackow E. Elevation of cardiac output and oxygen delivery improves outcome in septic shock. Chest 1992;102:216–220.

Tuxen DV. Permissive hypercapnic ventilation. Am J Respir Crit Care Med 1994;150: 870–874.

Yu M, Levy MM, Smith P, Takiguchi SA, Miyasaki A, Myers SA. Effect of maximizing oxygen delivery on morbidity and mortality rates in critically ill patients: a prospective, randomized, controlled study. Crit Care Med 1993;21:830–838.

Zapol WM, Snider MT, Hill D. Extracorporeal membrane oxygenation in severe acute respiratory failure. A randomized prospective study. JAMA 1979;242:2193–2196.

Experimental Pharmacotherapy

Abraham E, Park YC, Covington P, Conrad SA, Schwartz M. Liposomal prostaglandin E_1 in acute respiratory distress syndrome: a placebo-controlled, randomized, double-blind, multicenter clinical trial. Crit Care Med 1996;24:10–15.

Anzueto A, Baughman RP, Guntupalli KK, Weg JG, Wiedemann HP, Raventos AA, Lemaire F, Long W, Zaccardelli DS, Pattishall EN. Aerosolized surfactant in adults with sepsis-induced acute respiratory distress syndrome. N Engl J Med 1996;334(22):1417–1421.

Bernard GR, Luce JM, Sprung CL, Rinaldo JE, Tate RM, Sibbald WJ, Kariman K, Higgins S, Bradley R, Metz CA, Harris TR, Brigham KL. High-dose corticosteroids in patients with the adult respiratory distress syndrome. N Engl J Med 1987;317:1565–1570.

Chiche JD, Canivet JL, Damas P, Joris J, Lamy M. Inhaled nitric oxide for hemodynamic support after postpneumonectomy ARDS. Intensive Care Med 1995;21:675–678.

Craig J, Mullins D. Nitric oxide inhalation in infants and children: physiologic and clinical implications. Am J Crit Care 1995;4(6):443–450.

Fierobe L, Brunet F, Dhainaut JF, Monchi M, Belghith M, Mira JP, Dall'ava-Santucci J,

Dinh-xuan AT. Effect of inhaled nitric oxide on right ventricular function in adult respiratory distress syndrome. Am J Respir Crit Care Med 1995;151:1414–1419.

Fisher CJ Jr, Agoti JM, Opal SM, Lowry SF, Balk RA, Sadoff JC, Abraham E, Schein RMH, Benjamin E. Treatment of septic shock with the tumor necrosis factor receptor: Fc fusion protein. N Engl J Med 1996;334:1697–1702.

Frazee LA, Neidig JA. Ketoconazole to prevent acute respiratory distress syndrome in critically ill patients. Ann Pharmacother 1995;29:784–786.

Giacoia GP. Nitric oxide: a selective pulmonary vasodilator. South Med J 1995;88(1):33–41.

Gross NJ. Pulmonary surfactant: unanswered questions. Thorax 1995;50:325–327.

Günther A, Siebert C, Schmidt R, Ziegler S, Grimminger F, Yabut M, Temmesfeld B, Walmrath D, Morr H, Seeger W. Surfactant alterations in severe pneumonia, acute respiratory distress syndrome, and cardiogenic lung edema. Am J Respir Crit Care Med 1996;153: 176–184.

Hallman M, Maasilta P, Sipilä, Tahvanainen J. Composition and function of pulmonary surfactant in adult respiratory distress syndrome. Eur Respir J 1989;2(suppl 3):104S–108S.

Hamvas A, Wise PH, Yang RK, Wampler NS, Noguchi A, Maurer MM, Walentik CA, Schramm WF, Cole FS. The influence of the wider use of surfactant therapy on neonatal mortality among blacks and whites. N Engl J Med 1996;334:1635–1640.

Laurent T, Markert M, Feihl F, Schaller MD, Perret C. Oxidant-antioxidant balance in granulocytes during ARDS: effect of N-acetylcysteine. Chest 1996;109:163–166.

McCuthchan JA, Wolff JL, Zeigler EJ, Braude AL. Ineffectiveness of single-dose human antiserum to core glycolipid (E coli J5) for prophylaxis of bacteremia, Gram-negative infection, in patients with prolonged neutropenia. Schweiz Med Wochenschr Suppl 1993; 14:40–45.

Meduri GU, Chinn AJ, Leeper KV, Wunderink RG, Tolley E, Winer-Muram HT, Khare V, Eltorky M. Corticosteroid rescue treatment of progressive fibroproliferation in late ARDS: patterns of response and predictors of outcome. Chest 1994;105(5):1516–1527.

Meduri GU, Headley S, Tolley E, Shelby M, Stentz F, Postlethwaite A. Plasma and BAL cytokine response to corticosteroid rescue treatment in late ARDS. Chest 1995;108: 1315–1325.

Quinn AC, Petros AJ, Vallance P. Nitric oxide: an endogenous gas. Br J Anaesth 1995;74: 443–451.

Rossaint R, Slama K, Steudel W, Gerlach H, Pappert D, Veit S, Falke K. Effects of inhaled nitric oxide on right ventricular function in severe acute respiratory distress syndrome. Intensive Care Med 1995;21:197–203.

Rossaint R, Gerlach H, Schmidt-Ruhnke H, Pappert D, Lewandowski K, Steudel W, Falke K. Efficacy of inhaled nitric oxide in patients with severe ARDS. Chest 1995;107:1107–1115.

Sood SL, Balaraman V, Finn KC, Britton B, Uyehara CF, Easa D. Exogenous surfactants in a piglet model of acute respiratory distress syndrome. Am J Respir Crit Care Med 1996; 153:820–828.

Suter PM, Domenighetti G, Schaller MD, Laverriere MC, Ritz R, Perret C. N-acetylcysteine enhances recovery from acute lung injury in man: a randomized, double-blind, placebo-controlled clinical study. Chest 1994;105:190–194.

Veldhuizen RAW, McCaig LA, Akino T, Lewis JF. Pulmonary surfactant subfractions in patients with the acute respiratory distress syndrome. Am J Respir Crit Care Med 1995; 152:1867–1871.

Verder H, Robertson B, Greisen G, Ebbesen F, Albertsen P, Lundstrom K, Jacobsen T. Surfactant therapy and nasal continuous positive airway pressure for newborns with respiratory distress syndrome. N Engl J Med 1994;331:1051–1055.

Walmrath D, Günther A, Ghofrani HA, Schermuly R, Schneider T, Grimminger F, Seeger W. Bronchoscopic surfactant administration in patients with severe adult respiratory distress syndrome and sepsis. Am J Respir Crit Care Med 1996;154:57–62.

Weg JG, Balk Ra, Tharratt RS, Jenkinson SG, Shah JG, Zaccardelli D, Horton J, Pattishall EN. Safety and potential efficacy of an aerosolized surfactant in human sepsis-induced adult respiratory distress syndrome. JAMA 1994;272(18):1433–1438.

Williams JG, Maier RV. Ketoconazole inhibits alveolar macrophage production of inflammatory mediators involved in acute lung injury (adult respiratory distress syndrome). Surgery 1992;112:270–277.

Wright PE, Carmichael LC, Bernard GR. Effect of bronchodilators on lung mechanics in the acute respiratory distress syndrome (ARDS). Chest 1994;106:1517–1523.

Yu M, Tomasa G. A double-blind, prospective, randomized trial of ketoconazole, a thromboxane synthetase inhibitor, in the prophylaxis of the adult respiratory distress syndrome. Crit Care Med 1993;21(11):1635–1643.

Zapol WM, Hurford WE. Inhaled nitric oxide in adult respiratory distress syndrome and other lung diseases. Adv Pharmacol 1994;31:513–530.

Ziegler EJ, McCuthchan JA, Fierer J, Glauser MP, Sadoff JC, Douglas H, et al. Treatment of Gram-negative sepsis and shock with human antiserum to a mutant *Escherichia coli*. N Engl J Med 1982;307:1225–1230.

Ziegler EJ, Fisher CJ, Sprung CL, Straube RC, Sadoff JC, Foulke GE, Wortel CH, Fink MP, Dellinger P, Teng NNH, Allen IE, Berger HJ, Knatterud GL, LoBuglio AF, Smith CR, the HA-1A Sepsis Study Group. Treatment of Gram-negative bacteremia and septic shock with HA-1A human monoclonal antibody against endotoxin: a randomized, double-blind, placebo-controlled trial. N Engl J Med 1991;324:429–436.

Complications and Sequelae

Dever LL, Johanson WG Jr. Pneumonia complicating adult respiratory distress syndrome. Clin Chest Med 1995;16(1):147–153.

Elliott CG, Rasmusson BY, Crapo RO, Morris AH, Jensen RL. Prediction of pulmonary function abnormalities after adult respiratory distress syndrome (ARDS). Am Rev Respir Dis 1987;135:634–638.

Gammon RB, Shin MS, Groves RH. Clinical risk factors for pulmonary barotrauma: a multivariate analysis. Am J Respir Crit Care Med 1994;149:8–13.

Hudson LD. What happens to survivors of the adult respiratory distress syndrome? Chest 1994;105(3):123S–125S.

Koffef MH, Shapiro SD, Fraser VJ, Silver P, Murphy DM, Trovillion E, Hearns ML, Richards RD, Cracchilo L, Hossin L. Mechanical ventilation with or without 7-day circuit changes: a randomized controlled trial. Ann Intern Med 1995;123:168–174.

McHugh LG, Milberg JA, Whitcomb ME, Schoene RB, Maunder RJ, Hudson LD. Recovery of function in survivors of the acute respiratory distress syndrome. Am J Respir Crit Care Med 1994;150:90–94.

Papazian L, Bregeon F, Thirion X, Gregoire R, Saux P, Denis JP, Perin G, Charrel J, Dumon

JF, Affray JP, Gouin F. Effect of ventilator-associated pneumonia on mortality and morbidity. Am J Respir Crit Care Med 1996;154:91–97.

Pingleton SK. Barotrauma in acute lung injury: is it important? Crit Care Med 1995;23(2): 223–224.

Rouby JJ, Lherm T, de Lassale EM, Poete P, Bodin L, Finet JF, Callard P, Viars P. Histologic aspects of pulmonary barotrauma in critically ill patients with acute respiratory failure. Intensive Care Med 1993;19:383–389.

Schnapp LM, Chin DP, Szaflarski N, Matthay MA. Frequency and importance of barotrauma in 100 patients with acute lung injury. Crit Care Med 1995;23(2):272–278.

Sutherland KR, Steinberg KP, Maunder RJ, Milberg JA, Allen DL, Hudson LD. Pulmonary infection during the acute respiratory distress syndrome. Am J Respir Crit Care Med 1995; 152:550–556.

12 Mechanical Ventilation: ICU Management

Mari M. Goldner, John J. Marini, Paul L. Marino

Many clinicians find the process of mechanical ventilation (MV) intimidating. This is an entirely appropriate reaction in that one is influencing a critical body function in a manner that often is not at all physiologic and has considerable morbidity. At the same time, however, the practice of MV is undergirded by a finite set of fundamental principles based in physiology and physics. When the clinician can articulate and apply these principles, he or she can develop a ventilatory strategy that optimizes the patient's support and safety, and in the process gain insights into the underlying pathophysiology.

In this chapter the fundamental concepts are presented, woven in as they become implicit in the practical process of instituting, monitoring, and adjusting MV. This process can be outlined as follows:

- The need for respiratory assistance is recognized.
- Ventilatory support is begun.
- The effect of the initial ventilatory strategy is assessed and settings are adjusted to optimize benefit and minimize harm.
- Complications of MV are monitored and treated if found.
- Evidence that MV may be successfully discontinued is sought and MV is withdrawn.

INDICATIONS FOR MECHANICAL VENTILATION

Indications for MV should be separated from those related to airway intubation. A primary need for endotracheal intubation is present when the patency or hygiene of the upper or lower airway is jeopardized; causes include inability to protect the airway and the presence of excessive secretions or edema. Respiratory assistance is needed when the patient is unable to achieve adequate gas exchange; i.e., to maintain PaO_2 and pH in an acceptable range or when work of breathing (WOB) is excessive and unsustainable.

In general, hypoxemia is a more immediately life-threatening condition than is hypercarbia and/or respiratory acidosis because the body has relatively small oxygen stores and a fairly large buffering capacity. Hypercapnia that portends progressive alveolar hypoventilation (and therefore worsened hypoxemia) and acidosis accompanied by life-threatening metabolic derangements (e.g., hyperkalemia) or cardiovascu-

Table 12.1. Indications for Endotracheal Intubation

Current inability to protect the airway
CNS dysfunction
   Toxic/metabolic central respiratory depression
   Stroke
   Head trauma
Actual or potential airway compromise
   Excessive secretions
   Airway edema
      Inhalational injury
      Epiglottitis
      Anaphylaxis
      Facial or neck trauma

lar compromise (a controversial area) are indications for immediate respiratory support (Tables 12.1 and 12.2).

GOALS OF MECHANICAL VENTILATION

The goal of any mechanical ventilatory strategy is to provide adequate, noninjurious support of the patient. The term ''strategy'' will be used frequently throughout this chapter to emphasize the idea that each component of the ventilator settings is part of a plan, subject to ongoing assessment and revision, with specific objectives and considerations.

- Adequate oxygenation and ventilation;
- Stable hemodynamics;
- Noninjurious pressures and volumes;
- Nontoxic concentrations of oxygen.

Adequate Oxygenation and Ventilation

In general, it is desirable to maintain an oxygen saturation (SaO_2) above 90% and ideally above 92%; values lower than 90% risk desaturation with minor variations

Table 12.2. Indications for Assisted Ventilation

Lung failure (usually hypoxemic)	Bellows failure (usually hypercapnic)
Primary	Increased work of breathing
Pneumonia	Asthma, COPD exacerbation
Acute lung injury	Increased minute ventilation requirement
Secondary	Metabolic acidosis
Cardiogenic pulmonary edema	Increased dead space fraction
Pulmonary embolism	

in PaO_2. As will be discussed below, the ultimate goal is oxygen delivery, which is influenced by cardiac output and hemoglobin. For most patients, the desired $PaCO_2$ is that which is in the normal range for the patient and/or that which maintains a near physiologic pH. There may be times when the $PaCO_2$ is allowed to rise ("permissive hypercapnia") in the interests of noninjurious ventilatory patterns. During CO_2 retention, the pH is allowed to decrease but generally not to less than 7.15.

Stable Hemodynamics

The shift from negative to positive pressure breathing cycles significantly affects the loading conditions of the heart and frequently decreases cardiac output. Care must be taken to ensure that sufficient tissue perfusion and oxygen delivery are maintained during positive pressure ventilation (PPV).

Noninjurious Pressures

A major influence on current ventilator management is the increasing recognition that high distending pressures and perhaps large tidal swings of alveolar pressure can injure previously normal lung and that this effect may be compounded in the inhomogeneous environment of the injured lung. Airway pressures must be monitored carefully and settings tailored to avoid iatrogenic lung injury.

Nontoxic Concentrations of Oxygen

The harmful effects of high concentrations of inspired oxygen have long been recognized. The complex and dynamic balance between reactive molecular damage and reparative host defense in the injured lung is incompletely understood. Most clinicians strive for an FiO_2 less than 0.60 to avoid significant toxicity.

VENTILATION-PERFUSION RELATIONS

With these goals in mind, we will now address the principles most basic to ventilating a patient: what determines how the provision of inspired gas translates into the delivery of oxygen to and removal of CO_2 from the tissues.

The level of oxygen (PaO_2) yielded by a given FiO_2 is a function of the degree of the uniformity of distribution of ventilation and the degree of matching of ventilation and perfusion. Lung units that are empty of gas (as a result of atelectasis or flooding) require high pressures to open, and airflow takes the "path of least resistance." Therefore:

- Whether a lung unit is aerated at end expiration is extremely important in determining the ventilation it receives;
- Regional ventilation is a function of regional impedance to flow (i.e., regional resistance and compliance).

Distribution of blood flow is similarly affected by regional resistance in the blood vessels. This is a function of gravity, vasomotor tone, and other mechanical factors such as narrowing or tethering by adjacent lung volume and transpulmonary pressure. The body strives for optimal matching of ventilation and perfusion. Lung units that are ventilated but not perfused contribute to *dead space;* units that are perfused but not ventilated give rise to *shunt.* Hypoxic vasoconstriction is the body's defense against shunt; although regional alkalosis may encourage vasodilation, there is no mechanism to counteract dead space ventilation.

Ventilation and $PaCO_2$

The relationship between ventilation and $PaCO_2$ is governed by Equation 1. The practical implications of this equation are several. $PaCO_2$ is directly proportional to metabolic rate ($\dot{V}CO_2$) and inversely proportional to minute ventilation ($\dot{V}_E$). $\dot{V}_E$, and to a lesser extent $\dot{V}CO_2$, can thus be manipulated to effect the desired change in $PaCO_2$.

$$PaCO_2 = 0.863(\dot{V}CO_2)/[\dot{V}_E(1 - V_D/V_T)] \tag{1}$$

For a given $\dot{V}_E$, $PaCO_2$ varies directly with dead space. Because anatomic dead space does not vary in proportion to tidal volume (V_T), the dead space fraction increases as size of total V_T is decreased. In the presence of lung disease and/or increased extent of zone I (which can result from increasing V_T), alveolar dead space is increased sometimes to levels of 0.7 to 0.8.

Thoracic Pressure and Cardiac Function

A spontaneously breathing person generates cycles of negative pressure during inspiration that increase to zero (atmospheric) on expiration. The passive-ventilated patient receives cycles of positive inspiratory pressure that decrease to zero on expiration. In both cases these pressures (really the *transpulmonary* pressures) are transmitted to all intrathoracic structures. Venous return is a function of the pressure gradient from the peripheral blood vessels to the right atrium; this gradient is decreased when intrathoracic (and thus right atrial) pressure is increased. The afterload of the left ventricle (LV) is importantly influenced by the transmural pressure required to eject blood (LV transmural pressure = LV systolic pressure − intrathoracic pressure); hence an increase in intrathoracic pressure decreases the LV transmural pressure.

PPV, therefore, has several effects on cardiac function: decreased venous return and decreased LV afterload. There are also smaller and less predictable tendencies to increase LV preload (by "squeezing" blood out of the lungs) and variable effects on right ventricle (RV) afterload. In general, in patients with normal cardiac function and particularly in those starting out with diminished preload (e.g., with volume depletion or low vasomotor tone), PPV tends to decrease cardiac output. Patients with impaired cardiac function, on the other hand, may have augmented cardiac output with positive pressure as a result of more favorable loading conditions of the heart.

The effect on cardiac output is a key variable in the success of a ventilatory strategy because of its impact on oxygen delivery. The amount of oxygen delivered to tissues is expressed by the following equation:

$$DO_2 = 1.39(Hgb)(SaO_2)(cardiac\ output) + 0.003(PaO_2) \qquad (2)$$

It can be seen from this equation that ventilator settings that raise the PaO_2 at the expense of cardiac output may easily *decrease* O_2 delivery (important here is the position on the oxyhemoglobin dissociation curve; see Figure 12.2). The other impact of cardiac output on oxygenation is in determining mixed venous oxygen saturation ($SmvO_2$). If cardiac output is marginal or inadequate, tissues must extract more oxygen per milliliter of blood, lowering $SmvO_2$. As many cases of respiratory failure are accompanied by impaired gas exchange and impaired $\dot{V}/\dot{Q}$ relations, it may not be possible to fully saturate the blood before it exits the pulmonary circulation, thus lowering SaO_2.

INSTITUTING VENTILATORY SUPPORT
Noninvasive Ventilation

Not all MV requires endotracheal intubation; in some cases only a relatively brief period of moderate respiratory support is required to temporize until the underlying condition is improved. Noninvasive positive pressure ventilation (NPPV) involves the application of positive pressure through a tight sealing mask. This pressure can be delivered continuously (CPAP, continuous positive airway pressure), intermittently (IPPV, intermittent positive pressure ventilation), or both (i.e., CPAP with additional cyclic positive pressure excursions). When correctly applied to appropriate patients, NPPV can avoid the need for endotracheal intubation and its attendant risk of complications. Alternatively, NPPV can ease the transition to spontaneous ventilation of a recently extubated patient.

In addition to avoiding complications of endotracheal intubation, NPPV is generally more comfortable, tends to preserve the patient's own airway defense mechanisms, and allows the patient to speak and swallow. As the placement and removal of an endotracheal tube are not necessary, ventilatory support may be begun and withdrawn with greater flexibility than with conventional ventilation.

Mechanism of Action

• Decreased work of breathing;
• Increased efficiency of breathing;
• Support of the failing heart.

Decreased Work of Breathing

The inspiratory WOB has two components. First, any positive pressure remaining in the chest at end expiration (total PEEP, the sum of conventional PEEP and auto-

PEEP) must be counterbalanced (see Monitoring section for further discussion of auto-PEEP). Counterbalancing auto-PEEP or intrinsic PEEP (PEEPi) can account for up to 43% of the WOB in an exacerbation of obstructive lung disease. By decreasing the pressure gradient from distal to proximal airway at end expiration, CPAP reduces the work required of the inspiratory muscles to initiate inward flow.

The second component of inspiratory WOB is that required to draw fresh gas into the lungs. When there is high airflow resistance, "stiff" lungs, high $\dot{V}_E$ requirements, or weakened respiratory pump function, this load may result in respiratory failure. By giving a "boost" of positive pressure at the airway opening, the transpulmonary pressure is increased; consequently, the V_T entrained may be greater or the spontaneous work reduced.

Increased Efficiency of Breathing

When faced with an excessive inspiratory workload, the body's response is to decrease V_T and increase respiratory rate. Because the relative proportion of dead space ventilation (V_D/V_T) increases, this rapid shallow breathing tends to be inefficient. By increasing V_T, NPPV decreases V_D/V_T. Shallow breathing also promotes atelectasis, which impairs gas exchange through $\dot{V}/\dot{Q}$ mismatch; thus, NPPV also increases efficiency by improving $\dot{V}/\dot{Q}$ relations.

Support of the Failing Heart

The vicious synergism between cardiac and respiratory failure is frequently encountered in clinical practice. The effects of positive intrathoracic pressure on the loading conditions of the heart were discussed above. NPPV can initiate a beneficial synergy: as the heart is unloaded, pulmonary edema is decreased (because of decreased LV filling pressures plus redistribution of lung water). This improves airway resistance and lung compliance such that the large negative pleural pressure swings previously taxing the heart are no longer needed, and oxygenation and cardiac performance further improve.

Clinical Studies

Appropriate patient selection is crucial to the success of NPPV. As might be inferred from the effects of NPPV outlined above, this mode is best suited for a relatively stable patient whose main problem is pump failure, which is usually hypercapnic. Hypoxemic respiratory failure, particularly when caused by cardiogenic pulmonary edema and/or not expected to last longer than 24–48 hours, may also respond well.

Results of a recent large series of patients receiving NPPV are shown below (Meduri, 1996). Improvement tended to be proportional to the level of pressure applied; increased V_T, improved gas exchange, lower respiratory rate, and decreased diaphragmatic activity were documented. Overall, in experienced hands, endotra-

Table 12.3. Response to NPPV

Parameter	Hypoxemic Failure	Hypercapnic Failure	Hypercapnic Insufficiency	Refused Intubation	Total
No. (%)	41 (26)	52 (33)	22 (13)	26 (16)	158
Duration (hrs)[a]	26 (2–192)	22 (1–89)	22 (2–72)	31 (4–97)	25 (1–192)
ABG correction	20 (49)	31 (60)	13 (59)	15 (58)	88 (56)
ABG improvement	11 (26)	15 (29)	3 (14)	2 (8)	32 (20)
ABG no improvement	10 (24)	6 (11)	6 (27)	9 (35)	38 (24)
No. of intubations	14 (34)	15 (29)	10 (45)	NA	46 (35)
Intubated, died	5 (12)	1 (2)	4 (18)	NA	10 (6)
Complications[b]	8 (20)	6 (12)	3 (14)	3 (12)	25 (16)
Discontinue NPPV[c]	16	17	12	5	57 (36)
ICU mortality	9 (22)	1 (2)	4 (18)	2 (12)	25 (16)
Predicted mortality[d]	0.4 ± 0.19	0.26 ± 0.15	0.22 ± 0.19	0.40 ± 0.22	0.32 ± 0.19

(From Meduri GU, Turner RE, Abou-Shala N, et al. Noninvasive positive pressure ventilation via face mask: first-line intervention in patients with acute hypercapnic and hypoxemic respiratory failure. Chest 1996:183. Reprinted with permission.)
[a] Expressed as median and range (in parenthesis).
[b] Complications included facial skin necrosis in 20, nosocomial pneumonia in 1, auto-PEEP in 1, and gastric distension in 3.
[c] Reasons for discontinuing NPPV included inability to correct ABG values (20), inability to decrease dyspnea (7), intolerance to NPPV (6), hemodynamic instability (6), and secretion management (4).
[d] Predicted mortality by APACHE II score.
ABG, arterial blood gas. NPPV, noninvasive positive pressure ventilation.

cheal intubation can be avoided in up to 70% of patients in whom NPPV is used with subsequent decreased duration of MV and shorter ICU stay (Table 12.3).

Application of NPPV

NPPV can be given via nasal or full face mask. Nasal masks have the advantage of less dead space, less claustrophobia, and allow for better oral secretion clearance, speech, and oral intake. A full face mask tends to work better with extreme dyspnea (most of these patients tend to mouth breathe), bypasses nasal airway resistance, and does not depressurize when the mouth is opened.

In NPPV, the patient receives CPAP and/or an IPPV component. IPPV can be in the form of pressure support (most common) or mandatory ventilator breaths. When CPAP and IPPV are compared, each gives a comparable reduction in transdiaphragmatic pressure; however, CPAP reduces PEEPi more effectively than IPPV, and IPPV improves gas exchange more than CPAP. The combination of the two modalities seems to be superior to either applied alone (Table 12.4).

Meduri and coworkers have extensive experience in the area of NPPV; their algorithm for mask ventilation is shown below. Their points of emphasis include:

- Allow the patient to achieve full synchrony with the ventilator before strapping the mask in place.
- Use skin patches to reduce air leaks and prevent skin breakdown.
- The first 30–60 minutes of NPPV are crucial for troubleshooting problems, promoting patient comfort, monitoring for complications, and assessing response.

Table 12.4. Application of NPPV

1. Position the head of the bed at a 45° angle and place the harness behind the patient's head while explaining the modality to the patient.
2. Choose the correct mask size and type of cushion.
3. Connect the mask to the ventilator, similar to connecting an endotracheal tube.
4. Set initial ventilator settings: CPAP 0 cm H_2O, PSV 10 cm H_2O, and FiO_2 titrated to an O_2 saturation greater than 90%. Turn off the humidifier's heater and alarms.
5. Optional: apply wound care dressing on the nasal bridge.
6. Provide reassurance while holding the mask gently on the patient's face until the patient's respiration is in full synchrony with the ventilator.
7. Secure the mask with the harness. Avoid a tight fit, allowing enough space to pass two fingers beween straps and patient's face.
8. Adjust ventilator settings to CPAP 3–5 cm H_2O and PSV 10–25 cm H_2O to achieve V_T greater than or equal to 7 mL/kg and a respiratory rate less than 25 breaths/min. Set alarms on the ventilator (low pressure, high respiratory rate, and apnea) and backup rate.
9. Ask the patient to call for needs (repositioning the mask, pain or discomfort, expectoration, and oral intake) or development of complications (respiratory difficulties, abdominal distension, nausea, or vomiting).

From Meduri GU. Noninvasive positive pressure ventilation in patients with acute respiratory failure. Clin Chest Med 1996;17(3):539. Reprinted with permission.
CPAP, continuous positive airway pressure; PSV, pressure support ventilation.

Monitoring During NPPV

The monitoring of a patient receiving NPPV should be similar to that of an intubated patient (see Monitoring section below). Closer scrutiny may be required early in the course of NPPV because the patient does not necessarily have a secure airway or a guaranteed level of $\dot{V}_E$. As detailed by Meduri and colleagues, areas of special focus in NPPV include:

• Monitor for gastric distension;
• Monitor for leaks and skin pressure effects of mask;
• Monitor handling of oral secretions.

Conventional Mechanical Ventilation: The Initial Ventilatory Strategy

When it is determined that the patient requires intubation and MV, the clinician must select the initial ventilator settings. These include mode of ventilation, targeted V_T or airway pressure, minimum respiratory frequency, FiO_2, and desired PEEP level. As the major modes of ventilation require more lengthy discussion, we will begin with the other parameters.

Tidal Volume

Tidal volume (V_T) is generally chosen relative to the weight of the patient. In the past, tidal volumes in the range of 10 to 15 mL/kg (e.g., 700–1050 mL for a 70 kg patient) were used routinely. As the occurrence of barotrauma has been increasingly recognized, clinicians have moved toward smaller tidal volumes. A V_T of 8 to 10 mL/kg is now widely recommended, and in cases of "stiff" lungs, even smaller tidal volumes (4–6 mL/kg) may be used, as will be discussed later.

Frequency

The term *frequency* is used to refer to the respiratory rate set on the ventilator; since some patients generate spontaneous breaths, the total number of breaths per minute (respiratory rate) may exceed the set frequency. Although the choice of V_T is largely influenced by the size of the patient, a wide range of frequencies may be chosen in accordance with the physiologic needs and constraints of the patient. It is by setting the frequency that the clinician translates the chosen V_T into a level of $\dot{V}_E$ for the patient.

Minute Ventilation

$\dot{V}_E$ is the volume of gas moved in and out of the lungs in one minute. As was seen in Equation 1, $\dot{V}_E$ is a primary determinant of CO_2 elimination; the effects of $\dot{V}_E$ on oxygenation are important but indirect. Normal resting $\dot{V}_E$ is 4–6 L/min. In conditions of exercise (increased $\dot{V}CO_2$) and disease (increased V_D/V_T and/or increased $\dot{V}CO_2$), $\dot{V}_E$ requirements increase routinely to 10–12 L/min and may be as high as 20 or more. In addition, a number of CO_2-independent neurohumoral mechanisms may contribute to the patient's perceived need for $\dot{V}_E$—i.e., his or her respiratory drive (Table 12.5).

Inspired Oxygen Concentration

The FiO_2 should be set at the minimal level necessary to achieve an acceptable level of oxygen delivery while affording a safety margin against desaturation. A common clinical practice is to place the patient on 100% oxygen at the time of intubation and then to decrease FiO_2 fairly quickly (e.g., by increments of 10% every 10 minutes) following the patient's pulse oximetry as a guide, provided that a good correlation is noted between arterial blood gas (ABG) values and concurrent oximeter readings. A final saturation of 90–92% is generally adequate.

Table 12.5. Determinants of $\dot{V}_E$ Requirement

CO_2 production and acid-base status
Dead space fraction and efficiency of gas exchange
Neurohumoral mechanisms
Pain, anxiety
CNS dysfunction (stroke, meningitis)
Intrinsic lung processes
Edema, atelectasis, infarction

Mode of Ventilation

The mode of ventilation refers to the protocol that the ventilator uses to deliver gas to the patient. Each mode of ventilation is characterized by:

- How tidal gas delivery is determined;
- The response of the ventilator to patient respiratory efforts;
- The degree of clinician control over upper and lower limits on $\dot{V}_E$ and pressure.

Traditionally, ventilator modes have been classified according to the method of gas volume determination: in *flow-controlled, volume-cycled* modes, flow is controlled and a fixed V_T is set; in *pressure-regulated* modes, an applied pressure level is set. The reason for this distinction is that to expand the chest requires power—power in an amount equal to that required to overcome flow-resistive forces and any residual positive pressure remaining in the chest at end expiration (auto-PEEP). This relation is expressed in the modified equation of motion:

$$P = VR + \frac{V_T}{C} + PEEPi \qquad (3)$$

This equation shows that inspiratory pressure and flow are not independent variables; rather, they relate to each other via the impedance characteristics (compliance and resistance) of the system. Hence, the clinician can specify either the job to be done (i.e., expand the chest with a given flow profile to a given volume) or the available energy (i.e., apply a given pressure level for a given time interval), but not both. Volume-cycled ventilation (VCV) is an example of the former; pressure-regulated ventilation is an example of the latter.

Volume-cycled Ventilation

The modes of ventilation with which clinicians are usually most familiar—assist control ventilation (ACV) and synchronized intermittent mandatory ventilation (SIMV)—are both volume-cycled modes. In each of these modes there are several ways to characterize a breath: according to how it is triggered and according to how its structure (volume, flow, duration) is determined. The breath may be *ventilator-initiated* or it may be *patient-initiated.* The characteristics of the breath are either *mandatory,* i.e., clinician-mandated, or *spontaneous,* with volume, flow, and duration varying with the patient's inspiratory effort. All ventilator-initiated breaths are mandatory breaths; patient-initiated breaths may be mandatory or spontaneous. The key distinction between ACV and SIMV lies in the machine's response to patient-initiated breaths.

Assist Control Ventilation

ACV is the mode most commonly begun with when MV is instituted. In ACV, every patient-initiated breath is a mandatory breath, delivered with all the same flow characteristics as ventilator-triggered mandatory breaths. Well-adjusted ACV is a good mode to rest patients with because if flow demands are met, patient work is reduced to triggering the ventilator and no effort is required to draw gas through the circuit. It is important to meet the patient's flow demands for several reasons. First, if flow is perceived as too slow, the inspiratory effort may continue throughout the inspiratory phase, increasing WOB. Second, because in ACV every breath has the same architecture, an inappropriate flow rate will promote dyssynchrony.

While ACV is a good mode for patients with high ventilatory requirements, it can be disadvantageous, even dangerous, in patients with airflow obstruction. With ACV, a small increase in respiratory rate can translate into a large increase in $\dot{V}_E$, and significant dynamic hyperinflation (DH) may result. In a patient who is not closely monitored this can have serious consequences (hypotension, barotrauma), and, in general, ACV should not be used in the presence of severe airflow obstruction. A lesser but also important problem is the tendency to develop respiratory alkalosis, which is more common with ACV than with SIMV.

Synchronized Intermittent Mandatory Ventilation

In SIMV, the respiratory cycle can be thought of as divided into "windows" of time. Respiratory cycle length is determined by the set respiratory frequency; e.g., if the set frequency is 10, the respiratory cycle length is 6 seconds. At the beginning of the cycle, the mandatory breath window is open and the ventilator is poised to deliver a mandatory breath. If the patient makes an inspiratory effort, he or she will receive the preset V_T (this is a patient-triggered mandatory breath). Once the mandatory breath has been delivered, the mandatory breath window for that respiratory cycle closes and the spontaneous breath window opens. From this point until the end of the current respiratory cycle, an inspiratory effort yields only what the patient is capable of drawing from the ventilator (spontaneous breath). If the patient makes no inspiratory effort during the respiratory cycle, the ventilator gives a mandatory breath at the end of the cycle (ventilator-triggered mandatory breath) and no spontaneous breath window ever opens.

An advantage of SIMV is that it offers flexible support; the patient can trigger some, none, or all of the mandatory breaths, and the transition to weaning can be simply to turn down the SIMV rate. SIMV assures a secure minimum level of $\dot{V}_E$, but if the patient should become tachypneic, there is less likelihood of developing a respiratory alkalosis than with ACV because the spontaneous breaths in SIMV tend to be smaller than the mandatory breaths. Taking spontaneous breaths also tends to offset the hemodynamic impact of this mode.

The major disadvantage cited in SIMV is the tendency to increase WOB. The act of triggering the ventilator alone can impose significant WOB, and in SIMV, the patient must also pull the V_T for any desired spontaneous breaths. This workload can be minimized by an adequate preset level of $\dot{V}_E$ and/or augmenting spontaneous breaths with pressure support (see below). Some patients may find the variable tidal volumes and breath architecture (between mandatory and spontaneous breaths) unsettling.

Pressure-regulated Ventilation

Pressure Support Ventilation

Although it is often used in conjunction with SIMV, pressure support ventilation (PSV) is technically a pressure-regulated mode in that a pressure is set and V_T is variable. In PSV used alone, all breaths are spontaneous. When the patient makes an inspiratory effort, the ventilator pressurizes the system to a preset level and maintains that pressure level until the inspiratory effort ceases (usually recognized by a critical decrease in inspiratory flow rate). The effect of this pressurization is to give an inspiratory "boost," which augments V_T to a degree determined by the amount of pressure applied and the impedance of the respiratory system. Because the net effect of a given pressure support level is variable, it is generally best to think of PSV in terms of the V_T generated by the level rather than the absolute amount of pressure itself.

Low level PSV is that which results in a V_T of less than approximately 4 mL/kg. In conditions of respiratory muscle fatigue, pressure support in this range decreases WOB by allowing a decreased respiratory rate; the pressure support augments V_T such that the same $\dot{V}_E$ can be achieved at a lower respiratory rate.

In the range of pressure support associated with tidal volumes of 4 to 7 mL/kg, the effect of PSV is to decrease WOB by decreasing the patient's contribution to each V_T; V_T size tends to remain constant, but patient work decreases.

At high levels of pressure support, those resulting in tidal volumes of 7 to 9 mL/kg patient work is significantly offset, and any additional increases in pressure support level tend simply to increase the size of each V_T.

SIMV + Pressure Support

A common practice is to add a low level of pressure support to SIMV to take advantage of the guaranteed $\dot{V}_E$ and spontaneously breathing of SIMV while offsetting some of the imposed work. The pressure support level chosen should be that which results in an acceptable V_T, generally 300 mL or more. Pressure support may similarly be combined with pressure-controlled intermittent mandatory ventilation (discussed below) to smoothly support the spontaneous breaths with a waveform similar to that encountered during mandated breaths. Figure 12.1 shows a comparison of modes during ventilator-initiated and patient-initiated breaths.

Volume-assured Pressure Support (VAPS)

This newer mode is available on some ventilators, similar to SIMV + pressure support. In this mode, a pressure support level and a minimum V_T are chosen. If the patient effort is not sufficient to draw the minimum V_T, a constant flow breath begins to augment the V_T to the desired value.

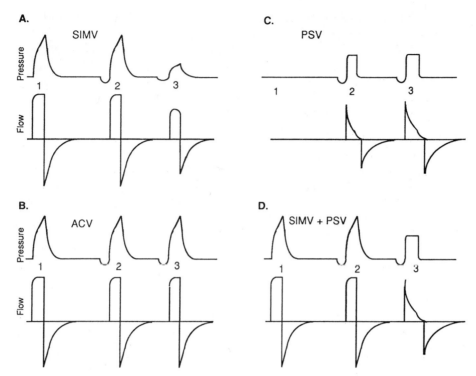

Figure 12.1. Comparison of pressure and flow waveforms during different modes of volume-cycled ventilation. In each panel, breath 1 is a ventilator-initiated mandatory breath, breath 2 is a patient-initiated mandatory breath, and breath 3 is a spontaneous breath. Note that in SIMV (**A**), the spontaneous breath has a different volume and architecture than the mandatory breaths; in ACV (**B**), all breaths are mandatory breaths. In PSV (**C**), there are no ventilator-initiated breaths and the V_T varies between breaths. The V_T of spontaneous breaths in SIMV + PSV (**D**) tend to be larger than in SIMV alone (**A,** breath 3).

Comparison of Modes

Work of Breathing

The degree of assistance provided by the ventilator (ratio of mandatory $\dot{V}_E$ to total $\dot{V}_E$; $\dot{V}E_m/\dot{V}_E$ tot) determines the WOB in SIMV. When $\dot{V}E_m/\dot{V}_E$ tot is low (< 0.5), WOB is higher in SIMV than in ACV. Provided there is good synchrony with the ventilator, WOB is generally less with ACV than with SIMV. The WOB in PSV varies with pressure support level as described above.

EFFECT ON ABG

Spontaneous breathing is associated with improved $\dot{V}/\dot{Q}$ relationships relative to passive ventilation, as a result of preferential ventilation of dependent lung regions with active diaphragm movement. Oxygenation may theoretically be improved with low level SIMV and PSV relative to ACV, although this difference might also be offset by an increased oxygen cost of breathing.

Because of higher $\dot{V}_E$, there is a tendency toward lower $PaCO_2$ and higher pH with ACV than with SIMV. Alterations in dead space fraction and CO_2 production may also play a role.

HEMODYNAMIC EFFECTS

As discussed earlier, positive intrathoracic pressure (from PPV and/or PEEP) tends to decrease RV preload and increase LV afterload, whereas negative intrathoracic pressure has the opposite effect. The net effect in an individual patient depends on the magnitude and duration of pressure swings, the functional status of the myocardium, and the volume status of the patient. There is a tendency toward higher cardiac output with SIMV than with ACV.

Pressure-controlled Ventilation

Although commonly used in neonatal ventilation, pressure-controlled ventilation (PCV) is infrequently the initial mode of ventilation in adult patients; rather, it is a mode used when a volume-cycled mode fails to meet oxygenation goals or generates undesirably high pressures. In PCV, the clinician sets the pressure that the ventilator will generate with each breath, the duration that the pressure will be applied, and the frequency of breaths; flow profile is always decelerating flow and peak flow rate is determined by the inspiratory time fraction. The duration of inspiration may be set as a fraction of the respiratory cycle or it may be set as an absolute number in seconds. The V_T generated in this mode, then, becomes a function of pressure level, inspiratory time, and, importantly, the impedance (resistance and compliance) of the respiratory system and the pressure gradient from airway to alveolus at the onset of inspiration. Thus, just as pressure varies breath to breath in VCV, so volume varies breath to breath in PCV.

PCV offers several potential advantages over VCV. For a given mean airway pressure, PCV tends to improve oxygenation, probably because of improved distribution of ventilation. PCV sets an upper limit on peak airway and thus maximal alveolar pressure, potentially limiting barotrauma.

Disadvantages of PCV include:

- Variable $\dot{V}_E$. There is no guaranteed minimum level of $\dot{V}_E$ in PCV; the clinician must depend on appropriately set and responded to ventilator alarms to warn that $\dot{V}_E$ has changed significantly.
- Need for sedation. Flow and I:E ratio may be nonphysiologic in PCV, and dyssynchrony may be problematic if the patient is not heavily sedated.
- Lack of clinician familiarity. Because most clinicians do not use this mode routinely, many may not have the appropriate reflex responses (e.g., if increased $\dot{V}_E$ is desired, increasing the frequency may have the opposite effect if PEEPi develops and V_T falls).

Special Modes of Ventilation

Inverse-ratio Ventilation

"Inverse ratio" refers to a lengthening of the inspiratory fraction of the duty cycle. Inverse-ratio ventilation (IRV) is an alternative mode for patients, usually with ARDS, in whom oxygenation is either inadequate or achieved only at potentially injurious levels of pressure or toxic concentrations of oxygen with a conventional ventilatory strategy. IRV can be applied with either volume- or pressure-cycled ventilation.

RATIONALE

The theory behind prolonging inspiratory time is as follows: a longer inspiratory time promotes gas mixing between alveolus and distal airways, and the increased alveolar "dwell time" increases the exposure of capillary blood to fresh gas. Extending inspiratory time also increases mean airway pressure without increasing alveolar pressure (provided there is no significant rise in PEEPi), thus promoting oxygenation through alveolar recruitment and the redistribution of lung water.

Drawbacks of IRV are similar to those seen with PCV: shortened expiratory time may result in DH, heavy sedation is almost always required for patient tolerance, and there may be deleterious hemodynamic consequences.

High-frequency Ventilation

In spontaneous breathing and conventional MV, gas delivery is accomplished by bulk flow. In high-frequency ventilation (HFV), very small tidal volumes (sometimes smaller than anatomic dead space) are delivered at high frequencies by jets or oscillators. Frequencies may be higher than 100 breaths per minute in adults and higher than 300 breaths per minute in infants. Proposed mechanisms for gas transport relate to the presence of several kinds of flow within the airway and principles of gas mixing within lung units.

RATIONALE

The unique flow characteristics of HFV are thought to enhance gas delivery and improve $\dot{V}/\dot{Q}$ relations in the heterogeneous environment of the acutely injured lung. The smaller pressure swings and lower peak pressures are believed to reduce the risk of barotrauma.

HFV requires a special ventilator and considerable experience to be applied and adjusted safely. Complications associated with HFV include inspissation of secretions and potentially severe tracheobronchitis as a result of the high flows and gas trapping.

MONITORING DURING MECHANICAL VENTILATION

Once the patient is settled on the initial ventilator settings, the clinician must evaluate both the efficacy and consequences of the initial strategy. Monitoring during MV is an ongoing process that involves interrogation of the ventilator and assessment of the patient to understand the effects of the current strategy and to plan and implement modifications of that strategy. The focus is on parameters of gas exchange and O_2 delivery, lung mechanics, and the state of the patient's respiratory neuromuscular function and WOB. The first stage of this assessment is relatively straightforward: assure that the ABCs of airway, breathing, and circulation are met.

Airway: Endotracheal Tube Position

Use of end-tidal CO_2 detection devices is a routine part of intubation in most institutions. The detection of exhaled CO_2 confirms placement within the airway with good sensitivity; however, it does not assure optimal positioning of the tube. A chest x-ray should be obtained immediately postintubation and the location of the tip of the endotracheal tube ascertained. The tip should be positioned 2–6 cm above the carina, keeping in mind head position at the time of the x-ray; the tip may rise or descend approximately 4 cm with extremes of neck extension and flexion, respectively.

Breathing: Adequacy of Gas Exchange and Oxygen Delivery

Arterial Blood Gas

An ABG should be checked within the first 30 minutes of instituting MV and periodically thereafter. Changes affecting oxygenation are largely complete within 10 minutes, whereas $PaCO_2$ changes occur more slowly (30–60 min).

Pulse Oximetry

Pulse oximetry provides a convenient noninvasive measurement of oxygenation using spectrophotometric principles to determine the SaO_2 of hemoglobin. Pulse oximetry can be useful in titrating FiO_2 provided that the clinician bears in mind the following principles:

- The shape of the oxyhemoglobin dissociation curve (Fig. 12.2) renders SaO_2 insensitive to significant changes in PaO_2 on the "flat portion" of the curve ($SaO_2 > 94\%$). An SaO_2 below 90% can represent dangerously low levels of PaO_2.
- Variation in skin pigmentation can influence SaO_2. Darker skin pigment may cause a falsely high measured SaO_2. The effect is variable, and correlation with ABG values should be obtained for each patient.
- Anemia and hyperbilirubinemia by themselves do not generally interfere with the accuracy of pulse oximetry.

Circulation: Hemodynamics

As discussed earlier, in a normal heart, cardiac output is sensitive to changes in preload and PPV tends to decrease cardiac output by decreasing venous return.

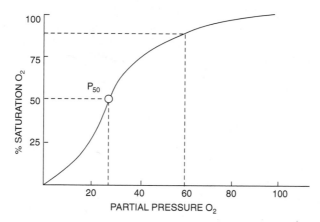

Figure 12.2. Oxyhemoglobin dissociation curve. Note the nonlinear relation of the partial pressure of oxygen in plasma (PaO_2) and the arterial oxygen saturation (SaO_2): at low PaO_2 (< 60 mm Hg) there is a greater change in SaO_2 for a given change in PaO_2 than at a higher PaO_2 (> 60 mm Hg).

Failing myocardium is more sensitive to changes in afterload, and cardiac output can be augmented by positive pressure-induced decreases in LV transmural pressure.

The level of mean airway pressure, as a best practical estimate of mean alveolar pressure, is most closely associated with the tendency toward hemodynamic compromise. The degree to which alveolar pressure is transmitted to the pleural space depends on the relative compliances of the lung and chest wall; the hemodynamic effect of a given change in mean airway pressure will be greater when the lungs are relatively compliant and/or the chest wall is relatively stiff. In a patient with volume depletion or low vasomotor tone (e.g., sepsis), the tendency for PPV to decrease filling pressures of the heart will be accentuated. The generation of negative pleural pressure by spontaneous inspiratory efforts tends to counter the effects of positive pressure.

Relevant Principles of Lung Mechanics

Having assured that gas exchange and hemodynamics are acceptable, the mechanical properties of the patient-ventilator system should be assessed. The pressure required to deliver a given V_T over a given inspiratory time is a function of the elastic and resistive properties of the system. In a ventilator, the system includes the ventilator circuit, endotracheal tube, patient airways, lung parenchyma, and chest wall.

Compliance

Compliance reflects the elasticity or stiffness of the respiratory system and is measured in milliliters per centimeter H_2O. Normal supine lung compliance is approximately 100 mL/cm H_2O; in ARDS the compliance may decrease to levels as low

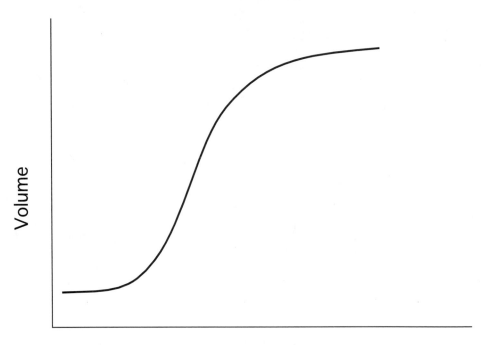

Transpulmonary Pressure

Figure 12.3. Pressure-volume (PV) curve of the normal respiratory system. Compliance equals the change in lung volume for a given change in distending pressure (i.e., dV/dP or the tangential slope of the PV curve at any point). dV/dP, change in volume/change in pressure.

as 20 mL/cm H_2O; i.e., the application of 1 cm H_2O pressure would only inflate the ARDS lung by 20 mL, whereas the same pressure applied to the normal lung would achieve a volume of 100 mL.

Compliance is greatest (i.e., greatest change in volume for a given change in pressure) in the midvolume range and lowest at high and low lung volumes (Fig. 12.3). At high volumes, the lung units may be overdistended and have little increase in volume for a given increase in pressure. At low volumes, some units are collapsed and require pressure to be opened; until the critical opening pressure is reached, increases in pressure yield little increase in volume.

Resistance

Resistance is impedance to flow. In ventilated patients there are two components to resistance: resistance of the endotracheal tube and resistance of the patient's airways. The relative contribution of each is variable. Resistance contributed by the endotracheal tube varies with endotracheal tube lumen size and gas flow rate; smaller tube diameter and higher flow rates increase resistance. Airway resistance may fluctuate and is significantly affected by lung volume; at higher volumes, airways are tethered open and resistance decreases. In patients with obstructive lung disease, airway resistance tends to outweigh endotracheal tube resistance.

The relationship between pressure, flow, and resistance is shown in Equation 4, where P = pressure, $\dot{V}$ = flow, and R = resistance. Note the parallel to the familiar physics equation governing flow of electrons, V = IR, where V = voltage, akin to pressure; I = current, akin to gas flow; and R = resistance.

$$P = \dot{V}R \qquad\qquad (4)$$

Intrinsic PEEP

Also known as auto-PEEP, PEEPi is present when a positive pressure gradient from the alveolus to the airway opening exists at end expiration. Most commonly this occurs as a result of incomplete exhalation caused by airflow obstruction and/or high $\dot{V}_E$; in this case, DH is said to be present. During DH, functional residual capacity (FRC, the end-expiratory or relaxed lung volume) progressively increases until a new steady state is reached at which the lung recoil pressure generated by each subsequent V_T is sufficient to drive full exhalation of that volume. PEEPi can exist in the absence of DH when there is ongoing active contraction of expiratory muscles at end expiration.

PEEPi has several important consequences:

- Lung compliance may decrease if DH shifts the position of the respiratory system up to a less favorable portion of the pressure-volume curve (closer to total lung capacity).
- The WOB and/or triggering the ventilator may be increased because of a need to counterbalance the PEEPi to initiate inspiratory flow.
- Hemodynamics may be adversely affected as with any other positive intrathoracic pressure, as previously described.

Ventilator-based Monitoring

The above principles come directly into play when we turn to assess the patient and the patient-ventilator interaction via the ventilator. The clinician should inspect the pressure readings and waveforms (if available) on every ventilated patient. The pressures noted on the ventilator may be within an acceptable range and formal calculations of compliance and resistance need not be made; in other cases, the readings may point to a problem that must be investigated and corrected.

Ventilator Pressures

PEAK PRESSURE

The peak airway pressure (Ppk) is the maximum pressure generated in the airway as the V_T moves into the system. This is the pressure generated by forcing a given flow through the airways and expanding the lungs and chest wall with the V_T. This pressure is therefore a function of flow rate and of the resistance and compliance of the system. Ppk is directly observable from the manometer and often from a digital display on the ventilator. In general, it is desirable to keep peak pressures below 45 cm H_2O. The potential adverse consequences of an elevated Ppk depend on the cause of the elevation and therefore the cause should always be determined. Most agree that high peak pressure as a result of increased airways resistance is less serious than high peak pressure resulting from decreased compliance because flow-resistive pressure is not directly transmitted to the alveoli, the site of barotrauma.

PLATEAU PRESSURE

The plateau pressure (Pplat) is the pressure present in the system at end inspiration; flow has come to zero, so all flow-resistive pressure is gone, and the pressure present is caused by the presence of that specific volume distending the lung and chest wall plus the level of any PEEPi present. Pplat is measured by setting an end-inspiratory pause of 1 second on the ventilator and noting the level at which the manometer plateaus during the pause (some ventilators also have a digital display). The presence of respiratory effort must be looked for (visually and by palpation of the abdominal muscles) because this will affect the observed Pplat value: ongoing active expiration will raise the observed Pplat and inspiratory effort will lower it.

INTRINSIC PEEP

PEEPi may be measured in many different ways, each with advantages and pitfalls. Detailed discussion of these methods is beyond the scope of this chapter. One traditional method for measuring PEEPi is to place an end-expiratory hold on the ventilator and determine the pressure level present at exactly the time that the next inspiration is supposed to begin. This method becomes unreliable in the actively breathing patient because it is affected by respiratory effort as described above. It has been recently suggested that in the presence of severe airflow obstruction, some airways close at end expiration and hence do not communicate with the airway opening, thereby "hiding" the positive pressure distal to the point of closure (Leatherman, 1996). Because the physical presence of this trapped gas reduces the number of available air channels and makes the surrounding lung region stiffer, the effective compliance of the lung is lowered. Changes in Pplat, therefore, can be used as a proxy for auto-PEEP. In patients with airflow obstruction, the presence of an elevated Pplat has been shown to be a reliable indicator of the presence of DH.

It is important to measure the Pplat and PEEP when trying to sort out the cause of increased peak pressure. An elevated Ppk may be caused by high flow rates, increased airways resistance, decreased respiratory system compliance, or a combination of these. The contribution of airways resistance is estimated by calculating the difference between the peak and plateau pressures. If the difference between Ppk and Pplat is greater than 10–15 cm H_2O, increased resistance is present. Resistance should then be formally calculated using Equation 5. Normal resistance is 2–6 cm H_2O/L/sec; the causes of elevated resistance are listed in Table 12.6.

$$R = (Ppk - \text{total PEEP})/\text{flow in liters per second} \qquad (5)$$

Table 12.6. Causes of Increased Resistance

Endotracheal tube
  High flow rate
  Small lumen
    Kinking
    Biting
    Secretions
Airways
  Bronchospasm
  Secretions
  Low lung volumes (uncommon)

An elevated Pplat indicates a decrease in the compliance of the system as a result of an abnormality in lung volume (high or low), lung parenchyma, or chest wall (including diaphragm/abdomen). As above, PEEPi will decrease the effective compliance, but not the actual lung tissue compliance. Because PEEPi must be measured (to obtain total PEEP), it will become clear if the increased Pplat is because of PEEPi. Compliance may be calculated by the following equation (see also Table 12.7):

$$C = \text{tidal volume in liters/Pplat} - \text{total PEEP} \qquad (6)$$

Pressure and Flow Tracings

A major advance in MV has been the provision of real-time tracings, allowing the clinician to observe the pattern of airway pressure and gas flow as well as the dynamic pressure-volume relationship in the ventilated patient. As will be discussed

Table 12.7. Causes of Decreased Compliance

Stiff lungs
  Edema
  Consolidation
  Fibrosis
  Atelectasis
  Lung volume close to RV or TLC
Stiff chest wall
  Kyphoscoliosis or other chest wall deformity
  Obesity
  Ascites or abdominal distention
External lung compression
  Pneumothorax
  Pleural effusion
Dynamic hyperinflation

---

shortly, each inspiratory flow pattern creates a characteristic flow and pressure tracing. Examination of the tracings for evidence of deviation from the ideal profile and assessment of the effect on the waveform of altering ventilator settings gives clues to lung mechanics, as well as to patient effort and synchrony. It is important for clinicians to be familiar with the waveforms showing overdistension, PEEPi, and dyssynchrony, shown in Figure 12.4.

Patient-based Monitoring

The interaction between the patient and the ventilator is key to the outcome of any ventilatory strategy. Areas to be assessed include:

- Can the patient trigger the ventilator easily?
- Is the patient's breathing in synchrony with the ventilator?
- Is the overall WOB acceptable?
- What has been the effect on hemodynamics and volume status, and how can they be optimized?

Patient-Ventilator Interaction

In assessing the patient-ventilator interaction, the first step is simply to look at the patient. Does the patient look comfortable? If the patient does not appear comfortable, does this seem to be related to or independent of the presence of MV? (This is not always easy to discern.)

TRIGGERING

Of importance here are both the *set* sensitivity and the *effective* sensitivity of the ventilator. A patient triggers the ventilator by making an inspiratory effort that decreases the level of either a base pressure or a base flow that the ventilator monitors constantly; when a threshold level of decrease is achieved, triggering occurs and the patient has access to fresh gas in the form of either a mandatory or a spontaneous breath. *Set sensitivity* refers to the threshold decrease set by the clinician (-2 cm H_2O is a standard setting); *effective sensitivity* may be higher in the presence of PEEPi. For example, if the patient has 8 cm H_2O of PEEPi and the set sensitivity is a -2 cm H_2O pressure decrease, that patient must pull down a total of 10 cm H_2O pressure to trigger the ventilator, hence the effective sensitivity is -10 cm H_2O. Adding a small amount of external PEEP can help restore the sensitivity of the system; adding 75% of the level of PEEPi is recommended, in this case, 6 cm H_2O. Additional causes of difficulty triggering the ventilator are a narrow endotracheal tube, airway obstruction, and bronchospasm.

FLOW DEMANDS

Depending on the patient's respiratory drive, the inspiratory flow rate may meet, exceed, or fall short of the demands of the patient. A patient who seems to tense abdominal muscles during inspiratory flow may be perceiving the inspiratory flow

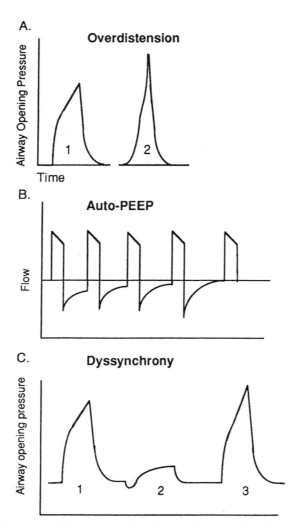

Figure 12.4. Common problems revealed in flow tracings. **A.** Overdistension: breath 1 has the ideal profile of a constant flow breath; breath 2 has an abrupt rise in pressure midway through the breath, signifying overdistension. **B.** Auto-PEEP: note that in breaths 1–3, expiratory flow does not come to zero before the next inspiration starts. As the respiratory rate slows, allowing longer expiratory time, expiratory flow comes to zero. **C.** Dyssynchrony: breath 1 has the ideal pressure profile of a constant flow breath. In breath 2, patient inspiratory effort has deformed the pressure profile by exerting negative pressure on the system. In breath 3, active expiratory effort resisting the mandatory breath deforms the profile by increasing pressure at the end of the inspiration.

rate as too high, and the patient should be reassessed at a lower flow rate or longer inspiratory time. A patient who continues a strong inspiratory effort well into inspiration needs a higher peak inspiratory flow. Potential solutions include:

- Increase set inspiratory flow rate;
- Change to decelerating flow pattern to give highest flow at the onset of inspiration; peak flow rate must be increased to avoid compromising expiratory time;
- Change to a pressure support mode that may be capable of generating higher initial flows, depending on the pressure set.

Cardiovascular Interactions

HEMODYNAMICS AND FLUID RETENTION

The immediate hemodynamic effects of PPV were reviewed above. Over the ensuing hours to days of MV, there is a tendency for most patients to retain fluid. This occurs for several reasons:

- Immobility;
- Decreased venous return stimulates atrial receptors and ADH secretion is increased;
- Positive pressure-induced decrease in cardiac output and/or blood pressure leads to alterations in renal blood flow, stimulating sodium and water reabsorption;
- Hypoalbuminemia is common among ventilated patients (cause unclear).

Fluid retention associated with MV is best managed by optimization of hemodynamics and judicious use of diuretics. If large amounts of fluid have been retained, the patient should be closely observed because detrimental fluid shifts may occur during the transition to spontaneous breathing.

TAILORING THE VENTILATORY STRATEGY

After making an initial assessment of the patient's hemodynamics, mechanics, and interaction with the ventilator, the next step is to tailor the ventilatory strategy according to the needs of the patient and the goals of the clinician.

PEEP

Positive end-expiratory pressure is an important tool in MV. The effects on ease of triggering and altering loading conditions of the heart were discussed earlier. The primary use of PEEP, however, is to improve oxygenation and lung mechanics by recruiting lung volume and redistributing lung water.

Recruitment of Lung Volume

PEEP increases the FRC of the respiratory system by recruiting collapsed or minimally ventilated terminal airspaces and further expanding already open lung units.

In the heterogeneous environment of lung injury, these processes may occur simultaneously and to varying degrees; PEEP helps to maintain the patency of "marginal" alveoli that might otherwise collapse at end expiration. To the extent that PEEP recruits lung units, compliance is increased; to the extent that alveolar overdistension occurs, compliance is worsened. The pressure-volume relationship of the respiratory system (compliance curve) constructed using airway opening pressure simply reflects their net effect.

Redistribution of Lung Water

PEEP redistributes edema fluid from the alveoli into the interstitial space by altering the balance of hydrostatic forces. Edema redistribution improves lung compliance and tends to offset surfactant inactivation by proteinaceous edema fluid.

Overall beneficial effects of PEEP include:

- Improved overall $\dot{V}/\dot{Q}$ matching by increased surface area for gas exchange, favorable redistribution of perfusion, and decreased shunt as a result of decreased cardiac output;
- Improved compliance;
- Decreased resistance (higher lung volumes).

Architecture of Gas Delivery

Inspiratory Flow Profile

In VCV, the clinician has several options for the pattern of gas flow during inspiration. The most commonly used flow profiles are *constant flow* (square wave), *decelerating flow* (decelerating ramp), and *sine wave* flow. Although it has been suggested recently that decelerating flow may be advantageous in the diseased lung, no clear overall advantage of one waveform over another has been shown. For the individual patient, however, one flow profile may serve the goals of the clinician or demands of the patient better than another.

CONSTANT FLOW

For a given V_T and inspiratory time, constant flow generates higher peak pressures and shorter inspiratory times than decelerating flow ("decel"). Because flow is constant, airflow resistance is constant, and therefore airway pressure tracings can be interrogated for information on lung compliance.

DECELERATING FLOW

Here flow rate is linearly decelerating, at a rate specific to the ventilator being used. For a given V_T, this flow pattern and peak flow rate will give a lower peak pressure and longer inspiratory time than will constant flow; inspiratory time can be shortened by increasing peak inspiratory flow rate. This flow profile "front loads" the breath, which may suit the demands of a patient with a high respiratory drive and may promote more even distribution among lung units with heterogeneous time constants.

Peak Inspiratory Flow Rate

The choice of inspiratory flow rate is especially important in patients who are spontaneously triggering the ventilator, particularly in those with a high respiratory drive. Ideally, the inspiratory flow rate should match the patient's demand to minimize patient WOB and maximize synchrony.

The usual range for inspiratory flow is 40–80 L/min. High flow rates (80–100 L/min) may be used to meet patients' flow demand and/or to shorten inspiratory time. Increases in peak pressure caused solely by an increase in inspiratory flow rate tend to dissipate in the large airways, are not transmitted to the alveoli, and therefore are unlikely to cause barotrauma. Low inspiratory flow rates are sometimes used to prolong inspiratory time, thus raising mean airway pressure (Fig. 12.5) and enhancing alveolar recruitment and gas mixing. Very slow rates of inspiratory flow, however, can restrict the expiratory time sufficiently to result in gas trapping.

I:E Ratio

The way in which inspiratory time and I:E ratio are determined varies among ventilators. In some, inspiratory time can be set as a fixed fraction of the respiratory cycle length (Ttot) so that the absolute value of inspiratory time will vary with breath frequency. In others, inspiratory time and time fraction are the result of clinician-set inspiratory flow rate, V_T, and breath frequency. Finally, if the absolute inspiratory time is set, expiratory time and I:E ratio vary with respiratory frequency.

Factors to consider when manipulating inspiratory time fraction include the presence and vigor of spontaneous breathing, the presence of airflow obstruction, and the oxygenation and hemodynamic responses to manipulating airway pressure. In a spontaneously breathing patient, I:E ratio should approximate the patient's own breathing pattern, which varies from approximately 0.25 at slow frequencies to approximately 0.5 during maximal effort. Inspiratory time remains relatively constant at 0.8–1.2 seconds. In the presence of significant airflow obstruction or high $\dot{V}_E$, inspiratory time fraction should be shortened to allow sufficient expiratory time. Hemodynamic compromise generally occurs in direct proportion to the level and duration of positive intrathoracic pressure; a shortened inspiratory time tends to mitigate hemodynamic effect. Conversely, in a passive patient, oxygenation is enhanced by prolonging inspiratory time and elevating mean airway pressure; peak flow rate, flow profile, and the addition of an inspiratory pause are all used to this end. Considerable sedation may be needed for patients to tolerate an extended inspiratory time.

Adjuncts to Mechanical Ventilation

In some patients, even optimally tailored ventilator settings are not sufficient to meet the needs of the patient or the goals of the clinician. A number of adjuncts are available to enhance oxygenation and promote CO_2 excretion.

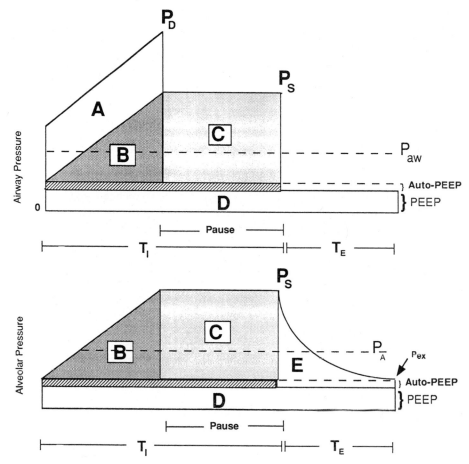

Figure 12.5. Schematic drawings of an idealized pressure tracing for one respiratory cycle during constant flow mechanical ventilation. **Top: A,** nonelastic (frictional); **B,** tidal elastic; **C,** pause; **D,** positive end-expiratory pressure (PEEP) component. The *cross-hatched area* corresponds to auto-positive end-expiratory pressure (auto-PEEP). Note that auto-PEEP adds to airway pressure only during inspiration since airway pressure decreases to the set PEEP level during exhalation. Bottom: **B, C, D,** and *cross-hatched areas* are as defined above; *E,* expiratory frictional component. P_D, peak dynamic pressure; P_S, peak static pressure; P_{aw}, mean airway pressure; P_A, mean alveolar pressure; *Pex*, end-expiratory alveolar pressure; T_I, inspiratory time; T_E, expiratory time. (From Marini JJ, Ravenscraft SA. Mean airway pressure: physiological determinants and clinical importance. I. Physiological determinants and measurements. Crit Care Med 1992;20:1461–1472. Reprinted with permission.)

Enhancing Oxygenation

In a patient who is difficult to oxygenate, one should begin with the simplest, least invasive maneuvers. The patient should be aggressively diuresed as indicated and tolerated, and the mechanics of the thoracic cavity should be optimized (i.e., any collections of air, pleural fluid, or ascites thought to infringe on ventilation should be evacuated). If this fails to improve oxygenation sufficiently, the following adjuncts should be considered.

MINIMIZE O_2 CONSUMPTION

- Avoid agitation and fever, which elevate $\dot{V}CO_2$;
- Maximize ventilator synchrony to minimize WOB;
- Optimize sedation to decrease respiratory drive;
- Consider neuromuscular blockade in refractory cases.

PRONE POSITIONING

For many years it has been known that some patients experience a significant improvement in oxygenation when they are placed in the prone position.

Mechanism

Although investigation is ongoing into the exact mechanisms of benefit in prone positioning, it is clear that $\dot{V}/\dot{Q}$ relationships improve in those who respond. CT studies demonstrate that previously atelectatic dorsal regions are better ventilated in the prone position, while blood flow to those regions is well-maintained. In animal models, shunt fraction is decreased and FRC is increased, and the gradient of pleural pressures is decreased. The sustained benefit from prone positioning suggests that the effect is not simply one of redistribution of atelectasis and edema.

Clinical Studies

Although the majority of patients placed prone have improved oxygenation, not all of them do; a small minority experience deterioration in oxygenation and hemodynamics. Patients who improve within the first 30 minutes are likely to show continued improvement at 120 minutes (Pappert).

Application

Prone positioning should be considered for hemodynamically stable patients in early ARDS who have significantly impaired oxygenation ($PaO_2/FiO_2 < 100$). Practical considerations in turning the patient include:

- Caution with the head, central lines, endotracheal and chest tubes.
- Appropriate support of the upper chest and pelvis with pillows to allow easy excursion of chest and abdomen and to decrease facial edema.
- Return of the patient to the supine position at least for a brief period once or twice daily for routine cares.

Complications

Facial edema and pressure injury to weight-bearing areas are the most frequent adverse sequelae of prone positioning. The potential morbidity of dislodging lines and tubes can be decreased with appropriate care. At present, it is not possible to predict which previously hemodynamically stable patient will deteriorate with turning.

NITRIC OXIDE

Previously called endothelium-derived relaxing factor, nitric oxide is a potent vasodilator produced both constitutively and inducibly by vascular endothelium. It is quickly inactivated by hemoglobin, to which it binds with high affinity. Inhaled nitric oxide is used experimentally as a selective pulmonary vasodilator. Delivered by the inhaled route, nitric oxide preferentially vasodilates ventilated regions, thus diverting blood from less well-ventilated areas and improving $\dot{V}/\dot{Q}$ matching. Nitric oxide also acts to decrease pulmonary artery pressure, which decreases RV afterload, helps restore adaptive vasoconstriction (further improving $\dot{V}/\dot{Q}$ relations), and may decrease formation of interstitial edema.

Clinical Studies

In patients with ARDS, nitric oxide has been shown to decrease pulmonary artery pressure, decrease intrapulmonary shunting, and increase PaO_2/FiO_2 ratio with no effect on mean arterial pressure or cardiac output and little apparent tachyphylaxis (Roissant). Nitric oxide has been used in adults with primary pulmonary hypertension, postchest surgery, and to relax hypercapnic pulmonary vasoconstriction. It has also been used in children, with persistent pulmonary hypertension of the newborn, congenital heart disease, and a variety of acute lung injury states.

Application

At present, nitric oxide is available only in experimental clinical trials by approved investigators. Nitric oxide is delivered through attachments to or within the ventilator circuit, at concentrations ranging from 2 to 80 parts per million. The circuit is equipped with a scavenging system to prevent escape into ambient air.

Adverse Effects

Toxicity issues regarding nitric oxide remain under investigation. Animal studies have shown no toxicity with prolonged exposure to low concentration; high-dose exposure can cause methemoglobinemia and pulmonary edema. There is also concern over the effect of oxidant radical formation. Rebound pulmonary vasoconstriction and hypoxemia may occur after long-term use, presumably as a result of suppressed constitutive enzymatic products of nitric oxide metabolism. Slow weaning of nitric oxide may be required in such patients.

AEROSOLIZED PROSTACYCLIN

The rationale for aerosolized prostacyclin is similar to that for inhaled nitric oxide. Prostacyclin, or PGI_2, is a potent vasodilator of both the pulmonary and systemic circulations. Delivered by the aerosolized route, via intermittent or continuous nebulization, PGI_2 acts preferentially in better ventilated regions. Aerosolized PGI_2 has been used in patients with primary and secondary pulmonary hypertension and in patients with ARDS. Walmrath and colleagues compared aerosolized PGI_2 to inhaled nitric oxide and found the drugs to be of equal efficacy in reducing shunt fraction and pulmonary artery pressure and in increasing the PaO_2/FiO_2 ratio. Any impact on ARDS mortality remains to be determined.

SURFACTANT REPLACEMENT THERAPY

A mainstay in the treatment of respiratory distress syndrome of the newborn (a condition of surfactant deficiency), surfactant replacement therapy (SRT) has also been used to treat adults with acute lung injury.

Mechanism

Patients with ARDS have been shown to have impaired surfactant function and production, as well as reduced total amount of surfactant. These alterations increase the tendency for alveolar flooding and collapse, and hence the tendency toward decreased lung compliance and ventilation-perfusion mismatching. The exogenous replacement of surfactant attempts to restore normal surface tension in lung units.

Clinical Studies

Although clearly life-saving in the newborn, the benefit of surfactant in the treatment of ARDS is less clear. While some randomized studies have shown survival benefit (Weg), others have not (Anzueto), and the role for SRT in ARDS remains to be defined. Its value may well depend on the nature of the surfactant used and on the mode and timing of its administration.

Application

Recombinant surfactant is given endotracheally, either instilled as liquid or nebulized. The large volumes of liquid required in adults (150–200 mL) are problematic and may result in clogging of ventilator filters.

PARTIAL LIQUID VENTILATION

Partial liquid ventilation (PLV) employs a dense liquid perfluorocarbon with high gas solubility and low surface tension to replace the lung-gas interface with lung-liquid and liquid-gas interfaces in the hope of improving oxygenation and decreasing shearing forces and barotrauma. This modality is called *partial* liquid ventilation because rather than filling the entire system with liquid, the lungs are filled to a volume equivalent to FRC. The patient is then ventilated with a conventional ventilatory mode.

Mechanism

Described by some as "liquid PEEP," it is proposed that the dense fluid recruits atelectatic lung units, particularly in dependent regions. This combined with a redistribution of blood flow away from dependent regions may improve $\dot{V}/\dot{Q}$ relationships. There is an impressive lavaging effect of the immiscible liquid within the alveoli and airway, enhancing secretion clearance. The possibility that the liquid may possess antiinflammatory properties is also being pursued.

Clinical Studies

Clinical studies have been performed in neonates and adults that have demonstrated increased lung compliance and improved oxygenation. A controlled comparison of efficacy and safety to a lung protective strategy has not yet been conducted.

Application

At present, liquid perfluorocarbon (such as Perflubron, Alliance Pharmaceuticals) is available only through clinical trials. The liquid is administered through intratracheal instillation in an amount approximately equal to FRC (estimated at 20–30 mL/kg body weight or judged achieved by the visualization of a meniscus in the endotracheal tube at end expiration). The appropriate amount to administer and optimal ventilator settings to use remain unclear.

Complications

The radiodense nature of the liquid completely opacifies the chest x-ray, rendering it almost useless for clinical use (Fig. 12.6). There is a suggestion of an increased pneumothorax rate among patients receiving PLV, although this may be related in part to the ventilatory strategy employed. Toxicity data is limited; thus far there are no known local or systemic adverse effects from short-term use or from entry of the fluid into the pleural space.

Enhancing CO_2 Removal

As with adjuncts to oxygenation, noninvasive measures should be undertaken in preference to invasive measures if CO_2 elimination must be enhanced.

MINIMIZE CO_2 PRODUCTION

- Treat fever. Metabolic rate increases approximately 10% for every 1 degree Celsius elevation in core body temperature.
- Optimize nutrition. Whatever the source of calories, overfeeding increases CO_2 production. Carbohydrates may be especially problematic because of their high respiratory quotient ($\dot{V}CO_2/\dot{V}O_2$).
- Minimize patient activity. Attention to sedation and WOB can decrease $\dot{V}CO_2$. Neuromuscular blockade of a vigorously breathing patient may reduce $\dot{V}CO_2$ by 25% or more.
- Minimize V_D/V_T. Assure that V_T is optimized; for the same $\dot{V}_E$, an inappropriately small or large V_T can increase dead space, as can the application of excessive PEEP.

TRACHEAL GAS INSUFFLATION

Tracheal gas insufflation (TGI) is the continuous or phasic delivery of fresh gas into the central airways near the main carina. TGI is used to increase the efficiency of alveolar ventilation and as part of a pressure-limiting strategy to enable the use of lower tidal volumes without excessive hypercapnia.

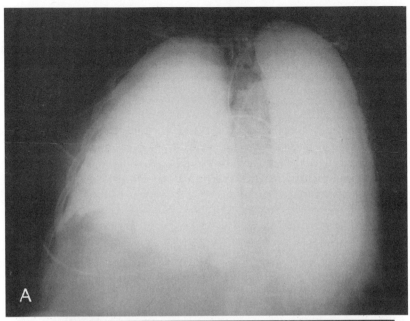

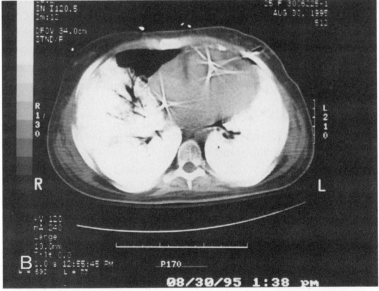

Figure 12.6. Chest radiograph (**A**) and CT scan (**B**) in a patient with ARDS treated with partial liquid ventilation. The extreme radiodensity of the perfluorochemical tends to impair imaging assessment. A small pneumothorax is evident in the left pleural space. No pneumothorax is present on the right. (From Marini JJ. Evolving concepts in the ventilatory management of acute respiratory distress syndrome. Clin Chest Med 1996;17(3):555–576. Reprinted with permission.)

Mechanism

By flushing the proximal dead space, the front of gas entering the alveoli in early inspiration has a decreased concentration of CO_2 and hence a more favorable gradient for CO_2 removal. Better gas mixing may also promote excretion.

Clinical Studies

As shown by Ravenscraft and colleagues, TGI can reliably decrease $PaCO_2$ by 15–25% or allow a decrease of up to 25% in $\dot{V}_E$, while maintaining $PaCO_2$ stable. Efficacy of TGI is proportional to the volume of fresh gas delivered during expiration rather than to the TGI flow rate itself. A small increment in PaO_2 is sometimes seen; this, however, is likely to be a consequence of increased mean airway pressure and/or FRC from TGI-induced increases in V_T or DH ("intrinsic PEEP"), neither of which is an intended effect of TGI.

Application

TGI may be applied using a specialized endotracheal tube or via a small catheter (e.g., a pediatric feeding tube) placed within the endotracheal tube, with its tip positioned just proximal to the carina. TGI flows less than 10 L/min are generally sufficient to achieve near optimal CO_2 elimination. Because TGI tends to increase end-expiratory lung volume, a careful assessment for overdistension and DH must be made when TGI is used, and ventilator settings must be adjusted accordingly.

TGI delivered solely during expiration (or even during just a portion of expiration) may be as effective as continuous TGI, possibly with less tendency toward hyperinflation. Other areas of ongoing investigation include the impact of shape and position of the insufflation catheter and the optimization of ventilator triggering during TGI.

Complications

Complications of TGI include DH, impaired ventilator triggering, secretion inspissation, and airway mucosal trauma resulting directly from the catheter or from its gas jet. Because of the potential for severe morbidity from incorrectly administered TGI, this technique should be used only by those experienced in its application.

EXTRACORPOREAL CO_2 REMOVAL

Extracorporeal CO_2 removal ($ECCO_2R$) is a method of accomplishing CO_2 elimination without the need to ventilate the lung with high pressure. Approximately 30% of cardiac output is diverted from a central vein to the extracorporeal circuit and exposed to fresh gas across a semipermeable membrane before returning to the right atrium. Oxygenation is accomplished by continuous tracheal insufflation of oxygen, and the lungs are ventilated at a low frequency to prevent atelectasis.

Mechanism

$ECCO_2R$ attempts to allow the lungs to rest and heal while providing adequate oxygenation and CO_2 removal for body tissues.

Clinical Studies

Because of the heterogeneity and bias in patient selection criteria, clinical studies are difficult to compare. Experienced centers report comparable survival between $ECCO_2R$ and conventional therapy (Morris). Because of recent progress in implementing low pressure ventilatory strategies without $ECCO_2R$, further investigation will help define the role, if any, for $ECCO_2R$ in lung protection.

Complications of Mechanical Ventilation

The varied complications of MV can be severe, even fatal. These complications can be categorized as those related to the placement and presence of the endotracheal tube and those related to the process of ventilation.

Endotracheal Tube-related Complications

INTUBATION

Although intubation is accomplished smoothly and safely in the majority of cases, there are many well-recognized complications.

Trauma

Injury to the cervical spinal cord may occur in the setting of an unrecognized neck fracture or intrinsic bony or ligamentous weakness. Laryngeal trauma may include vocal cord hematoma or paralysis. Pharyngeal mucosal trauma is most common after blind nasal intubation and may lead to mediastinal and/or subcutaneous emphysema. Retropharyngeal infection may complicate pharyngeal trauma and occasionally progresses to life-threatening mediastinitis.

Hypoxia

Hypoxia may result from prolonged unsuccessful attempts at intubation or from unrecognized malpositioning of the endotracheal tube (e.g., in the esophagus). Many practitioners routinely use disposable CO_2 detectors to confirm endotracheal placement; this may be unreliable in cases such as prolonged resuscitation.

Hypotension

Hypotension occurs commonly immediately after intubation. There are usually multiple causes, including the hemodynamic effects of the process prompting intubation and the vasodilating effects of sedating and paralyzing medications. Moreover, elevations of pleural pressure resulting from the loss of cyclically negative intrathoracic pressure of spontaneous breathing and/or the presence of DH can impede venous return.

An indwelling endotracheal tube may malfunction, irritate adjacent structures, circumvent host defenses, or compromise secretion clearance.

Mechanical Complications

ENDOTRACHEAL TUBE MALFUNCTION

Endotracheal tubes may become kinked or obstructed with secretions; cuff balloon rupture may occur, necessitating tube replacement.

TISSUE INJURY

Although less common since the advent of low pressure cuffs, the force exerted by the endotracheal tube on adjacent structures may interfere with mucosal perfusion. The resulting injury is generally proportional to the level and duration of inflation pressure, but this is unpredictable and injury may begin within hours of intubation. Laryngeal ulceration is relatively common and may rarely lead to granuloma formation or stricture.

Tracheal injury occurs most commonly at the site of the endotracheal tube cuff; other frequent sites of trauma are at the tube tip and at points of contact with suction catheters. Ulceration is the most common form of injury, although now seen much less than previously thanks to softer endotracheal tube cuffs, lower cuff pressures, and cuff pressure monitoring. Rarely, ulceration may progress to tracheal stenosis or tracheomalacia; tracheo-esophageal fistula occurs rarely, usually in the setting of ventilation via tracheostomy.

Infectious Complications

SINUSITIS

Sinus abnormalities complicate approximately 40% of all intubations sustained for ventilatory support and occur more frequently in patients with a nasotracheal tube. Clinically significant sinusitis develops in 2–20% of patients intubated for more than 5 days; the incidence is highest in patients who are immunocompromised or who have sustained a head injury. The most common aerobic pathogens are *Staphylococcus epidermidis* and Gram-negative rods. Diagnosis may be made clinically and confirmed with radiographic imaging (CT is more sensitive and specific than are plain films) and needle aspiration procedures. Treatment involves removal of nasal tubes, application of a vasoconstricting nasal spray to promote drainage, and antibiotics when appropriate.

VENTILATOR-ASSOCIATED PNEUMONIA

Ventilator-associated pneumonia (VAP) is defined as bacterial pneumonia developing in a patient who has undergone MV for at least 48 hours. The pathogenesis of VAP has been summarized as follows:

• Although the oropharynx teems with microbes, the upper airway is normally sterile below the vocal cords, swept clean by the mucociliary escalator, and protected by an effective cough. Bypassing the upper airway with an endotracheal tube seriously impairs these defenses while facilitating inoculation of the lower airway and lungs with high concentrations of potential pathogens (John J. Marini, M.D., unpublished communication).

Table 12.8. Predispositions to Ventilator-associated Pneumonia

Sinusitis	Coexisting nasogastric tube
Poor dentition	Lengthy period of ventilation
Immobilization	High gastric pH
Immune compromise	Condensate within ventilator tubing
Supine position	Frequent ventilator circuit disconnections

- While the overall rate of VAP is approximately 20–40%, increasing in direct proportion to the number of days of MV, some groups are at particularly high risk (Table 12.8). VAP is most often caused by an inoculum of pathogens entering via the airway, particularly in liquid secretions.

MICROBIOLOGY

An etiologic agent may not be found in up to 50% of patients with VAP, and, as discussed below, the recovery of a potential pathogen does not assure that the organism isolated is causative of the pneumonia or that bacterial pneumonitis is even present. A recent American Thoracic Society consensus statement provides a useful organizational framework for the diagnosis and management of nosocomial pneumonia, which is applicable to VAP (American Thoracic Society). Pneumonias are classified as early (within 5 days of admission) or late (developing 5 days or more after admission); risk factors such as underlying illnesses and use of devices and medications that alter host defenses are considered; and severity of illness (mild-to-moderate or severe) is assessed. Based on the intersection of these criteria, likely pathogens can be identified.

Common pathogens in early nosocomial pneumonia of any severity are enteric Gram-negative bacilli and methicillin-sensitive *Staphylococcus aureus*. Mild-to-moderate pneumonia in the patient with risk factors may be caused by the same "core" pathogens, but anaerobes, *Legionella,* and *Pseudomonas* must also be considered. A severe pneumonia occurring after 5 days of hospitalization may be caused by any of the pathogens just mentioned plus *Pseudomonas* and methicillin-resistant *S. aureus* (see Chapter 7).

DIAGNOSIS

The literature addressing the diagnosis of VAP is vast and conflicting. This area of research is fueled by findings that clinical judgment (using conventional laboratory and radiologic tools) may lead to inappropriate diagnoses and therapies in 30 to 60% of cases. Most studies invoke fever, leukocytosis, purulence of tracheal secretions, appearance of CXR infiltrates, and increased oxygen requirements; they differ in their selection of adjuncts to diagnosis, their gold standards for diagnosis, and their findings regarding the importance of these adjuncts.

Adjuncts to the diagnosis of VAP include endotracheal aspiration, and sampling of the distal airway may be performed with a "protected specimen" brush. Directed catheters are available that by virtue of their shape tend to enter either the right or

Table 12.9. Noninfectious Causes of Fever and Pulmonary Infiltrates (From Meduri, 1995)

Atelectasis	Pulmonary embolus
Proliferative phase of ARDS	Pulmonary hemorrhage
Bronchiolitis obliterans with organizing pneumonia	Gastric aspiration

From Meduri GU. Diagnosis and differential diagnosis of ventilator-associated pneumonia. Clin Chest Med 1995. Reprinted with permission.

the left mainstem bronchus and thus can be passed blindly. Protected specimen brushes may also be passed bronchoscopically. The addition of bronchoalveolar lavage via either the bronchoscope or a wedged catheter significantly enlarges the sampling area. At present no firm consensus exists regarding the role of invasive testing in the diagnosis of VAP.

The preponderance of the literature suggests that *quantitative* bacteriologic techniques increase specificity in the diagnosis of VAP; a colony count of $\geq 10^4$ colony forming units (CFU) per milliliter of processed sample is generally required to support the diagnosis of VAP. Cultures obtained off antibiotics or on a stable antibiotic regimen (no change in 24 hours) have a reasonable yield; a change in the antibiotic regimen within the 24 hours prior to obtaining the culture significantly reduces sensitivity.

DIFFERENTIAL DIAGNOSIS OF VAP

Crucial to the workup of suspected VAP is recognition that there are important noninfectious causes of fever and pulmonary densities in the mechanically ventilated patient. Major noninfectious causes are listed in Table 12.9. These diagnoses require rigorous exclusion of infection and often necessitate special radiologic techniques or biopsy procedures, occasionally including open lung biopsy.

Complications of Positive Pressure Ventilation

Barotrauma and Volutrauma: Stretch-induced Injury

Ventilator-induced lung injury (VILI) represents a spectrum of injury ranging from overt tissue rupture and air leaks to more subtle histopathologic changes and alterations in lung mechanics that may be difficult to distinguish from the underlying disease process. The incidence of VILI is unclear, in part because the underlying disease may mask its true incidence and also because much of the available data was obtained during an era in which higher pressures were employed, no longer reflecting current practice. Risk factors for barotrauma are listed in Table 12.10.

Table 12.10. Risk Factors for Barotrauma

Necrotizing lung pathology	Duration of ventilation
Nonhomogeneous parenchymal disease	Minute ventilation requirement
Secretion retention	High peak cycling pressure
Young age	High mean alveolar pressure

PATHOGENESIS

It is known that high ventilatory pressures and excessive regional lung volumes can damage previously normal lungs. This potential for harm is compounded by the heterogeneous nature of acute lung injury. Differences in the regional impedance to lung inflation lead to unevenly distributed ventilation and the simultaneous existence of collapsed and overdistended lung units.

Although the distinction between *barotrauma* and *volutrauma* (i.e., pressure-induced and volume-induced lung injury) is not a clear one, the latter term implies tissue damage without extra-alveolar gas. Tissue damage routinely observed after ventilating normal animals with plateau pressures > 35 cm H_2O is reduced if the chest is bound prior to such ventilation (thus reducing the *transalveolar* pressure). This protection suggests that the *volume* achieved rather than the pressure itself is responsible for the tissue damage. Ventilatory patterns that favor high cyclical shearing forces as a result of repetitive opening and closing of marginally recruited alveoli are strongly associated with lung injury.

High peak inspiratory pressures disrupt the alveolar epithelium, causing increased permeability and impaired surfactant production and function. Concomitantly, these high pressures damage the microvasculature by increasing microvascular pressure and endothelial permeability. The net effect is to promote alveolar flooding and impair surfactant. Increased surface tension promotes atelectasis and increases vulnerability to cyclic opening and closure. Diffuse alveolar damage (DAD), a final common pathway of such injury, is manifested by granulocyte infiltration, hyaline membrane formation, and proteinaceous edema with subsequent fibroblast proliferation and fibrosis.

PULMONARY AIR LEAKS

Abnormal gas collections caused by MV are thought to be more directly attributable to pressure induced injury (i.e., barotrauma). Air leaks occur when gas released from overdistended alveoli dissects along the bronchovascular sheaths, generally toward the hilum. *Tension pneumothorax* is a dreaded consequence of alveolar rupture; *tension gas cysts,* which may progress to devastating systemic gas embolism, are another potentially devastating complication. More commonly air leaks take the form of pneumomediastinum, pneumopericardium, or interstitial or subcutaneous emphysema.

Careful scrutiny of the chest radiograph or CT for evidence of barotrauma is mandatory in mechanically ventilated patients at increased risk. Particular attention must be paid to the hila and mediastinum for evidence of abnormal gas collections. Pneumothorax may present atypically in supine patients. Two characteristic radiographic signs of pneumothorax in the supine patient are the presence of an abnormal lucency overlying the lung or upper abdomen as the gas tracks to the most anterior region and the ''deep sulcus sign'' as a result of free pleural gas along the diaphragmatic recess (Fig. 12.7).

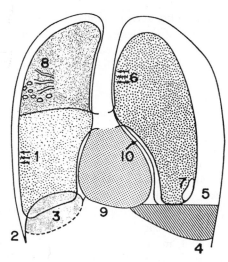

Figure 12.7. Radiographic signs of barotrauma: *1*, visible visceral pleural line; *2*, deep sulcus sign; *3*, radiolucency localized to the upper abdomen; *4*, inverted hemidiaphragm; *5*, air-fluid level; *6*, mediastinal shift; *7*, subpleural air cyst; *8*, interstitial emphysema; *9*, complete diaphragm sign; *10*, pneumomediastinum. (From Marini JJ. Respiratory medicine for the house officer. 2nd ed. Baltimore: Williams & Wilkins, 1987. Reprinted with permission.)

Oxygen Toxicity

High concentrations of oxygen inhaled over long periods of time are potentially injurious to the lung. Toxicity increases exponentially as FiO_2 rises above 0.6.

PATHOGENESIS

Increased concentrations of oxidizing free radicals overwhelm antioxidant defense mechanisms and result in cellular injury via lipid peroxidation, enzyme inhibition, and DNA strand breakage. O_2 toxicity may manifest in several different ways.

An *alveolar-capillary leak* syndrome has been noted in humans and animals after exposure to 100% oxygen for brief periods. Direct hyperoxic injury to the alveolar-capillary endothelium leads to increased permeability, edema, and inflammation. This may result in *diffuse alveolar damage,* the final common pathway of many toxic insults to the lung. DAD begins with an inflammatory exudative phase and progresses to a fibrotic phase. Nash and colleagues have shown that brief (16-hour) exposure to high FiO_2 in humans did not affect inflammatory response as revealed in bronchoalveolar lavage fluid; however, longer (48-hour) exposure in animals provoked more significant histologic inflammation than did hyperventilation, although pressures induced by hyperventilation were not specified.

Oxygen toxicity may promote *microatelectasis* via several mechanisms. Atelectasis may result from hyperoxic injury to the surfactant-generating type II pneumocyte, with increased surface tension and altered permeability leading to alveolar collapse.

Absorption atelectasis is an entity seen particularly in low $\dot{V}/\dot{Q}$ regions; here there is a net loss of gas as the rate of O_2 absorption exceeds replenishment by CO_2; the low concentration of nitrogen in the inspired gas cannot maintain alveolar patency.

Mucociliary transport is impaired by high concentrations of oxygen, impairing host defenses in the injured lung.

CLINICAL IMPLICATIONS

There are several clinical subgroups in which O_2 toxicity is clearly deleterious. Bronchopulmonary dysplasia (BPD) is a well-described consequence of high inspired oxygen concentrations administered in the treatment of respiratory distress syndrome of the newborn. Fortunately, the incidence of this complication has dropped dramatically with the advent of surfactant replacement therapy. Because patients who have received *bleomycin* chemotherapy are highly susceptible to the injurious effects of high FiO_2 and can sustain irreversible fibrosis, every effort should be made to avoid a high FiO_2 in these patients.

With these exceptions, it is not clear how susceptible the human lung is to oxygen toxicity and how that susceptibility is modified (increased or decreased) by disease. While it is advisable to avoid an FiO_2 greater than 0.6, this is not always possible to do. Although there is not full agreement on the subject, many investigators believe that high ventilatory pressures may be more harmful in most patients than high FiO_2.

WEANING

In most intubated patients, discontinuation of MV is accomplished easily as the cause of respiratory failure resolves. The remaining patients require a more tailored program of progressive withdrawal of ventilatory support.

Assessing Readiness to Wean
Physiologic Considerations

There are three major factors influencing the ability to sustain spontaneous breathing:

- The relationship of respiratory load to the strength and endurance of the respiratory musculature;
- Oxygenation;
- Cardiovascular performance.

Other important clinical variables include hemoglobin concentration, temperature, nutritional status, electrolyte balance, adequacy of sleep, and psychological factors.

The interaction between the mechanical load and the capacity of the respiratory neuromuscular system is generally the most important determinant of ventilator dependence. Discontinuation of MV is rarely contemplated in patients with significantly impaired oxygenation; cardiovascular factors will be discussed below. The load on the respiratory system per liter of ventilation is influenced by the imposed load of the ventilator circuit and the intrinsic load, airway resistance, lung compliance, and PEEPi. The product of $\dot{V}_E$ and work per liter of ventilation determines the power required. Ventilatory drive, muscular strength, thoracic configuration, and DH are the main determinants of the ability of the ventilatory pump to satisfy this requirement.

The ability to protect the airway and to clear secretions frequently determines the ability to sustain spontaneous respiration. Although difficult to assess fully in the intubated patient, secretion clearance is an important consideration in all for whom extubation is contemplated. Consequently, the volume and characteristics of secretions, the vigor of oropharyngeal reflexes, and the strength of the patient's cough should be carefully assessed prior to extubation.

Predictive Indices

A number of physiologic indices are used to predict weaning outcome. No single index is definitive, but when used in combination these measurements can be useful to suggest that MV may be discontinued successfully and to follow a patient's progress toward weaning:

- Respiratory rate $\leq$ 35 breaths per minute;
- $\dot{V}_E \leq$ 10–15 L/min, depending on body size;
- Maximal inspiratory pressure more negative than -30 cm H_2O;
- Vital capacity $>$ 10–15 mL/kg;
- Frequency/tidal volume ratio $<$ 100 breaths/min/L.

This index of "weanability" has the highest positive (78%) and negative (95%) predictive values of any single index yet described. As an example, a patient with a respiratory rate of 24/min and V_T of 400 mL has a ratio of 24/0.4 = 60.

Modes of Weaning

The three modes of weaning in most widespread use are T-piece trials, SIMV weaning, and pressure support weaning. Regardless of the mode chosen, it is crucial that:

- Signs of respiratory insufficiency and patient distress are recognized and monitored. These signs include tachypnea (respiratory rate $>$ 35/min) and irregular or rising tachycardia, diaphoresis, agitation, and panic.
- The patient is allowed to rest adequately should signs of respiratory distress develop. Adequate rest may require increased ventilator support at night to facilitate sleep. Overt respiratory muscle fatigue prolongs the weaning process; it takes at least 24 hours to recover from even a moderate level of respiratory muscle fatigue.

T-piece Trials

In a T-piece trial, the patient is disconnected from the ventilator and the endotracheal tube is attached to a T-shaped piece of tubing through which humidified gas flows.

A CPAP of 0 cm H_2O without pressure support serves a similar function when the ventilator circuit remains attached. Use of a T-piece offers the advantage of minimal imposed resistance by the circuit; drawbacks include the absence of ventilator monitoring and ventilatory backup should the patient's level of ventilation fall significantly. In addition, some patients (particularly those with chronic obstructive pulmonary disease, CHF, and psychologic ventilator dependence) may find the transition from fully assisted ventilation to unsupported T-piece breathing disturbingly abrupt.

The duration of the T-piece trial is not standardized and may last from minutes to hours. The ability to comfortably sustain breathing for 2 hours on a T-piece correctly predicted sustained ventilator independence in 88% of patients in one study.

SIMV Weaning

In this mode, the frequency of machine breaths is gradually decreased. The rate of decrease is guided by clinical assessment and in some instances by blood gases. Patients who tolerate 2–4 machine breaths per minute for 1–2 hours can usually be extubated successfully.

In flow-controlled SIMV, as the patient assumes a progressively active role, the WOB may rise exponentially (rather than linearly) as the machine breath rate is decreased. If the patient's flow demand exceeds the flow supplied by the ventilator, patient effort continues throughout inspiration, and the proportion of work performed by the ventilator decreases for each machine breath. The use of pressure-controlled machine cycles in SIMV better maintains the machine's work proportion per breath.

Advantages of SIMV weaning are that the patient's respiratory output can be monitored and backed up by the ventilator and that the larger machine breaths may help to avoid or reverse atelectasis. A disadvantage of SIMV weaning is that the demand valve circuit imposes an increased WOB; this may be offset to some degree by the addition of a low level (e.g., 5 cm H_2O) of pressure support or by utilizing flow triggering.

Pressure Support Weaning

In pressure support weaning, the level of pressure support is gradually lowered so that the patient assumes an increasing share of the respiratory workload. The rate of pressure support reduction should be guided by the total respiratory rate rather than by V_T. This mode promotes the efficiency of each breath, offsets the ventilator-imposed WOB (although unfortunately to an unpredictable degree), and allows the patient full control over respiratory rate and breath architecture. One drawback of pressure support weaning is that with conventional PSV, no minimum level of $\dot{V}_E$ is assured.

Although some patients may tolerate weaning from 5 cm H_2O pressure support, others may fail when MV is discontinued after reaching this ostensibly low level of respiratory support. This is most likely to occur in weak patients with compliant lungs and high respiratory rates for whom the 5 cm H_2O support with each breath performed a substantial fraction of the WOB. In patients such as these, pressure support should be decreased to very low levels before extubation is undertaken.

Comparison of Modes

Many wise and experienced clinicians share the opinion that weaning is simply a process that distinguishes patients who do need a ventilator from those who don't. While this underscores the need to resolve the underlying process, it has recently become clear that for a subset of patients, the weaning mode does make a difference.

In a recent major study of patients who had failed initial T-piece trials, pressure support weaning was more successful (i.e., higher proportion of patients extubated and shorter mean duration of weaning) than SIMV or T-piece weaning. Pressure support gives the patient the ability to draw additional power from the ventilator with increasing respiratory frequency and promotes greater efficiency of breathing. For the patient with marginal respiratory reserve, this may make a significant difference in the duration of weaning.

Progress in weaning can be made only as fast as the clinician allows it to be made. An inherent advantage of T-piece trials is that a patient who is ready for extubation can declare so in a matter of 2 hours. In busy clinical practice, it is all too easy to pass over the patient who is doing well on a given level of pressure support or SIMV rate and not to regularly reassess the patient throughout the day and decrease the ventilatory support as rapidly as might be physiologically possible. One reasonable approach is to use a 2-hour T-piece trial initially; if the patient clearly well tolerates the trial clinically (with or without ABG measurement, a controversial topic), extubation may be considered. If the trial is not well tolerated, the clinician may consider repeating the trial later or proceeding directly to a pressure support wean as outlined above.

Causes of Difficulty in Weaning

A meticulous investigation should be made regarding the specific cause(s) of weaning difficulty (Table 12.11). Most of the variables listed below can be deduced from the physiologic principles already outlined; two deserve special attention.

Impaired Cardiac Status

Cardiac ischemia is a major and often undetected cause of failure to wean. Clinicians are sometimes puzzled by weaning failure that occurs in the setting of acceptable respiratory-based weaning parameters. One recent study revealed that in a medical/cardiac ICU with a 49% prevalence of coronary artery disease, 6% of patients had ECG evidence of ischemia during weaning. Among those failing initial attempts at weaning, the prevalence of ischemia was 22%.

MECHANISMS

As the patient assumes an increasing share of the breathing workload, cardiac output and intrapleural pressure rise, boosting the afterload to the left ventricle. In the study

Table 12.11. Causes of Difficulty in Weaning

Imposed loads	Dynamic hyperinflation
Demand valve	Respiratory muscle weakness
Narrow endotracheal tube	Myopathy, neuropathy
Respiratory system factors	Phrenic nerve injury, other diaphragm dysfunction
Increased airway resistance	Nutritional factors
Bronchospasm	Nonrespiratory factors
Secretions	Poor cardiac status
Decreased respiratory system	Metabolic disturbance
compliance	Hypermetabolism (disease, fever, overfeeding)
Intrinsic lung disease	Acid-base, electrolyte disturbance (esp.
Atelectasis	hypophosphatemia)
Suboptimal positioning	Sleep deprivation
Obesity, abdominal distension	Anxiety

Adapted from Slutsky AS, et al. Mechanical ventilation. Consensus statement of the American College of Chest Physicians. Chest 1993.

cited above, heart rate-blood pressure product rose significantly among all patients during weaning. If LV performance deteriorates, LVEDP (left ventricular end-diastolic pressure) and therefore PCWP (pulmonary capillary wedge pressure) and interstitial edema increase, lung compliance worsens, and a vicious cycle of deterioration begins (Fig. 12.8).

In a patient with unexplained failure to wean, occult ischemia or heart failure should be considered. Attention should be paid to weaning-induced changes in heart rate, blood pressure, PCWP, and ECG. A full 12-lead ECG and/or echocardiogram should be obtained during the weaning attempt itself. Diuresis, afterload reduction, and ischemia prophylaxis may enable successful withdrawal of ventilatory support.

Sleep Disturbance

ICU patients frequently have markedly deranged sleep–wake cycles and are often frankly sleep-deprived. This takes a toll on both physical and emotional endurance. Careful attention should be paid to the sleep hygiene of patients exhibiting difficulty weaning, and increased ventilator support at night should be given to help assure

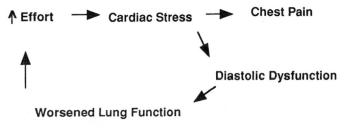

Figure 12.8. The cycle of weaning failure during cardiac stress.

adequate rest. Scheduled anxiolytics and hypnotics may improve sleep quality and duration.

Tracheostomy

The development of high volume, low pressure endotracheal tube cuffs has altered the practice of performing a tracheostomy on patients ventilated for longer than 14 days. As both prolonged MV and tracheostomy are associated with a small but significant risk of tracheal injury, the decision to perform a tracheostomy should be based on patient comfort and mobility, the ongoing requirement for bronchial hygiene or MV, the need to bypass the larynx, or the need to establish a secure airway.

A tracheostomy offers several advantages. Comfort, communication, and mobility are all enhanced by tracheostomy. For many patients and their families this is of significant psychological benefit and may enhance clinical outcome in ways that cannot be readily quantified. Nutrition is generally believed to be improved following tracheostomy, although the benefits of oral intake may be offset by a possible increase in aspiration risk and occasional difficulty with swallowing and glottis function.

The presence of the tracheostomy tube incurs many of the same risks as does the endotracheal tube (tracheal injury and subsequent stenosis, vocal cord trauma, fistulae formation, etc.). Tracheal dilatation and stenosis occur more commonly after tracheostomy. Mortality and major morbidity from the operative procedure are each less than 1%; the incidence of minor problems (e.g., minor hemorrhage, subcutaneous and mediastinal emphysema and infection) is generally less than 10%.

Decisions on timing of tracheostomy thus require an individualized assessment of risks and benefits. One reasonable approach has been outlined by Heffner (1994): at the end of 7 days of intubation, the patient is assessed. Translaryngeal intubation is continued if it appears likely that the patient will be extubated within the next 7 days and there is no other compelling reason to secure a permanent airway. If, however, it seems evident that the patient will require MV for more than 14 days, an early tracheostomy is performed to allow patients and family to benefit from the advantages listed above for as much of the hospital course as possible.

VENTILATION IN SPECIFIC SETTINGS
Mechanical Ventilation during ARDS

While mortality from ARDS remains discouragingly high, its incidence appears to be waning (see Chapter 11). This decrease may in part owe to the recent shift toward ventilatory strategies that promote healing of the injured lung. Modification of ventilatory patterns in ARDS stems from the recognition that:

• The aeratable capacity of the lung in ARDS may be extremely small (perhaps only one-third normal). Hence, conventional tidal volumes may require injurious transalveolar pressures and alveolar overdistension in these areas of relatively normal compliance.

• Damage may be caused by the cyclic opening and closing of atelectatic lung regions. Injurious shear forces may occur if end-expiratory tidal pressures fall below a certain opening pressure (Pflex, see below).

Ventilator Management

A *lung protective strategy* strives to avoid overdistension while maintaining alveolar patency throughout the respiratory cycle. This is accomplished through a pressure-targeted ventilation and the acceptance, when necessary, of supranormal levels of $PaCO_2$ (permissive hypercapnia).

Pressure-targeted Ventilation

The static pressure-volume curve of the recently injured lung has two regions of inflection (Fig. 12.9). The lower inflection zone, "Pflex," represents the pressure above which the slope of the pressure-volume curve (i.e., the lung compliance) no longer improves with each volume increment. The upper inflection zone is characterized by the upper deflection point (UDP), the point at which lung compliance

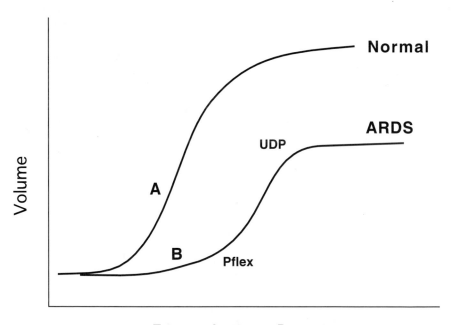

Figure 12.9. The pressure-volume curve of the respiratory system during lung injury. In the injured lung (curve B), lower and upper inflection zones, Pflex, and UDP can be seen. Compliance is lower and FRC (lung volume at transpulmonary pressure = 0) is smaller than in the injured lung.

abruptly decreases, presumably because overdistension begins to outweigh recruitment. The pressure targets in one popular lung protective strategy are to use a PEEP level that keeps the minimum pressure (i.e., end-expiratory pressure) above Pflex and a V_T that ensures a Pplat below the UDP (generally, but not invariably, 35 cm H_2O). Ideally this prevents both tidal derecruitment at end expiration and tidal overdistension at end inspiration.

Permissive Hypercapnia

In the interests of reducing transalveolar pressures, $\dot{V}_E$ is maintained at a relatively low level, resulting in an increase in $PaCO_2$. Acute elevations in $PaCO_2$ may increase sympathetic tone, increase pulmonary vascular resistance, and impair CNS and cardiovascular function. When the rate of rise of $PaCO_2$ is relatively slow, however (e.g., less than 10 mm Hg/hr, keeping pH above 7.15–7.20 and $PaCO_2 \leq 80$), hypercapnia is generally well tolerated. One recent study measured the hemodynamic effects of a rapid rise in $PaCO_2$ 40–59 mm Hg over 30–60 minutes). Of the 11 patients studied, none experienced significant cardiovascular compromise. Shunt fraction increased, perhaps because of increased cardiac index as a result of decreased systemic vascular resistance (SVR). Five patients needed a mean 13% increase in FiO_2. The oxyhemoglobin dissociation curve was shifted to the right as expected with acidosis, but O_2 extraction did not increase (Thorens).

CO2 retention generally requires deep sedation and may be complicated by cardiovascular deterioration (elevated $PaCO_2$ can cause myocardial depression and either hypertension or hypotension) and later depression of respiratory drive as a result of compensatory metabolic alkalosis. Important contraindications to permissive hypercapnia include elevated intracranial pressure, overt cardiovascular dysfunction, and significant pulmonary hypertension. Beta-adrenergic blocking agents should not be used in permissive hypercapnia because profound hypotension may result from impaired sympathetic vasoconstriction. Uncorrected hypovolemia, significant preexisting metabolic acidosis, and refractory hypoxemia are relative contraindications to permissive hypercapnia.

Other Adjuncts in Therapy of ARDS

Prone positioning has been used successfully in early ARDS and in some cases can dramatically improve oxygenation. Prolonging inspiratory time by adding an end-inspiratory pause or by decreasing expiratory flow may enhance oxygenation (see discussion of Inverse-Ratio Ventilation). PLV may be employed in the context of an approved clinical trial.

Mechanical Ventilation During Severe Airflow Obstruction

During exacerbations of asthma and COPD, airways resistance is greatly increased, with consequent decreased expiratory flow and potential for significant DH. Inspiratory flow resistance alone can elevate peak pressures; an elevated Pplat in the setting of airflow obstruction strongly suggests DH. The ventilator monitor may reveal a concave expiratory flow-volume curve as flow decreases exponentially with decreasing lung volume. The persistence of expiratory flow until the onset of inspiration (Fig. 12.4*B*) suggests DH.

Estimation of Dynamic Hyperinflation

Quantitation of DH in this setting can be difficult. In a passive patient, an expiratory hold may be placed on the ventilator and the pressure read from the manometer at exactly the time the next inspiration was due to be delivered. The patient must be completely relaxed when using the airway occlusion technique because active expiration may cause overestimation of DH and unrecognized inspiratory effort can lead to its underestimation. An insufficient end-expiratory occlusion time will underestimate DH, as will an excessively compliant ventilator circuit.

Because prematurely closed airways may not transmit the trapped pressures distal to them, the occlusion technique may be misleading in the measurement of PEEPi. In this setting, the Pplat may be the best proxy for PEEPi. While exact quantitation of PEEPi may not be possible, one can follow the trends in Pplat as reflecting trends in PEEPi when V_T and external PEEP are held constant. If quantitation of PEEPi itself is desired, one approach is to measure the Pplat and then to allow a period of apnea by decreasing the respiratory frequency to 8 breaths/min. The difference between the initial Pplat and the Pplat on the *first* breath after the apnea equals the PEEPi.

Ventilator Management

The principal determinants of DH are $\dot{V}_E$ and, to a lesser extent, inspiratory time fraction (because $T_I/Ttot$ determines $T_E/Ttot$). The approach to ventilating the severely flow-limited patient, therefore, is to decrease $\dot{V}_E$ and extend expiratory time, a strategy known as *controlled hypoventilation*. As in ARDS, permissive hypercapnia is often a consequence of this lung protective strategy.

DECREASE $\dot{V}_E$

No formula can replace time at the bedside working to understand the flow demands and characteristics of the individual patient. In general, small to moderate tidal volumes should be used (e.g., 6–8 mL/kg) in conjunction with modest ventilatory frequency (e.g., 8–12 breaths/min). To achieve a desired $\dot{V}_E$, decreasing the V_T rather than the respiratory frequency may be more effective because patients with extremely slow terminal expiratory flows may have a greater reduction in DH via a reduced V_T than an extended expiratory time.

The assist control mode should **not** be used in a patient with severe airflow obstruction if there is any chance of spontaneous breathing because the patient can quickly and easily develop dangerous levels of DH by frequent triggering of mandatory breaths. The ventilator high pressure alarm tends to be relatively insensitive to

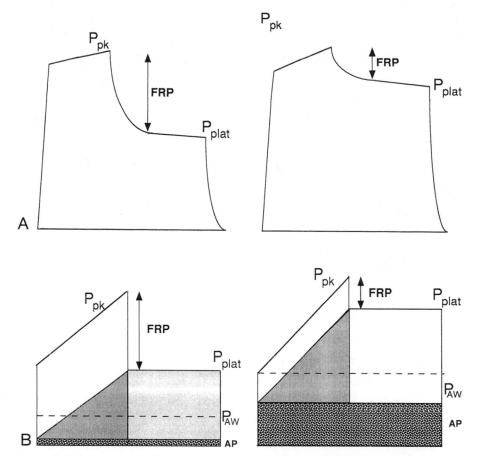

Figure 12.10. Airway opening pressures with a change in auto-PEEP (*AP*). Note that the peak airway pressure (*Ppk*) does not change significantly despite a large change in auto-PEEP and mean airway (P_{AW}) pressure. Flow-resistive pressure has decreased as a result of greater airway caliber at higher lung volumes. Because AP is present throughout the respiratory cycle, mean *alveolar* pressure may be higher than mean airway pressure. *FRP,* flow resistive pressure; *Pplat,* plateau pressure.

the development of DH since the rise in peak pressure because of increased DH may be offset by a fall in inspiratory flow-resistive pressure as the higher lung volume tethers airways open (Fig. 12.10).

EXTEND EXPIRATORY TIME

Expiratory time is maximized by making inspiratory time as short as possible. Inspiratory flow rates should be relatively high; rates as high as 100 L/min can be used safely. Increasing inspiratory flow rate will increase peak pressure because of an increase in inspiratory flow-resistive pressure—this is not pressure that is transmitted to the alveoli and should not by itself cause barotrauma. This is a different situation than that seen with ARDS, in which there are clearly injurious effects of high inspiratory pressures as a result of low lung compliance and/or excessive V_T.

MEDICAL MANAGEMENT

The patient will require heavy sedation to suppress respiratory drive because $PaCO_2$, a major determinant of respiratory drive, frequently rises with hypoventilation. Many clinicians find that the combination of a benzodiazepine and a narcotic are synergistic in producing sedation and decreased respiratory drive and that their simultaneous use is more effective than higher dose use of either agent alone. Propofol may also be a useful agent in this setting, particularly if it appears that the patient may improve quickly. Neuromuscular blocking agents should be used sparingly because of the risk of prolonged muscle weakness associated with the combined use of high-dose steroids and paralytics.

It is assumed that the patient will be receiving aggressive inhaled bronchodilator therapy and parenteral steroids; their use is detailed in Chapter 3. Mention should be made, however, of the role of metered dose inhalers (MDIs) in the intubated patient. Direct comparison of MDIs with conventional nebulizer treatment has shown the two delivery modes to be of equal efficacy in reducing airflow resistance. Drug delivery may also be increased with MDIs because little aerosolized medication is lost during exhalation with the MDI, compared with the nebulizer. Eight to ten or more puffs should be used per MDI administration, titrated to response.

Complications of Mechanical Ventilation During Airflow Obstruction

The two major complications of MV during severe airflow obstruction are DH and barotrauma. Life-threatening DH and tension pneumothorax can present similarly, and it is important to consider each of these processes in a patient experiencing a sudden deterioration characterized by hypotension and increased peak and plateau pressures. In this event, the patient should be given a trial of apnea: disconnect the patient from the ventilator, wait 30–40 seconds, and reassess hemodynamics. If the hypotension was caused by DH, there should be significant improvement in blood pressure; if no improvement follows the apnea and the clinical picture and physical examination is consistent with pneumothorax, strong consideration should be given to empiric needle decompression and chest tube placement.

BIBLIOGRAPHY

Albert RK, Leasa D, Sanderson M, et al. The prone position improves arterial oxygenation and reduces shunt in oleic acid-induced acute lung injury. Am Rev Respir Dis 1987;135: 628–633.

Al-Saady N, Bennet ED. Decelerating inspiratory flow waveform improves lung mechanics and gas exchange in patients on intermittent positive pressure ventilation. Intensive Care Med 1985;11:68–75.

Amato MBP, Barbas CSV, Bonassa J, et al. Volume-assured pressure support ventilation. A new approach for reducing muscle workload during acute respiratory failure. Chest 1992; 102:1225–1234.

Amato MBP, Barbas CSV, Medeiros DM, et al. Beneficial effects of the "open lung approach" with low distending pressures in acute respiratory distress syndrome. Am J Respir Crit Care Med 1995;152:1835–1846.

American Thoracic Society. Hospital-acquired pneumonia in adults: diagnosis, assessment of severity, initial antimicrobial therapy, and preventative strategies. A consensus statement. Am J Respir Crit Care Med 1995;153:1711–1725.

Anzueto A, Baughman RP, Guntupalli KK. Aerosolized surfactant in adults with sepsis-induced acute respiratory distress syndrome. N Engl J Med 1996;334:1417–1421.

Bradley TD, Holloway RM, McLaughlin PR, et al. Cardiac output response to continuous positive airway pressure in congestive heart failure. Am Rev Respir Dis 1992;145:377–382.

Brochard L, Rauss A, Benito S, et al. Comparison of three methods of gradual weaning from ventilatory support during weaning from mechanical ventilation. Am J Respir Crit Care Med 1994;150:896–903.

Brunet F, Mira JP, Belghith M, et al. Extracorporeal carbon dioxide removal technique improves oxygenation without causing overinflation. Am J Respir Crit Care Med 1994;149: 1557–1562.

Bryan CL, Jenkinson SG. Oxygen toxicity. Clin Chest Med 1988;9:141–152.

Chastre J, Fagon JY. Invasive diagnostic testing should be routinely used to manage ventilated patients with suspected pneumonia. Am J Respir Crit Care Med 1994;150:570–574.

Chatila W, Ani S, Guaglianone D, et al. Cardiac ischemia during weaning from mechanical ventilation. Chest 1996;109:1577–1583.

Clutton-Brock J. Two cases of poisoning by contamination of nitrous oxide with the higher oxides of nitrogen during anaesthesia. Br J Anaesth 1967;39:388–392.

Culpepper JA, Rinaldo JE, Rogers RM. Effect of mechanical ventilatory mode on tendency towards respiratory alkalosis. Am Rev Respir Dis 1985;132:1075–1077.

Davis WB, Rennard SI, Bitterman PB. Pulmonary oxygen toxicity: early reversible changes in human alveolar structures induced by hyperoxia. N Engl J Med 1983;309:878–883.

Dhand R, Jubran A, Tobin M. Bronchodilator delivery by metered-dose inhaler in ventilator-supported patients. Am J Respir Crit Care Med 1995;151:1827–1833.

Dreyfuss D, Basset G, Soler P, et al. Intermittent positive pressure hyperventilation with high inflation pressures produce pulmonary microvascular injury in rats. Am Rev Respir Dis 1985;132:880–884.

Fagon J-Y, Chastre J, Hance AJ, et al. Evaluation of clinical judgment in the identification and treatment of nosocomial pneumonia in ventilated patients. Chest 1993;103:547–553.

Fiehl F, Perret C. Permissive hypercapnia—how permissive should we be? Am J Respir Crit Care Med 1994;150:1722–1737.

Froese AB, Bryan AC. High frequency ventilation. Am Rev Respir Dis 1987;135:1363–1374.

Fuhrman BP, Paczan PR, DeFrancis M. Perfluorocarbon-associated gas exchange. Crit Care Med 1991;19:712–722.

Gattinoni L, Agostoni A, Pesenti A. Treatment of acute respiratory failure with low frequency positive pressure ventilation and extra-corporeal removal of CO_2. Lancet 1980;2:292–295.

Gattinoni L, Pesenti A, Avalli L, et al. Pressure-volume curve of total respiratory system in acute respiratory failure: computed tomographic study. Am Rev Respir Dis 1987;136: 730–736.

Gay PC, Patel HG, Nelson SB, et al. Metered dose inhalers for bronchodilator delivery in intubated, mechanically ventilated patients. Chest 1991;99:66–71.

Gregory TJ, Gadek JE, Weiland JE, et al. Survanta supplementation in patients with acute respiratory distress syndrome (ARDS). Abstract. Am Rev Respir Dis 1994;149:A567.

Groeger JS, Levinson MR, Carlon GC. Assist-control versus synchronized intermittent mandatory ventilation during acute respiratory failure. Crit Care Med 1989;17:607–612.

Heffner JE. Timing of tracheotomy in ventilator-dependent patients. Clin Chest Med 1991; 12:611–625.

Heffner JE, Casey K, Hoffman C. The care of the mechanically ventilated patient with a tracheotomy. In: Tobin MJ, ed. Principles and practice of mechanical ventilation. New York: McGraw-Hill, 1994.

Hirschl RB. Laboratory and clinical experience with liquid ventilation in respiratory failure. Respir Care 1996;41.

Hirschl RB, Tooley R, Parent AC, Johnson K, Bartlett RH. Improvement of gas exchange, pulmonary function, and lung injury with partial liquid ventilation. A study model in the setting of severe respiratory failure. Chest 1995;108:500–508.

Hudson LD, Hurlow RS, Craig KC, Pierson DJ. Does intermittent mandatory ventilation correct respiratory alkalosis in patients receiving assisted mechanical ventilation? Am Rev Respir Dis 1985;132:1071–1074.

Jubran A, Tobin MJ. Noninvasive oxygen monitoring. In: Cheng EY, Lund N, eds. Problems in critical care. Philadelphia: Lippincott, 1992.

Jubran A, Van De Graaff WB, Tobin MJ. Variability of patient-ventilator interaction in patients with chronic obstructive pulmonary disease. Am J Respir Crit Care Med 1995; 152:129–136.

Kakmarek RM. Management of the patient-mechanical ventilator system. In: Pierson DJ, Kakmarek RM, eds. Foundations of respiratory care. New York: Churchill Livingston, 1992.

Kolobow T, Moretti MP, Fumagalli R, et al. Severe impairment in lung function induced by high peak airway pressure during mechanical ventilation. An experimental study. Am Rev Respir Dis 1987;135:312–315.

Kramer N, Meyer TJ, Meharg J, et al. Randomized, prospective trial of noninvasive positive-pressure ventilation in acute respiratory failure. Am J Respir Crit Care Med 1995;151: 1799–1806.

Laghi F, D'Alfonso N, Tobin MJ. Pattern of recovery from diaphragm fatigue over 24 hours. J Appl Physiol 1995:539–546.

Langer M, Mascheroni D, Marcolin R, et al. The prone position in ARDS patients. A clinical study. Chest 1988;94:103–107.

Leach CL, Greenspan JS, Rubenstein SD, et al. Partial liquid ventilation with perflubron (LiquiVent): a pilot safety and efficacy study in premature newborns with severe RDS who have failed conventional therapy and exogenous surfactant. Presented at the American Academy of Pediatrics Meeting, Dallas, TX, 1994.

Leatherman JW. Mechanical ventilation in obstructive lung disease. Clin Chest Med 1996; 17(3):577–590.

Leatherman JW, Ravenscraft SA, Iber C, et al. High peak inflation does not predict barotrauma during mechanical ventilation of status asthma. Am Rev Respir Dis 1989;139:154A.

Leatherman JW, Ravenscraft SA. Low measured intrinsic positive end-expiratory pressure in mechanically ventilated patients with severe asthma: hidden auto-PEEP. Crit Care Med 1996;24:541–546.

Lodato RF. Oxygen toxicity. In: Tobin MJ, ed. Principles and practice of mechanical ventilation. New York: McGraw-Hill, 1994.

MacIntyre NR. Respiratory function during pressure support ventilation. Chest 1986;89: 677–683.

MacIntyre NR. High frequency ventilation. In Tobin MJ, ed. Principles and practice of mechanical ventilation. New York: McGraw-Hill, 1994.

MacIntyre NR. New modes of ventilation. Clin Chest Med 1996;17(3):411–422.

Mador MJ. Assist-control ventilation. In: Tobin MJ, ed. Principles and practice of mechanical ventilation. New York: McGraw-Hill, 1994.

Mancebo J. Weaning from mechanical ventilation. Eur Respir J 1996;9.

Manthous CA, Hall JB, Kushner R, et al. The effect of mechanical ventilation on oxygen consumption in critically ill patients. Am J Respir Crit Care Med 1995;151:210–214.

Marcy TW. Inverse ratio ventilation. In: Tobin MJ, ed. Principles and practice of mechanical ventilation. New York: McGraw-Hill, 1994.

Marcy TW, Marini JJ. Respiratory distress in the ventilated patient. Clin Chest Med 1994: 55–74.

Marini JJ. Respiratory medicine for the house officer. 2nd ed. Baltimore: Williams & Wilkins, 1987.

Marini JJ. Pressure-controlled ventilation. In: Tobin MJ, ed. Principles and practice of mechanical ventilation. New York: McGraw Hill, 1994.

Marini JJ. Tracheal gas insufflation: a useful adjunct to ventilation? Thorax 1994;49:735–737.

Marini JJ. Evolving concepts in the ventilatory management of acute respiratory distress syndrome. Clin Chest Med 1996;17(3):555–576.

Marini JJ, Culver BH. Systemic air embolism consequent to mechanical ventilation in ARDS. Ann Intern Med 1989;110(9):699–703.

Marini JJ, Ravenscraft SA. Mean airway pressure: physiological determinants and clinical importance. I. Physiological determinants and measurements. Crit Care Med 1992;20: 1461–1472.

Marini JJ, Ravenscraft SA. Mean airway pressure: physiological determinants and clinical importance. II. Clinical implications. Crit Care Med 1992;20:1604–1616.

McCulloch TM, Bishop MJ. Complications of translaryngeal intubation. Clin Chest Med 1991;12(3):507–521.

McKibben AW, Ravenscraft SA. Pressure-controlled and volume-cycled mechanical ventilation. Clin Chest Med 1996;17:395–410.

Meduri GU. Diagnosis and differential diagnosis of ventilator-associated pneumonia. Clin Chest Med 1995;16:61.

Meduri GU. Noninvasive positive pressure ventilation in patients with acute respiratory failure. Clin Chest Med 1996;17:513–553.

Meduri GU, Mauldin GL, Wunderink RG, et al. Causes of fever and pulmonary densities in patients with clinical manifestations of ventilator-associated pneumonia. Chest 1994;106: 221–235.

Meduri GU, Turner RE, Abou-Shala N, et al. Noninvasive positive pressure ventilation via face mask: first-line intervention in patients with acute hypercapnic and hypoxemic respiratory failure. Chest 1996;109:179–193.

Morris AH, Wallace CJ, Menlove RL, et al. Randomized clinical trial of pressure-controlled inverse ratio and extracorporeal CO_2 removal for adult respiratory distress syndrome. Am J Respir Crit Care Med 1994;149:295–305.

Nahum A, Shapiro R. Adjuncts to mechanical ventilation. Clin Chest Med 1996;17(3): 491–512. Nahum A, Ravenscraft SA, Nakos G, et al. Effect of catheter flow direction on CO_2 removal during tracheal gas insufflation in dogs. J Appl Physiol 1993;75:1238–1246.

Nakos G, Zakinthinos S, Kotanidou A, et al. Tracheal gas insufflation reduces the tidal volume while PaCO$_2$ is maintained constant. Intensive Care Med 1994;20:407–413.

Nash G, Blennerhassett JB, Pontoppidan H. Pulmonary lesions associated with oxygen therapy and artificial ventilation. N Engl J Med 1967;267:357–368.

Niederman MS, Torres A, Summer W. Invasive diagnostic testing is not needed routinely to manage suspected ventilator-associated pneumonia. Am J Respir Crit Care Med 1994;150: 565–569.

Oda H, Nogami H, Kusumoto, et al. Long-term exposure to nitric oxide in mice. J Jpn Soc Air Pollut 1976;11:150–160.

Olschewsski H, Walmrath D, Schermuly R, et al. Aerosolized prostacyclin and Iloprost in severe pulmonary hypertension. Ann Intern Med 1996;124:820–824.

Pappert D, Rossaint R, Slama K, et al. Influence of positioning on ventilation-perfusion relationships in severe adult respiratory distress syndrome. Chest 1994;106:1511–1516.

Parker JC, Hernandez LA, Peevy KJ. Mechanisms of ventilator-induced lung injury. Crit Care Med 1993;21:131–143.

Pelosi P, Crosi M, Calappi E, et al. The prone position during general anesthesia minimally affects respiratory mechanics while improving functional residual capacity and increasing oxygen tension. Anesth Analg 1995;80:955–960.

Pinsky MR, Summer WR. Augmentation of cardiac function by elevation of intrathoracic pressure. J Appl Physiol 1983;54:950–955.

Ravenscraft SA. Tracheal gas insufflation: adjunct to conventional mechanical ventilation. Respir Care 1996;41(2):105–111.

Ravenscraft SA, Burke WC, Nahum A. Tracheal gas insufflation augments CO$_2$ clearance during mechanical ventilation. Am Rev Respir Dis 1993;148:345–351.

Roissant R, Falke KJ, Lopez BS, et al. Inhaled nitric oxide for the adult respiratory distress syndrome. N Engl J Med 1993;328:399–405.

Rossi A, Ranieri VM. Positive end-expiratory pressure. In: Tobin MJ, ed. Principles and practice of mechanical ventilation. New York: McGraw-Hill, 1994.

Salord F, Gaussorgues P, Marti-Flich J, et al. Nosocomial maxillary sinusitis during mechanical ventilation: a prospective comparison of orotracheal versus the nasotracheal route for intubation. Intensive Care Med 1990;16:390–393.

Schuster DP. A physiologic approach to initiating, maintaining, and withdrawing mechanical ventilatory support during acute respiratory failure. Am J Med 1990;88:268–278.

Shapiro BA, Cane RD, Harrison RA. Positive end-expiratory pressure in acute lung injury. Chest 1983;83:558–563.

Slutsky AS, et al. Mechanical ventilation. Consensus statement of the American College of Chest Physicians. Chest 1993;104:1833–1859.

Solis R, Anselmi C, Lavietes M. Rate of decay or increment of PaO$_2$ following a change in supplemental oxygen in mechanically ventilated patients with diffuse pneumonia. Chest 1993;103:554–556.

Stauffer JL, Olson DE, Petty TL. Complications and consequences of endotracheal intubation and tracheotomy: a prospective study of 150 critically ill adults. Am J Med 1981;70:65–76.

Thorens J-B, Lolliet P, Ritz M, et al. Effects of rapid permissive hypercapnia on hemodynamics, gas exchange, and oxygen transport and consumption during mechanical ventilation for the acute respiratory distress syndrome. Intensive Care Med 1996;22:182–191.

Torres A, Aznar R, Gatell JM, et al. Incidence, risk, and prognosis factors of nosocomial pneumonia in mechanically ventilated patients. Am Rev Respir Dis 1990;142:523–528.

Tutuncu AS, Faithful NS, Lachman B. Intratracheal perfluorocarbon administration combined with mechanical ventilation in experimental respiratory distress syndrome: dose-dependent improvement of gas exchange. Crit Care Med 1993;21(7):962–969.

Walmrath D, Schneider T, Schermuly R, et al. Direct comparison of inhaled nitric oxide and aerosolized prostacyclin in acute respiratory distress syndrome. Am J Respir Crit Care Med 1996;153:991–996.

Weg JG, Balk RA, Tharratt RS, et al. Safety and potential efficacy of an aerosolized surfactant in human sepsis-induced adult respiratory distress syndrome. JAMA 1994;272:1433–1438.

Wilcox DT, Glick PL, Karamanoukian HL, et al. Perfluorocarbon-associated gas exchange improves pulmonary mechanics, oxygenation, ventilation, and allows nitric oxide delivery in the hypoplastic lung congenital diaphragmatic hernia lamb model. Crit Care Med 1995; 23:1858–1863.

Yang KL, Tobin MJ. A prospective study of indexes predicting the outcome of trials of weaning from mechanical ventilation. N Engl J Med 1991;134:1107–1108.

Zapol WM, Rimar S, Gillis N, et al. Nitric oxide and the lung. Am J Respir Crit Care Med 1994;149:1375–1380.

13 Pulmonary Embolism

M. Gabriel Khan, Lucy B. Palmer

INCIDENCE

In the United States, the incidence of pulmonary embolism has been estimated to exceed 650,000 cases per year. A common and difficult clinical problem, pulmonary embolism is the third most frequent cause of death in the United States.

- Pulmonary embolism accounts for up to 100,000 deaths annually, and approximately 33% of the deaths occur within 1 hour of the onset of symptoms.
- The diagnosis is not suspected in more than 50% of the patients who die.
- Approximately 10% of patients with pulmonary embolism will die in the first hour, and another 20% will die later in the course of the illness.
- When a timely diagnosis is made, more than 90% of patients will survive.
- When pulmonary embolism is overlooked, more than 30% of cases will result in death. Prevention, early diagnosis, and treatment of this serious disease are vital.

PATHOGENESIS

Pulmonary emboli arise from a number of sites, but the primary sources are the deep iliofemoral and thigh veins. Other sites include the pelvic veins and, less commonly, the right atrium and ventricle. The calf veins do not usually give rise to significant emboli but may extend upward in approximately 15% of cases.

Risk factors include any processes that increase venous stasis, damage the intima of the venous system, or cause a hypercoagulable state. Certain clinical conditions present particularly high risk for pulmonary embolism. Patients with these conditions must be considered for prophylactic measures, and a diagnostic workup must be initiated promptly if there are any symptoms of pulmonary embolism. High-risk clinical conditions and underlying factors include:

- History of thromboembolic disease;
- Prolonged anesthesia associated with surgery;
- Surgery or injury to the lower extremities or hip;
- Surgical treatment triggers an increase in factor VIII, a decrease in protein C activity, and an increase in platelet adhesiveness;
- Immobilization after a fracture or surgery or myocardial infarction;
- Pregnancy (particularly postpartum) or use of estrogen-containing compounds;
- Congestive heart failure;

- Malignancy (Trousseau's syndrome). Tumor cells appear to interact with thrombin and plasmin-generating systems. Some cancers cause a decrease in platelet antithrombin and antithrombin III activity and an increase in fibrinogen. In patients with deep venous thrombosis (DVT) and ill-defined risk factors, it is advisable to assess the following: a thorough history and physical examination, abdominal ultrasound, serum carcinoembryonic antigen, fecal occult blood, prostate-specific antigen in men, and mammography in women.
- Street drugs that increase platelet count and adhesiveness;
- Obesity;
- Hypercoagulable diathesis: Protein C, S, or antithrombin III deficiency, polycythemia, and thrombocythemia are implicated in less than 15% of cases of DVT; rarely, high levels of factor V or factor VII may be underlying factors.
- Patients with primary or secondary antiphospholipid syndrome: Assess for anticardiolipin IgG, IgM.

PATHOPHYSIOLOGY

The effects of pulmonary emboli on gas exchange are multifold:

- Increase in alveolar dead space: There is ventilation of the dead space that receives no blood flow;
- Bronchoconstriction and loss of alveolar surfactant in the area of the embolus;
- Hyperventilation;
- Hypoxemia.

Hypoxemia has been attributed to multiple causes, including increased shunt (both intrapulmonary and intracardiac, in cases of patent foramen ovale), widening of the arterio-venous O_2 difference caused by acute changes in cardiac output secondary to right heart failure, increased perfusion to low V/Q units secondary to elevated pulmonary pressures, and atelectasis associated with the loss of surfactant.

Hemodynamic effects of pulmonary emboli depend not only on the size of the embolus but also on the patient's baseline cardiopulmonary status. Normal individuals can tolerate an embolic event of substantial size without significant changes in pulmonary artery pressures. Pulmonary hypertension may occur when 30% or more of the vascular bed is obstructed. In patients with significant underlying pulmonary vascular disease, however, smaller emboli can result in cor pulmonale if acute elevations of the mean pulmonary arterial pressure exceed 40 mm Hg. Pulmonary hypertension appears to be caused by not only decreased cross-sectional area of the vascular bed but also pulmonary artery constriction, which may result from hypoxemia and neural and humoral factors. In a patient with no preexisting cardiopulmonary disease, shock is caused by obstruction of more than 50% of the pulmonary circulation.

PROGNOSIS

The prognosis for patients with pulmonary embolism is usually excellent if they survive the first hour and the diagnosis is made. The degree and rate of resolution are most abnormal in patients with underlying cardiopulmonary disease. Recurrent thromboembolism is uncommon in patients with an acute presentation of pulmonary embolism if treated appropriately. The rate of resolution has been examined using hemodynamic, angiographic, and scan abnormalities.

- Hemodynamic improvement may be minimal the first week after a large embolus.
- Most scans and angiograms will show significant improvement in 3 weeks.
- Complete angiographic resolution can occasionally occur as soon as 7 days after the embolic event.
- There will be minimal further resolution after 2–3 months.
- With underlying cardiopulmonary disease, complete resolution may never occur.

DIAGNOSIS
Clinical Hallmarks

The diagnosis of pulmonary embolism should be strongly considered in patients who manifest one or more of the following clinical patterns.

Acute Unexplained Dyspnea

- Patients present with dyspnea, tachypnea, and tachycardia; these three findings may be transient. Tachypnea and tachycardia are sustained in patients with massive embolism.
- Unexplained sudden syncope with shortness of breath.
- Patients frequently have sustained a large embolus or have underlying cardiopulmonary disease.

Pulmonary Infarction

- Patients usually have sustained, submassive embolus.
- Most patients will have pleuritic chest pain, dyspnea, hemoptysis, and chest x-ray infiltrate. At least three out of four of these findings are usually present.

Other common findings, including fever, occasional friction rub, mild wheeze, and/or crepitations, may be detected on auscultation. Leukocytosis may also occur, but there is a conspicuous absence of band cells that are virtually always present in patients with a bacterial pneumonia, which is frequently the main differential diagnosis.

A small pleural effusion with blunting of the costophrenic angle and pleural-based consolidation are frequent. Large effusions with bronchial breathing, which may persist for some weeks, occasionally occur. The effusion is often blood-tinged or frankly hemorrhagic and has the qualities of an exudate; however, up to 20% of cases yield a transudative pattern. When an exudative effusion is present, a pH less than 7.2 suggests infection. When requesting pH of the pleural aspirate, it is crucial to use the same technique for collecting and transporting the pleural aspirate as is used for arterial blood gas analysis (see Chapter 9).

Because lung parenchyma is oxygenated by the airways as well as by the pulmonary and bronchial circulation, infarction usually occurs when there is damage to two of the three supplies. Therefore, pulmonary infarction occurs more commonly in patients with underlying cardiopulmonary disease. After an infarct, the necrosis of intra-alveolar septae with dense hemorrhage undergoes slow resolution with fibrosis and scar formation, as opposed to complete resolution in patients with no underlying disease.

Acute Cor Pulmonale and Cardiogenic Shock

Massive emboli cause obstruction or large filling defects in two or more lobar arteries. If greater than 70% of the pulmonary vascular cross-sectional area is obstructed, this results in acute pulmonary hypertension exceeding 40–45 mm Hg. Acute right ventricular dilatation and failure supervene, but blood pressure may be temporarily preserved because of an increase in systemic vascular resistance caused by adrenergic reflexes. Over one-half of deaths caused by thromboembolic disease result from massive pulmonary embolism, which is responsible for the majority of deaths that occur within the first hour after the onset of symptoms. The mortality rate of patients with massive pulmonary embolism and shock is approximately 33%. Symptoms and signs include the following:

- Presyncope or syncope, especially associated with shortness of breath;
- Abrupt unexplained severe dyspnea and signs that may simulate an acute exacerbation of chronic obstructive lung disease;
- Oppressive central chest pain (usually nonpleuritic);
- Marked apprehension, restlessness, anxiety;
- Clouding of consciousness, urinary incontinence, hiccups, and, rarely, seizures;
- Cold, clammy skin;
- Signs of cardiogenic shock;
- Intensified pulmonic component of the second heart sound, accompanied by wide physiologic splitting of the second heart sound caused by prolonged right ventricular ejection.

Chronic Cor Pulmonale in Patients with Recurrent Pulmonary Embolism or with an Undetermined Cause

While most pulmonary emboli resolve over weeks, residual obstruction persists in a small group of patients, resulting in pulmonary hypertension and cor pulmonale. This may be secondary to persistent major vessel obstruction or to recurrent small emboli or possible in situ thrombosis. In patients with major vessel obstruction, the diagnosis is often not made at the time of the initial embolic event. Clinical features include the following:

- Patients present with increasing dyspnea and fatigue, as well as signs of right ventricular failure. These symptoms appear to be caused by pulmonary hypertension, which causes further vessel damage.
- The perfusion scan may reveal large bilateral perfusion defects without ventilation abnormality.
- Right heart catheterization and pulmonary angiography are required for diagnosis.

Diagnostic Pitfalls

Certain symptoms and signs, while nonspecific, are sensitive and, when combined with significant risk factors (Tables 13.1–13.3), increase the likelihood of pulmonary embolism. Tables 13.1 and 13.2 show the most commonly demonstrated signs and symptoms in the National Heart, Lung, Blood Institute's Prospective Investigation of Pulmonary Embolism Diagnosis (PIOPED), a large multicenter study examining the accuracy of lung scans compared with pulmonary angiography.

- Dyspnea and pleuritic pain are the most common symptoms.
- Tachypnea and crepitations are the most common findings on physical examination.

Combining the results of clinical diagnosis (clinical probability) and lung scanning can greatly increase the accuracy of diagnosis in certain settings and help direct decision-making as soon as the result of the lung scan is available. Figure 13.1 gives an algorithm for the diagnosis and management of suspected pulmonary embolism.

In PIOPED, when a clinical impression of high probability of pulmonary embolism was combined with a high probability scan, the condition was present in 96% of the cases. Conversely, if both scan and clinical impression were low probability

Table 13.1. Symptoms: No Preexisting Cardiac or Pulmonary Disease

	Pulmonary Embolism N = 117 Number (%)	No Pulmonary Embolism N = 248 Number (%)
Dyspnea	85 (73)	178 (72)
Pleuritic pain	77 (66)	146 (59)
Cough	43 (37)	89 (36)
Leg swelling	33 (28)	55 (22)
Leg pain	30 (26)	60 (24)
Hemoptysis	15 (13)	20 (8)
Palpitations	12 (10)	44 (18)
Wheezing	10 (9)	28 (11)
Anginalike pain	5 (4)	15 (6)

No significant differences were seen.
From Stein PD, Terrin ML, Hales CA, et al. Clinical, laboratory, roentgenographic, and electrocardiographic findings in patients with acute pulmonary embolism and no preexisting cardiac or pulmonary disease. Chest 1991;100:60. Reprinted with permission.

Table 13.2. Signs of Acute Pulmonary Embolism: No Preexisting Cardiac or Pulmonary Disease

	Pulmonary Embolism N = 117 Number (%)	No Pulmonary Embolism N = 248 Number (%)
Tachypnea (20/min)	82 (70)	169 (68)
Crackles	60 (51)	98 (40)[a]
Tachycardia (> 100 min)	35 (30)	59 (24)
Fourth heart sound	28 (24)	34 (14)[a]
Increased P_2	27 (23)	33 (13)[a]
Deep venous thrombosis	13 (11)	27 (11)
Diaphoresis	13 (11)	20 (8)
Temperature > 38.5	8 (7)	29 (12)
Wheezes	6 (5)	21 (8)
Homan's sign	5 (4)	6 (2)
Right ventricular lift	5 (4)	6 (2)
Pleural friction rub	3 (3)	6 (2)
Third heart sound	3 (3)	11 (4)
Cyanosis	1 (1)	5 (2)

[a] $p < 0.05$.

From Stein PD, Terrin ML, Hales CA, et al. Clinical, laboratory, roentgenographic, and electrocardiographic findings in patients with acute pulmonary embolism and no preexisting cardiac or pulmonary disease. Chest 1991;100:60. Reprinted with permission.

for embolism, the diagnosis was correctly excluded in 96% of the cases. For example, if a patient presents with sudden pleuritic pain and becomes hypoxemic on the fifth postoperative day and the chest x-ray shows a small area of atelectasis, the diagnosis of pulmonary embolism is likely. If the scan is high probability, it is not necessary for the workup to proceed. This is a logical approach, but, unfortunately, it does

Table 13.3. Risk Groups for Thromboembolism

Risk Group	Incidence of Venous Thrombosis (%)	Incidence of Fatal PE (%)
Medical patients	15	1
General and gynecologic surgery	15–20	1
Neurologic surgery	15–20	1
Urologic surgery	15–20	5
Total knee replacement	40–70	5
Hip replacement	40–70	1–2
Hip fracture	40–70	1–5

Data from Hyers T, Hull R, Weg J. Second American College of Chest Physicians Conference on antithrombotic therapy, antithrombotic therapy for venous thromboembolic disease. Chest 1989;95:38S. Reprinted with permission.

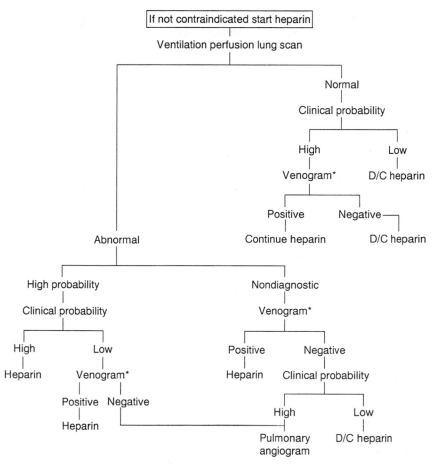

Figure 13.1. Algorithm for the management of suspected pulmonary embolism. *D/C,* discontinue; *, femoral venography (see text).

not embrace many scenarios that may be encountered, and the assignment of high probability and low probability to clinical assessment is still subjective. In PIOPED, the majority of assessments were intermediate, with 20–79% likelihood of pulmonary embolism.

Laboratory Tests

Complete blood count and blood chemistries are nonspecific. As mentioned above, leukocytosis may be present. Lactate dehydrogenase may be elevated in approximately 70% of cases, but this is a nonspecific and delayed finding. Plasma D-dimer ELISA is a useful screening test in patients with suspected PE who are more than 1 week postoperative or who have no coexisting acute illness, including acute myocardial infarction. In patients with pulmonary embolism, some fibrin clot is broken down to D-dimers that are assayed. The test is sensitive but nonspecific. Plasma D-dimer levels less than 500 ng/mL are rarely observed in patients with pulmonary angiographic evidence of pulmonary embolism.

Chest X-Ray

Numerous radiographic abnormalities have been described. None of them, however, are specific or sensitive (see Chapter 1, Fig. 1.15).

- Atelectasis;
- Pleural effusion;
- Elevated hemidiaphragm;
- Pleural-based consolidation (Hampton's hump);
- Pulmonary artery enlargement;
- Abrupt vessel cutoff (knuckle sign); abrupt tapering of the lower lobe branches;
- Area of hyperlucency: oligemia (Westermark's sign);
- Dilatation of azygos vein;
- Enlargement of any chamber of the heart.

Arterial Blood Gas (ABG)

The most common abnormalities of the arterial blood gas include:

- Hypoxemia: PaO_2 less than 80 mm Hg or less than age predicted is present in more than 70% of cases but is nonspecific. More than 13% of patients with proven pulmonary embolism have a PaO_2 greater than 80 mm Hg, on room air, especially if the blood sample is drawn several hours after the event. The alveolar-arterial (A-a) gradient exceeds 20 mm Hg in up to 80% of patients with proven pulmonary embolism, but as with hypoxemia, this is nondiagnostic.
- Respiratory alkalosis: This is a common finding and is usually present, even in patients with chronic obstructive pulmonary disease and CO_2 retention. CO_2 retention from pulmonary emboli is seen only in the setting of massive emboli.

Swan-Ganz Catheter

Many patients who present with severe hypoxemia while in the intensive care unit setting may have a Swan-Ganz catheter in place. Elevated pulmonary artery pressures and the inability to obtain a good wedge tracing may suggest a massive embolus. If the embolus is massive and sufficient to cause right ventricular failure and decreased cardiac output, pulmonary artery pressures may be only moderately elevated.

Electrocardiogram

- Sinus tachycardia is common but too nonspecific to assist in diagnosis.
- A pattern of acute cor pulmonale: S_1-Q_3-T_3 (T-wave inversion in 3) with lead 2

following the pattern in lead 1 rather than lead 3; Q waves in leads 3 and AVF but not in lead 2, a finding that is unlike inferior infarction.

- S_1-S_2-S_3.
- Qr in V_1.
- Right axis deviation.
- Right ventricular strain pattern: Inverted T waves V_1 to V_3 or V_4 with prominent S waves in V_5, V_6 caused by right ventricular dilatation.
- Transient incomplete or complete right bundle branch block.
- Nonspecific ST segment or T-wave inversion (in up to 33% of patients).
- ST segment depression V_4–V_6 (may be caused by poor coronary perfusion in patients with ischemic heart disease).
- ST segment elevation in V_1, AVR, and lead 3.

These findings are uncommon and nonspecific but may occur suddenly; their transient appearance increases the likelihood of pulmonary embolism. Patterns of acute right heart strain should raise the concern of a large embolic event. With massive pulmonary embolism causing syncope, acute unexplained shortness of breath, or shock, one or more of the listed ECG changes occur. Thus, the ECG requires careful scrutiny.

Lung Scan

The first-line investigation for patients with suspected pulmonary embolism is a ventilation/perfusion scan, except for patients with acute cor pulmonale pattern and/ or cardiogenic shock, in whom emergency pulmonary angiography is essential. It must be emphasized that the lung scan may not be useful in many patients with underlying cardiopulmonary disease who will have an indeterminate scan. The PIO-PED study did reveal, however, that the specificity of a high probability scan in patients with prior cardiopulmonary disease was similar to that in patients with no underlying disease (97% versus 98%). Many radiologists request a scan prior to angiographic study to guide their injection and permit a selective study if appropriate. The perfusion scan should be performed first because a normal scan will usually negate the need for further workup. The following rules govern the properly interpreted lung scan report. (See Table 13.4 for definition of scans in the PIOPED study.)

Normal Scans. A normal scan associated with a normal chest x-ray usually indicates the absence of pulmonary embolism. Although some investigations have revealed a 2–4% incidence of positive pulmonary angiograms, studies show that patients with normal scans who have negative studies of their lower extremities for venous thrombosis have an excellent prognosis without anticoagulation. In this setting, it is likely that a clot undetected by a scan is not clinically significant.

Nondiagnostic Lung Scans. Recent data from large multicenter studies suggest that nondiagnostic lung scans should include all scans other than normal and high probability scans. Previously, scans have been rated in compartments of likelihood of pulmonary embolus. With the exception of high probability and normal scans, these terms are frequently misleading and may be dangerous because of the high frequency of low probability scans in patients with angiographic pulmonary embo-

Table 13.4. PIOPED Central Scan Interpretation Categories and Criteria

High Probability

≥ Two large (> 75% of a segment) segmental perfusion defects without corresponding ventilation or x-ray abnormalities.

≥ Two moderate segmental (≥ 25% and ≤ 75% of a segment) perfusion defects without matching ventilation or chest x-ray abnormalities and one large mismatched segmental defect.

≥ For moderate segmental perfusion defects without ventilation or chest x-ray abnormalities.

Intermediate Probability (Indeterminate)

Not falling into normal, very low, low, or high probability categories.

Borderline high or borderline low.

Difficult to categorize as low or high.

Low Probability

Nonsegmental perfusion defects (e.g., very small effusion causing blunting of the costophrenic angle, cardiomegaly, enlarged aorta, hila, and mediastinum, and elevated diaphragm).

Single moderate mismatched segmental perfusion defect with normal chest x-ray.

Any perfusion defect with a substantially larger chest x-ray abnormality.

Large or moderate segmental perfusion defects involving no more than four segments in one lung and no more than three segments in one lung region with matching ventilation defects either equal to or larger in size, and chest x-ray either normal or with abnormalities substantially smaller than perfusion defects.

> Three small segmental perfusion defects (< 25% of a segment) with a normal chest x-ray.

Very Low Probability

≤ Three small segmental perfusion defects with a normal chest x-ray.

Normal

No perfusion defects present.

Perfusion outlines exactly the shape of the lungs as seen on the chest x-ray (hilar and aortic impressions may be seen, chest x-ray and/or ventilation study may be abnormal).

From The PIOPED investigators: Value of the ventilation/perfusion scan in acute pulmonary embolism. JAMA 1990;263:2755. Reprinted with permission.

lism. Both PIOPED and a large series by Hull have shown that pulmonary emboli may be present in 25–40% of patients with low probability scans (Table 13.5). The terms intermediate and low probability scans are misleading and should not be used. Intermediate and low probability scans should be classified as nondiagnostic and dictate the need for further investigations (Fig. 13.1).

High Probability Scans. These scans reveal multiple segmental perfusion defects with ventilation mismatch. These scans are specific but lack sensitivity, which can be as low as 40%. In the PIOPED study, sensitivity of these scans was 97%, but only 102 of 251 patients (41%) with positive angiograms had high probability scans. Similarly, in an investigation by Hull, only 52 of 98 patients (41%) with pulmonary embolism by angiogram had high probability scans.

Table 13.5. Lung Scan and the Incidence of Pulmonary Embolus

Lung Scan Report	Pulmonary Embolism Present[a]	
	Ref. 5	Ref. 11
Normal	2%	4%
High probability	57%	88%
Nondiagnostic	42%	16–33%

[a] Differences between these two large clinical studies are most likely due to different definitions of subgroups of scans.
Ref. 5—Hull RD, Raskob GE. Low probability lung scan findings: a need for change. Ann Int Med 1991;174:142.
Ref. 11—Pioped Investigators: Value of the ventilation-perfusion scan in acute pulmonary embolism. JAMA 1990;203:2753.

Femoral Venography and Venous Studies

Above-the-knee DVT is present in 70–90% of patients with angiographic pulmonary embolism. Thus, evaluation of the lower extremities is often warranted in decision making in patients suspected of having pulmonary embolism. Femoral venography remains the gold standard against which other methods are measured.

Because screening of patients with asymptomatic DVT is not specific with the available noninvasive tests, venography is strongly advisable, particularly for the assessment of patients with suspected pulmonary embolism and to be certain of the need for continued heparin therapy. Thus, Figure 13.1 advocates venography and not ultrasonography or impedance plethysmography; the latter lacks sensitivity and specificity. Real-time B-mode compression ultrasonography is a useful test for patients with symptomatic proximal DVT; this can be supplemented by Doppler flow-detection ultrasonic imaging (duplex scanning) but is of no value for calf vein thrombi. Thus these noninvasive tests are fraught with medicolegal scenarios.

Echocardiography

Echocardiography can identify patients with right ventricular overload caused by pulmonary embolism. Echocardiographic signs include:

- Right ventricular dilatation;
- Right ventricular hypokinesis with sparing of the apex;
- Abnormal interventricular septal motion;
- Tricuspid regurgitation;
- Lack of decreased inspiratory collapse of the inferior vena cava;
- Pulmonary artery dilatation.

Pulmonary Angiography

Pulmonary angiography is the final step necessary in properly selected patients. Pulmonary angiography is performed to confirm or exclude the diagnosis of pulmonary embolism in the following situations:

- Nondiagnostic lung scan with a negative femoral venogram or impedance plethysmography and remaining suspicion of pulmonary embolism;
- As an emergency procedure for diagnostic confirmation prior to embolectomy in patients with acute cor pulmonale pattern and/or cardiogenic shock. In this setting, lung scan is not indicated.
- High probability scan in a patient with a history of pulmonary emboli (these scans have less specificity in this group);
- High probability scan with a high risk of bleeding.

The risks of angiography include:

- Allergic reaction to contrast material. The procedure can be carried out, if strongly warranted, using premedication with corticosteroids and antihistamine with epinephrine standby.
- Cardiac perforation (occurs in up to 0.3% of patients, but is virtually nonexistent in experienced hands).
- Arrhythmias (usually easily controlled).
- Depression of myocardial contractility may precipitate heart failure within minutes to 1 hour of the procedure in patients with left ventricular dysfunction. Also, a large volume of contrast material is required and imposes an osmotic load; thus, intravenous (IV) furosemide may be required.
- Pulmonary hypertension may be exacerbated by the procedure, but selective injections are often possible and are well tolerated.
- The morbidity rate is 2–4%; the mortality rate is less than 0.2%.

THERAPY

The algorithm given in Figure 13.1 does not cover all scenarios but directs logical decision making and ensures appropriate management. Another approach recommended by other authors is illustrated in Figure 13.2. This strategy uses noninvasive studies that are nonspecific and that may not be appropriate for the management of life-threatening conditions such as pulmonary embolism.

Heparin

Heparin (5,000–10,000 units) is given as an IV bolus if there is no contraindication to anticoagulant therapy. The bolus is followed immediately by an initial continuous infusion of heparin: 1520 U/hour in patients without known risks of bleeding and 1280 U/hour in those with risk of bleeding (Table 13.6). The activated partial throm-

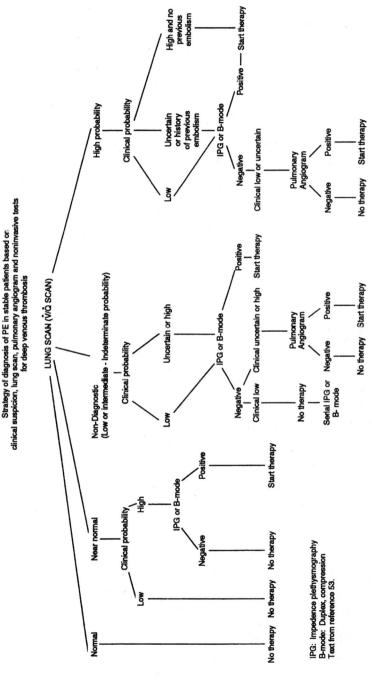

Figure 13.2. Strategy for diagnosis of pulmonary embolism in stable patients based on clinical suspicion, lung scan, pulmonary angiogram, and noninvasive tests for deep venous thrombosis. *IPG*, impedance plethysmography; *B-mode*, duplex, compression ultrasound. (From Arroliga AC, Matthay MA, Matthay RA. Pulmonary thromboembolism and other pulmonary vascular diseases. In: George RB, Light RW, Matthay MA, Matthay RA, eds. Chest medicine: essentials of pulmonary and critical care medicine. 3rd ed. Baltimore: Williams & Wilkins, 1995:279. Reprinted with permission.)

Table 13.6. Continuous Infusion Heparin[a]

Rate (mL/hr)	Units (/hr)	Units (/24 hrs)
21	840	20,160
25	1000	24,000
28	1120	26,880
30	1200	28,800
32	1280	30,720
34	1360	32,640
36	1440	34,560
38	1520	36,480
40	1600	38,400
42	1680	40,320
44	1760	42,240
46	1840	44,160
48	1920	46,080
50	2000	48,000

[a] For each heparin order, specify both the rate of flow and the dose in units per hour.
20,000 units of heparin in 500 mL of 5% dextrose in water. If noncardiac, dilute in 0.9% saline. 1 mL equals 40 units.
Commence with No. 5, 1280 units/hr and adjust to maintain activated PTT at 1.5–2.5 times the upper limit of the control value (usual therapeutic range 60–85 seconds).

boplastin time (PTT) is done 6 hours later and the infusion adjusted to maintain the PTT 1.5–2 times the patient control level. Heparin is usually continued for 5–10 days; warfarin (Coumadin) is started between the second and fifth day. The International Normalized Ratio (INR) should be in the therapeutic range of 2 to 3 for 48 hours prior to the discontinuation of heparin.

The mean dose of the heparin infusion that is required to prolong the PTT to 1.5 times control is approximately 33,000 U/24 hours (1360/hour). Most patients require from 24,000 to 36,480 U/24 hours (1520/hour). Less than 20% of patients require 36,000–42,000 U/24 hours to achieve the therapeutic goal of 1.5 to 2.5 times the upper limit of normal of the control PTT value.

The platelet count should be done on the third day of heparin administration, then daily. Heparin-induced thrombocytopenia (HIT) usually begins between 3 and 15 days after commencement of heparin, and in approximately 0.4% of these patients, serious arterial or venous thrombosis occurs. Warfarin is continued for 3–6 months. In some patients with ongoing risk factors, prolonged therapy may be required.

Thrombolytic Agents

Thrombolytic therapy is of value to restore circulation in patients with hemodynamic compromise in the setting of massive emboli or shock. Streptokinase, urokinase, and tissue-type plasminogen activator (t-PA) are the three agents currently available.

Despite their ability to accelerate the early rate of resolution, there has been no proven benefit in long-term morbidity or mortality compared with heparin therapy alone. The unknown benefits must be weighed against the significant bleeding risks associated with the use of these agents. Despite early speculation that t-PA might be associated with less bleeding, early investigations have not shown this to be true.

The current indication for thrombolytic agent use is massive pulmonary embolism and hemodynamic compromise.

Dosage: The two most commonly used agents are streptokinase and urokinase.

- Streptokinase: 250,000 U over 30 minutes IV, then infusion of 100,000 U for 12–24 hours followed by IV heparin.
- Urokinase: 4,400 IU/kg as a loading dose over 10 minutes, followed by 4,400 IU/kg for 12 to 24 hours followed by IV heparin.
- t-PA: 100 mg as a continuous peripheral IV infusion over 2 hours.

After 3 hours of treatment with either agent, testing should be done to ensure a "lytic state." This can be monitored with a number of tests, including *euglobulin* lysis time, fibrinogen level, fibrinogen degradation products, prothrombin time, or PTT. This testing is not used to adjust dosing but to determine whether systemic fibrinolysis has been achieved. If it has not, the patient may need to be rebolused.

Pulmonary Embolectomy

Pulmonary embolectomy in the setting of an acute embolus is a controversial treatment reserved for patients with massive embolism and hypotension who have not responded to conventional therapy. The mortality is approximately 50%, which most likely reflects the severity of the process being treated (frequently these patients have already arrested and are requiring cardiopulmonary resuscitation). This option is a viable one in only a few institutions. Pulmonary embolectomy may be done surgically or by a transvenous catheter, which removes the clot via suction. When pulmonary embolectomy is performed, the patient must also have placement of a vena caval filter.

Inferior Vena Cava Barrier

Inferior vena cava barrier is a useful intervention that prevents the migration of large clots. Currently, the ideal method is transvenous insertion of a filter device that permits blood flow to prevent occlusion and long-term complications. There are numerous types and sizes of devices available, and these vary from institution to institution.

Indications include:

- Patients recovering from life-threatening pulmonary embolism to prevent further massive embolism;
- Contraindication for anticoagulants;

* Recurrent emboli during adequate anticoagulation;
* Patients undergoing pulmonary embolectomy.

PREVENTION IN PATIENTS AT RISK

Patient populations have been stratified into risk categories for DVT and pulmonary emboli. Methods of prevention are modified for the individual clinical groups and their risk of bleeding.

* For patients at low to moderate risk, low-dose heparin should be given (5,000 units subcutaneously every 8–12 hours starting at the time of risk).
* Neurosurgical procedures, major knee surgery, and urologic surgery should be treated with intermittent pneumatic compression.
* Patients undergoing hip surgery should be treated with adjusted-dose heparin to keep PTT in the upper half of normal range or with warfarin to prolong the pro-thrombin time to 1.3–1.5 times control (INR 2 to 3).
* Hip fracture patients should receive prophylactic therapy to achieve an INR 2 to 3.
* In some high-risk patients, there may be a role for combined modalities (e.g., pneumatic compression and anticoagulation).

BIBLIOGRAPHY

Bell WR, Simon GL, DeMets DL. The clinical features of submassive and massive pulmonary emboli. Am J Med 1977;62:35.

Caracci BF, Rumbolo PM, Mainini S, et al. How accurate are ventilation-perfusion scans for pulmonary embolism? Am J Surg 1988;156:477.

Cruickshank MK, Levine MN, Hirsh J, et al. A standard heparin nomogram for the management of heparin therapy. Arch Intern Med 1991;151:333.

Dalen JE, Alpert JS. Natural history of pulmonary embolism. Prog Cardiovasc Dis 1975;42:259.

Dantzker PR, Bower JS. Clinical significance of pulmonary function tests: alterations in gas exchange following pulmonary thromboembolism. Chest 1982;81:495.

Hirsh J. Antithrombotic therapy in deep vein thrombosis and pulmonary embolism. Am Heart J 1992;123:1115.

Hirsh J. Heparin. N Engl J Med 1991;324:1565.

Hirsh J. The optimal duration of anticoagulant therapy for venous thrombosis. N Engl J Med 1995;332:1710.

Hull RD, Raskob GE. Low-probability lung scan findings: a need for change. Ann Intern Med 1991;174:142.

Hull RD, Hirsh J, Carter CJ, et al. Pulmonary angiography, ventilation lung scanning and venography for clinically suspected pulmonary embolism with abnormal perfusion lung scan. Ann Intern Med 1983;98:891.

Hyers JM, Hull RD, Weg JE. Antithrombotic therapy for venous thromboembolic disease. Chest 1989;95:375.

McBride K, LaMorte WW, Menzoian JO. Can ventilation-perfusion scans accurately diagnose pulmonary embolism. Arch Surg 1986;121:754.

Meyer G, Sors H, Charbonnier B, et al. Effects of intravenous urokinase versus alteplase on total pulmonary resistance in acute massive pulmonary embolism: a European multicenter double-blind trial. J Am Coll Cardiol 1992;19:239.

Moser KM. Venous thromboembolism. Am Rev Respir Dis 1990;141:235.

Moser KM, Spragg RG, Utley J, et al. Chronic thrombotic obstruction of major pulmonary arteries. Ann Intern Med 1983;99:299.

PIOPED Investigators: Value of the ventilation-perfusion scan in acute pulmonary embolism. JAMA 1990;263:2753.

Stein PD, Athanasoulis C, Alavi A, et al. Complications and validity of pulmonary angiography in acute pulmonary embolism. Circulation 1992;85:462.

Stein PD, Coleman RE, Gottschalk A, et al. Diagnostic utility of ventilation/perfusion lung scans in acute pulmonary embolism is not diminished by pre-existing cardiac or pulmonary disease. Chest 1991;100:604.

Stein PP, Terrin ML, Hales CA, et al. Clinical laboratory, roentgenographic and electrocardiographic findings in patients with acute pulmonary embolism and no pre-existing cardiac or pulmonary disease. Chest 1991;100:598.

Weinmann EE, Salzman EW. Deep vein thrombosis. N Engl J Med 1994;331:1630.

14 Pulmonary Hypertension and Cor Pulmonale

M. Gabriel Khan

PULMONARY HYPERTENSION

Primary and secondary pulmonary hypertension are important causes of pulmonary heart disease, cor pulmonale. The expertise of both pulmonologist and cardiologist is usually required to manage these life-threatening conditions. Primary pulmonary hypertension (PPH) is a rare disease that is often fatal; this devastating disease occurs with particular frequency in young women.

Because PPH is rare, accounting for less than 0.1% of all cases of pulmonary hypertension, it will be discussed after considering the more important causes of secondary pulmonary hypertension (Fig. 14.1).

Pathophysiology

Normal resting peak systolic pulmonary artery pressure at sea level ranges from 20 to 25; the mean is 12–16 mm Hg, and the end-diastolic ranges from 6 to 10 mm Hg. The pulmonary circulation is a low-resistance circuit. Normally, an arteriovenous pressure gradient of only 2–10 mm Hg exists to circulate the cardiac output through the low-resistance pulmonary vascular channels. Pulmonary hypertension exists when pulmonary vascular resistance increases and the pulmonary artery systolic and mean pressures at rest are consistently above 30 and 20 mm Hg, respectively.

Causes of Pulmonary Hypertension

Pulmonary hypertension may be caused by several disease states, including the following:

- Physiologic from all causes of hypoxemia;
- Diseases, primarily of the lung parenchyma, that also affect the pulmonary vascular bed;
- Vascular involvement in systemic disease;
- Pulmonary thromboembolism;
- All causes of left ventricular failure; mitral stenosis or regurgitation, left atrial myxoma, and pulmonary veno-occlusive disease;

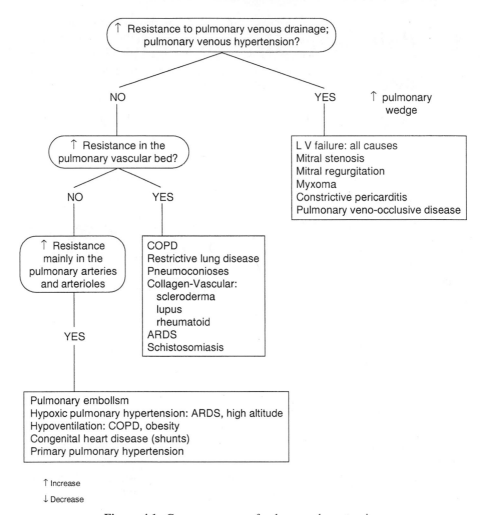

Figure 4.1. Common causes of pulmonary hypertension.

• Congenital heart disease, left-to-right shunts;
• PPH.

Figure 14.1 presents an algorithmic approach derived from considering the parts of the pulmonary circulation in which increased resistance to blood flow actuates pulmonary hypertension. Except when the diagnosis is clinically obvious, it is advisable to first exclude pulmonary venous hypertension that results in an increase in pulmonary wedge pressure.

Clinical Features

Mild pulmonary hypertension (pulmonary artery pressure 40/20, mean greater than 25 mm Hg) is usually asymptomatic. Moderate pulmonary hypertension with pulmonary artery pressure of 50–60 (systolic) and 25–30 (diastolic) (mean greater than 40 mm Hg) may cause dyspnea on exertion and easy fatigability. These symptoms occur more commonly with severe pulmonary hypertension (pulmonary artery pressure greater than 80/35, mean greater than 55 mm Hg). Tachypnea and occasional chest pain, presyncope, syncope, and, rarely, sudden death may also occur.

Symptoms and signs may be caused by the underlying diseases listed in Figure 14.1. Common findings include the following:

- A giant A wave in the jugular venous pulse;
- A left parasternal lift or heave caused by right ventricular hypertrophy;
- A parasternal, palpable systolic pulsation in the left intercostal space;
- An accentuated, pulmonary component of the second heart sound;
- An ejection click caused by dilatation of the main pulmonary artery;
- A fourth heart sound at the lower left sternal border; with severe pulmonary hypertension or cor pulmonale, a right-sided S_3 that increases on inspiration;
- An early decrescendo diastolic murmur maximal in the second left intercostal space caused by pulmonary regurgitation;
- A murmur of tricuspid regurgitation with prominent V waves if the tricuspid valve annulus is dilated;
- Finally, signs of right heart failure; jugular venous pressure 4–12 cm.

Investigations

Chest X-ray and Electrocardiogram

- X-ray evidence of dilatation of the main, right, and left pulmonary arteries with attenuation of peripheral branches (see Chapter 1 and Fig. 14.2);
- Electrocardiogram (ECG): peaked P waves in leads II, III, and AVF caused by right atrial enlargement; S_1Q_3, $S_1S_2S_3$, an S wave in V_5, or an R/S ratio in V_5 or V_6 of less than 1; right axis deviation, right ventricular hypertrophy, and ST segment depression with T-wave inversion in leads $V_1–V_3$.

Echocardiography

Echocardiographic evaluation is extremely useful in detecting causes of left heart failure, left atrial enlargement, mitral stenosis, myxoma, elevation of the pulmonary artery pressure, right ventricular hypertrophy, tricuspid regurgitation, enlargement of cardiac chambers, or shunts.

Lung Scan

The lung scan is not diagnostic and must be analyzed in conjunction with a probability clinical assessment (see Chapter 13 and Fig. 13.1).

In the absence of chronic obstructive lung disease, lung scans help in differentiating pulmonary embolism from PPH.

- Normal lung scan or diffuse mottling, salt and pepper pattern, and no segmental defects strongly suggest PPH if other causes of secondary pulmonary hypertension are excluded.
- One or more segmental or larger defects suggest pulmonary embolism (Fig. 13.1).

Pulmonary Angiography

If pulmonary embolism versus PPH cannot be resolved by the aforementioned systematic clinical approach and the investigations outlined, pulmonary angiogram is advisable to exclude chronic pulmonary embolism. Also, fiberoptic angioscopy can verify the presence of thrombi in the pulmonary arteries and evaluate their accessibility for removal.

Lung Biopsy

- In patients with moderate to severe pulmonary hypertension, transbronchial biopsy may cause significant bleeding and is contraindicated;
- Sampling errors are common;
- May be useful to confirm the type of interstitial lung disease causing pulmonary hypertension.

Therapy

Treatment of secondary pulmonary hypertension entails adequate management of the underlying disease. Hypoxemia must be corrected. If the PaO_2 is less than 55 mm Hg at rest, oxygen is advisable for at least 15 hours daily.

Nifedipine Extended Release

(Procardia XL)

Nifedipine may cause a decrease in pulmonary artery pressure, especially in patients with collagen vascular disease. The response to calcium antagonists is variable. A dose of nifedipine (20–180 mg daily) may be required. Some patients respond, while others do not. If an acute response occurs with a reduction in pulmonary artery pressure, a salutary long-term response usually can be expected.

Digoxin

Digoxin is indicated for the management of atrial fibrillation with a ventricular response greater than 90/min at rest or greater than 100/min on mild activities, such as walking 100 feet or more. A trial of the drug is advisable in patients with left or right heart failure and sinus rhythm.

Furosemide

Patients with right heart failure caused by pulmonary hypertension that is triggered by increased resistance in the vascular bed or pulmonary arteries benefit from small doses of furosemide (20–40 mg daily). In these patients, larger doses of diuretics have a propensity to precipitate electrolyte imbalance, especially hypochloremic metabolic alkalosis. Occasionally, acetazolamide may be given 3 days weekly, if needed, for correction of this electrolyte abnormality. Caution is necessary because this combination may cause hypokalemia.

Pulmonary thromboembolism is a major cause of pulmonary hypertension and is discussed in Chapter 13.

PRIMARY PULMONARY HYPERTENSION

PPH is extremely rare. The incidence is approximately two cases per million population. Thus, only a few medical centers have gained adequate experience in managing the condition. PPH is perhaps the most devastating disease encountered in cardiopulmonary medicine. This is particularly so because the disease affects young adults. There is invariably progressive elevation of pulmonary vascular resistance and pulmonary artery pressure, which causes right ventricular failure and death. The diagnosis is entertained only after exclusion of all causes of secondary pulmonary hypertension, particularly recurrent pulmonary embolism.

Etiology

PPH occurs most often in children and young adults. A marked frequency has been observed in the Indian subcontinent. A National Registry report of 187 patients indicated that 63% of patients were women (mean age 36 ± 15). In the Mayo Clinic follow-up study of 120 patients, 73% were female, the mean age was 34 years, and, in two families, PPH occurred in two brothers.

The etiology of PPH is unknown. There is strong evidence that points to an abnormality in the pulmonary vascular endothelium. Endothelial injury and dysfunction are key factors. Increased pulmonary vascular reactivity and vasoconstriction commonly observed in patients with PPH indicates that a marked vasoconstrictive tendency is an important pathogenic factor in predisposed individuals. Hypovasodilatation appears to be the result of loss of endothelial cell integrity. Decreased endothelium-derived relaxing factor (EDRF) may result in hypovasodilatation. The resultant vasoconstriction may enhance the secretion of the potent vasoconstrictor endothelin, particularly in the presence of platelet aggregation.

The following associations have been noted as possible factors or aggravating mechanisms:

- Thromboembolism and amniotic fluid embolism. Occult thromboembolism may cause slow progressive pulmonary hypertension with clinical manifestations only in the terminal stage of illness and is difficult to exclude as a cause of clinically diagnosed PPH. In some studies, up to 50% of patients diagnosed with PPH were found to have thromboembolism. Occult thromboembolism is not the underlying process, however, in the majority of patients with PPH.

- The pulmonary vasculature reveals intense intimal proliferation that results in almost complete occlusion in some arteries. The intimal fibrosis may be a protective reaction to some form of endothelial injury in susceptible subjects. The role of several growth factors, including those derived from platelets and fibroblasts, is being investigated.
- Most patients with PPH have plexogenic arteriopathy similar to that observed in Eisenmenger's syndrome and in cases in which severe pulmonary hypertension and death were caused by appetite suppressants. Most children in the Indian subcontinent present in the late teenage years and die within 5 years, with an aggressive plexiform arteriopathy, arteritis, and fibrinoid necrosis affecting the small muscular pulmonary arteries of undetermined cause.
- Recent studies have estimated that elevated plasma concentrations of endothelin-1 are associated with pulmonary hypertension. Endothelin is a potent vasoconstrictor; endothelin ETA receptor antagonists reportedly reduce pulmonary artery pressure in experimental animals.
- Approximately 6% of cases are familial. Familial cases have been reported with autosomal dominant inheritance. The occurrence of familial PPH strongly supports a genetic susceptibility.
- Toxic cooking oil syndrome.
- The anorexic agent (aminorex fumarate). In Europe, PPH occurred in 0.2% of individuals ingesting this agent, which is no longer available. French investigators reported a cluster of cases of PPH among individuals who had used derivatives of fenfluramine, a serotonin reuptake inhibitor, in the early 1990s. A recent study showed that the use of fenfluramine and dexfenfluramine as obesity pills was associated with an increased risk of PPH, in particular when these agents were used for more than 3 months. Fenfluramine dexfenfluramine and aminorex may be implicated in the causation of the disease; experimentally these agents have been shown to cause potassium channel blockade with consequent pulmonary vasoconstriction. These agents decrease serotonin uptake.
- Raynaud's phenomenon was reported in 8.2% of cases in the 1991 National Registry and in 10% of cases in the Mayo Clinic study. In families of patients with PPH, Raynaud's phenomenon may occur in members not affected by PPH. This suggests that vasospasm in pulmonary arteries may be a factor. This association deserves investigative exploration. The association may be related, however, to the presence of undetected collagen-vascular or autoimmune disease.
- A defect in the nitric oxide synthase system may be implicated and deserves intensive study. Vascular endothelial cells synthesize nitric oxide from L-arginine. Nitric oxide is a potent vasodilator now known to be the endothelium-derived relaxing factor. Patients with PPH appear to be deficient in the endothelial-derived vasodilator prostacyclin and nitric oxide. The circulatory system is believed to be in a state of active vasodilatation under the influence of many factors, including prostacyclin and nitric oxide. Thus, systemic and pulmonary hypertension may be envisaged as a state of hypovasodilatation. In patients with PPH, this pathophysiologic mechanism may be confined, perhaps genetically, to the pulmonary arterioles.
- Prolonged intense pulmonary vasoconstriction causes pulmonary hypertension and

pathologic changes, including plexogenic pulmonary arteriopathy and fibrinoid necrosis. It is of interest that inhaled nitric oxide administered to patients with PPH resulted in a marked decrease in pulmonary vascular resistance, equal to that achieved with IV prostacyclin.

- In a study of PPH in children, five of eighteen patients died within five years of diagnosis. The mean survival time was 29 months. Right heart failure was the principal cause of death. Autopsy of these patients showed marked enlargement and hypertrophy of the right side of the heart and great dilatation of the pulmonary artery. The small pulmonary arterioles showed medial hypertrophy and marked intimal proliferation that narrowed the vessel lumen. No plexiform lesions were identified; no thromboemboli were found in large or small pulmonary arteries. The main pulmonary artery showed fewer, shorter, and more irregular elastic fibers than did the aorta. This finding indicates that PPH in these individuals was acquired after birth.

- Badesch et al. reported four patients with PPH who had hypothyroidism and low titer-positive antinuclear antibody; this may suggest an underlying autoimmune process. Two of these patients had Raynaud's phenomenon. An autoimmune process may cause an abnormality in the pulmonary vascular endothelium, increased vascular reactivity, and vasoconstriction.

Clinical Features

The most common clinical findings derived from the Mayo Clinic study and the National Registry include the following:

- Progressive dyspnea (66%); decreased exercise tolerance may be incapacitating;
- Fatigue and weakness (20%);
- Presyncope, syncope (13%);
- Dizziness (20%);
- Raynaud's phenomenon (10%);
- Exertional chest pain (10%) caused by right ventricular myocardial ischemia and/ or distension of the major pulmonary arteries;
- A left parasternal heave caused by right ventricular hypertrophy;
- A palpable systolic pulsation caused by a dilated pulmonary artery;
- A large A wave in the jugular venous pulse;
- A loud pulmonic component of the second heart sound (93%) and a closely split second heart sound;
- A right ventricular 4th heart sound;
- A pulmonary ejection click;
- Tricuspid regurgitation (40%);
- Enlargement of the main pulmonary arteries on chest radiograph (90%).

Prognosis in the Mayo Clinic study was poor; only 21% of patients survived 5 years. The results from the National Prospective Registry recruitment and follow-up of 144 patients indicated survival rate at 1 year (68%), 3 years (48%), and 5 years (34%). Mortality was closely associated with three variables:

Table 14.1. Median Survival for Patients with Primary Pulmonary Hypertension Compared with Three Hemodynamic Variables[a]

Hemodynamic Variable	Median Survival Time in Months
Mean pulmonary artery pressure	
$\geq$ 85 mm Hg	12
< 55 mm Hg	48
Mean right arterial pressure	
$\geq$ 20 mm Hg	1
< 10 mm Hg	46
Mean cardiac index	
< 2 l/min/m^2	17
$\geq$ 4 l/min/m^2	43

[a] Modified from Ann Intern Med 1991;115:343.

- Mean pulmonary artery pressure;
- Mean right atrial pressure;
- Mean cardiac index as shown in Table 14.1.

Investigations

Figure 14.2 shows radiologic features of severe pulmonary hypertension of uncertain cause.

Because the clinical features, ECG, chest radiograph, echocardiography, and lung scan do not serve to distinguish all cases of PPH from secondary pulmonary hypertension, right heart catheterization and pulmonary angiogram are virtually always required prior to labeling the patient as having PPH. In addition, the pathologic lesions of PPH appear to be indistinguishable from those found in patients with secondary pulmonary hypertension caused by congenital heart disease, appetite-suppressing agents, and scleroderma.

Indications for right heart catheterization and pulmonary angiography include the following:

- If the history, physical, and chest x-ray are not in keeping with secondary pulmonary hypertension;
- Echocardiographic assessment shows the absence of left heart disease and the presence of unexplained moderate to severe pulmonary hypertension; enlargement of the right atrium and ventricle;
- The presence of normal arterial blood gases;
- A normal lung scan; salt and pepper pattern or diffuse patchy perfusion abnormalities are observed;
- Exclusion of chronic pulmonary embolism, which is a conflicting diagnosis requiring pulmonary angiography.

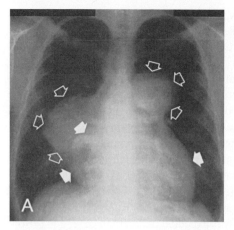 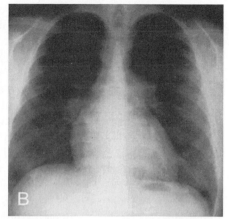

Figure 14.2. Dilatation of the pulmonary arteries in primary pulmonary hypertension. A 17-year-old male patient presented with severe pulmonary hypertension of uncertain cause (i.e., primary pulmonary hypertension). A chest x-ray film (**A**) revealed massive dilatation of the central pulmonary arteries (*open white arrows*) and right ventricular enlargement (*solid white arrows*) that had not been present three years earlier (**B**). There was no evidence of congenital heart disease. Pulmonary angiography showed no sign of chronic thromboembolic disease or veno-occlusive disease. The pulmonary arterial pressure was 106/58 mm Hg (mean 76), with a mean right atrial pressure of 9 mm Hg, cardiac output of 5.4 L/min, and pulmonary vascular resistance of 17.5 Wood units. Calcium antagonists had no effect on pulmonary hemodynamics. Because of a progressive increase in the pulmonary-artery diameter and recent clinical deterioration with repeated episodes of syncope, a heart–lung transplantation has been recommended. (From Lang IM, Kneussl MP. Dilatation of the pulmonary arteries in primary pulmonary hypertension. N Engl J Med 1996;334:302. Massachusetts Medical Society. Reprinted with permission.)

Therapy

Calcium Antagonists

Symptomatic patients with moderate to severe pulmonary hypertension may show a partial response to calcium antagonists. Nifedipine has advantages over verapamil and diltiazem because these agents may cause a worsening of right heart failure.

Titrated high doses of nifedipine extended release (180–240 mg daily) and diltiazem (up to 720 mg daily) have been shown to cause substantial reduction in pulmonary artery pressure in some patients with PPH, but diltiazem may worsen right heart failure. Reduction in pulmonary artery pressure and pulmonary vascular resistance persisted at 1 year in at least 4 of 13 patients treated with nifedipine. Five of the thirteen individuals failed to respond to massive doses of these agents. This variability in response has been documented in other small studies.

Adenosine is effective in predicting the response of calcium antagonists. Adenosine has a half-life of less than six seconds, and minor adverse effects are thus transient. Among 17 of 64 patients with proven PPH who responded to treatment, the dose of nifedipine ranged from 120 to 240 mg daily. Although only a small number responded to calcium antagonists, they had markedly better survival (94% at 5 years) compared with patients who did not respond. Improvement in quality of life and functional class was observed. Digoxin was administered to all patients taking calcium antagonists.

Note: Caution is necessary. Calcium antagonists should not be administered to patients with marginal hemodynamic status. It is necessary to document accurate baseline hemodynamics prior to the trial of calcium antagonists. Deaths have been caused by nifedipine in patients with severe PPH. A relevant case report describes a 17-year-old previously healthy woman who had dyspnea for nine months. Cardiac index was 1.8 L/min, wedge pressure 17 mm Hg, BP 95/52, CVP 17 mm Hg, heart rate 115/min. The patient was given 20 mg of nifedipine and 37 minutes later, the BP dropped to 86/52, CVP rose to 26, electromechanical dissociation ensued, and resuscitation was unsuccessful. Calcium antagonists should not be given to all patients with PPH because a salutary response is expected in less than 25%, and serious harm may ensue in many. Patients who do not show a marked dramatic hemodynamic response to calcium antagonists do not appear to benefit from long-term therapy. Calcium antagonists should not be administered without hemodynamic guidance.

Calcium antagonists are contraindicated in patients with the following:

- Central venous pressure greater than 12 mm Hg;
- Heart rate greater than 100;
- Cardiac index less than 2 L/min/m^2.

Nifedipine has been shown to partially prevent acute pulmonary vasoconstriction caused by hypoxemia. Calcium antagonists are known to cause ventilation perfusion derangements, however, and may provoke hypoxemia in some patients.

Digoxin

Digoxin is advisable in all patients administered calcium antagonists and in all patients with right heart failure.

Prostacyclin

Prostacyclin (epoprostenol) has an extremely short half-life (several minutes) and is administered as a continuous infusion, which should not be suddenly discontinued. This agent is effective and has a role in controlling elevated pulmonary hemodynamics for weeks to months in properly selected patients considered for lung transplantation. In a study of 22 patients, hemodynamic and clinical benefits were maintained up to 18 months with continuous prostacyclin infusion. A multicenter 12-week prospective randomized study by Barst et al. showed that continuous intravenous infusion of epoprostenol (prostacyclin) was superior to conventional therapy and caused an improvement in survival. In the 41 epoprostenol-treated patients, pulmonary artery pressure improved and the median distance walked in 6 minutes rose from 315 meters at baseline to 362 meters at 12 weeks; conventional therapy caused a decrease from 270 meters at baseline to 204 meters at 12 weeks. No patients died in the treated group versus eight deaths in the group randomly assigned to conventional therapy. In some less critically ill patients, prostacyclin therapy may delay the need for transplantation indefinitely. Prostacyclin causes improvement in most patients and can be used in class III and IV patients, whereas calcium antagonists may cause deleterious effects in many and salutary effects in less than 25%. Thus, prostacyclin is currently the treatment of choice for class III and IV patients.

Other Agents

Pepke-Zaba et al. observed the acute effects of inhaled nitric oxide compared with continuous IV prostacyclin in eight patients with severe pulmonary hypertension. Prostacyclin caused significant reduction in pulmonary and systemic vascular resistance. Inhaled nitric oxide showed a similar decrease in pulmonary vascular resistance but, as expected, had no effect on systemic vascular resistance as a result of rapid inactivation of nitric oxide by hemoglobin.

Further developments are anticipated in the research of phenomena that involve vasoconstriction and hypovasodilatation, which appear to have escaped homeostatic control.

Endothelin-1 concentration is increased in patients with PPH. Thus, endothelin ETA receptor antagonists are being tested. Anticoagulants are recommended in all patients with PPH. In the Mayo Clinic study, survival improved in some patients with this form of therapy.

Transplantation

Heart–lung, double lung, or, preferably, single lung transplantation has a role in properly selected patients. Single lung transplantation reportedly is as effective as double lung transplantation in the majority of patients with PPH. Obliterative bronchiolitis remains a major problem in more than 33% of patients, the majority of whom require high-dose corticosteroids. In a study of single lung transplant carried out in 12 patients for pulmonary hypertension, 11 patients survived up to 22 months. The 3-month hemodynamic report indicated a reduction of pulmonary artery systolic pressure from 92 ± 7 mm Hg to 29 ± 6 mm Hg ($p = 0.001$). In specialized centers, these procedures continue, with hope for improved survival and relief of suffering for some patients.

COR PULMONALE

Heart disease secondary to lung disease is classified as cor pulmonale (pulmonary heart disease). Right ventricular hypertrophy or right heart failure may occur as a result of severe pulmonary hypertension caused by a number of diseases affecting the pulmonary vascular bed or arteries, as outlined earlier in this chapter. The most common causes of cor pulmonale are long-standing severe chronic bronchitis, emphysema, and restrictive lung disease (see Chapters 5 and 6); patients in this category usually show PaO_2 less than 55 mm Hg when they are free from an exacerbation of the disease. Hypoxia is a potent stimulus for vasoconstriction and pulmonary hypertension. Pulmonary embolism is discussed in Chapter 13; a rare cause of PPH was discussed earlier in this chapter.

Pulmonary hypertension and right ventricular hypertrophy develop in up to 25% of patients, and right heart failure is manifest in approximately 10% of these individuals.

Notable findings include:

- Increased shortness of breath on minimal exertion;
- Easy fatigability at rest;
- Tachypnea;
- Pursed lip expiration;
- Paradoxical abdominal breathing and constant use of accessory muscles of respiration;
- Asterixis and chemosis; engorgement of blood vessels in the fundi caused by hypercapnia and, rarely, papilledema;
- Central cyanosis with warm peripheries is the usual finding; the occurrence of added peripheral cyanosis with cold peripheries indicates that right heart failure has supervened.

Radiologic features are shown in Figure 1.18A-B in Chapter 1.

In patients with cor pulmonale, cardiac murmurs may be difficult to detect. In particular, it is easy to miss the murmur of significant mitral regurgitation. Echocardiography is recommended to exclude significant mitral regurgitation if doubt exists in a patient with right heart failure and chronic obstructive pulmonary disease. Bothersome shortness of breath may be improved with the addition of ACE inhibitors in patients in whom valve repair or replacement is not feasible. Surgery may be contraindicated because of the terminal respiratory status.

ECG commonly shows:

- Poor R-wave progression in V_2 to V_4 that may mimic old anterior infarction;
- P pulmonale (P $\geq$ 2.5 mm in leads 2, 3, or AVF);
- Low voltage precordial leads; R/S ratio, equal to or less than 1 in V_5 or V_6.

Therapy

Bronchodilators

The treatment of exacerbation of chronic bronchitis with bronchodilators, albuterol (salbutamol), ipratropium, and pulsed corticosteroid therapy may produce temporary symptomatic relief (see Chapter 5). Cessation of smoking, breathing exercises, efficient physiotherapy, and advice on nutrition are necessary.

Oxygen

Correction of hypoxemia with continuous oxygen administration (minimum 15 hours daily) to keep the PaO_2 greater than 60 mm Hg may provide a modest improvement in survival. Long-term oxygen therapy is advisable in patients with cor pulmonale and PaO_2 less than 55 mm Hg. If right heart failure is present or the hematocrit is above 55% with PO_2 56–59 mm Hg, continuous (15h/day) oxygen therapy is recommended.

Monitor blood gases to maintain the pH in the normal range and adequate oxygenation without increasing the $PaCO_2$.

Digoxin

Digoxin is advisable in the management of atrial fibrillation with uncontrolled ventricular response but should be given if left heart failure occurs, and it may benefit some patients with right heart failure in sinus rhythm. ACE inhibitors are not useful.

Furosemide

At low doses, furosemide is given for bothersome bilateral pitting edema.

Dosage: 20–40 mg daily for a few days, then alternate-day therapy is preferred. Edema should be allowed to subside gradually over weeks. The edema improves with the slow correction of hypoxemia. It must be reemphasized that diuretics commonly precipitate hypochloremic metabolic alkalosis in these patients, and acetazolamide (250 mg three times daily) given 3 days weekly once or twice monthly may be required. Alkalosis causes hypoventilation, and this complication must be avoided.

BIBLIOGRAPHY

Abenhaim L, Moride Y, Brenot F, et al. Appetite-suppressant drugs and the risk of primary pulmonary hypertension. N Engl J Med 1996;335:609.

Badesch DB, Wynne KM, Bonvallet S, et al. Hypothyroidism and primary pulmonary hypertension: an autoimmune pathologic link? Ann Intern Med 1996;119:44.

Barst RJ, Rubin JL, Long WA, et al. A comparison of continuous intravenous epoprostenol (prostacyclin) with conventional therapy for primary pulmonary hypertension. N Engl J Med 1996;334:296.

D'Alonzo GE, Barst RJ, Ayres SM, et al. Survival in patients with primary pulmonary hypertension. Results from a National Prospective Registry. Ann Intern Med 1991;115:343.

Fuster V, Steele PM, Edwards WD, et al. Primary pulmonary hypertension national history and the importance of thrombosis. Circulation 1984;70:580.

Okada M, Yamashita C, Okada M, et al. Endothelin receptor antagonists in a beagle model of pulmonary hypertension: contribution to possible potential therapy. J Am Coll Cardiol 1995;25:1213.

Pasque MK, Trulock EP, Kaiser LR, et al. Single-lung transplantation for pulmonary hypertension. Three-month hemodynamic follow-up. Circulation 1991;84:2275.

Pepke-Zaba J, Higenbottam TW, Dinh-Xuan AT, et al. Inhaled nitric oxide as a cause of selective pulmonary vasodilatation in pulmonary hypertension. Lancet 1991;338:1173.

Pietra GG, Edwards WD, Kay JM, et al. Histopathology of primary pulmonary hypertension. A qualitative and quantitative study of pulmonary blood vessels from 58 patients in the

National Heart, Lung, and Blood Institute Primary Pulmonary Hypertension Registry. Circulation 1989;80:1148.

Rich S, Dantker DR, Ayres SM, et al. Primary pulmonary hypertension. A national prospective study. Ann Intern Med 1987;107:216.

Rich S, Kaufmann E. High-dose titration of calcium channel-blocking agents for primary pulmonary hypertension: guidelines for short-term drug testing. J Am Coll Cardiol 1991; 18:1323.

Rich S, Kaufmann E, Levy PS. The effect of high dosease of calcium-channel blockers on survival in primary pulmonary hypertension. N Engl J Med 1992;327:76.

Rubin LT. Primary pulmonary hypertension. Chest 1993;104:236.

Rubin LJ, Mendosa J, Hood M, et al. Treatment of primary pulmonary hypertension with continuous intravenous prostacyclin (epoprostenol): results of a randomized trial. Ann Intern Med 1990;112:486.

Sandoval J, Bauerle O, Gomez A, et al. Primary pulmonary hypertension in children: clinical characterization and survival. J Am Coll Cardiol 1995;25:466.

Schrader BJ, Inbar S, Kaufmann L, et al. Comparison of the effects of adenosine and nifedipine in pulmonary hypertension. J Am Coll Cardiol 1992;19:1060.

15 Lung Cancer and the Solitary Pulmonary Nodule

Thomas W. Shields

LUNG CANCER

Lung cancers may be divided into three major categories: non-small cell carcinomas, small cell carcinomas, and carcinoids (Table 15.1). Other malignant tumors are infrequently encountered and are of less clinical importance. Some clinicians have combined small cell tumors and carcinoids into the category of neuroendocrine (NE) tumors (Table 15.2) because of similar embryologic derivation, pathologic features, and observed functional activities (expression of amine precursor uptake and decarboxylation cell properties). Nonetheless, because the investigation, staging, and therapeutic management of these two tumor types are so different, they should be considered as separate entities rather than as NE tumors.

DIAGNOSTIC INVESTIGATION

Radiographic Studies

Radiographic Features on Standard Radiographs

The radiographic findings caused by carcinoma of the lung result from the tumor itself, from changes in the pulmonary parenchyma distal to an obstructed bronchus (atelectasis, infection, or both), and from spread of the tumor to extrapulmonary, intrathoracic sites (hilar and mediastinal lymph nodes, pleura, chest wall, and other mediastinal structures). The findings vary with the location, cell type, and length of time that the tumor has been present.

The chest x-ray is abnormal in 97–98% of all patients with lung cancer. The abnormality is most suggestive of tumor in more than 80% of these patients.

Early Radiographic Features

The early radiographic signs of lung tumors are listed in Table 15.3. The incidence of these early features in a screening program revealed a peripheral nodule or mass in 33%, a peripheral "infiltrate" in 25%, and a hilar enlargement in 28% of patients. Atelectasis or a pleural effusion each occurred in 3% of patients, and obstructive emphysema was seen in only 1%.

617

Table 15.1. Histologic Classification of Lung Carcinoma

Squamous cell—Epidermoid—Carcinoma
  Spindle cell (squamous) variant
Adenocarcinoma
  Acinar adenocarcinoma
  Papillary adenocarcinoma
  Bronchoalveolar carcinoma
  Solid carcinoma with mucous formation
Large cell undifferentiated carcinoma
  Giant cell variant
  Clear cell variant
Undifferentiated small cell carcinoma
  Oat cell—typical small cell—carcinoma
  Intermediate—polygonal, fusiform—cell type
  Combined—mixed—cell type
Adenosquamous carcinoma
Carcinoid tumor
  Typical
  Atypical
Other tumors

From Shields TW. Lung cancer and the solitary pulmonary nodule. In: Khan MG, ed. Cardiac and pulmonary management. Philadelphia, PA: Lea & Febiger, 1993. Reprinted with permission.

Usual Radiographic Manifestations

The radiographic features are classified as hilar, pulmonary parenchymal, and intrathoracic extrapulmonary (Table 15.4). The incidences of the initial presenting radiographic findings are presented in Table 15.5.

Special Radiographic Studies

In addition to the standard x-rays of the chest taken with the patient in the posteroanterior and lateral positions, other x-rays can be obtained with the patient in the right or left anterior oblique, the lordotic, or other special positions to delineate further

Table 15.2. Neuroendocrine Carcinomas of the Lung

Carcinoid tumors—"typical" carcinoids
Well-differentiated cell type—"atypical" carcinoids
Intermediate cell type—polygonal or fusiform small cells
Small cell type—"typical" or oat cells

From Shields TW. Lung cancer and the solitary pulmonary nodule. In: Khan MG, ed. Cardiac and pulmonary management. Philadelphia, PA: Lea & Febiger, 1993. Reprinted with permission.

Table 15.3. Early Radiologic Findings in Lung Cancer

Homogeneous parenchymal density
   Nodular or linear-shaped
Nonhomogeneous parenchymal density
Cavitation within a solid mass
Local infiltration along a blood vessel
Segmental consolidation or atelectasis
Enlargement of the hilar area
Pleural effusion
Obstructive emphysema

From Shields TW. Lung cancer and the solitary pulmonary nodule. In: Khan MG, ed. Cardiac and pulmonary management. Philadelphia, PA: Lea & Febiger, 1993. Reprinted with permission.

any suspected lesion. Other radiographic studies, such as standard tomography, 55° oblique tomography, bronchography, contrast study of the esophagus, angiography, azygography, and pneumomediastinography, are rarely indicated.

Conventional Tomography

Conventional tomography is indicated only to evaluate a solitary pulmonary nodule (SPN). The study is not included in the routine evaluation of the patient with lung cancer.

Table 15.4. Radiologic Abnormalities Associated with Lung Cancer

Region	Type of Involvement
Hilus	Hilar enlargement without discrete mass
	Hilar mass
	Perihilar mass
Parenchyma	Small peripheral mass 3 cm or less, distinct or indistinct border
	Large peripheral mass greater than 3 cm
	Bronchial obstruction
	Atelectasis, consolidation, or obstructive pneumonitis (loss of lung volume)
	Lung abscess with thick irregular wall
	Localized obstructive emphysema
Intrathoracic extrapulmonary structures	Mediastinal mass or widening
	Chest wall invasion with bony destruction
	Pleural effusion
	Paralyzed, elevated hemidiaphragm

From Shields TW. Lung cancer and the solitary pulmonary nodule. In: Khan MG, ed. Cardiac and pulmonary management. Philadelphia, PA: Lea & Febiger, 1993. Reprinted with permission.

Table 15.5. Radiographic Findings in 200 Patients with Lung Cancer

Tumor in the periphery of the lung	39.5%
Hilar tumor	19.5%
Atelectasis	13.5%
Pleural effusion	7.0%
Hilar invasion	5.0%
Normal	4.0%
Infiltrative shadow in the periphery	3.0%
Other	8.5%

Adapted from Amemiya R, Oho K. X-ray diagnosis of lung cancer. In: Hayata Y, ed. Lung cancer diagnosis. New York: Igaku-shoin, 1982.

Computed Tomography

Computed tomography (CT) is almost routinely performed in patients suspected of having lung cancer. Thin-section CT through the hilar area or helical CT technique may be superior to standard CT with contrast infusion.

Advantages

• Permits evaluation of the size of the superior mediastinal lymph nodes as well as of the subcarinal lymph nodes (Table 15.6, Fig. 15.1, Fig. 15.2);

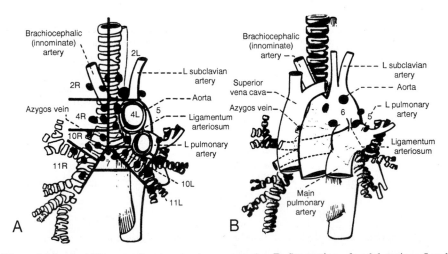

Figure 15.1. A, ATS map of regional pulmonary nodes. **B,** Separation of nodal stations 5 and 6 requires anterior thoracostomy. (From the American Thoracic Society. Tisi GM, Fiedman PJ, Peters RM, et al. Clinical staging of primary lung cancer. Am Rev Respir Dis 1983;127:659. Reprinted with permission.)

Table 15.6. Proposed Definitions of Regional Nodal Stations for Prethoracotomy Staging

X	Supraclavicular nodes.
2R	Right upper paratracheal (suprainnominate) nodes: Nodes to the right of the midline of the trachea, between the intersection of the caudal margin of the innominate artery with the trachea, and the apex of the lung. (Includes highest R mediastinal node.) (Radiologists may use the same caudal margin as in 2L.)
2L	Left upper paratracheal (supra-aortic) nodes: Nodes to the left of the midline of the trachea between the top of the aortic arch and the apex of the lung. (Includes highest L mediastinal node.)
4R	Right lower paratracheal nodes: Nodes to the right of the midline of the trachea between the cephalic border of the azygos vein and the intersection of the caudal margin of the brachiocephalic artery with the right side of the trachea. (Includes some pretracheal and paracaval nodes.) (Radiologists may use the same cephalic margin as in 4L).
4L	Left lower paratracheal nodes: Nodes to the left of the midline of the trachea between the top of the aortic arch and the level of the carina, medial to the ligamentum arteriosum. (Includes some pretracheal nodes.)
5	Aortopulmonary nodes: Subaortic and para-aortic nodes, lateral to the ligamentum arteriosum or the aorta or left pulmonary artery, proximal to the first branch of the LPA.
6	Anterior mediastinal nodes: Nodes anterior to the ascending aorta or the innominate artery. (Includes some pretracheal and preaortic nodes.)
7	Subcarinal nodes: Nodes rising caudal to the carina of the trachea but not associated with the lower lobe bronchi or arteries within the lung.
8	Paraesophageal nodes: Nodes dorsal to the posterior wall of the trachea and to the right or left of the midline of the esophagus. (Includes retrotracheal, but not subcarinal, nodes.)
9	Right or left pulmonary ligament nodes: Nodes within the right or left pulmonary ligament.
10R	Right tracheobronchial nodes: Nodes to the right of the midline of the trachea from the level of the cephalic border of the azygos vein to the origin of the right upper lobe bronchus.
10L	Left peribronchial nodes: Nodes to the left of the midline of the trachea between the carina and the left upper lobe bronchus, medial to the ligamentum arteriosum.
11	Intrapulmonary nodes: Nodes removed in the right or left lung specimen plus those distal to the main stem bronchi or secondary carina. (Includes interlobar, lobar, and segmental nodes.)[a]

From the American Thoracic Society. Tisi GM, Fiedman PJ, Peters RM, et al. Clinical staging of primary lung cancer. Am Rev Respir Dis 1983;127:659. Reprinted with permission.
[a] Postthoracotomy staging: Nodes could be divided into stations 11, 12, and 13 according to the AJC classification.

- Better than 55° oblique tomography for evaluation of hilar lymph nodes;
- Good for demonstrating vertebral body invasion; less effective for rib cage or direct mediastinal invasion;
- May reveal presence of small, undetected pleural effusion;
- May suggest encirclement of vital structures by the tumor (Fig. 15.3).

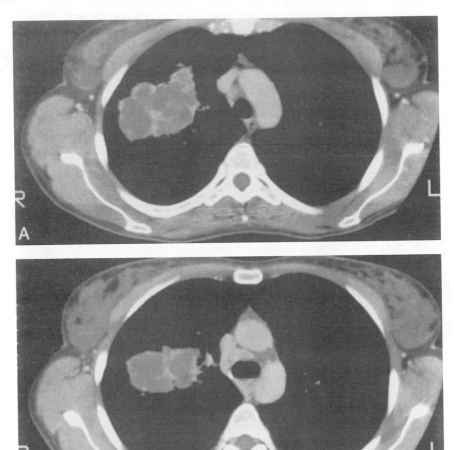

Figure 15.2. CT scans of the chest of a patient with a carcinoma of the right upper lobe with enlarged paratracheal nodes (station 2-Naruke map) (**A**) and in the superior tracheobronchial region (station 4) at the level of the azygos vein (**B**). Both nodes were positive for metastatic tumor at mediastinoscopy. (From Shields TW, ed. General thoracic surgery. 4th ed. Baltimore, MD: Williams & Wilkins, 1994. Reprinted with permission.)

Lymph nodes in the superior mediastinum normally measure less than 1 cm in the short axis of the node. In the subcarinal area, normal lymph nodes may measure as large as 1.5 cm. The threshold size for nodal enlargement in the various stations is shown in Table 15.7.

Disadvantages

- Cannot differentiate between inflammatory tissue and tumor;
- Of little or no value in the identification of the inferior mediastinal lymph nodes (paraesophageal and pulmonary ligament stations);

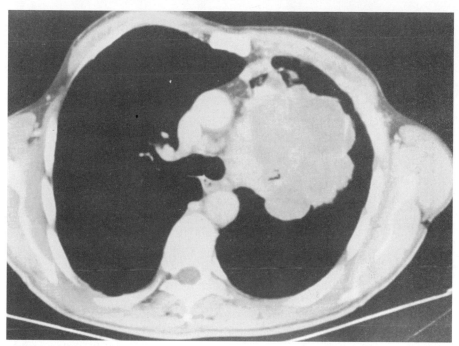

Figure 15.3. CT scan of a large tumor of the left upper lobe with direct invasion of the aortic window is an extension to the trachea at the level of the bifurcation. (From Shields TW, ed. General thoracic surgery. 4th ed. Baltimore, MD: Williams & Wilkins, 1994. Reprinted with permission.)

Table 15.7. Threshold Sizes for Nodal Enlargement

Region	Short-axis Measurement above which Node is Considered Enlarged (mm)
2R	7
2L	7
4R	10
4L	10
5	9
6	8
7	11
8R	10
8L	7
10R	10
10L	7

From Glazer GM, Gross BH, Quint LE, et al. Normal mediastinal lymph nodes: number and size according to American Thoracic Society mapping. AJR 1985;144:261. Reprinted with permission.

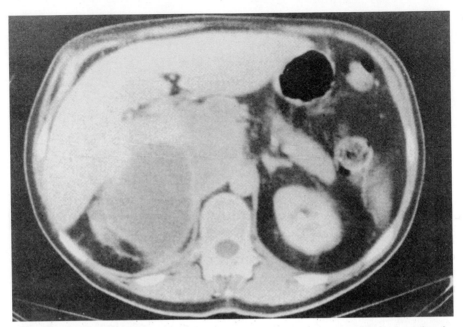

Figure 15.4. CT scan of the upper abdomen of a patient with a carcinoma of the lung showing a large asymptomatic mass of the right adrenal gland. Percutaneous fine-needle biopsy revealed the presence of metastatic carcinoma. (From Shields TW, ed. General thoracic surgery. 4th ed. Baltimore, MD: Williams & Wilkins, 1994. Reprinted with permission.)

- Evaluation of parietal, mediastinal, or diaphragmatic pleural invasion is difficult;
- Invasion of mediastinal structures is difficult to determine.

When obvious invasion or encirclement of a mediastinal structure is absent and the tumor mass only abuts the structure, the CT must be considered indeterminate even in the absence of a fat plane. When contact with the mediastinum is 3 cm or less, when contact with the aorta is less than 90°, or when mediastinal fat is present between the mass and the mediastinal structure, the tumor can be resected. In 75% of such patients, mediastinal invasion is absent; in the remaining 25%, only limited focal invasion is present.

A CT scan of the thorax should include the upper abdomen—even in asymptomatic patients—because a small incidence of occult metastasis to either the liver or the adrenals may be suggested (Fig. 15.4).

Magnetic Resonance Imaging

The role of magnetic resonance imaging (MRI) in evaluating the patient with lung cancer has yet to be determined.

Advantages

- Requires no contrast material;
- May be obtained in sagittal and coronal planes;

- More accurate than CT in showing chest wall invasion and extrathoracic spread; especially good in evaluating superior sulcus tumors;
- May be more valuable than CT in demonstrating invasion of mediastinal structures.

Disadvantages

- Poor spatial resolution;
- Longer scan times;
- Thicker image slices;
- Inability to detect presence of calcium in pulmonary nodules or lymph nodes.

As with CT scanning, controversy persists regarding the value of MRI in the determination of metastatic involvement of mediastinal lymph nodes. Some authors have suggested that T_1 relaxation values may differentiate benign and malignant lymph node tissue, but such postulation has not gained universal acceptance. Most clinicians believe that relaxation time measurements of mediastinal lymph nodes will prove to have limited value in assessing the presence of mediastinal lymph node metastatic disease.

Ultrasonography

- May be used to detect the presence and extent of pleural or pericardial effusions;
- May detect the presence of metastasis to liver or adrenal glands.

Transesophageal Endoscopic Ultrasonography

- May be used to evaluate the mediastinal lymph nodes.

Advantages

- Identifies a greater proportion of lymph nodes present in the aortic window and subcarinal areas than does standard CT.
- May identify nodes in the paraesophageal (posterior) area and in the pulmonary ligament regions in the inferior mediastinum that are not identified by CT scan.
- May be used to guide transesophageal fine-needle aspiration of suspicious lymph nodes, especially in the aortopulmonary window and subcarinal regions.

Disadvantages

- Nodes in anterior mediastinum or right paratracheal area cannot be adequately visualized.
- Cannot distinguish metastatically involved nodes from normal lymph nodes, although, at times, the contour and echo characteristics of the lymph node may suggest metastatic involvement.

Transbronchoscopic Ultrasonography

Transbronchoscopic ultrasonography is a new technique now being evaluated in assisting fine-needle aspirations of enlarged mediastinal lymph nodes.

Positron Emission Tomography

Cancer cells are characterized by having a higher glycolytic rate than normal cells; active inflammatory cells may also have an increased rate, but to a lesser extent than malignant cells. By the use of positron emitter substances such as the glucose analogue [2-^{18}F]fluoro-2-deoxy-D-glucose (FDG), both primary and metastatic malignant lesions may be identified by positron emission tomography (PET). Various technical and economic problems are still being solved, but in evaluating primary pulmonary lesions and their metastatic spread, PET with FDG appears to be a promising modality. It is best used in conjunction with standard CT or MRI or, better yet, with "anatometabolic" imaging by fusion of FDG PET with CT or MRI. The use of C-11 methionine PET has also been suggested but it does not appear to be as specific as FDG.

Advantages

- Specific uptake by primary malignant lung lesions greater than 1 cm in size in 80–90% of cases.
- Significant uptake in metastatically involved mediastinal nodes in more than 90% of instances, regardless of the size of the involved lymph node.
- Enlarged mediastinal lymph nodes that have no uptake on FDG PET can be assumed to be free of metastatic tumor.
- Whole-body tomography may identify extrathoracic metastatic deposits in bone, liver, and adrenal areas in as many as 11% of asymptomatic patients.

Disadvantages

- Eventual cost of the procedure.
- There may be increased uptake in active inflammatory tissues, such as tuberculosis, abscess, and granulomas. Quantitative standard uptake value (SUV) is less than that of malignant tissue. SUV is less for primary lung lesion than for metastatic lesion in the mediastinal nodes.
- Cardiac muscle has increased uptake and may obscure adjacent malignant foci.
- Difficult to identify exact location or lymph node group involved by PET scan alone.

Sputum Cytology

With appropriate cytologic study of several sputum specimens, tumor cells are found in 45–90% of patients. Cell type agrees with the final histologic diagnosis in approximately 85% of patients. The accuracy of such testing is approximately 90–100% for small cell carcinoma, 92–96% for squamous cell carcinoma, and 87–97% for adenocarcinoma. The undifferentiated carcinomas, the poorly differentiated epidermoid carcinomas, and combined carcinomas are more difficult to type correctly.

Cytologic studies are most often positive in patients with large tumors that involve a major bronchus. Peripheral lesions frequently do not communicate with a bronchus, thus the diagnostic results are less rewarding. Bronchial brushing or biopsy may be carried out to improve the yield.

A few patients with carcinoma of the lung but without a pulmonary lesion revealed on chest x-rays are identified because of an incidental finding of tumor cells in the sputum during a screening examination. At least 75% of these findings are from squamous cell lesions. These occult lung carcinomas may represent a readily identifiable lesion of the bronchus on bronchoscopic examination, but in approximately 25% of patients, the primary lung tumor is not initially identified by bronchoscopy and biopsy of a visualized lesion. Complete examination of the oropharynx and esophagus is required to rule out other orodigestive tumors; repeated bronchoscopy with brushing of individual lobes is then necessary. Approximately 50% of this subset of patients requires 2–5 examinations before localization is obtained. The examinations should be spaced at 8- to 12-week intervals.

Tumor Markers

Tumor markers have little clinical value in the diagnosis of lung cancer (Table 15.8). They are of some value in determining the possible response to therapy and the prognosis of small cell lung carcinoma.

Radionuclide Studies

Radionuclide scanning of the lung is satisfactory for identifying the primary tumor but is not diagnostic. Scanning with ^{67}Ga may identify metastatic tumor deposits in the mediastinal lymph nodes as well as at distant sites. The use of ^{67}Ga scans for detection of possible mediastinal lymph node involvement has been supplanted by CT evaluation of the mediastinum. Other scans also are more efficient for detecting distant metastases.

The use of radionuclide-labeled monoclonal antibodies for identifying primary lung tumors, regional metastases, and tumor recurrences is under active investigation. Immunoscintigraphy may detect 75% of the primary lung tumors and may identify tumor spread that CT imaging failed to identify.

Ventilation and perfusion scans are useful in evaluating preoperative and predicting postoperative pulmonary function in poor-risk candidates for surgical resection. A predicted postoperative forced expiratory volume in one second (FEV_1) of 40% is the lowest allowable limit for pneumonectomy.

Bronchoscopy and Transbronchial Needle Aspiration

The tracheobronchial tree in all patients suspected of having a tumor of the lung should be examined with either the rigid or the flexible fiberoptic bronchoscope.

Table 15.8. Tumor Markers in Lung Cancer

Substance	Frequency of Occurrence in		
	Non-small Cell	Small Cell	Carcinoid
Polypeptide hormones			
ACTH[a]	+	+ +	+
ADH (arginine vasopressin)[a,b] neurophysins	±	+ +	±
Calcitonin[b]	+	+ + +	+
Bombesin (gastrin-releasing peptides)	+	+ + +	+
Human chorionic gonadotropin	+	+	
Parathyroid hormone	+	−	
Enzymes			
Dopa decarboxylase	−	+ +	
Neuron-specific enolase	−	+ +	+
Histaminase	−	+ +	
Creatine kinase	−	+ +	
Synaptophysin	−	+ +	+
Biogenic amines			
Serotonin	−	+ +	+
5-Hydroxytryptophan	−	+	
Histamine	−	+	
Tumor-associated antigens			
Carcinoembryonic antigen[b]	+ +	+ +	
Morphologic markers			
Electron-dense granules	±	+ +	+
Specific chromosome abnormality	−	+	

From Shields TW. Lung cancer and the solitary pulmonary nodule. In: Khan MG, ed. Cardiac and pulmonary management. Philadelphia, PA: Lea & Febiger, 1993. Reprinted with permission.
[a] Clinical syndrome associated with elevated marker level.
[b] Clinically useful for monitoring therapy.

- Permits direct visualization or positive biopsy findings in 25–50% of patients.
- Positive biopsy is more frequent in squamous and large cell undifferentiated tumors than in adenocarcinomas. Small cell tumors are readily identified. Centrally located suspected carcinoid tumors should be biopsied.
- Length of normal bronchus proximal to the tumor should be noted.
- Rigidity or loss of mobility of either the main-stem bronchus or the bronchus intermedius suggests metastatic lymph node disease.

Transbronchial fine-needle aspiration is indicated when rigidity is present and when enlarged mediastinal lymph nodes are identified by CT examination, even though endobronchial abnormality is not present. The sensitivity of fine-needle aspiration of enlarged lymph nodes in patients with non-small cell carcinoma may be as high as 82%. A positive aspiration obviates the more invasive diagnostic procedure of mediastinal exploration. Overall, aspiration is most often positive in the presence of right upper lobe endobronchial lesions and in the presence of mediastinal lymph nodes more than 1 cm in size. Increased yield may be obtained by guidance by transbronchoscopic ultrasound.

Percutaneous Transthoracic Needle Aspiration

Needle aspiration of a suspected carcinoma of the lung is often performed without indication.

Indications

- In the patient with an undiagnosed but clinically nonresectable tumor;
- In a patient who is not a medical candidate or who refuses resection of an otherwise resectable tumor and in whom a tissue diagnosis cannot be obtained by other means.

Complications

- A postaspiration pneumothorax is seen in 25% of patients.
- Of these patients, approximately 25% (6% of all patients) require a closed tube thoracostomy.
- Hemoptysis occurs infrequently.

Contraindications

- A hemorrhagic diathesis;
- Pulmonary hypertension;
- Severe emphysema with multiple bullae.

Needle biopsy of the pleura (usually with a cutting needle) in the presence of pleural effusion is positive for tumor in 60–75% of patients with proven bronchial carcinoma.

Thoracoscopy and Video-assisted Thoracoscopy

Thoracoscopic examination of the pleural space infrequently is indicated in patients with suspected bronchial carcinoma. A cytologically undiagnosed pleural effusion is the most frequent indication. Direct visualization of the lung and directed biopsy of an indeterminate mass by use of thoracoscopy may be of value, especially in the patient in whom a standard thoracotomy is contraindicated. In patients with a solitary indeterminate pulmonary nodule, video-assisted thoracoscopic surgical removal of the nodule has become the procedure of choice, supplanting the use of percutaneous or bronchoscopic directed fine-needle aspiration of the nodule. When the nodule proves to be a malignant lesion, at present the standard procedure is conversion to an open thoracotomy and the appropriate surgical resection carried out. Video-assisted major pulmonary resections (lobectomy or pneumonectomy) are still considered investigational. It has been suggested that video-assisted thoracoscopic visualiz-ation of the pleural space be done immediately prior to thoracotomy. Previously undetected pleural seeding or locally nonresectable extension of the tumor beyond the lung would contraindicate the planned thoracotomy. The efficacy of this proce-dure is undetermined because such findings are identified in less than 5% of patients believed to have resectable disease at the completion of appropriate preoperative evaluation.

Supraclavicular Lymph Node Biopsy

Any palpable cervical lymph nodes should be excised or aspirated for histologic study; most of these are involved by tumor. Biopsy of nonpalpable lymph nodes in the scalene area is not indicated except in specific instances. It has been recom-mended primarily in patients with central adenocarcinomas (although all cell types could be considered) that have superior mediastinal metastatic lymph node involve-ment who are candidates for neoadjuvant therapy protocols. Metastatic involvement of the scalene nodes would preclude such an aggressive therapeutic approach.

Mediastinal Lymph Node Biopsy

The most valuable invasive diagnostic procedure other than a thoracotomy is a prethoracotomy mediastinal exploration. The choice of a standard mediastinoscopy, an extended cervical mediastinoscopy, an anterior mediastinotomy, or a combination of these procedures depends on the location of the enlarged mediastinal lymph node(s) as demonstrated on the CT scan. It has been suggested that a video-assisted thoracoscopic surgical exploration may readily be substituted for an anterior medias-tinotomy when the latter procedure is indicated.

Indications

- Mediastinal lymph nodes 1 cm or greater in size in patients with known non-small cell carcinoma;
- Multiple lymph nodes of normal size in patients with adenocarcinoma;
- In patients with potentially resectable central tumors in whom a tissue diagnosis has not been established;
- All potential surgical candidates with known small cell carcinoma.

Results

- 60–65% of enlarged mediastinal lymph nodes in patients with non-small cell carcinoma contain metastatic tumor;
- 35–40% of enlarged lymph nodes in non-small cell carcinoma are only inflamma-tory or hyperplastic without tumor.

Routine mediastinal exploration has a positive yield of metastatic disease of 34%. Only 7–15% of lymph nodes of normal size (in the absence of associated enlarged lymph nodes with tumor) contain "occult" metastasis. Metastatic involvement of lymph nodes of normal size is more common in adenocarcinoma than in squamous carcinoma; the incidence in small cell tumors is highest.

The policy of foregoing a mediastinal exploration based on clinical (bronchoscopic and radiologic) findings without CT examination is inappropriate except in patients with a small peripheral tumor with normal hilar and mediastinal shadows. The incidence of mediastinal node involvement is approximately 5–10% in these patients. In more than 90% of patients, a complete resection can be done. In most other patients who are believed to have no nodal involvement or at most only lobar or hilar disease but in whom mediastinal node disease is discovered at thoracotomy, a complete resection can be accomplished in only 50%. Similarly, in patients with enlarged mediastinal nodes identified by CT scan but with no prethoracotomy exploration and in whom metastatic disease is identified at thoracotomy, only a 50% complete resection rate can be obtained. In either of these two situations, an excessively high incidence of inappropriate thoracotomies has therefore been done. Thus, with the exception noted, all patients with a potentially resectable carcinoma should undergo a CT scan, and all those in whom enlarged mediastinal nodes are identified should be evaluated by a preoperative mediastinal exploration. In patients with enlarged nodes that are negative on a FDG PET scan, thoracotomy can be done without a prior mediastinal exploration.

Investigation for Distant Metastases

CT scans of the brain and upper abdomen and radionuclide bone scans are the preferred diagnostic procedures for determining the presence of extrathoracic metastatic disease.

Indications

- Presence of symptoms or physical or laboratory findings (elevated alkaline phosphatase or LDH levels) suggestive of metastatic disease in any extrathoracic organ system in patients with non-small cell tumors or carcinoids.
- In all patients, symptomatic and asymptomatic, with small cell tumors.
- Brain scans in patients with adenocarcinoma and involved mediastinal nodes who are potential candidates for neoadjuvant therapy protocols. A positive finding would negate such a therapeutic approach.

Routine "metastatic" evaluation is not indicated in asymptomatic patients with non-small cell tumors. Yield of useful information from a routine brain CT scan is less than 1%; from an upper abdominal CT scan, 1–3%; from a bone CT scan, less than 4%.

STAGING

Once the diagnosis has been established and the extent of the disease determined, the disease should be staged by one of two morphologic classifications. In addition,

Table 15.9. Karnofsky Scale of Performance Status

Condition	Percentage	Comments
A: Able to carry on normal activity and to work. No special care is needed.	100	Normal, no complaints, no evidence of disease
	90	Able to carry on normal activity, minor signs or symptoms of disease
	80	Normal activity with effort, some signs or symptoms of disease
B: Unable to work. Able to live at home, care for most personal needs. A varying degree of assistance is needed.	70	Cares for self, unable to carry on normal activity or to do active work
	60	Requires occasional assistance, but is able to care for most needs
	50	Requires considerable assistance and frequent medical care
C: Unable to care for self. Requires equivalent of institutional or hospital care. Disease may be progressing rapidly.	40	Disabled, requires special care and assistance
	30	Severely disabled, hospitalization indicated although death not imminent
	20	Hospitalization necessary, very sick, active supportive treatment necessary
	10	Moribund, fatal processes progressing rapidly
	0	Dead

From Shields TW, ed. General thoracic surgery. 4th ed. Baltimore, MD: Williams & Wilkins, 1994: 1128. Reprinted with permission.

the functional status should be determined, usually by the Karnofsky and Burchenal's classification (Table 15.9). A clinical-severity staging, which takes into consideration the clinical features presented by the patient, has been suggested. This staging system may give a better guide to the individual patient's prognosis, especially in those with advanced disease.

Non-Small Cell Lung Carcinoma

The morphologic staging system is most appropriate in determining the treatment options and the prognosis in patients with non-small cell lung cancer. The extent of tumor is codified by the descriptor T, the presence of lymph node metastases by the descriptor N, and the status of distant metastasis by the descriptor M (Table 15.10). The combinations of the TNM designations are separated into four stage categories to denote the extent of the disease process (Table 15.11). These categories can be determined at the completion of the diagnostic evaluation (clinical), at the time of thoracotomy (surgical), or by examination of the resected specimen (pathologic).

Problems with Present Classification

- T1N0M0 can be classified as stage IA and T2N0M0 as stage IB because of significant difference in survival;

Table 15.10. New International Staging System: TNM Classification

Primary Tumor (T)	
TX	Tumor proven by the presence of malignant cells in bronchopulmonary secretions but not visualized roentgenographically or bronchoscopically, or any tumor that cannot be assessed as in a retreatment staging.
T0	No evidence of primary tumor.
Tis	Carcinoma in situ.
T1	A tumor that is 3.0 cm or less in greatest diameter, surrounded by lung or visceral pleura, and without evidence of invasion proximal to a lobar bronchus at bronchoscopy.[a]
T2	A tumor more than 3.0 cm in greatest diameter, or a tumor of any size that either invades the visceral pleura or has associated atelectasis or obstructive pneumonitis extending to the hilar region. At bronchoscopy, the proximal extent of demonstrable tumor must be within a lobar bronchus or at least 2.0 cm distal to the carina. Any associated atelectasis or obstructive pneumonitis must involve less than an entire lung.
T3	A tumor of any size with direct extension into the chest wall (including superior sulcus tumors), diaphragm, or the mediastinal pleura or pericardium without involving the heart, great vessels, trachea, esophagus, or vertebral body, or a tumor in the main bronchus within 2.0 cm of the carina without involving the carina.
T4	A tumor of any size with invasion of the mediastinum or involving heart, great vessels, trachea, esophagus, vertebral body, or carina, or presence of malignant pleural effusion.[b]
Nodal Involvement (N)	
N0	No demonstrable metastasis to regional lymph nodes.
N1	Metastasis to lymph nodes in the peribronchial or the ipsilateral hilar region or both, including direct extension.
N2	Metastasis to ipsilateral mediastinal lymph nodes and subcarinal lymph nodes.
N3	Metastasis to contralateral mediastinal lymph nodes, contralateral hilar lymph nodes, and ipsilateral or contralateral scalene or supraclavicular lymph nodes.
Distant Metastasis (M)	
N0	No (known) distant metastasis.
M1	Distant metastasis present. Specify site(s).

From Mountain CF. A new international staging system for lung cancer. Chest 1986;89(Suppl):225S. Reprinted with permission.

[a] The uncommon superficial tumor of any size with its invasive component limited to the bronchial wall, which may extend proximal to the major bronchus, is classified as T1.

[b] Most pleural effusions associated with lung cancer result from tumor. Cytopathologic examination of pleural fluid (on more than one specimen) in a few patients is negative for tumor, however, and the fluid is nonbloody and is not an exudate. When these elements and clinical judgment dictate that the effusion is not related to the tumor, the patient should be staged as T1, T2, or T3, excluding effusion as a staging element.

Table 15.11. New International Staging System Stage Grouping

TX N0 M0	An occult carcinoma with bronchopulmonary secretions containing malignant cells, but without other evidence of the primary tumor or evidence of metastasis to the regional lymph nodes or distant metastasis.
Stage 0	
Tis N0 M0	Carcinoma in situ.
Stage I	
T1 N0 M0	A tumor that can be classified T1 or T2 without any metastasis to
T2 N0 M0	nodes or distant metastasis.
Stage II	
T1 N1 M0	Any tumor classified as T1 or T2 with metastasis to the lymph
T2 N1 M0	nodes in the peribronchial or ipsilateral hilar region only.
Stage IIIA	
T3 N0 M0	A tumor that can be classified as T3 without nodal metastasis or
T3 N1 M0	with metastasis limited to the peribronchial, ipsilateral hilar, and
T1 N2 M0	ipsilateral mediastinal lymph nodes. T1 and T2 tumors that have
T2 N2 M0	metastasized to the level of the ipsilateral mediastinal lymph
T3 N2 M0	nodes only are also included.
Stage IIIB	
Any T, N3 M0	Any tumor more extensive than T3 or any tumor with
T, any N, M0	supraclavicular or contralateral mediastinal lymph node involvement, or any tumor with a malignant pleural effusion, but without evidence of distant metastasis.
Stage IV	
Any T, any N, M1	Any tumor with distant metastatic spread.

From Mountain CF. A new international staging system for lung cancer. Chest 1986;89(suppl):225S. Reprinted with permission.

- Classification of N2 disease as stage IIIA;
- How to classify tumors with satellite tumor nodules;
- How to classify patients with two primary synchronous tumors;
- Classification of patients without evident pleural involvement but positive cytologic pleural lavage at thoracotomy.

Most patients with N2 disease have nonsurgical disease. Only a 2% long-term salvage rate is reported in patients with N2 disease confirmed prior to thoracotomy. "Occult" N2 disease discovered at thoracotomy may be resected, resulting in long-term salvage rates of 30–45%. The overall salvage rate in patients with N2 disease is no more than 5–8%; patients with evident N2 disease should be classified as having stage IIIB disease.

Patients with satellite nodules, synchronous tumors, or positive pleural lavage have salvage rates of 18–22%. All these manifestations should be classified as stage IIIA disease, although there are some exceptions to this generalization.

Small Cell Lung Carcinoma

The morphologic staging of small cell lung cancer is less detailed. It is generally only categorized as limited or extensive disease. Limited disease is defined as disease confined to the ipsilateral hemithorax with or without contralateral hilar or ipsilateral supraclavicular lymph node involvement. Extensive disease is any disease that extends beyond these limits.

Patients with limited disease that is clinically a potential surgical lesion should be further staged regarding their T and N status.

Carcinoid Tumors

Carcinoid tumors should be staged by the International Staging System. No extensive preoperative staging procedures are indicated. A CT scan of the chest is necessary only when radiographic evidence suggests mediastinal lymph node enlargement. The tumors are classified postoperatively as typical or atypical, with or without lymph node metastasis.

Functional Status

The performance status of most surgical candidates is less important than the morphologic stage because almost all have a Karnofsky score of 80 or higher. In patients with stage IIIB or IV non-small cell tumors or in patients with small cell carcinomas, functional status is important relative to the patient's response to therapy and prognosis. The lower the Karnofsky score, the poorer the outcome for each.

TREATMENT

Treatment options consist of surgical resection, radiation therapy, chemotherapy, supportive medical care, or a combination of these options. Surgical resection should be considered in all patients when it can completely remove all tumor and is curative in intent. A palliative (more rightly called "incomplete") resection confers no benefit in the outcome of the disease and must be avoided. Radiation therapy and chemotherapy may be used with either intent but most often are palliative in result. Neoadjuvant therapy (chemo or radiation therapy or both) followed by surgical excision remains investigational.

The selection of the appropriate therapeutic approach depends on the cell type of the tumor, the stage of the disease, the medical condition of the patient, and at times the presence or absence of symptoms.

Surgical Therapy

NON-SMALL CELL LUNG CARCINOMA

Surgical resection is the most effective therapy for non-small cell carcinoma of the lung, even though it is applicable to fewer than one-fourth of all new patients seen.

Surgical candidates are primarily most of the patients with stage I or II disease and a few patients with stage IIIA disease. Patients with stage IIIB or IV disease are considered as potential surgical patients only in exceptional situations.

Contraindications to Definitive Surgical Resection

Based on the Extent and Location of the Tumor

- Extensive N2 disease;
- N3 or T4 disease;
- M1 disease.

Controversy persists regarding whether resection should be carried out for some patients with N2 disease discovered by a prethoracotomy mediastinal exploration. N2 disease in one nodal station (low superior mediastinal [stations 3, 4, or 5] or subcarinal [station 7], preferably in only 1 lymph node and without capsular invasion or fixation) may be considered as potential surgical disease.

Tumors involving a main-stem bronchus within 2 cm of the tracheal carina (T3) or involving the tracheal carina or encroaching on the tracheal wall (T4) are generally nonresectable. Rarely, a small tumor without lymph node involvement can be removed by a main-stem bronchoplastic procedure or a tracheal sleeve pneumonectomy.

On rare occasions, solitary brain metastasis identified in a patient with a resectable lung carcinoma may be excised, followed by whole-brain irradiation. Resection of the lung tumor then may be considered. The primary disease should preferably be stage I, but certainly no more advanced than stage II. Some centers, however, will consider this approach in stage IIIA disease. The excision of the primary tumor and a solitary adrenal metastasis may be considered in selected patients.

Based on Medical Status of Patient

- FEV_1 reduced to $< 1L$;
- Predicted postoperative $FEV_1 < 30\%$;
- Postoperative carbon monoxide diffusion capacity (DL_{CO}) $< 40\%$;
- Decrease in oxygen saturation during maximal exercise $> 2\%$;
- VO_2max with exercise < 10 mL/kg/min;
- Presence of hypoxia at rest or after mild exercise;
- Presence of hypercapnia, $CO_2 > 45$ mm Hg;
- Recent myocardial infarction (within 3 months);
- Uncontrolled heart failure;
- Uncontrollable arrhythmia.

The patient history and electrocardiogram (ECG) are sufficient to evaluate the patient's cardiac status when both are normal. When the ECG is abnormal, when an arrhythmia is present, or when the patient has a history of angina, of a previous myocardial infarct, or of controlled failure, a stress test should be performed. When the stress test is normal, other studies need not be done. If the stress test is not completed or is equivocal, a ^{201}Tl scan to evaluate myocardial perfusion should be done. When either the stress test or the ^{201}Tl scan is abnormal, a coronary angiogram should be obtained. When a patient is a candidate for myocardial revascularization or other cardiac procedures and has a resectable lung cancer, both procedures should be done at the same time, when possible.

Advanced age alone does not preclude surgical resection. Acceptable mortality rates and satisfactory long-term survival have been obtained in patients 80 years of age and older.

Based on Thoracotomy Findings

* Metastatic seeding of the parietal pleura;
* Undetected T4 disease (direct involvement of vertebral body, vena cava, aorta, heart);
* Extensive N2 disease with extracapsular growth and/or fixation to surrounding structures;
* Inability to safely control the blood supply to the lung;
* Required resection more than can be tolerated by the patient.

The percentage of patients in whom one or more of these local contraindications are found varies with the preoperative selection of the patients and the aggressiveness of the individual surgeon in the operative management. A nonresection rate should be no higher than 5–10%.

Definitive Surgical Resection

The goal of a definitive surgical resection is the complete removal of all gross and microscopic tumor within the involved hemithorax. Anything less must be regarded as an incomplete resection and should be avoided.

Lung tissue preservation without compromising the adequacy of the tumor removal is recommended. Lobectomy and pneumonectomy and their modifications (bilobectomy, sleeve resection) are the standard procedures. A properly selected segmentectomy is appropriate, but lesser resections (wedge resection or even a more limited local resection) should be considered as a compromise necessitated by the patient's pulmonary or cardiac status. Any of these operations may be combined with the en bloc resection of an involved adjacent nonvital structure.

A lobectomy is the most common operative procedure (Table 15.12). Radiographic occult tumors that have been localized only by bronchial brushing or by biopsy of a suspicious mucosal lesion generally require a lobectomy, but some occult tumors necessitate a bilobectomy or pneumonectomy because of their location.

All procedures should be accompanied by sampling of the ipsilateral superior mediastinal and subcarinal lymphatic stations or by a standard, systematic mediastinal lymph node dissection. The latter has become the preferred procedure by most; however, there is no evidence that a radical lymph node dissection is of any benefit over the former. Its primary value is that it better defines the extent of N2 disease when present than does only nodal sampling.

The advantages of a lobectomy are that it permits conservation of lung parenchyma

Table 15.12. Operative Procedures in Non-Small Cell Carcinoma of the Lung

Operations	Approximate Frequency (%)	Operative Mortality (%)
Lobectomy	62	3
Bilobectomy	6	4
Sleeve Lobectomy	1	5
Pneumonectomy	25	6
Segmentectomy	3	2
Lesser Resection	3	< 1

From Shields TW. Lung cancer and the solitary pulmonary nodule. In: Khan MG, ed. Cardiac and pulmonary management. Philadelphia, PA: Lea & Febiger, 1993. Reprinted with permission.

and is better tolerated in the long term than is a pneumonectomy. The 30-day postoperative mortality is approximately 3%. In patients older than 70 years of age, the mortality may be increased. A sleeve lobectomy for excision of a tumor involving the upper lobe orifice may be done to negate the necessity of a pneumonectomy. This may also be done in a patient with a peripheral lesion with a positive node at the junction of the lobar bronchus with the main-stem bronchus.

A standard pneumonectomy is required when a lobectomy or one of its modifications is not sufficient to remove the local disease or its metastases to the lobar or hilar lymph nodes. In properly selected patients, the mortality rate is approximately 6%. The late development of pulmonary hypertension and subsequent ventilatory disability, however, are additional disadvantages of the procedure, particularly in older patients.

In patients with small peripheral tumors without lymph node involvement (T1N0), segmentectomy has been advocated to preserve more functional lung tissue in older patients and in those with major defects in pulmonary function. The mortality rate is low (2–5%). A wedge resection or even a local cautery or laser excision of a small lesion without lymph node involvement can be done as a compromise procedure. The local recurrence rate after segmentectomy or lesser procedure is more than that observed after a lobectomy. Video-assisted thoracoscopic surgical resection of small (< 2 cm) peripherally located carcinomas has been reported. This may be an option in the management of a poor-risk patient but should not be considered as standard practice. No long-term survival data are available, and the incidence of local recurrence is not known.

Extended resections to excise T3 lesions extending into the parietal pleura, chest wall, diaphragm, or pericardium are indicated when all of the disease can be removed by the procedure. Mediastinal lymph node involvement decreases markedly the value of any extended procedure. Resection of the vena cava or other great vessels in the chest is rarely indicated.

When the tumor involves the apex of the chest and adjacent structures (superior sulcus tumor), and vertebral body invasion or Horner's syndrome are not present, an en bloc resection may be carried out. Preoperative irradiation is used initially.

Radiation therapy in the range of 35–45 Gy should be given preoperatively. If no evidence of distant spread occurs 1 month after completion of this therapy, resection is undertaken. When lymph nodes are positive or when extensive vertebral bony involvement is present, resection is contraindicated. In such instances, additional irradiation is given after thoracotomy.

Results of Surgical Treatment

The overall 5-year salvage rates after surgical resection vary from as low as 7.5% to as high as 45%; the average figures are usually between 20 and 35%. The prognosis after resection primarily depends on the postsurgical TNM classification of the tumor (Table 15.13).

Adjuvant Therapy

Depending on the stage of the disease at the time of resection, 28 to more than 75% of patients with lung carcinoma die from metastases or local recurrence of the carcinoma. Some form of adjuvant therapy would appear to be indicated in most patients. Unfortunately, with few exceptions the use of irradiation, chemotherapy, or immunotherapy has not been successful to date.

Preoperative Irradiation

- No benefit relative to survival;
- Some patients may be harmed by its use;
- Absence of tumor after irradiation has no effect on survival;
- Routine use contraindicated.

Table 15.13. Survival Relative to TNM Classification

TNM Subset	Clinical		Surgical	
	No.	% Surviving	No.	% Surviving
T1N0M0	591	61.9	429	68.5
T2N0M0	1,012	35.8	436	59.0
T1N1M0	19	33.6	67	54.1
T2N1M0	176	22.7	250	40.0
T3N0M0	221	7.6	57	44.2
T3N1M0	71	7.7	29	17.6
Any N2M0	497	4.9	168	28.8
Any M1	1,166	1.7	—	—
Total	3,753		1,436	

From Mountain CE. A new international staging system for lung cancer. Chest 1986;89(suppl):225S. Reprinted with permission.

Postoperative Irradiation in Stage II and Stage III

- Reduction of local recurrence observed;
- No survival benefit;
- Timing of irradiation, immediate versus delayed, is undetermined.

Chemotherapy

- Prolongation of disease-free interval in stage II and stage IIIA adenocarcinoma;
- A recent report of oral administration of tegafur (FT) plus uracil (UFT) 400 mg/kg/day for 1 year (postoperatively) with or without cisplatin and vindestine increased the rate of long-term survival in completely resected patients compared with a control group that received no adjuvant therapy (64.1% versus 49.0%);
- Consensus is that routine use is not indicated.

Immunotherapy

- No indication for its use at present.

Neoadjuvant Therapy. Recent interest has grown in the use of preoperative chemotherapy with or without radiation therapy in marginally resectable or nonresectable stage IIIA and IIIB disease, particularly in those with known N2 involvement, in an attempt to convert the local disease into a resectable lesion. The more common regimens have used cisplatin and fluorouracil infusion with 30–40 Gy of irradiation. A critical analysis of the present status of neoadjuvant therapy for stage IIIA non-small cell lung cancer reveals response rates to cisplatin-based chemotherapy of approximately 50%, regardless of the actual regimen used. The addition of radiation therapy does not appear to be of any major benefit and may complicate the technical aspects of the operative procedure. The addition of irradiation may increase the toxicity to doxorubicin and mitomycin-C. Serious toxicity consisting of profound neutropenia, mitomycin lung toxicity, and esophagitis is observed. A 3.2% mortality rate from the adjuvant therapy is reported. Several complete local responses have been reported (no tumor present in the resected specimen) and, in other patients, tumors initially thought to be unresectable could be removed. The relationship of this local control to long-term survival remains unknown; however, several recent randomized studies have shown benefit of neoadjuvant therapy plus resection over surgical resection alone in patients with stage IIIA N2 disease.

SMALL CELL LUNG CARCINOMA

Surgical resection is applicable to only 5–8% of all patients with small cell lung cancer. The surgical candidates are those with stage I disease, selected stage IIIA non-N2 patients, and possibly stage II disease. Chemotherapy is an integral part of the multimodality approach and may be given either preoperatively or postoperatively. Local irradiation to the chest in patients with positive lymph nodes may be indicated postoperatively. The efficacy of postoperative prophylactic cranial irradia-

Table 15.14. Survival in Surgically Resected Small Cell Lung Cancer

Stage	Toronto Study[a] (%)	International Society of Chemotherapy Lung Study[b] (%)
I	71	60
II	38	36
IIIA	18	33
Total	36	47

From Shields TW. Lung cancer and the solitary pulmonary nodule. In: Khan MG, ed. Cardiac and pulmonary management. Philadelphia, PA: Lea & Febiger, 1993. Reprinted with permission.
[a] 5-year survival—initial chemotherapy followed by surgical resection.
[b] 4-year survival—initial resection followed by chemotherapy.

tion is under question because of observed neurologic defects in long-term survivors. Because the rate of brain relapse is only 15% in stage I disease, some authors negate its routine use. Long-term survival in surgically treated patients with small cell cancer is shown in Table 15.14.

CARCINOID TUMORS

Typical carcinoid tumors are managed with the most conservative surgical resection possible. Lymph nodes should be removed when grossly abnormal. Bronchoscopic resection is contraindicated except as a palliative measure. Atypical carcinoids, although of greater malignant potential, are managed in the same manner. The long-term survival rate for patients with typical carcinoids is more than 90%; for those with atypical tumors, the rate is 50%.

Endobronchial Management of Lung Cancer

Recurrent tumor obstructing the lower trachea or main-stem bronchi may be coagulated endoscopically to prevent death from strangulation. The development of laser technique has made the endoscopic approach more satisfactory.

Both carbon dioxide (CO_2) and neodymium-YAG lasers can be used to remove obstructing cancerous tissue. Phototherapy with hematoporphyrin derivative has also been evaluated experimentally.

Laser Therapy

Laser therapy is more suitable than phototherapy. YAG laser is better than CO_2 laser because it can be used with the flexible fiberscope, its light wavelength is not absorbed appreciably by either water or blood, and its energy can penetrate several millimeters. The CO_2 laser requires rigid-tube endoscopy, its depth of penetration is less than 1 mm, and its efficacy relies on an absolutely dry field.

The YAG laser produces a thermal necrosis that debulks the tumor, and it controls any superficial bleeding. The technique is not without danger. Bleeding from perforation of a large vessel may occur, as may late hemorrhage from tumor necrosis.

Indications for YAG Laser Therapy

- The airway obstruction is unresponsive to other reasonable therapy;
- The lesion protrudes into the bronchial lumen without obvious extension beyond the cartilage;
- The axial length of the endobronchial component of the tumor is < 4 cm;
- The bronchoscopist can see the bronchial lumen;
- Functioning lung tissue exists beyond the obstruction.

Satisfactory palliation of severe obstruction or hemoptysis may occur in 79% of patients with advanced malignant tumors involving the trachea or main-stem bronchi by the use of the YAG laser.

Brachytherapy with endobronchial implantation of a radiation source is usually indicated after completion of the laser therapy.

Bronchoscopic Phototherapy with Hematoporphyrin Derivative (HpD-PT)

This method can be used to manage an advanced, previously treated tumor causing significant airway obstruction. HpD-PT has not been as successful as either CO_2 or neodymium-YAG lasers. Clinical trials are being carried out to define its usefulness and to improve its technique.

In a small subset of patients with radiographic occult lesions, bronchoscopic phototherapy has been successfully used as the primary treatment method. The lesion must be confined to the mucosa or be an in situ carcinoma less than 3 cm^2 in surface area.

Endoscopic Management of Carcinoid Tumors

Most of the growth of an endobronchial carcinoid occurs outside the involved bronchial lumen. Endoscopic removal results in an incomplete excision in almost all patients. This technique is recommended only in patients in whom surgical resection of the tumor is contraindicated.

Endobronchial Stents

Metallic expandable (Gianturco) stents and polyethylene-covered expandable metal stents have been used to obtain and maintain a patent bronchial lumen in selected patients with proximal obstructing tumors. At present, the main indication for their use in the cancer patient is a short life expectancy.

Radiation Therapy

Non-Small Cell Lung Carcinoma

The role of radiation therapy as a curative treatment method for patients with lung cancer is minor. In potentially operable good-risk candidates who do not undergo resection, a reported 22.5% 5-year survival rate was obtained following a radiation dose of 40–55 Gy. In poor-risk patients (elderly patients with poor pulmonary or cardiac function), a survival rate of only 6% was reported. In patients with nonresectable extensive stage IIIA and IIIB disease, the long-term survival rate is reduced to 3%. Although greater survival rates (10–16%) have been published, irradiation clearly has little to offer as a curative treatment. A selective approach to its use should be practiced. The use of radiation therapy as the sole therapeutic method in superior sulcus tumors, however, has been suggested to be efficacious, with a projected 5-year survival rate of 23%.

As a palliative method to decrease symptoms or to relieve the patient of symptoms (Table 15.15), irradiation produces results better than those afforded by any other palliative therapeutic intervention. Radiation therapy is the mainstay of treatment for the patient with nonresectable symptomatic non-small cell carcinoma.

Small Cell Lung Carcinoma

Thoracic irradiation is considered by most clinicians to have a valuable role in the multimodality management of localized small cell lung carcinoma. The best regimen for its use with intensive chemotherapy remains unresolved. In patients with extensive disease, radiation therapy is primarily used as a palliative measure to control persistent or recurrent symptoms.

Table 15.15. Palliation of Symptoms in Patients Following Radiation Therapy

Symptom	Percentage[a]
Hemoptysis	84 to 95
Chest pain	61 to 72
Dyspnea	60
Atelectasis	
SCLC	57
Non-SCLC	15

From Weisenburger TH. Non-small cell lung cancer: definitive radiotherapy and combined modality therapy. In: Roth JA, Ruckdeschel JC, Weisenburger TH, eds. Thoracic oncology. Philadelphia: WB Saunders, 1989. Reprinted with permission.
[a] Percentage of patients experiencing palliation.
SCLC, small cell lung cancer.
Non-SCLC, non-small cell lung cancer.

Bronchial Carcinoid Tumors

These tumors are resistant to irradiation. Its use is rarely indicated for recurrent or metastatic disease.

Chemotherapy

Non-Small Cell Lung Carcinoma

Chemotherapy, other than possibly neoadjuvant therapy, has no role as a curative treatment method. Its use as a palliative method in nonresectable disease is controversial. Randomized trials of multidrug therapy, particularly cisplatin-based regimens, have shown some superiority over supportive care alone. The aggregate median survival is approximately 2 months greater in the chemotherapy-treated groups. The qualitative impact on survival is undetermined, but the toxic effects, as well as costs of the chemotherapy, are well known. Its use, other than in clinical trials, should be discouraged except in the few symptomatic, advanced-stage patients with a good initial performance status who cannot be enrolled in an appropriate clinical trial.

Small Cell Lung Carcinoma

Multidrug chemotherapy, with or without local irradiation, is the treatment of choice in all but the few patients with localized disease. It is most effective in patients with limited-stage disease and in those with disseminated disease who still have a good performance status.

Limited-Stage Disease

Frequently used chemotherapy combinations are listed in Table 15.16. No best combination is as yet known. The response rates are 70–90%. The value of late intensification therapy, the use of alternating noncross-resistant drugs, and the duration of

Table 15.16. Frequently Used Chemotherapy Combinations for Small Cell Lung Cancer

Chemotherapy Combination	Abbreviation
Cyclophosphamide, Adriamycin (doxorubicin), vincristine	CAV
Cyclophosphamide, methotrexate, lomustine (CCNU)	CMC_N
Etoposide (VP-16), cisplatin	VpP
Cyclophosphamide, Adriamycin (doxorubicin), etoposide (VP-16)	CAVp
Cyclophosphamide, Adriamycin (doxorubicin), etoposide (VP-16), cisplatin	CAVpP
Etoposide (VP-16), carboplatin	VpCP

From Feld R, Ginsberg RJ, Payne DG. Treatment of small cell lung cancer. In: Roth JA, Ruckdeschel JC, Weisenburger TH, eds. Thoracic oncology. Philadelphia, PA: WB Saunders, 1989. Reprinted with permission.

therapy are still under investigation. Although treatment of 12 to 24 months (with maintenance therapy considered essential) was standard in the past, currently six courses of chemotherapy with adjuvant thoracic irradiation appear to be as satisfactory as prolonged treatment regimens. The timing and radiation dosage are under intensive investigation. Prophylactic cranial irradiation is usually recommended for the complete responders. This therapeutic intervention decreases the number of brain relapses but does not prolong survival. Neurologic toxicities in patients with long-term survival are forcing a reevaluation of the use of radiation and of the manner in which it is given.

Extensive Disease

Similar chemotherapeutic regimens are used in the management of patients with extensive disease. Response rates of 50 to 75% are achieved. Local thoracic and prophylactic cranial irradiation is not used routinely. Either may be used in patients who have obtained a complete response to the chemotherapy. Radiation therapy in patients with extensive disease is most often used as a palliative measure for the management of uncontrolled or recurrent symptoms.

TREATMENT RESULTS

In patients with localized disease, survival rates equal to or more than 2 years are reported to be between 15 and 43%. Five-year survival rates have varied between 5 and 20%. Significant favorable independent variables for prolonged survival are listed in Table 15.17.

In patients with extensive disease, survival rates of 1 year or more are reported to be between 21 and 42%. Survival rates of 2 or more years are 3 to 19%; 5-year survival is rarely observed in this group (< 1%). Similar favorable prognostic factors as recorded for patients with limited disease appear to be applicable to patients with extensive disease. Prognostic factors with a negative effect on survival are listed in Table 15.18.

Table 15.17. Favorable Factors for Survival in Limited Small Cell Lung Cancer

Good performance status
Female sex
70 years of age or younger
No pleural effusion
Tumor confined to lung
Normal LDH value
"Classic" growth pattern (vs. "variant") in culture

From Shields TW. Lung cancer and the solitary pulmonary nodule. In: Khan MG, ed. Cardiac and pulmonary management. Philadelphia, PA: Lea & Febiger, 1993. Reprinted with permission.

Table 15.18. Negative Prognostic Factors for Survival of Patients with Small Cell Lung Cancer with Extensive Disease

---

Poor performance status
Weight loss
More than one site of distant metastasis
Liver or brain metastasis
Local extension beyond the lung
Increase CEA, LDH, neuron-specific enolase
Variant growth pattern in culture

From Shields TW. Lung cancer and the solitary pulmonary nodule. In: Khan MG, ed. Cardiac and pulmonary management. Philadelphia, PA: Lea & Febiger, 1993. Reprinted with permission.

Carcinoid Tumors

The use of chemotherapy in patients with local recurrent or metastatic disease is experimental. Because of the neuroendocrine similarities between the atypical carcinoid tumors and the small cell tumors, similar treatment regimens may be attempted in these patients.

Immunotherapy

At present, immunotherapy appears to have no place in the therapeutic management of patients with lung cancer.

THE SOLITARY PULMONARY NODULE

A solitary pulmonary nodule is most often an incidental finding on a routine radiographic examination of the chest in an asymptomatic patient. It may be identified in either the posteroanterior or the lateral view and is frequently identified in only one of these views. Lordotic, oblique, and stereoscopic views may be profitably used to define an indistinct or questionable lesion.

Radiographic Limits of Visibility

The lower limit of radiographic visibility is between 6 and 7 mm. Such small lesions frequently are identified only when located in an intercostal space at a distance from the chest wall, diaphragm, or mediastinum. Lesions as small as 3 mm may be identified, but such SPNs are recognized only in retrospect.

Experimentally, 3-mm disks with sharp borders may be visualized, but once the borders become rounded or ill-defined, this low limit of visibility is lost. Because most pulmonary nodules are spherical, the presence of an SPN usually is not appreciated until it is 1 cm in size.

Definition

The definition of an SPN is controversial.

Typical Features

- Spherical or ovoid in shape and relatively well demarcated;
- May be associated with other pulmonary disorders but should be distinct from them;
- Surrounded by air-containing lung but may be located just beneath the visceral pleura;
- Margins may be sharply demarcated or ill-defined;
- Margins may be smooth, umbilicated, nodular, or spiculated;
- Some clinicians inappropriately exclude nodules that contain readily recognizable calcifications on the standard radiologic views;
- Cavitation may be present, but a thin-walled lesion containing air or an air-fluid level is best considered a pulmonary cavitary;
- May be associated with small satellite nodules;
- Invasion into the chest wall, diaphragm, or mediastinum should be absent;
- Grossly discernible mediastinal lymphadenopathy should not be present.

Table 15.19. Causes of Solitary Pulmonary Nodule

Neoplasms	Inflammatory Lesions	Malformations
Primary carcinoma	Tuberculoma and	Arteriovenous
Solitary metastasis	tuberculous lesions	malformations
Hamartoma	Histoplasmosis	Vascular endothelioma
Primary sarcoma	Coccidioidomycosis	Sequestrated segment
Bronchial carcinoid	*Cryptococcus*	Traumatic Lesions
Reticulosis	Nonspecific granuloma	Hematoma
Fibroma	Chronic lung abscess	Hernias
Myxoma	Lipoid pneumonia	Cysts
Neurogenic tumor	Massive fibrosis	Bronchogenic
Lipoma	Rheumatoid granuloma	Pericardial
Myoblastoma	Gumma	Dermoid
Hibernoma	Mycetoma	Teratoma
Solitary fibrous tumor	Parasitic Lesions	Pulmonary Infarct
of the pleura	*Echinococcus granulosus*	Rounded Atelectasis
Leiomyoma	*Ascaris lumbricoides*	
Plasmocytoma	*Dirofilaria immitis*	
Sclerosing		
hemangioma		
Thymoma		
Endometriosis		
Sugar tumor		

Adapted from Bateson EM. Analysis of 155 solitary lung lesions illustrating the differential diagnosis of mixed tumors of the lung. Clin Radiol 1965;16:60.

Table 15.20. Incidence (%) of Common Types of Solitary Pulmonary Nodules

Malignant	
Primary carcinoma of the lung	28
Carcinoid tumor	2
Metastatic tumor	10
Benign	
Infectious granuloma	50
Noninfectious granuloma	2
Benign tumors	2
Miscellaneous	6

From Lillington GA. Pulmonary nodules: solitary and multiple. Clin Chest Med 1982;3:361. Reprinted with permission.

The most controversial feature is the size of the lesion. Many series have included any lesion as large as 6 or even 8 cm in diameter, but more recent reports consider only lesions 4 cm or less in size as SPNs. A suggested cutoff of 3 cm would conform to the size of a T1 lesion in the various classifications of carcinoma of the lung. SPNs larger than 3 cm in size in most reported surgical series are usually malignant, with the exceptions of a large noncalcified granuloma or a hamartoma.

Etiology

An SPN is an important finding because it may represent an early carcinoma of the lung. The percentage these primary lung tumors represent in a series of SPNs varies with the population pool from which the series is derived. The percentage may be as low as 5% in a routine radiographic survey of all adults in a geographic catchment area to as high as 75% in a highly selected, surgically resected group. The other causes of an SPN are other tumors (benign or metastatic), granulomas, other inflammatory processes, vascular lesions, and miscellaneous lesions (Table 15.19). A typical distribution of the major causes is shown in Table 15.20.

Malignant Solitary Peripheral Nodules
Primary Lung Tumors

Most solitary peripheral malignant primary lung tumors are either adenocarcinomas, including the bronchioalveolar subtype, or squamous cell tumors. Large cell and small cell undifferentiated tumors are less frequently observed. Bronchial carcinoids, both typical and atypical cell types, are less commonly present.

Solitary Metastatic Nodule in Lung

Of all SPNs, 10% are metastatic tumors. Only 1–2% of metastatic tumors to the lung, however, occur as solitary nodules. The incidence is 2% for adenocarcinoma of the colon and 1.2% for breast carcinoma.

A patient with a previous or concurrent (unless uncontrolled) squamous cell primary extrapulmonary tumor rarely has a solitary metastasis to the lung. A new SPN in such patients, except for a small incidence of a granulomatous or other benign lesion, is usually a second primary tumor in the lung, regardless of the cell type of the lung tumor.

In patients with an extrapulmonary primary adenocarcinoma, the possibility that the new SPN is a metastatic lesion is approximately 50%; a few benign lesions have been observed.

In patients in whom the original extrapulmonary tumor was a sarcoma or a melanoma, the new SPN is almost always a metastatic lesion; infrequently it may be a benign lesion and rarely a new primary lung carcinoma.

Other Malignant Lung Tumors

Primary malignant lung tumors, such as soft tissue sarcomas (fibrosarcoma, leiomyosarcoma, and other mesenchymal derived tumors) and pulmonary blastomas (embryoma), may occur as an SPN.

Benign Pulmonary Lesions

Granulomas

Infectious granulomas comprise the largest percentage of SPNs—approximately 50% or more. The cause of the infectious granulomas varies with the geographic area of the population under review.

In the catchment area of the Mississippi River Valley and its tributaries, histoplasmosis is the common cause; in the Southwest, coccidioidomycosis is the more common cause. In Europe, tuberculosis is the most common cause of the SPN. Cryptococcosis may be encountered but has no specific geographic distribution.

Parasitic lesions rarely are causes of pulmonary granulomas, but lesions caused by *Echinococcus granulosus, Ascaris lumbricoides,* and *Dirofilaria immitis* have been reported.

Noninfectious granulomas, such as lipoid pneumonia, rheumatoid granuloma, resolving hematoma, rounded atelectasis, and pulmonary infarct, have appeared as an SPN.

Benign Lung Tumors

Hamartomas are the most common benign tumors that occur as SPNs (2–5%). They comprise 77% of all benign lung tumors. Slow growth of these tumors may be observed. Occasionally, benign mesenchymal tumors of the lung, such as fibromas, lipomas, and leiomyomas, occur as SPNs. Rarely, a neurogenic tumor or a clear cell tumor (a sugar tumor) may occur in this manner.

Vascular Lesions

A solitary pulmonary arterio-venous fistula is one of the vascular lesions that should be considered in the differential diagnosis of an SPN. Other lesions to be considered are a sclerosing hemangioma, an endothelioma, and a pulmonary infarct.

Benignancy Versus Malignancy

Criteria of Malignancy

No single criterion identifies a malignant SPN.

Suggestive Features

- A patient older than 40 years (the risk increases with advancing age);
- A history of smoking;
- A history of a previous malignancy elsewhere;
- The absence of calcification;
- An ill-defined, umbilicated, or spiculed ("corona radiata") margin;
- A large size;
- Contrast enhancement with iodized compound on high-resolution CT (HRCT);
- Positive FDG PET study.

Only 4–15% of T1 carcinomas are smaller than 1 cm in diameter, whereas more than 53% are larger than 2 cm.

Criteria of Benignancy

As with malignancy of an SPN, no one criterion establishes benignancy with absolute certainty.

Suggestive Features

- Rapid or slow or no rate of growth;
- Specific types of calcification;
- Density of the SPN;
- A fatty density within the nodule;
- Characteristic shape of a scar on tomographic examination;
- No or minimal contrast enhancement with iodized compound on HRCT;
- Negative FDG PET study.

Rate of Growth of SPN

The absence of growth over a 2-year period as established by retrospective review of previous available chest x-rays may be considered as almost an absolute criterion of benignancy. Rare examples of a primary adenocarcinoma behaving in this manner have been noted.

With the availability of previous chest x-rays, the rate of growth (the "doubling time") can be estimated. A 25% increase in the diameter of the SPN represents approximately a doubling of the volume of the mass. A 3- to 5-mm increase in the diameter of an SPN represents approximately one doubling time of an initial 1-cm to 2-cm SPN, respectively. A rapid doubling time (less than 36 days) or a slow doubling time (more than 465 days) can be accepted as representative of a benign process. Doubling times between 36 and 465 days can occur in either a benign or malignant SPN.

Presence of Calcification

The presence of a central nidus, laminar layers, diffuse homogeneous distribution, or "popcorn" distribution (observed in some hamartomas) of calcification on radiologic examination (including conventional or computed tomography) can be accepted as denoting benignancy. Eccentric or dystrophic calcification regardless of its size cannot be considered as signifying a benign lesion. Either type of calcification can occur in a primary lung tumor. Calcification may occur in a bronchial carcinoid (30% on CT) and in some metastatic lesions (osteogenic sarcoma, chondrosarcoma, mucinous adenocarcinomas of the endometrium, and, rarely, some lesions from the gastrointestinal tract).

Density of Nodule

Many benign granulomas that appear to be noncalcified by conventional radiographic studies contain microcalcifications, which increase the density of an SPN. Malignant lesions do not contain microcalcifications and their density is less. The density can be evaluated by computed tomographic densitometry, which is measured in Hounsfield units (HU).

- Density is estimated by averaging density numbers within the nodule and deriving a representative CT number expressed in HU.
- A mean CT number more than 164 HU is presumed to represent a granulomatous lesion.
- Of all indeterminate (noncalcified) nodules eventually proved to be benign, 60% had CT numbers of this magnitude.
- CT densitometry is most effective in SPNs measuring less than 3 cm in diameter with smooth or lobulated borders.

Initially these results could not be confirmed by other investigators because of differences in the technique, the equipment used, and the variations that could be attributed to the size of the patient and the location of the nodule. The development of a reference phantom that could reduce the sources of densometric error and provide a standard independent of scanner variations has overcome this problem. In a multicenter study, CT densitometry could be generalized in any scanner once

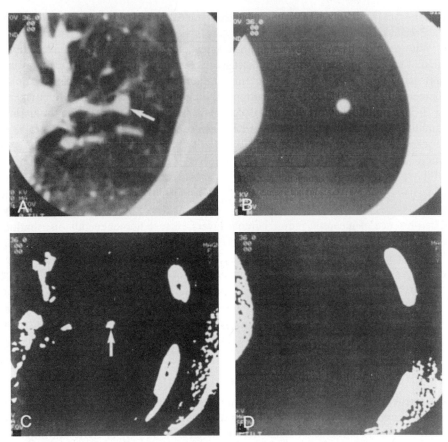

Figure 15.5. CT phantom nodule study. **A,** HRCT shows a small nodule (*arrow*) in the left lung. **B,** CT image of the phantom shows reference nodule corresponding to the site and position of the patient's nodule. **C,** CT image of the patient's nodule is compared with **D,** the image of the phantom nodule at the window setting at which the phantom nodule disappears. Persistent density of the patient's nodule indicates the presence of calcification and is consistent with a benign lesion. (From Shields TW, ed. General thoracic surgery. 4th ed. Baltimore, MD: Williams & Wilkins, 1994. Reprinted with permission.)

standardization was achieved. In two studies, 30–35% of the noncalcified, indeterminate SPNs were found to be more attenuating (higher density) than the phantom. Benignancy was confirmed in these SPNs by long-term follow-up examination (Fig. 15.5). The use of a reference phantom has not lived up to its expectations, however, and is now infrequently done.

Fat Within a Nodule

CT examination may reveal tissue consistent with the density of fat. This finding may be seen in one-third of hamartomas and in the rare lipoid pneumonias. Fatty tissue is not found in malignant lesions. Some authors have suggested that the SPN can be considered a benign lesion when fatty tissue is identified on CT.

Shape and Size

A well-demarcated, smoothly marginated SPN or an SPN with a bosselated margin, especially of less than 1 cm in size, frequently is a benign lesion, but malignancy cannot be ruled out. Some authors have suggested, however, that if the SPN is linear in shape, consistent with scarring, the lesion can be considered benign. This determination is best made by conventional tomography. There should be no nodularity or irregularities. The SPN may be angular in shape, with smooth tapering margins ending in points. Another variation is an SPN consisting of a conglomeration of multiple tiny nodules. In one study, all 38 uncalcified SPNs characterized by these features were proved to be benign. Further corroboration of this observation is necessary.

The finding of vascular connections to a SPN suggests the possibility of an arteriovenous fistula or an embolus; contrast enhancement CT or angiographic studies can confirm the vascular nature of the SPN.

Evaluation of the Patient with a Solitary Pulmonary Nodule

History

- Age of the patient is most important. Only 1–3% of SPNs are malignant in patients 35 years of age or younger. In patients older than 50 years of age, approximately 50% of SPNs are malignant, and the incidence increases with advancing age.
- A history of smoking markedly increases the possibility that the SPN is malignant.
- Acute respiratory symptoms may suggest the presence of an inflammatory process.
- A granuloma is more common in an immunocompromised host.
- Symptoms or other findings related to another organ system suggest the possibility of a primary tumor in a site other than the lung.
- Hemoptysis is unusual with an SPN and suggests the possibility of a radiographically unidentified endobronchial lesion.
- A history of a previous malignancy raises the possibility that the SPN is a solitary metastasis or a new primary lung tumor.
- An SPN in an asymptomatic patient negates an extensive search for an occult primary tumor. The incidence of an SPN representing a metastasis from a truly occult tumor is less than 0.5%.

Physical Examination

Examination of the thorax should be complete to rule out the possibility that the observed radiographic mass is not a skin or readily palpated bone or soft tissue tumor. The supraclavicular fossa should be evaluated for the presence of cervical lymphadenopathy. The thyroid, breasts, prostate, and testes should be examined for the presence of an asymptomatic mass.

Sputum Cytology and Skin Tests

Sputum cytology may be obtained but is only infrequently positive for tumor (< 5%) in a malignant SPN. When positive, the cytologic cell type may agree with the final histologic diagnosis in 85–90% of cases.

Skin tests for tuberculous or fungal infections are of little or no value in evaluating an SPN. At best, if negative, they render the diagnosis of a specific granuloma unlikely. A positive skin test has no relevant value in the management of the patient.

Radiographic Studies

Standard Radiographic Studies

If the SPN possibly could represent a nipple shadow, nipple markers with repeat radiographs should be obtained. When the SPN is indistinct, radiographs in other positions (lordotic, oblique views) may be helpful. The SPN should be examined for features highly suggestive of malignancy or benignancy, and any chest x-rays taken should be compared with available previous chest x-rays. When the nature of the SPN can be determined with reasonable certainty at this point, a therapeutic decision can be made. The indeterminate nodule requires further evaluation.

The pulmonary hilar and mediastinal shadows should be critically examined. If both these areas are normal, CT evaluation of the mediastinum for the presence of enlarged nodes is unnecessary.

Conventional Tomography

The indeterminate SPNs should be evaluated by conventional tomography guided by appropriate location by low kV fluoroscopy. If characteristic benign calcification or a linear shape (scar) is present, the SPN may be considered benign. If neither of these features is present, the SPN remains indeterminate.

Computed Tomography

The remaining indeterminate SPNs should be evaluated by standard CT (8- to 10-mm sections), by high-resolution tomography (1- to 2-mm sections), or by HRCT with contrast enhancement.

Standard Computed Tomography

Standard CT is recommended for:

• Patients with an extrathoracic primary tumor;
• Presence of abnormal or obscured hilar or mediastinal shadows;
• Indeterminate SPNs larger than 2 cm in size.

Patients with a previous history of a metachronous primary tumor or a synchronous primary tumor outside the chest should be evaluated to determine the presence of multiple lesions. Multiple lesions are identified by CT in 45% of such patients; 80% of these are metastatic nodules (the others are small benign granulomas or small intrapulmonary lymph nodes).

In patients with an associated abnormal or obscured hilar or mediastinal shadows, CT permits investigation of the mediastinum for the presence of enlarged lymph nodes as well as further examination of the nodule.

HRCT Densitometry and Contrast Enhancement

- Permits identification of unsuspected calcification within a benign SPN that may have been undetected by previous examinations.
- Calcification must be distributed in what has been described as a benign pattern.
- Particular caution is necessary in interpreting the calcifications in a lesion in a patient with a known extrathoracic malignant tumor because some of these may be calcified. Rarely a primary tumor will contain dystrophic calcifications.
- When calcification is not visually evident, it had been suggested that the density of the lesion should be compared with a reference densitometry phantom; however, as noted, this is now only infrequently done.
- The use of HRCT with iodinated contrast material will result in significant greater enhancement of a malignant noncalcified SPN than that observed in a granulomatous or benign neoplastic nodule (Fig. 15.6). The suggested recommended dose

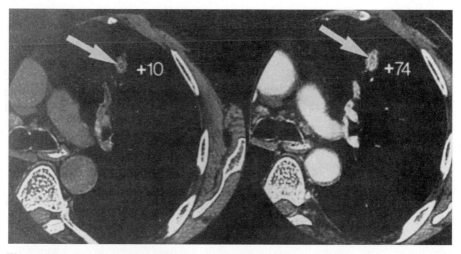

Figure 15.6. CT scan (2-mm collination) in a 78-year-old man with a squamous cell carcinoma of the left upper lobe. Nodule enhanced 64 HU from 10 HU on the precontrast image (*left*) to 74 HU on the 60-second postcontrast image (*right*). Note region of interest used to measure mean attenuation (*arrows*). (From Swenson SJ, Brown LR, Colby TV, Weaser AL. Pulmonary nodules: CT evaluation of enhancement with iodinated contrast material. Radiology 1995;194:393–398. Reprinted with permission.)

is 420 mg I/kg in an injection of 100 mL of nonionic solution at a rate of 2 mL/sec. HRCT images of the nodule are obtained before and after the injection. In a large series of patients, malignant lesions were enhanced by a value of 40 HU (range 20–108 HU), whereas granulomatous and benign neoplastic nodules were enhanced by a value of 12 HU (range: 4–58 HU). The enhancement is believed to be the result of greater vascularity of the malignant lesions, this being more prominent in the periphery of the nodule rather than in its center. A threshold value of 20 HU was observed in the malignant nodules, although enhancement of 16–24 HU can be considered as being indeterminate. At the threshold value of 20 HU, sensitivity was 100%, specificity was 76.9%, positive predictive value was 90.2%, negative predictive value was 100%, and accuracy was 92.6%. The important feature of this procedure is that when no or only minimal enhancement occurs (less than 15 HU), the nodule can be considered benign and need not be removed. Nodules enhanced more than 20 HU should be removed.

Detection of Malignancy with FDG PET

Positron emission tomography with FDG for the identification of malignant indeterminate SPNs is now under investigation. Focal hypermetabolism (increased uptake of FDG) is an indication of malignancy, whereas no increase in metabolism (no increased FDG uptake) is seen in most benign lesions. Some increased uptake may occur in active inflammatory masses, but quantitatively the uptake is less than that seen in malignant lesions.

Advantages

• Noninvasive technique;
• False–negative findings rare;
• Avoids surgical removal of benign nodules.

Disadvantages

• Availability and possibly cost;
• False–positive findings in 10–15%;
• Mass must be at least 1 cm or greater in size to be evaluated by FDG PET.

Despite these radiographic studies and the use of FDG PET, some SPNs will remain indeterminate. Additional diagnostic studies should be used in a selective manner to resolve the nature of the lesion. Video-assisted thoracoscopic surgical excision or, if necessary, thoracotomy may be the final diagnostic procedure.

Bronchoscopic Examination

Bronchoscopic evaluation with transbronchoscopic biopsy or aspiration of an SPN of the size defined (≤ 3 cm) is not indicated as a separate procedure. Results are positive in fewer than 20% of the patients with malignant nodules. This evaluation may be considered in larger lesions (> 3 cm), but otherwise the bronchoscopic examination of the tracheobronchial tree need be done only at the time of operation if one is indicated.

Transthoracic Fine-needle Aspiration Biopsy

Routine Fine-needle Aspiration

Routine fine-needle aspiration of an SPN is not needed to prove a preoperative diagnosis in nodules believed to be malignant. The argument that the SPN may represent a small cell carcinoma and that this procedure would rule out a resection is not valid. Recent reports from North America, Europe, and Japan have shown that excellent results can be obtained by primary resection of stage I small cell tumors followed by aggressive chemotherapy; projected 62–73% 5-year survival rates have been reported. The rare occurrence of development of tumor in the needle tract after a fine needle aspiration of a malignant SPN has been recorded, thus further negating the unnecessary routine use of the procedure.

Aspiration performed to attempt to establish a benign diagnosis in the indeterminate SPN is controversial. Although some authors report that benignancy can be established in 85% of truly benign lesions, several reports have emphasized a false–negative yield (the lesion subsequently proved to be malignant) in as many as 30–35% of indeterminate SPNs diagnosed as not being malignant.

Selective Fine-needle Aspiration

A fine-needle biopsy may be justified in a few clinical settings.

Indications

- Patient's refusal of a recommendation for operation: Patient refuses resection of an SPN unless a preoperative diagnosis of tumor is established or the patient desires some other therapeutic (radiation therapy) management.
- Medical condition precludes operative intervention: The presence of insufficient pulmonary function, noncorrectable cardiac contraindications, or a recent myocardial infarction carries a prohibitive operative risk. When a diagnosis of malignancy is obtained, other therapy may be recommended.
- Suspected hamartoma: Indicated if the appearance is suggestive of a hamartoma but neither calcification nor fatty tissue is identified on HRCT. Although often attended with an increased risk of postoperative pneumothorax, confirmation of diagnosis negates an unnecessary thoracotomy.
- Immunocompromised patient: Indicated when attempting to identify a specific opportunistic inflammatory process, such as cryptococcus, an atypical mycobacterial, or fungal infection.
- Patient with a previous malignant melanoma: Rules out the remote possibility of

a secondary primary lung tumor that should be resected. If a benign lesion is identified, the resection is not indicated because its removal has little or no influence on the subsequent longevity of the patient. Removal of a metastatic melanoma is controversial.

Metastatic Evaluation

A "metastatic" evaluation (brain, upper abdominal, and bone scans) is contraindicated in the asymptomatic patient with an SPN. The rate of discovery of an occult metastasis is too small (1–3%) to justify the "metastatic" evaluation.

Video-assisted Thoracoscopic Removal

The video-assisted surgical resection of a peripherally located small (< 3 cm) indeterminate SPN has become the procedure of choice for diagnosis. Although techniques have been described for the resection of more centrally located SPNs deep within the lung substance, such lesions are best resected by an open thoracotomy.

Thoracotomy

The ultimate diagnostic procedure is thoracotomy with resection of the indeterminate SPN. With the appropriate preoperative evaluation, no more than 25–35% of the resected SPNs should be benign; the other SPNs are malignant tumors.

Other Diagnostic Options
Artificial Intelligence

Computer-aided diagnosis of an SPN by discriminant analyses or based on the use of the Bayesian theorem has been reported as useful. The data in these studies, however, are unique to the given institutional study pattern and are not applicable to all situations. Refinement of such analyses may result in wide applicability for all patients in the future.

Period of "Watchful Waiting"

The periodic observation of an indeterminate SPN by serial chest x-rays to determine whether the nodule is growing at a malignant rate is unacceptable in most situations. The exceptions are an SPN in patients under the age of 35 years who have never smoked cigarettes, SPNs discovered in association with an acute lower respiratory infection, and SPNs less than 1 cm in size (with a well-defined, smooth border) in nonsmokers who are high operative risks because of concurrent cardiac, pulmonary, or other life-threatening comorbid conditions.

Recommended Plan of Management

Several optional courses can be taken in the management of the patient with an asymptomatic SPN. The selection of one over another depends on the age of the patient, the availability of previous chest x-rays, the radiographic characteristics of the nodule, and a history or the presence of a primary extrathoracic malignancy.

Age of Patient

In patients under the age of 35 years, a period of observation is justified unless the radiographic characteristics strongly support a presumptive diagnosis of tumor (large size, spiculated or markedly ill-defined borders, and the absence of calcification or fatty tissue). Radiographs should be obtained at 3-month intervals for a least 2 years. If growth is observed, transthoracic fine-needle biopsy may be justified to establish a diagnosis. If tumor is present or the diagnosis remains in doubt, video-assisted surgical resection or thoracotomy is indicated.

Availability of Previous Chest X-rays or Doubling Time

If previous chest x-rays reveal no growth over a 2-year period or if more recent films show a rapid doubling time (< 30 days) or slow growth (> 465 days), the lesion may be considered benign and should be observed at periodic intervals. If the doubling time falls between these two extremes, further radiographic evaluation of the SPN is indicated.

Nonavailability of Previous Chest X-rays or Indeterminate Doubling Time

If the SPN is noncalcified on the standard radiographic views, fluoroscopic evaluation and conventional tomography should be done to identify any typically benign pattern of calcification within the nodule. A linear benign shape of the mass may also be discerned by this examination. If neither is demonstrated, standard CT or HRCT should be carried out to identify any "typical" calcification pattern or the presence of fatty tissue within the mass. A pulmonary arterio-venous malformation may be identified by its vascular connections as well as by its pattern of enhancement on dynamic CT imaging. If none of these features is present, HRCT with infusion of an iodinated compound to determine the presence of contrast enhancement should be obtained. If the lesion can be presumed to be benign by any of these studies, periodic radiographic reevaluation of the mass can be recommended. If the nodule remains "indeterminate," video-assisted thoracoscopic surgery or thoracotomy and resection should be carried out.

Synchronous or Metachronous Primary Extrathoracic Malignancy

The approach to a patient with an SPN who has a history of a previous extrathoracic neoplasm or in whom the SPN was discovered at the time of evaluation should be tailored to the type and site of the extrathoracic primary tumor and to the clinical situation existing at the time of the discovery of the SPN.

Clinical Status of Patient

The extrathoracic tumor must be controlled or controllable locally, and no evidence of metastases to other sites should be present or detectable. The potential sites of other metastatic involvement vary with the type of original primary tumor and must be appropriately evaluated. For example, a patient with breast or prostatic cancer should have a radionuclide bone scan, and a patient with colon carcinoma should have an abdominal CT study to evaluate the liver and the local site of resection to rule out recurrence. If available, tumor markers (α-fetoprotein and human chorionic gonadotropin levels for patients with nonseminomatous testicular tumors, acid phosphatase in a patient with prostatic cancer) should be obtained. Radioactive iodine uptake study should be done in a patient with a previous thyroid carcinoma. If any of these studies is positive, resection is best delayed, and the patient should be managed with chemotherapy, hormonal therapy, or irradiation (radioactive ^{131}I) as indicated.

Radiographic Evaluation

All potential surgical patients should undergo conventional CT of the chest for evaluation of the presence of multiple nodules. When multiple nodules are present, the lesions can be assumed to be metastatic. The management of multiple pulmonary metastases is not germane to this presentation.

If the nodule is solitary, HRCT with contrast enhancement should be done; the absence of contrast enhancement or minimal enhancement suggests benignancy of the nodule. If this criterion for benignancy is not met, prompt resection is indicated.

Cell Type of Original Primary Tumor

All potential solitary metastases, with the exceptions previously noted, should be resected. Some authors have questioned the efficacy of this procedure in actually improving the patient's ultimate prognosis. This question is unanswerable. The most compelling reason for resecting an SPN in patients with a previous squamous cell primary tumor is that the SPN most often represents a new primary lung cancer; in patients with a previous adenocarcinoma, the possibility is 50%. In patients with a previous sarcoma, on the other hand, the SPN rarely represents a primary lung cancer.

Prognosis

Radiographic Observation

Solitary nodules that have met the radiographic or at times the cytologic criteria of benignancy should be observed periodically over a period of time because these lesions rarely eventually prove to be malignant. The prognosis is near 100% for long-term survival in these patients.

Prospective observation for growth of small lesions is to be condemned except in nonsmoking patients under the age of 35 years or in those whose clinical condition or personal beliefs negate resection. Watchful waiting, which may permit the growth of a lung cancer, increases the likelihood of locoregional and distant metastasis. An increased size of a malignant SPN also has an unfavorable effect on the patient's prognosis.

SURGICAL RESECTION

Benign Nodule

The prognosis after resection is excellent.

Primary Lung Tumor

The resection of a primary malignant SPN of the lung results in an overall 60–70% 5-year survival rate. The smaller the lesion, the better the prognosis. Nodules smaller than 1 cm have an 80% long-term survival rate, those between 1 and 2 cm have a 74% rate, and those larger than 2 cm have a 51% survival rate. In some series, the survival rates for each of the size categories have been reported to be 10–20% higher.

Metastatic Malignant Solitary Pulmonary Nodule

The resection of a solitary pulmonary metastasis results in overall long-term survival rates of 20–30%.

BIBLIOGRAPHY

Aberg T, Malmberg KA, Nilsson B, Nou E. The effect of metastasectomy: fact or fiction? Ann Thorac Surg 1980;30:378.

Albain KS, Crowley JJ, Livingston RB. Long-term survival and toxicity in small cell lung cancer. Chest 1991;99:1425.

Albertucci M, DeMeester TR, Rothberg M, et al. Surgery and the management of peripheral lung tumor adherent to the parietal pleura. J Thorac Cardiovasc Surg 1992;103:8–13.

Armstrong JG, Minski BD. Radiation therapy for medically inoperable stage I and II non-small cell lung cancer. Cancer Treat Rev 1989;16:247.

Arroliga AC, Buzaid AC, Matthay RA. Which patients can safely undergo lung resection. J Respir Dis 1991;12:1080–1086.

Backer CL, Shields TW, Lockhart CG, et al. Selective preoperative evaluation for possible N2 disease in carcinoma of the lung. J Thorac Cardiovasc Surg 1987;93:337.

Black WC, Armstrong P, Daniel TM. Cost effectiveness of chest CT in T1N0M0 lung cancer. Radiology 1988;167:373.

Bleyer WA. Hobson's choice in CNS radioprophylaxis of small cell lung cancer (editorial). Int J Radiat Oncol Biol Phys 1988;15:783.

Bourguet P, Dazord L, Desrues B, et al. Immunoscintigraphy of human lung squamous cell carcinoma using an iodine-131 labelled monoclonal antibody (P066). Br J Cancer 1990; 61:230.

Buhr J, Berghauser KH, Moor H, et al. Tumor cells in intraoperative pleural lavage. An indicator for the poor prognosis of bronchogenic carcinoma. Cancer 1990;65:1801.

Burt M, Wronski M, Arbit E, et al. Resection of brain metastases from non-small cell lung carcinoma. Results of therapy. J Thorac Cardiovasc Surg 1992;103:399–441.

Calhoun P, Feldman PS, Armstrong P, et al. The clinical outcome of needle aspiration of the lung when cancer is not diagnosed. Ann Thorac Surg 1986;41:592.

The Canadian Lung Oncology Group. Investigation for mediastinal disease in patients with apparently operable lung cancer. Ann Thorac Surg 1995;60:1382–1389.

Casey JJ, Stempel BG, Scanlon EF, Fry WA. The solitary pulmonary nodule in the patient with breast cancer. Surgery 1984;96:801.

Caskey CL, Templeton PA, Zerhouni EA. Current evaluation of the solitary pulmonary nodule. Radiol Clin North Am 1990;28:511.

Chang AE, Schaner EG, Conkle DM, et al. Evaluation of computed tomography in the detection of pulmonary metastases. Cancer 1979;43:913.

Chin R, Ward R, Cappellari JC, Keyes J, Haponik EF. Mediastinal node (N2) involvement by PET-FDG scanning in non-small cell lung carcinoma (NSCLC): pathologic correlation. Chest 1994;106:89S.

Conill C, Astudillo J, Verger E. Prognostic significance of metastases to mediastinal levels in resected non-small cell lung carcinoma. Cancer 1992;72:1199–1202.

Cooper JD, Pearson FG, Todd TRJ, et al. Radiotherapy alone for patients with operable carcinoma of the lung. Chest 1985;87:289.

Coppage L, Shaw C, Curtis AM. Metastatic disease to the chest in patients with extrathoracic malignancy. J Thorac Imaging 1987;2:24.

Cortese DA. Endobronchial management of lung cancer. Chest 1986;89:234S.

Cummings SR, Lillington GA, Richard RJ. Estimating the probability of malignancy in solitary pulmonary nodules: a Bayesian approach. Am Rev Respir Dis 1986;134:449.

Cummings SR, Lillington GA, Richard RJ. Managing solitary pulmonary nodules. The choice of strategy is a "close call." Am Rev Respir Dis 1986;134:453.

Curran WJ Jr, Stafford PM. Lack of apparent difference in outcome between clinically staged IIIA and IIIB non-small cell lung cancer treated with radiation therapy. J Clin Oncol 1990; 8:409.

Dales RE, Stark RM, Raman S. Computed tomography to stage lung cancer. Approaching a controversy using meta-analysis. Am Rev Respir Dis 1990;141:1096.

Deschamps C, Pairolero PC, Trastek VF, et al. Multiple primary lung cancers: results of surgical treatment. J Thorac Cardiovasc Surg 1990;99:769.

Deslauriers J, Brisson J, Cartier R, et al. Carcinoma of the lung: evaluation of satellite nodules as a factor in influencing prognosis after resection. J Thorac Cardiovasc Surg 1989;97: 504.

Dewan NA, Gupta NC, Redepenning LS, Phalen JJ, Frick MP. Diagnostic efficacy of PET-FDG imaging in solitary pulmonary nodules: potential role in evaluation and management. Chest 1993;104:997–1002.

Diggs CH, Engler JE, Prendergast EJ, Kramer K. Small cell carcinoma of the lung. Treatment in the community. Cancer 1992;69:2075–2083.

Eagan RT, Rund C, Lee RE, et al. Pilot study of induction therapy with cyclophosphamide, doxorubicin, and cisplatin (CAP) and chest irradiation prior to thoracotomy in initially inoperable stage III MO non-small cell lung cancer. Cancer Treat Rep 1987;71:895.

Edell ES, Cortese DA. Bronchoscopic phototherapy with hematoporphyrin derivative for treatment of localized bronchogenic carcinoma: a 5-year experience. Mayo Clin Proc 1987; 62:8.

Edwards FH, Schaefer PS, Cohen AJ, et al. Use of artificial intelligence for preoperative diagnosis of pulmonary lesions. Ann Thorac Surg 1989;48:556.

Feinstein AR, Wells CK. A clinical-severity staging system for patients with lung cancer. Medicine (Baltimore) 1990;69:1.

Feld R. Chemotherapy as adjuvant therapy for completely resected non-small cell lung cancer: have we made progress. J Clin Oncol 1996;14:1045–1047.

Feld R, Ginsberg RJ, Payne DG. Treatment of small cell lung cancer. In: Roth JA, Ruckdeschel JC, Weisenburger TH, eds. Thoracic oncology. Philadelphia, PA: WB Saunders, 1989.

Glazer HS, Kaiser LR, Anderson DJ, et al. Indeterminate mediastinal invasion in bronchogenic carcinoma: CT evaluation. Radiology 1989;173:37.

Goldstein MS, Rush M, Johnson P, Sprung CL. A calcified adenocarcinoma of the lung with very high CT numbers. Radiology 1984;150:785.

Goldstraw P. The practice of cardiothoracic surgeons in the perioperative staging of non-small cell lung cancer. Thorax 1992;47:1–2.

Gross DH, Glazer GM, Orringer MB, et al. Bronchogenic carcinoma metastatic to normal-sized lymph nodes: frequency and significance. Radiology 1988;166:71.

Gupta NC, Frank AR, Dewan NA, et al. Solitary pulmonary nodules: detection of malignancy with PET with 2[F-18]fluoro-2-deoxy-D-glucose. Radiology 1992;184:441–444.

Harpole DH Jr, Johnson CM, Wolf WG, et al. Analysis of 945 cases of pulmonary metastatic melanoma. J Thorac Cardiovasc Surg 1992;103:743–750.

Harrow EM, Oldenburg FA, Lingenfelter MS, Smith AM Jr. Transbronchial needle aspiration in clinical practice. A five-year experience. Chest 1989;96:1268.

Heavey LR, Glazer GM, Gross BH, et al. The role of CT in staging radiographic T1N0M0 lung cancer. AJR 1986;146:285.

Huston J III, Muhm JR. Solitary pulmonary nodule evaluation with a CT reference phantom. Radiology 1987;163:481.

Huston J III, Muhm JR. Solitary pulmonary nodule evaluation with a CT reference phantom. Radiology 1989;170:653.

Ichinose Y, Hara N, Ohta M, et al. Preoperative examination to detect metastasis is not advocated for asymptomatic patients with stages I and II non-small cell lung cancer. Preoperative examination for lung cancer. Chest 1989;96:1104.

Ichinose Y, Hara N, Ohta M, et al. Brain metastases in patients with limited small cell lung cancer achieving complete remission. Correlation with TNM staging. Chest 1989;96:1332.

Ichinose Y, Yano T, Asho H, et al. Prognostic factors obtained by pathologic examination in completely resected non-small cell lung cancer: an analysis in each pathologic stage. J Thorac Cardiovasc Surg 1995;110:601–605.

Ishida T, Yokoyama H, Kaneko S, et al. Long-term results of operation for non-small cell lung cancer in the elderly. Ann Thorac Surg 1990;50:919.

Israel RH, Poe RH. The solitary pulmonary nodule: what to do, and why. J Respir Dis 1992; 13:308–318.

Izbicki JR, Passlick B, Karg O, et al. Impact of radical systematic mediastinal lymphadenectomy on tumor staging in lung cancer. Ann Thorac Surg 1995;59:209–214.

Izbicki JR, Thetter O, Habekost M, et al. Radical systematic mediastinal lymphadenectomy in non-small cell lung cancer: a randomized controlled trial. Brit J Surg 1994;81:229–235.

Johnson BE, Becker B, Goff WB III, et al. Neurologic, neuropsychologic, and computed cranial tomography scan abnormalities in 2- to 10-year survivors of small cell lung cancer. J Clin Oncol 1985;3:1659.

Johnson DH, Einhorn LH, Bartolucci A, et al. Thoracic radiotherapy does not prolong survival in patients with locally advanced, unresectable non-small cell lung cancer. Ann Intern Med 1990;113:33.

Karrer K, Shields TW, Denk H, et al. The importance of surgical and multimodality treatment for small cell bronchial carcinoma. J Thorac Cardiovasc Surg 1989;97:168.

Kerrigan DC, Spence PA, Crittenden MC, Tripp MD. Methylene blue guidance for simplified resection of a lung lesion. Ann Thorac Surg 1992;53:163–164.

Khouri NF, Meziane MA, Zerhouni EA, et al. The solitary pulmonary nodule. Assessment, diagnosis, and management. Chest 1987;91:128.

Klastersky J, Feld R, Kleisbauer JP, Rocmans P. Treatment of N2 non-small cell lung cancer (NSCLC). Chest 1989;96(suppl):835.

Klein JS, Webb WR. The radiologic staging of lung cancer. J Thorac Imag 1991;7:29–47.

Kormas P, Bradshaw JR, Jeyasingham K. Preoperative computed tomography of the brain in non-small cell bronchial carcinoma. Thorax 1992;47:106–108.

Kreisman H, Wolkove N, Quoix E. Small cell lung cancer presenting as a solitary pulmonary nodule. Chest 1992;101:225–231.

Kubota K, Matsuzawa T, Ito M, et al. Differential diagnosis of lung tumor with positron emission tomography: a prospective study. J Nucl Med 1990;31:1927–1932.

Kubota K, Matsuzawa T, Fujiwara T, et al. Comparison of C-11 methionine and F-18–fluoro-deoxyglucose for differential diagnosis of lung tumors. J Nucl Med 1989;30:788–779.

Kuhlman JE, Fishman EK, Kuhajda FP, et al. Solitary bronchioalveolar carcinoma: CT criteria. Radiology 1988;167:379.

Lad T, Rubinstein L, Sadeghi A. The benefit of adjuvant treatment for resected locally advanced non-small cell lung cancer. J Clin Oncol 1988;6:9.

Landreneau RJ, Hazelrigg SR, Ferson PF, et al. Thoracoscopic resection of 52 pulmonary lesions. Ann Thorac Surg 1992;54:800–807.

Landreneau RJ, Hazelrigg SR, Mack MJ, et al. Thoracoscopic mediastinal lymph node sampling. Useful for mediastinal lymph node stations inaccessible by cervical mediastinoscopy. J Thorac Cardiovasc Surg 1992;106:554–558.

Landreneau RJ, Herlan DB, Johnson JA, et al. Thoracoscopic neodymium: yittrium-aluminum garnet laser-assisted pulmonary resection. Ann Thorac Surg 1992;52:1176–1178.

Lauer RC, Fleck JF, Antony A, Einhorn LH. Is prophylactic cranial irradiation indicated in small cell lung cancer? In Proceedings of the American Society of Clinical Oncology (New Orleans). Vol 7. Philadelphia, PA: WB Saunders, 1988.

Lee JD, Ginsberg RJ. Pretreatment lung cancer staging for combined modality therapy: the role of ipsilateral scalene lymph node biopsy. Ann Thorac Surg. In press.

Lewis RJ, Caccavale RJ, Sisler GE. Video-assisted thoracic surgical resection of malignant lung tumors. J Thorac Cardiovasc Surg 1992;104:1679–1687.

Little AG, Stitik FP. Clinical staging of patients with non-small cell lung cancer. Chest 1990;97:1431.

Lung Cancer Study Group (prepared by Ginsberg RJ and Rubinstein LV). Randomized trial of lobectomy versus limited resection for T1N0 non-small cell lung cancer. Ann Thorac Surg 1995;60:615–623.

Mack MJ, Gordon MJ, Postma TW, et al. Percutaneous localization of pulmonary nodule for thoracoscopic lung resection. Ann Thorac Surg 1992;53:1123–1124.

Magilligan DJ Jr, Duvernoy BS, Malik G, et al. Surgical approach to lung cancer with solitary cerebral metastasis: twenty-five years' experience. Ann Thorac Surg 1986;42:360.

Martini N, Bains MS, Burt ME, et al. Incidence of local recurrence and second primary tumors in resected stage I lung cancer. J Thorac Cardiovasc Surg 1995;109:120–129.

Massard G, Moog R, Wihlm JM, et al. Bronchogenic cancer in the elderly: operative risk and long-term prognosis. Thorac Cardiovasc Surgeon 1996;44:40–45.

Mathisen DJ, Grillo HC. Carinal resection for lung cancer. J Thorac Cardiovasc Surg 1991; 102:16.

Mathisen DJ, Wain JC, Wright C, et al. Assessment of preoperative accelerated radiotherapy and chemotherapy in stage IIIA (N_2) non-small cell lung cancer. J Thorac Cardiovasc Surg 1996;111:123–133.

McLoud TC, Bourgouin PM, Greenberg RW, et al. Bronchogenic carcinoma: analysis of staging in the mediastinum with CT by correlative lymph node mapping and sampling. Radiology 1992;182:319–323.

Miller JD, Gorenstein LA, Patterson A. Staging: The key to rational management of lung cancer. Ann Thorac Surg 1992;53:170–178.

Mills SE, Cooper PH, Walker AN, Kron IL. Atypical carcinoid of the lung: a clinicopathologic study of 17 cases. Am J Surg Pathol 1982;6:643.

Mountain CF. A new international staging system for lung cancer. Chest 1986;89(suppl): 225S.

Murren JR, Buzaid AC, Hait EH. Critical analysis of neoadjuvant therapy for stage IIIA non-small cell lung cancer. Am Rev Respir Dis 1991;143:889.

Nathan MH, Collins VP, Adams RA. Differentiation of benign and malignant nodules by growth rate. Radiology 1962;79:321.

Naunheim KS, Kesler KA, D'Orazio SA. Thoracotomy in the octogenarian. Ann Thorac Surg 1992;51:547–551.

Neff TA. The science and humanity of the solitary pulmonary nodule. Am Rev Respir Dis 1986;134:433.

Nesbitt JC, Putnam JB Jr, Walsh GL, et al. Survival in early-stage non-small cell lung cancer. Ann Thorac Surg 1995;60:466–472.

Okumura M, Ohshima S, Kotake Y, et al. Intraoperative pleural lavage cytology in lung cancer patients. Ann Thorac Surg 1991;51:599.

Patz EF, Lowe VL, Hoffman JM, et al. Focal pulmonary abnormalities: evaluation with F-18 fluorodeoxyglucose PET scanning. Radiology 1993;188:487–490.

Payne WS, Bernatz PE, Pairolera PE, et al. Localization and treatment of radiographically occult lung cancer. In: Delarue NC, Eschapasse H, eds. Lung Cancer. Philadelphia, PA: WB Saunders, 1985.

Penketh AR, Robinson AA, Barber V, Flower CD. Use of percutaneous needle biopsy in the investigation of solitary pulmonary nodules. Thorax 1987;42:967.

Pogrebniak HW, Strovroff M, Roth JA, Pass HI. Resection of pulmonary metastasis from malignant melanoma: results of a 16-year experience. Ann Thorac Surg 1988;46:20.

Read RC, Schaefer RF, North W, Walls R. Diameter, cell type, and survival in stage I primary non-small cell lung cancer. Arch Surg 1988;123:446.

Reed JG, Rubin SA, Schnodig VJ. Interventional procedures used for diagnosing and treating lung cancer. J Thorac Imaging 1991;7:48–56.

Rege SD, Hoh CK, Glaspy JA, et al. Imaging of pulmonary mass lesions with whole-body positron emission tomography and fluorodeoxyglucose. Cancer 1993;72:82–90.

Rosengart TK, Martini N, Ghosn P, Burt M. Multiple primary lung carcinomas: prognosis and treatment. Ann Thorac Surg 1991;52:772–779.

Rotte KH, Meiske W. Results of computer-aided diagnosis of peripheral bronchial carcinoma. Radiology 1977;125:583.

Schenk DA, Strollo PI, Pichard JS, et al. Utility of the Wang 18-gauge transbronchial histology needle in the staging of bronchogenic carcinoma. Chest 1989;96:272.

Schulten M, Heiskell CA, Shields TW. The incidence of solitary pulmonary metastasis from carcinoma of the large bowel. Surg Gynecol Obstet 1976;143:727.

Scott WJ, Gobar LS, Hauser LG, et al. Detection of scalene lymph node metastases from lung cancer: positron emission tomography. Chest 1995;107:1174–1176.

Scott WJ, Gobar LS, Terry JP, et al. Mediastinal lymph node staging of non-small cell lung cancer. A prospective comparison of computed tomography and positron emission tomography. J Thorac Cardiovasc Surg 1996;111:642–648.

Scott WJ, Schwabe JL, Gupta NC, et al. Positron emission tomography of lung tumors and mediastinal lymph nodes using [18F]Fluorodeoxyglucose. Ann Thorac Surg 1994;58: 698–703.

Seyfer AE, Walsh DS, Graeber GM, et al. Chest wall implantation of lung cancer after thin-needle aspiration biopsy. Ann Thorac Surg 1989;48:284.

Shepherd FA, Evans WK, Feld R, et al. Adjuvant chemotherapy following surgical resection for small cell carcinoma of the lung. J Clin Oncol 1988;6:832.

Shepherd FA, Ginsberg RJ, Patterson A, et al. A prospective study of adjuvant surgery after chemotherapy for limited small cell lung cancer. A University of Toronto Lung Oncology Group Study. J Thorac Cardiovasc Surg 1989;97:177.

Shepherd FA, Laskey J, Evans WK, et al. Cushing's syndrome associated with ectopic corticotropin production and small cell lung cancer. J Clin Oncol 1992;10:21–27.

Shields TW. The use of mediastinoscopy in lung cancer: the dilemma of mediastinal lymph nodes. In: Kittle CF, ed. Current controversies in thoracic surgery. Philadelphia, PA: WB Saunders, 1986.

Shields TW. The "incomplete" resection. Ann Thorac Surg 1989;47:487.

Shields TW. Behavior of small bronchial carcinomas. Ann Thorac Surg 1990;50:691.

Shields TW. The significance of ipsilateral mediastinal lymph node metastasis (N2 disease) in non-small cell carcinoma of the lung. A commentary. J Thorac Cardiovasc Surg 1990; 99:48.

Shields TW. General thoracic surgery. 4th ed. Baltimore, MD: Williams & Wilkins, 1994.

Shirakusa T, Tsutsui M, Iriki N, et al. Results of resection for bronchogenic carcinoma in patients over the age of 80. Thorax 1989;44:189.

Siegelman SS, Khouri NF, Scott WW Jr, et al. Pulmonary hamartoma: CT findings. Radiology 1986;160:313.

Siegelman SS, Zerhouni EA, Leo FP, et al. CT of the solitary pulmonary nodule. AJR 1980; 135:1.

Stewart JG, MacMahon H, Vyborny CJ, Pollak ER. Dystrophic calcification in carcinoma of the lung: demonstration by CT. AJR 1987;148:29.

Sugarbaker DJ, Strauss GM. Advances in surgical staging and therapy of non-small cell lung cancer. Semin Oncol 1993;20:163–172.

Sugio K, Ishida T, Kaneko S, et al. Surgically resected lung cancer in young adults. Ann Thorac Surg 1992;53:127–131.

Swenson SJ, Brown LR, Colby TV, Weaver AL. Pulmonary Nodule: CT evaluation of enhancement with iodinated contrast material. Radiology 1995;194:393–398.

Talton B, Constable W, Kersh C. Curative radiotherapy in non-small cell carcinoma of the lung. Int J Radiol Oncol Biol Phys 1990;19:15–21.

Valk PE, Pounds TR, Hopkins DM, et al. Staging non-small cell lung cancer by whole-body positron emission tomographic imaging. Ann Thorac Surg 1995;60:1573–1582.

Van Houtte P, Rocmans P, Smets P, et al. Postoperative radiation therapy in lung cancer: a controlled trial after resection of curative design. Int J Radiat Oncol Biol Phys 1980;6:983.

Vokes EE, Bitran JD, Vogelzang NJ. Chemotherapy for non-small cell lung cancer. The continuing challenge. Chest 1991;99:1326. Editorial.

Wada H, Hitomi S. Teramatsu T, and the West Japan Study Group for lung cancer surgery. J Clin Oncol 1996;14:1048–1054.

Wahl RL, Quint LE, Cieslak RD, et al. "Anatometabolic" tumor imaging: fusion of FDG PET with CT or MRI to localize foci of increased activity. J Nucl Med 1993;34:1190–1197.

Wahl RL, Quint LE, Greenough RL, et al. Staging of mediastinal non-small cell lung cancer with FDG PET, CT, and fusion images: preliminary prospective evaluation. Radiology 1994;191:371–377.

Warren WH, Faber LP, Gould VE. Neuroendocrine neoplasms of the lung. A clinicopathologic update. J Thorac Cardiovasc Surg 1989;98:321.

Webb WR. The role of magnetic resonance imaging in the assessment of patients with lung cancer: a comparison with computed tomography. J Thorac Imaging 1989;4:65.

Webb WR, Gatsonis C, Zerhouni EA, et al. CT and MR imaging in staging non-small cell bronchogenic carcinoma: report of the Radiologic Diagnostic Oncology Group. Radiology 1991;178:705–713.

Wiersema MJ, Hassig WH, Hawes RH, Wonn MJ. Mediastinal lymph node detection with endosonography. Gastrointest Endosc 1993;39:788–793.

Wilkins EW, Grillo HC, Moncure AC, Scannel JG. Changing times and surgical management of bronchopulmonary carcinoid tumors. Ann Thorac Surg 1984;38:339.

Winning AJ, McIvor J, Seed WA, et al. Interpretation of negative results in fine-needle aspiration of discrete pulmonary lesions. Thorax 1986;41:875.

Wolfe WG, Sabiston DC Jr. Management of benign and malignant lesions of the trachea and bronchi with the neodymium-yttrium-aluminum-garnet laser. J Thorac Cardiovasc Surg 1986;91:40.

Yamashita K, Matsunoka S, Tsuda T, et al. Solitary pulmonary nodule: preliminary study of evaluation with incremental dynamic CT. Radiology 1995;184:340.

Yashar J, Weitberg AB, Glicksman AS, et al. Preoperative chemotherapy and radiation therapy for stage IIIa non-small cell carcinoma of the lung. Ann Thorac Surg 1992;53:440–444.

Zerhouni EA, Boukadoum M, Siddiky MA, et al. Standard phantom for quantitative CT analysis of pulmonary nodules. Radiology 1983;194:767.

Zerhouni EA, Stitik FP, Siegelman SS, et al. Computed tomography of the pulmonary nodule: a national cooperative study. Radiology 1986;160:319.

Zhang H, Yin W, Zhang L, et al. Curative radiotherapy of early operable non-small cell lung cancer. Radiother Oncol 1989;14:89–94.

Index

Page numbers followed by *f* refer to illustrations; page numbers followed by *t* refer to tables.

COVERS DIAGNOSIS AND TREATMENT IN A HEARTBEAT.

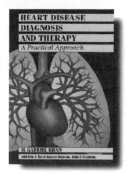

HEART DISEASE DIAGNOSIS AND THERAPY:
A Practical Approach

M. Gabriel Khan, MD, FRCP (London), FRCP(C), FACC
With special contributions by: Eric J. Topol, MD, FACC;
Sanjeev Saksena, MD, FACC; and John F. Goodwin, MD, FRCP (Lond), FACC

Now there's a practical answer to getting the clinical information you need without wading through "compressed" cardiology texts. **Heart Disease Diagnosis and Therapy** uses a straightforward, clinically focused style that's highlighted by bullets for quick access to relevant information.

With no unwanted anatomy, physiology, historical background, or pathology, there's plenty of space for a detailed discussion of key clinical topics. You'll find • myocardial infarction • angina • arrhythmias • heart failure • valvular heart disease • cardiomyopathies • hypertension. A practical chapter on preoperative management will help you screen cardiac patients for non-cardiac surgery.

Heart Disease Diagnosis and Therapy gives you a highly illustrated approach with proven decision making strategies and appropriate algorithms, all in an accessible format. Tear off the attached order form and send for your copy today.
1996/650 pages/149 illustrations/04614-4

Please send me _____ copies (04614-4)

Preview this text for a full month. If you're not completely satisfied,
return it within 30 days at no further obligation (US only).

PAYMENT OPTIONS:

TO ORDER OR FOR PRICING INFORMATION CALL TOLL FREE:
Call: 800-638-0672
FAX: 800-447-8438

IN CANADA
Call:800-665-1148

FROM OUTSIDE THE US AND CANADA:
Call 410-528-4223
Fax: 410-528-8550

INTERNET
E-mail: custserv@wwilkins.com
Home page: http://www.wwilkins.com

CA, IL, MA, MD, NY, and PA residents please add state sales tax. Prices subject to change without notice.

☐ Check enclosed (Plus $5.00 handling)
☐ Bill me (plus postage and handling)
☐ Charge my credit card (plus postage and handling)
    ☐ MasterCard   ☐ VISA   ☐ Am Express   ☐ Discover

_____   _____
card #   exp. date

_____
signature/p.o.#

_____
name

_____
address

_____
city/state/zip

_____
phone #   fax #

_____
specialty/profession

Williams & Wilkins
A Waverly Company

BUSINESS REPLY MAIL

FIRST CLASS PERMIT NO. 724 BALTIMORE, MD.

POSTAGE WILL BE PAID BY ADDRESSEE

Williams & Wilkins
P.O. Box 1496
Baltimore, Maryland 21298-9724

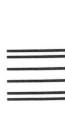